An Evidence-Based Approach to the Treatment and Care of the Older Adult With Cancer

Edited by
Diane G. Cope, PhD, ARNP, BC, AOCNP
Anne M. Reb, MSN, NP

Oncology Nursing Society
Pittsburgh, Pennsylvania

ONS Publishing Division
Publisher: Leonard Mafrica, MBA, CAE
Director, Commercial Publishing: Barbara Sigler, RN, MNEd
Technical Editor: Angela Klimaszewski, MSN, RN
Production Manager: Lisa M. George, BA
Staff Editor: Lori Wilson, BA
Copy Editor: Amy Nicoletti, BA
Graphic Designer: Dany Sjoen

An Evidence-Based Approach to the Treatment and Care of the Older Adult With Cancer

Library of Congress Control Number: 2005938450

ISBN 1-890504-58-0

Publisher's Note

This book is published by the Oncology Nursing Society (ONS). ONS neither represents nor guarantees that the practices described herein will, if followed, ensure safe and effective patient care. The recommendations contained in this book reflect ONS's judgment regarding the state of general knowledge and practice in the field as of the date of publication. The recommendations may not be appropriate for use in all circumstances. Those who use this book should make their own determinations regarding specific safe and appropriate patient-care practices, taking into account the personnel, equipment, and practices available at the hospital or other facility at which they are located. The editors and publisher cannot be held responsible for any liability incurred as a consequence from the use or application of any of the contents of this book. Figures and tables are used as examples only. They are not meant to be all-inclusive, nor do they represent endorsement of any particular institution by ONS. Mention of specific products and opinions related to those products do not indicate or imply endorsement by ONS.

ONS publications are originally published in English. Permission has been granted by the ONS Board of Directors for foreign translation. (Individual tables and figures that are reprinted or adapted require additional permission from the original source.) However, because translations from English may not always be accurate or precise, ONS disclaims any responsibility for inaccuracies in words or meaning that may occur as a result of the translation. Readers relying on precise information should check the original English version.

Printed in the United States of America

Oncology Nursing Society
Integrity • Innovation • Stewardship • Advocacy • Excellence • Inclusiveness

Contributors

Editors

Diane G. Cope, PhD, ARNP, BC, AOCNP
Nurse Practitioner
Florida Cancer Specialists
Fort Myers, Florida
Chapter 1. Cancer and the Aging Population
Chapter 17. Symptom Management of Diarrhea and Constipation

Anne M. Reb, MSN, NP
Research Nurse Manager, United States Military Cancer Institute
Henry M. Jackson Foundation
Walter Reed Army Medical Center
Washington, District of Columbia
Chapter 3. Physiology of Aging
Chapter 5. Cancer Screening in the Older Adult

Authors

Marie Aberle, MS, APRN-BC, BNSc, RN, AOCN®
Acute Care Nurse Practitioner
Blood and Marrow Transplant Clinic
Methodist Healthcare System
San Antonio, Texas
Chapter 10. The Older Adult With Lung Cancer

Deborah T. Berg, RN, BSN
Medical Science Liaison
Genentech BioOncology
San Francisco, California
Chapter 8. The Older Adult With Colorectal Cancer

Stewart M. Bond, RN, MSN, AOCN®
Doctoral Candidate
UNC School of Nursing
University of North Carolina at Chapel Hill
Chapel Hill, North Carolina
Chapter 16. Symptom Management of Mucositis

Deborah A. Boyle, RN, MSN, AOCN®, FAAN
Practice Outcomes Nurse Specialist
Project Leader, Gero-Oncology and Survivorship Nursing Studies Program
Banner Good Samaritan Medical Center
Phoenix, Arizona
Foreword; Chapter 7. The Older Adult With Breast Cancer

Ronni Chernoff, PhD, RD
Associate Director, Geriatric Research Education and Clinical Center
Central Arkansas Veterans Healthcare System
Professor, Geriatrics
Donald W. Reynolds Center on Aging and Department of Geriatrics
University of Arkansas for Medical Sciences
Little Rock, Arkansas
Chapter 18. Nutritional Care of the Older Adult With Cancer

Kimberly Christopher, PhD, RN, OCN®
Associate Professor and Chair
Department of Adult and Child Nursing
University of Massachusetts Dartmouth
North Dartmouth, Massachusetts
Chapter 25. Older Adults and Cancer Survivorship

Nessa M. Coyle, PhD, NP, FAAN
Supportive Care Program
Pain and Palliative Care Service
Department of Neurology
Memorial Sloan-Kettering Cancer Center
New York, New York
Chapter 19. Symptom Management of Pain

Georgia M. Decker, RN, MS, CS ANP, AOCN®
Founder and Nurse Practitioner
Integrative Care
Albany, New York
Chapter 22. Complementary and Alternative Therapies

Susan Derby, MA, CGNP, ACHPN
Nurse Practitioner
Pain and Palliative Care Service
Memorial Sloan-Kettering Cancer Center
New York, New York
Chapter 19. Symptom Management of Pain

Nancy M. Gardner, PhD
Assistant Professor
College of Nursing
Rutgers, The State University of New Jersey
Newark, New Jersey
Chapter 17. Symptom Management of Diarrhea and Constipation

Marilyn L. Haas, PhD, RN, CNS, ANP-C
Nurse Practitioner
Mountain Radiation Oncology
Asheville, North Carolina
Chapter 14. The Older Adult Receiving Radiation Therapy

Marilyn Tuls Halstead, RN, PhD
Associate Professor and Graduate Program Director
Department of Nursing
Towson University
Towson, Maryland
Chapter 23. Spiritual Care of the Older Adult With Cancer

Sarah H. Kagan, PhD, RN, APRN, BC, AOCN®
Associate Professor of Gerontological Nursing
University of Pennsylvania
Gerontology Clinical Specialist
Hospital of the University of Pennsylvania
Secondary Faculty, Department of Otorhinolaryngology: Head and Neck Surgery
University of Pennsylvania
Philadelphia, Pennsylvania
Chapter 9. The Older Adult With Head and Neck Cancer

Alice S. Kerber, MN, RN, AOCN®
Clinical Nurse Specialist
Cancer Screening and Community Outreach
Saint Joseph's Hospital
Atlanta, Georgia
Chapter 24. Legal and Ethical Issues

Cheryl D. Kosits, RN, MSN, OCN®, CCRC
Nurse Case Manager
Moores Cancer Center
University of California, San Diego Medical Center
San Diego, California
Chapter 12. The Older Adult With Non-Hodgkin Lymphoma

Sandra W. McLeskey, PhD, RN
Professor
School of Nursing
University of Maryland
Baltimore, Maryland
Chapter 10. The Older Adult With Lung Cancer

Sandra A. Mitchell, CRNP, MScN, AOCN®
Predoctoral Fellow, Department of Nursing
Oncology Nurse Practitioner
National Cancer Institute, National Institutes of Health
Bethesda, Maryland
Doctoral Student
Distance Education PhD Program, Cancer Research
University of Utah College of Nursing
Salt Lake City, Utah
Chapter 13. The Older Adult With Hematologic Malignancies and Disorders

Kathleen Murphy-Ende, RN, PhD, AOCNP
Nurse Practitioner
University of Wisconsin Hospital and Clinics
Madison, Wisconsin
Chapter 21. Palliative Care of the Older Adult With Cancer

Holly C. Nilsson, BA, RN
Master's Student
School of Nursing
Saint Louis University
Saint Louis, Missouri
Chapter 23. Spiritual Care of the Older Adult With Cancer

Maureen E. O'Rourke, RN, PhD
Associate Clinical Professor of Nursing
University of North Carolina, Greensboro
Greensboro, North Carolina
Adjunct Assistant Professor of Medicine
    Hematology/Oncology
Wake Forest University
Winston-Salem, North Carolina
*Chapter 11. The Older Adult With Prostate
    Cancer*

Janine A. Overcash, PhD, ARNP, BC
Gerontological Nurse Practitioner
College of Nursing
University of South Florida
Tampa, Florida
Chapter 4. Comprehensive Geriatric Assessment

Judith K. Payne, PhD, RN, AOCN®
Assistant Professor, Oncology Program
Duke University School of Nursing
Durham, North Carolina
Chapter 2. Research Issues and Priorities

Rowena N. Schwartz, PharmD, BCOP
Associate Professor of Pharmacy and Thera-
    peutics
School of Pharmacy
University of Pittsburgh
Pittsburgh, Pennsylvania
Chapter 6. Pharmacologic Issues

Judith A. Shell, PhD, LMFT, RN
Medical Family Therapist
Marriage and Family Therapist
Osceola Cancer Center
Kissimmee, Florida
*Chapter 20. Sexuality Care of the Older Adult
    With Cancer*

Janet H. Van Cleave, MSN, ACNP-CS,
    AOCN®
Acute Care Nurse Practitioner
The Mt. Sinai Medical Center of New York
    City
New York, New York
Doctoral Student
Yale University School of Nursing
New Haven, Connecticut
*Chapter 15. The Older Adult With Myelosuppres-
    sion and Anemia*

To my husband, Steve, and, son Adam, for their constant love and support of all my oncology nursing endeavors.
—*Diane Cope*

To my parents, Richard and the late Alice Noone Reb, for their ongoing love and inspiration. With gratitude and affection.
—*Anne Reb*

We would also like to express our sincere gratitude to all of the expert authors who made this book a reality. Their contributions are invaluable as we work toward collaborative research and evidence-based practice to improve the future healthcare needs of older adults with cancer.

Contents

Chapter 9. The Older Adult With Head and Neck Cancer   167

Chapter 10. The Older Adult With Lung Cancer   185

Chapter 11. The Older Adult With Prostate Cancer   225

Chapter 12. The Older Adult With Non-Hodgkin Lymphoma   251

Chapter 13. The Older Adult With Hematologic Malignancies and Disorders   277

Chapter 14. The Older Adult Receiving Radiation Therapy 311

Chapter 15. The Older Adult With Myelosuppression and Anemia 325

Chapter 16. Symptom Management of Mucositis 349

Chapter 21. Palliative Care of the Older Adult With Cancer   465

Chapter 22. Complementary and Alternative Therapies   485

Chapter 23. Spiritual Care of the Older Adult With Cancer   529

Chapter 24. Legal and Ethical Issues   561

Foreword

In 1980, I assumed my first oncology clinical nurse specialist position in a large tertiary care medical center in Phoenix. We had weekly interdisciplinary rounds that proved instructive as well as effective in addressing unmet patient needs and readying families for discharge. Following one such round, I had one of those "ah-ha" moments. Almost every patient we discussed that morning was an older person. Makes sense, I thought, living in the epicenter of retirement. Yet this revelation fostered my curiosity. If this was the case, Arizona must be unique in its cancer and aging affiliation.

With the help of a dedicated librarian colleague, we began searching multiple databases to analyze Arizona's cancer incidence and prevalence rates specific to older adults. What we found was both revealing and disconcerting. Arizona was characterized by a comparable predominance of cancer in older adults to the rest of the nation. Regardless of geography, cancer was a disease of the aging, with the majority of malignancies diagnosed in Americans older than age 65. Additionally, cancer was disproportionately diagnosed in a relatively small subset of Americans. More than half of all malignancies occurred in only 12% of the populace (Lew, 1976; Peterson & Kennedy, 1979). Never in my 12 years of clinical practice nor graduation from an oncology-specific clinical nurse specialist program had I heard these statistics. Why was this the case? I could not be only one of a handful of professionals specializing in oncology who was aware of this reality. Yet, in truth, it seemed I was.

In the early 1980s, the late and esteemed Dr. Paul Carbone from the University of Wisconsin and colleague Dr. Colin Begg were credited with revealing widespread ageism, particularly within the ranks of medical oncology. Their critique of 21 Eastern Cooperative Oncology Group clinical trials in eight different cancer primary sites affirmed extensive bias toward the older adult based solely on chronologic age (Begg & Carbone, 1983). Stereotyping prevailed, and physiologic age was not considered in decision making about appropriateness of antineoplastic therapies for the older adult. Exclusion, underdosing, and therapy substitution predominated when cancer treatment for the older adult was scrutinized. These findings soon were followed by comparable examples within the ranks of surgical and radiation oncology.

Shortly following this time, a collaborative effort to plan a working conference to synthesize existing data on cancer in the older adult and to identify knowledge gaps relative to this special population was initiated. In concert with medical oncologist Dr. Paul Carbone and surgical oncologist Dr. W. Bradford Patterson, Rosemary Yancik, PhD, formerly with the National Cancer Institute (NCI) and now with the National Institute on Aging (NIA), organized the conference "Perspectives on Prevention and Treatment of Cancer in the Elderly." What resulted was a significant initial effort to educate cancer professionals about the knowledge gap characteristic of cancer in the older adult. The first edited text on this topic was hence published in 1983 (Yancik, Carbone, Patterson, Steel, & Terry, 1983).

Around this same time, I submitted an abstract for the 1982 Oncology Nursing Society (ONS) Congress in St. Louis, MO, on the application of the ONS Standards of Practice to the care of the older adult with cancer. Although it was not accepted, this exercise further heightened my sense of concern over the global avoidance of this patient population. Speaking and writing on the subject enhanced my sense of empowerment to champion the older adult agenda. During the late 1980s and 1990s, various nursing authors began to publish on topics related to cancer and the older adult (Kagan, 2004). In 1992, ONS supported this much-needed advocacy stance by becoming the first professional specialty organization to take a position on the unmet needs of the older adult with or at risk for cancer (Boyle et al., 1992).

Twenty-five years have passed since my initial inquiries in this area, and this reality in cancer care is only beginning to garner focused attention. In 2001, NIA and NCI organized a workshop to provide a forum for leaders to address research priorities in the integration of aging and cancer research focused on people aged 65 and older (NIA, 2005). In 2003, ONS received a grant from the John A. Hartford Foundation to assist with a needs assessment to determine possibilities for inclusion of an older adult focus within the organization. That same year, the American Society of Clinical Oncology developed a gero-oncology continuing education curriculum for medical oncologists. They also funded several fellowships in gero-oncology coordinated and taught by geriatricians and oncologists. Recently, ONS updated its position on cancer in the older adult and collaborated on such with the Geriatric Oncology Consortium (Oncology Nursing Society & Geriatric Oncology Consortium, 2004). Kagan (2004) proposed a working definition of gero-oncology as reference to the assessment, management, and evaluation of the unique needs of the older adult with, or at risk for, cancer. Based on the premise of heterogeneity and the deliberative consideration of the interface between the aging process and cancer, this special focus was noted to "occur within the contextual paradigm of a life mostly lived" (Kagan). Yet, advances in technology and supportive care have contributed to the fact that older adults are living longer with cancer and other chronic illnesses and may have several years of life ahead. Kagan called for shifting the perspective from individual-level research in cancer and aging to family and community-level research to address an aging society's needs in cancer care and break down the ageism bias in healthcare disparities.

Finally, a more secure base was being established to support the growing voices of activism and more concerted efforts to counter bias and prejudice. Proof of moving forward is substantiated by this significant text, spearheaded by two champions of caring for older adults with cancer, Diane Cope and Anne Reb, with contributions by many dedicated colleagues with well-established interests in gero-oncology. I implore you, as readers of this text, to do one of the following. Take at least one key new piece of information and make it yours. In patient care discussions, force the integration of this new knowledge into care planning. Use these chapters in journal club forums. Locate an article referenced in this text, and post it for colleagues to read. Ask new questions of older adult patients and their caregivers that you have never asked before. Share these findings in charting, interdisciplinary deliberations, and scholarly writing. Make competency in gero-oncology nursing mandatory in your setting. Realize its necessity for your professional growth now and in the future.

I consider oncology nurses to be ambassadors for older adults. Patient advocacy responsibilities abound in considering the silence of elder-specific articulated need in cancer care. Become determined to foster activism in the public health venue. Engagement also can occur at home, in your community, within work, through professional education, via the media, and by having a political voice. As we give newfound recognition to the evolving epidemic of cancer in the aging, we must be cognizant of our roots and our own sensitivity deficits. Although well intended in our plans for nursing care, we must remember that older patients have been young, but the majority of caregivers have never been old. Highly specialized and individually tailored older adult care represents a new frontier in the field of oncology. Let it be known that geriatric oncology nursing is finally coming of age.

References

Begg, C.B., & Carbone, P.P. (1983). Clinical trials and drug toxicity in the elderly: The experience of the Eastern Cooperative Oncology Group. *Cancer, 52,* 1986–1992.

Boyle, D.A., Engelking, C., Blesch, K., Dodge, J., Sarna, L., & Weinrich, S. (1992). Oncology Nursing Society position paper on cancer and aging: The mandate for oncology nursing. *Oncology Nursing Forum, 19,* 913–933.

Kagan, S. (2004). Gero-oncology nursing research. *Oncology Nursing Forum, 31,* 293–299.

Lew, E.A. (1976). Cancer in old age. *CA: A Cancer Journal for Clinicians, 28,* 2–6.

National Institute on Aging. (2005). *Cancer burden for persons 65 years and older.* Retrieved June 21, 2005, from http://www.nia.nih.gov/ResearchInformation/ConferencesAndMeetings/ WorkshopReport/ExecutiveSummary.htm

Oncology Nursing Society & Geriatric Oncology Consortium. (2004). *Oncology Nursing Society and Geriatric Oncology Consortium joint position on cancer care in the older adult.* Retrieved June 28, 2005, from http://www.ons.org/publications/positions/Geriatric.shtml

Peterson, B.A., & Kennedy, B.J. (1979). Aging and cancer management: Clinical observations. *Cancer, 29,* 322–332.

Yancik, R., Carbone, P.P., Patterson, W.B., Steel, K., & Terry, W.D. (1983). *Perspectives on prevention and treatment of cancer in the elderly.* New York: Raven Press.

Deborah A. Boyle, RN, MSN, AOCN®, FAAN
Practice Outcomes Nurse Specialist
Project Leader, Gero-Oncology and
Survivorship Nursing Studies Program
Banner Good Samaritan Medical Center
Phoenix, Arizona

CHAPTER 1

Cancer and the Aging Population

Diane G. Cope, PhD, ARNP, BC, AOCNP

Introduction

A significant increase in the number of older adults in the United States is projected in the coming decades. Older adults, defined as people aged 65 years and older, possess greater cancer incidence and mortality rates compared to younger people. Approximately 60% of all cancers occur in the older adult population, resulting in an incidence rate that is 10 to 11 times higher than in the younger population (Ershler, 2003; Yancik & Ries, 2004). The risk of developing cancer is 8%–9% in people age 40–59, with a dramatic increase in risk of 20%–30% in people older than 60 years of age (Malik, 2004). Additionally, cancer mortality rates are higher for older adults, with approximately 70% of all cancer deaths occurring in people older than 65 (Ershler). With the steady growth in the aging population and the higher rates of cancer incidence in this group, healthcare providers need to be cognizant of this substantial public health concern that will be occurring in the near future and begin to focus attention on evidence-based approaches to the treatment and care of the older adult with cancer. This chapter will discuss the projections for the aging population, the epidemiologic trends of cancer in older adults, and future implications for healthcare providers caring for the older adult.

Aging Population

In 2000, an estimated 35 million people in the United States were age 65 or older, accounting for approximately 13% of the total population (Misra, Seo, & Cohen, 2004). This represents a tenfold increase since 1900, when only 3 million people were age 65 or older. In 2011, the baby boom generation, or those people born between 1946 and 1964, which comprises approximately 75 million individuals, will begin to turn 65. By 2030, it is projected that approximately 70 million people, or 20% of the population, will be older than 65 (U.S. Census Bureau, 1996). The fastest growing segment of the population is the older adult group age 85 and older. This reflects the improved life expectancy that is projected to increase 10 years by 2050. In 2000, an estimated 2% of the population was age 85 or older; however, this age group is projected to expand to almost 80 million, or 5% of the population, by 2050 (U.S. Census Bureau) (see Figure 1-1).

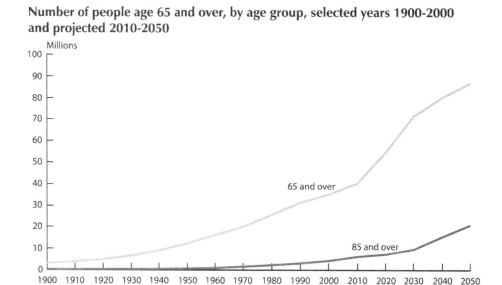

Number of people age 65 and over, by age group, selected years 1900-2000 and projected 2010-2050

Note: Data for 2010-2050 are projections of the population.
Reference population: These data refer to the resident population.
Source: U.S. Census Bureau, Decennial Census and Projections.

Figure 1-1. Aging Demographics

Note. From "Older Americans 2004: Key Indicators of Well-Being," by the Federal Interagency Forum on Aging-Related Statistics, 2005. Retrieved February 3, 2005, from http://www.agingstats.gov/chartbook2004/population.html

Cancer and Aging

Incidence Rates

Cancer is the leading cause of death in the United States in individuals younger than 85 years of age (Jemal et al., 2005). Cancer has been described as a disease of the older adult, with approximately 60% of all cancers occurring in people older than age 65 (Yancik & Ries, 2000). The increased incidence occurs up to the age of 85 years and declines after age 95 (Yancik & Ries, 1998). The increase in cancer incidence and mortality rates with increasing age also was supported in a recent annual report on the status of cancer (1973–1999) highlighting the impact of age on cancer burden (Edwards et al., 2002) (see Figure 1-2). A review of incidence data from the Surveillance, Epidemiology, and End Results Program, the National Program of Cancer Registries, the North American Association of Central Cancer Registries, and mortality data from the National Center for Health Statistics found that cancer rates for people 50–64 years of age were 7–16 times higher than rates for younger people (Edwards et al.). There was a two- to threefold increase in incidence rates in people age 65–74 compared to those in the 50–64 year age group. During the period of 1995–1999, the overall cancer incidence rate was stable, although specific age-related changes were noted. For men younger than 50, lung and colorectal cancer rates decreased, but prostate cancer rates increased. For men age 50 and older, a decrease in colorectal cancer incidence occurred for the 50–64 and 65–74 age groups, with an increase in prostate cancer occurrence for men aged 50–64. Lung cancer rates decreased for all of the older age groups. During the period of 1992–1999, cancer incidence rates decreased in African American men and stabilized during 1995–1999 for white men.

For women during the period of 1987–1999, an increase in overall incidence occurred because of increases in breast cancer rates for women 50–64 years of age and increases in lung cancer rates for women 65–74 years of age. Colorectal cancer rates decreased in women younger than 50 but increased in women older than 75 (Edwards et al., 2002).

Prostate, breast, lung, and colorectal cancers are the four most frequently occurring cancers in adults older than 50 (Edwards et al., 2002) (see Figure 1-3). For men older than 50, other frequently occurring malignancies are bladder cancer and non-Hodgkin lymphoma, with increased incidence of pancreatic cancer and leukemias

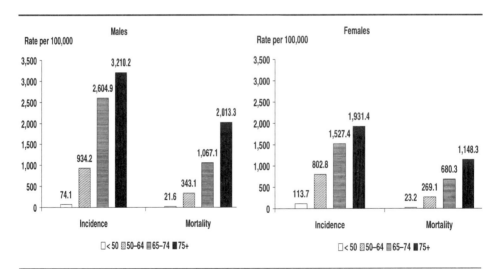

Figure 1-2. Average Annual Cancer Incidence and Mortality Rates for All Cancers by Gender and Age, 1995–1999

Note. From "Annual Report to the Nation on the Status of Cancer, 1973–1999, Featuring Implications of Age and Aging on U.S. Cancer Burden," by B.K. Edwards, H.L. Howe, L.A. Ries, M.J. Thun, H.M. Rosenberg, R. Yancik, et al., 2002, *Cancer, 94,* p. 2770. Copyright 2002 by the American Cancer Society and Wiley-Liss. Reprinted with permission.

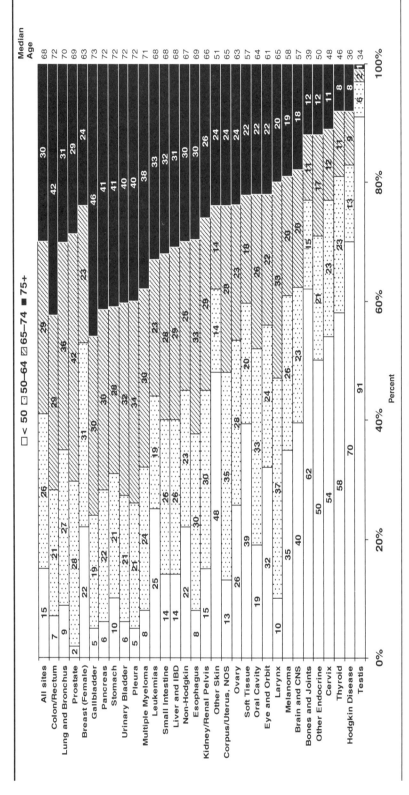

Figure 1-3. Age Distribution and Median Age for the Incidence of Major Cancers

Note. From "Annual Report to the Nation on the Status of Cancer, 1973–1999, Featuring Implications of Age and Aging on U.S. Cancer Burden," by B.K. Edwards, H.L. Howe, L.A. Ries, M.J. Thun, H.M. Rosenberg, R. Yancik, et al., 2002, *Cancer, 94*, p. 2782. Copyright 2002 by the American Cancer Society and Wiley-Liss. Reprinted with permission.

in people age 75 and older (Edwards et al.; Kennedy, 2001). For women older than 50, other frequently occurring malignancies are uterine cancer and non-Hodgkin lymphoma, with increased incidences of pancreatic cancer and leukemias also noted for those 75 and older (Edwards et al.; Kennedy).

Mortality Rates

Since 1950, cancer-related mortality rates have decreased in younger individuals but increased for individuals aged 65 years or older (Misra et al., 2004). A 4% decrease in cancer mortality rates occurred between 1971 and 1990, with an additional 7.7% reduction between 1991 and 1995 for people younger than 65. However, cancer mortality for people older than 65 increased by 15% between 1971 and 1990, with an additional 0.6% increase between 1991 and 1995. The increase in the number of cancer deaths reported for the older age group is reflected in the growth of the aging population (Yancik & Ries, 2004). For men 40 years of age and older, the most common cause of cancer-related death is lung cancer, followed by colorectal cancer for men 40–79 years of age and prostate cancer for men 80 years of age and older (Jemal et al., 2005).

Additional information from the latest annual report on the status of cancer (Edwards et al., 2002) indicated that during the period of 1993–1999, a decrease in mortality rates of 1% per year occurred for all cancers. The decrease was reflected in all age groups for men and women, except for women older than 75. Lung cancer mortality rates decreased for men in all age groups and for women younger than 65. Prostate cancer mortality rates decreased in all age groups except for men older than 75. Breast cancer mortality rates decreased for women younger than 65, with increases noted for African American women older than 75. Overall, cancer mortality rates for all sites combined decreased in women younger than 75 years of age, except for lung cancer, which decreased in women younger than 65. Figure 1-2 highlights mortality rates for all age groups during the period of 1995–1999. Males, in general, have higher mortality rates, partly because of increased tobacco use (Yancik & Ries, 2004).

The type of cancer also may influence mortality rates in older adults. Historically, cancers in the older adult are believed to be less aggressive (Repetto & Balducci, 2002). Certain cancers, however, have been found to present and act differently in older versus younger people. Older women with breast cancer have more indolent tumors that are better differentiated and possess a higher concentration of hormone receptors (Balducci, 2003). The decreased levels of sex hormones in older adults contributes to a hormonal environment that is less likely to stimulate growth of the breast cancer. In contrast, acute myeloid leukemia (AML) in older patients is associated with an approximate 70% higher prevalence of multidrug resistance (MDR-1) gene expression in comparison to younger patients, who present with approximately a 15%–20% multidrug resistance. The higher prevalence of the MDR-1 gene results in a decreased sensitivity to chemotherapy (National Comprehensive Cancer Network, 2004). Furthermore, the number of normal hematopoietic stem cells may be decreased because of the involvement of early pluripotent hematopoietic progenitors in the older adult (Balducci; Balducci & Lyman, 1997; Repetto & Balducci). As a result, AML is more difficult to treat in the older adult and is associated with a poorer prognosis and an increased risk of recurrence (Balducci & Extermann, 2001).

Survival Rates

Despite the increase in cancer incidence, mortality rates have shown a slight decrease during the period 1995–1999 in older adults. This may be attributed to improvements in treatment and supportive care. Consequently, relative survival rates or the ratio of the observed survival rate to the expected rate for a group of people from the general population for lung, colorectal, breast, and prostate cancers are not affected by age. However, observed five-year survival rates, the reflection of total mortality in a patient group regardless of cause, are lower for older adults, especially people age 75 or older, in comparison to younger adults (Edwards et al., 2002) (see Figure 1-4). Overall, women have better survival rates for cancer tumors common to both men and women (Yancik & Ries, 2004).

Future Implications

According to Edwards et al. (2002), if current cancer incidence rates were applied to the population projections for the next five decades, the number of patients with cancer would double from 1.3 million to 2.6 million between 2000 and 2050 because of population growth and aging (see Figure 1-5). Furthermore, a 12% increase in the cancer population is expected in adults age 75 and older, with a projection of 1,102,000 people by 2050 (Edwards et al.). For adults age 85 and older, cancer incidence rates are estimated to increase fourfold by 2050. These projections have a direct impact on future health care in research, practice, and educational settings. The following discussion will address the numerous issues related to each of these settings in caring for the older adult with cancer.

Research Implications

Given the projected population growth in the older age group and the increased cancer incidence rates, more research activities are needed involving the older adult with cancer. Research areas should include care across the cancer continuum, social support issues, quality-of-life factors, and survivorship. Several organizations are now emphasizing older adult cancer issues as research priorities. Currently, the National Cancer Institute (NCI) and the National Institute on Aging (NIA), both part of the National Institutes of Health (NIH), are funding a five-year, approximately $25 million grant program for eight research centers that will focus on cancer and aging to facilitate and expedite research in this area (NIH, 2004). Seven research areas were identified at a recent NIA/NCI workshop: patterns of care; treatment efficacy and tolerance; effects of comorbidity; prevention, risk assessment, and screening; psychosocial issues and medical effects; palliative care, end-of-life care, and pain relief; and the biology of aging and cancer. Results of the Oncology Nursing Society (ONS) Year 2005 Research Priorities Survey identified 20 research priorities: quality of life, decision making about treatment in advanced disease, patient/family education, decision making about treatment, pain, tobacco use and exposure, screening/early detection of cancer, prevention/risk reduction, palliative care, evidence-based practice, nurses as advocates, fatigue/lack of energy, cancer recurrence, curative treatment/care, patient outcomes of cancer care, cognitive impairment/mental status changes, late effects of treatment, hospice/end of life, initial cancer diagnosis, and ethical

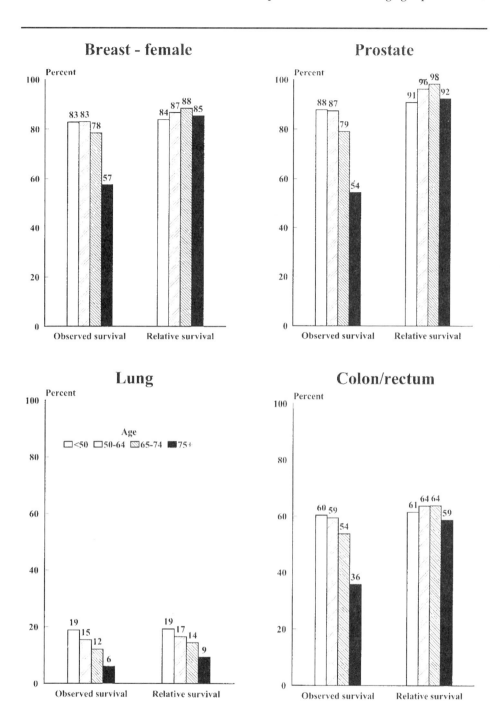

Figure 1-4. Five-Year Observed and Relative Survival Rates

Note. From "Annual Report to the Nation on the Status of Cancer, 1973–1999, Featuring Implications of Age and Aging on U.S. Cancer Burden," by B.K. Edwards, H.L. Howe, L.A. Ries, M.J. Thun, H.M. Rosenberg, R. Yancik, et al., 2002, *Cancer, 94,* p. 2785. Copyright 2002 by the American Cancer Society and Wiley-Liss. Reprinted with permission.

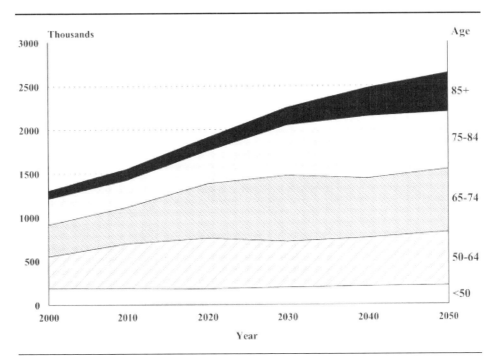

Figure 1-5. Projected Number of Cancer Cases for 2000–2050

Note. From "Annual Report to the Nation on the Status of Cancer, 1973–1999, Featuring Implications of Age and Aging on U.S. Cancer Burden," by B.K. Edwards, H.L. Howe, L.A. Ries, M.J. Thun, H.M. Rosenberg, R. Yancik, et al., 2002, *Cancer, 94,* p. 2786. Copyright 2002 by Wiley Interscience. Reprinted with permission.

issues (Berger et al., 2005). The National Institute of Nursing Research (2004) also highlighted the need for further research in the areas of chronic illness, including supporting family caregivers, end-of-life and palliative care issues, health promotion and disease prevention, quality of life, and symptom management. Many of these areas apply directly to the older adult with cancer and will be important research activities with the aging population. Nurses can play a key role in research activities and focus on specific areas of nursing practice and nursing outcomes. Although the nursing profession has taken a lead role in symptom management research, clinical studies specifically targeting older adults are lacking. Research areas specific to older adults with cancer that are lacking evidence-based data are detailed in Chapter 2. Furthermore, nurses can play a pivotal role in facilitating participation by the older adult in clinical trials.

Clinical Practice Implications

Because of the many physical and psychosocial factors surrounding the older adult with cancer, care for these individuals can be challenging. However, given the projected population changes in numbers of older adults within the next few decades, professional organizations are now recognizing the paucity of empirical evidence and are calling for greater attention to care of the older adult with cancer.

Recently, ONS and the Geriatric Oncology Consortium published a joint position on cancer care in the older adult (ONS, 2004). This position highlights requisite areas necessary to care for the older adult with cancer and the great need for empirical evidence to guide practice.

A major issue is the existence of comorbidities. The older adult is at higher risk for not only cancer but also other chronic health problems such as heart disease, hypertension, diabetes, and chronic obstructive pulmonary disease. Four out of five individuals 65 years of age or older have one or more coexisting comorbidities (Yancik, Ganz, Varricchio, & Conley, 2001). In addition, many older adults may possess other geriatric abnormalities such as deficits in self-care, malnutrition, metabolic disorders, depression, limitations in mobility and functional status, and cognitive impairments. Healthcare providers will need to possess astute assessment skills and address not only side effects of cancer and treatment but also be knowledgeable of other confounding diseases and their treatments. Nurses are in a key position to conduct comorbidity and functional assessments to identify limitations of the older adult, to facilitate treatment for reversible conditions identified by these assessments, and to make appropriate referrals for social support and community resources.

The cost of cancer and cancer treatment presents other challenges for the older adult. Retirement often is associated with limited income and financial resources. Economic status should be assessed and discussed with the older adult, and estimated costs of treatment should be reviewed prior to the initiation of treatment. Indirect costs of treatment, such as transportation and medications, also must be considered.

Educational Implications

To provide expert care, nurses and other healthcare providers will require formal training and educational programs focusing on the unique characteristics of the older adult with cancer. Oncology nurses will require a strong foundation in geriatric assessment, aging changes, and symptom management. Furthermore, nurses should have a broad knowledge base regarding other comorbidities and medical disorders that may be present in the older adult with cancer that can affect cancer and treatment.

Because of this need for geriatric nursing education, programs are now being developed to assist nurses in acquiring knowledge pertaining to the care of the older adult. One publication by the Hartford Geriatric Nursing Initiative and the American Association of Colleges of Nursing (2004) is intended to assist nurse educators in integrating geriatric nursing content into curricula. A second program, Nurse Competence in Aging, is a new initiative that is specifically targeting 400,000 practicing nurses who belong to specialty nursing organizations in an effort to improve the quality of health care of older adults through integration of gerontology content and knowledge (Scholder, Kagan, & Schumann, 2004). This project is a five-year, $5 million initiative that is being funded by the Atlantic Philanthropies.

Educational strategies specific for the older adult also are critical. In a review of patient education literature over a 10-year period, Chelf et al. (2001) found that patients with cancer want information about their illness; prefer discussion and education from their physician, although they found nurses and written materials to be important; identify high reading levels in printed materials; and suggest that other resources, such as the Internet, videotapes, audiotapes, and telephone contact, may help to improve cancer education. This review, however, did not discuss patient education specifically for the older adult. Clearly, further research addressing patient education and the special needs, such as sensory impairments, of the older adult are important for the future.

Conclusion

The projected growth of the older adult population has a direct impact on health care and the specialty of oncology. Healthcare providers need to address many research, practice, and education issues involving the older adult with cancer that have received minimal attention in the past. Additional research and greater focus on the older adult with cancer will produce much-needed evidence-based practice approaches.

The author acknowledges Anne Reb, MSN, NP, for her thoughtful contributions to this chapter.

References

Balducci, L. (2003). New directions in treating elderly patients with cancer. *ADVANCE, 1*(4), 1–2.

Balducci, L., & Extermann, M. (2001). A practical approach to the older patient with cancer. *Current Problems in Cancer, 25,* 6–76.

Balducci, L., & Lyman, G.H. (1997). Cancer in the elderly. Epidemiologic and clinical implications. *Clinics in Geriatric Medicine, 13,* 1–14.

Berger, A.M., Berry, D.L., Christopher, K.A., Greene, A.L., Maliski, S., Swenson, K.K., et al. (2005). Oncology Nursing Society year 2005 research priorities survey. *Oncology Nursing Forum, 32,* 281–290.

Chelf, J.H., Agre, P., Axelrod, A., Cheney, L., Cole, D.D., Conrad, K., et al. (2001). Cancer-related patient education: An overview of the last decade of evaluation and research. *Oncology Nursing Forum, 28,* 1139–1147.

Edwards, B.K., Howe, H.L., Ries, L., Thun, M.J., Rosenberg, H.M., Yancik, R., et al. (2002). Annual report to the nation on the status of cancer, 1973–1999, featuring implications of age and aging on U.S. cancer burden. *Cancer, 94,* 2766–2792.

Ershler, W.B. (2003). Cancer: A disease of the elderly. *Journal of Supportive Oncology, 1,* 5–10.

Hartford Geriatric Nursing Initiative & American Association of Colleges of Nursing. (2004, March). *Nurse practitioner and clinical nurse specialist competencies for older adult care.* Retrieved October 15, 2004, from http://www.aacn.nche.edu/Education/pdf/APNCompetencies.pdf

Jemal, A., Murray, T., Ward, E., Samuels, A., Tiwari, R.C., Ghafoor, A., et al. (2005). Cancer statistics, 2005. *CA: A Cancer Journal for Clinicians, 55,* 10–30.

Kennedy, B.J. (2001). Aging and cancer. *Primary Care and Cancer, 21,* 9–11.

Malik, S.A. (2004). The impact of aging on chemotherapy. *Clinical Lung Cancer, 5,* 243–244.

Misra, D., Seo, P.H., & Cohen, H.J. (2004). Aging and cancer. *Clinical Advances in Hematology and Oncology, 2,* 457–465.

National Comprehensive Cancer Network. (2004). *Senior adult oncology.* Retrieved October 15, 2004, from http://www.nccn.org/professionals/physician_gls/PDF/senior.pdf

National Institute of Nursing Research. (2004). *Mission statement.* Retrieved October 15, 2004, from http://ninr.nih.gov/ninr/research/diversity/mission.html

National Institutes of Health. (2004). *Integrating aging and cancer research.* Retrieved October 15, 2004, from http://grants2.nih.gov/grants/guide/pa-files/PA-02-169.html

Oncology Nursing Society. (2004). *Oncology Nursing Society and Geriatric Oncology Consortium joint position on cancer care in the older adult.* Retrieved October 15, 2004, from http://www.ons.org/publications/positions/Geriatric.shtml

Repetto, L., & Balducci, L. (2002). A case for geriatric oncology. *Lancet Oncology, 3,* 289–297.

Scholder, J., Kagan, S., & Schumann, M.J. (2004). Nurse competence in aging overview. *Nursing Clinics of North America, 39,* 429–442.

U.S. Census Bureau. (1996). *Population projections of the United States by age, sex, race, and Hispanic origin: 1995 to 2050.* Retrieved October 15, 2004, from http://www.census.gov/prod/1/pop/p25-1130/p251130a.pdf

Yancik, R., Ganz, P., Varricchio, C.G., & Conley, B. (2001). Perspectives on comorbidity and cancer in older patients: Approaches to expand the knowledge base. *Journal of Clinical Oncology, 19,* 1147–1151.

Yancik, R., & Ries, L.A. (1998). Cancer in the older person: Magnitude of the problem. In L. Balducci, G.H. Lyman, & W.B. Ershler (Eds.), *Comprehensive geriatric oncology* (pp. 95–104). Amsterdam, Australia: Harwood Academic.

Yancik, R., & Ries, L.A. (2000). Aging and cancer in America: Demographics and epidemiologic perspectives. *Hematology/Oncology Clinics of North America, 14,* 17–23.

Yancik, R., & Ries, L. (2004). Cancer in older persons: An international issue in an aging world. *Seminars in Oncology, 31,* 128–136.

CHAPTER 2

Research Issues and Priorities

Judith K. Payne, PhD, RN, AOCN®

Introduction and Background

Although cancer occurs in people of every age, it is fundamentally a disease of aging. As discussed in Chapter 1, the majority of patients with cancer in the United States are older than 70. Several theoretical reasons exist as to why cancer incidence increases in the older adult: accumulation of random genetic mutations leading to oncogene activation or amplification or decreased tumor-suppressor gene activity; lifetime carcinogen exposure; age-related alterations in the immune system (decreased immune surveillance); hormonal alterations or exposure; and long latency periods (Beers & Berkow, 2000–2005; Denduluri & Ershler, 2004). Understanding the theoretical underpinnings of cancer in the older adult is important because much of nursing research is driven by disease manifestations or response to accompanying treatment modalities; related functional and quality-of-life issues; or delivery of healthcare services.

The primary goal of nursing research is to develop a scientific knowledge base for nursing practice. This is critically important in the older adult population, specifically in an underserved and vulnerable patient population such as geriatric oncology. Older adults with cancer face a host of symptoms from the effects of treatment as well as the tumor, in addition to other age- and health-related problems. However, the conduct of research is of little value unless findings are used in practice to improve patient care. Contributions of nursing to improve patient outcomes can be optimized by the use of evidence-based practice (EBP) guidelines and research-based nursing treatments (Lo-Biondo-Wood & Haber, 2002; Payne, 2002). The term *EBP* has become widely adopted in recent years by the nursing profession (Estabrooks, 1998). Most researchers agree that although the terms *research utilization* and *EBP* are sometimes used interchangeably, they are not the same (Goode & Titler, 1996; Payne, 2002; Rutledge & Grant, 2002; Titler, Mentes, Rakel, Abbott, & Baumler, 1999). Adopting a commonly used definition, EBP is the conscious and judicious use of the current "best" evidence in the care of patients and delivery of healthcare services. Research utilization is a subset of EBP that focuses on the application of research findings. LoBiondo-Wood and Haber described EBP as a broader term that not only encompasses research utilization but also includes use of case reports and expert opinion in deciding the practices to be used in health care. According to Rutledge and Grant, EBP defines care that integrates best scientific evidence with clinical expertise, knowledge of pathophysiology, knowledge of psychological issues, and decision-making preference of patients. The Oncology Nursing Society (ONS, 2004) rendered the position that EBP affirms that making clinical decisions based on best evidence, either from the research literature or clinical expertise, improves the quality of care and the patient's quality of life.

The purpose of this chapter is to describe existing research, including evidence-based research and practice in the care of the older adult with cancer, and to discuss the unique challenges researchers face in attempting to develop theory and nursing science specific to this population. This chapter also will lay the foundation for thinking about current healthcare trends that support the importance of and critical need for knowledge in older adults with cancer. The latter part of the chapter outlines future directions in the research agenda that may foster collegial and professional consensus on oncology research issues in the older adult.

Scope of the Problem

As the population ages, cancer is becoming more of a problem for the older adult. The study of cancer and aging has emerged as a critical issue in oncologic care (Lichtman, 2004). Despite the magnitude of this problem, exploration of the unique problems associated with cancer in the older adult has only recently begun (Muss, Cohen, & Lichtman, 2000). Opportunities for conducting research in this population continue to grow and reflect the increasing awareness of the incidence of cancer in older adults. Kagan (2004) said the "knowledge generated by genomics and other areas in molecular biology suggests that we must separate more delicately defined issues of aging, and more sophisticated investigation is needed to build understanding of the phenomena that make cancer in older adults unique, intriguing, and multifaceted" (p. 297). Kagan's main thesis is that among the most pressing issues facing gero-oncology research are the requisite translations of knowledge into realistic evidence-based care with delineated outcomes, while overcoming ageism and planning for care delivery in an extremely fragmented and constrained healthcare environment. At present, gerontologic research does not consistently offer clear evidence on the question of the quality of functioning in advanced older age, and the picture is complex with counteracting forces and processes.

Perhaps the most obvious reason that geriatric oncology research lags behind research involving younger patients with cancer is that researchers have largely avoided including older adults in large multisite clinical trials, especially those that involve pharmaceuticals, invasive procedures, or innovative treatments. The literature describes reasons why healthcare providers tend to ignore older adults when recruiting subjects to clinical trials, which often are different from the reasons given by many older patients for not participating in research trials (Payne, 2003; Schilsky, 2004). Barriers identified as important to patient recruitment and enrollment from both the physicians' perspective and from older adults' perspective are discussed more thoroughly later in the chapter, and a list of identified barriers are included in Table 2-1.

Perhaps most alarming is that while enrollment in cancer trials is low for all adult patient groups (< 3%), racial and ethnic minorities as well as older adults were less likely to enroll in cooperative group cancer trials than were Whites and non-elderly

Table 2-1. Barriers to Patient Enrollment in Clinical Trials

Barrier	Patient Perspective	Physician Perspective
Lack of resources for additional travel expenses	X	
Patients want to be included in the treatment arm, and researchers cannot guarantee because of randomization.	X	
Reluctance of physicians to offer clinical trial participation to older adults because of presence of comorbidity		X
Caregiver burden is high, and caregivers are not always available.	X	
Additional time required by physician or nurse to explain possible treatments and obtain informed consent		X
Studies are poorly designed and not tailored to older adults with cancer.		X
Appropriate protocols are not available.		X
Distrust, fear of health care and research	X	
Lack of community and individual awareness of research protocols available	X	
Physicians lack understanding regarding value of clinical trials.		X
Research is not cost effective for the private practice physician.		X

(Morrow, Hickok, & Burish, 1994; Murthy, Krumholz, & Gross, 2004; Payne, 2003). This problem is reflective of current healthcare policy that does not adequately fund studies to provide the extra resources required for older adults seeking participation in clinical trials.

Historical Perspective

Until recently, limited knowledge has existed on how antineoplastic agents and other medications affect disease or symptom states in the older adult, specifically older patients with cancer. However, to obtain information about the benefits from usual dosages of chemotherapy compared to potential higher toxicity rates in the older adult patient, the Cancer and Leukemia Group B has designed trials specifically for patients aged 65 and older that have examined pharmacokinetics and tolerance of commonly used chemotherapy drugs, quality of life of older patients, and effectiveness of and adherence to oral chemotherapy in older women with stage II breast cancer (Schilsky, 2004). Increasingly, pharmacokinetic data are now available on a broad spectrum of chemotherapy agents, and many seem to benefit older patients (Balducci, 2003; Lichtman, 2004). Most promising are several new agents, including capecitabine, pegylated liposomal doxorubicin, weekly taxanes, vinorelbine, and gemcitabine, that appear to be well tolerated even in frail patients and may provide effective palliation of symptoms (Lichtman, 2004). Although aging occurs on a continuum, it is a highly individualized process and does not always predict the physiologic decline in an individual. Several physiologic processes occur with aging that affect the pharmacokinetics (absorption, distribution, metabolism, and excretion) of most antineoplastic agents (Lichtman, 2003; Sledge et al., 2003). According to Lichtman (2003), the volume of distribution of drugs is a function of body composition, and because fat content doubles in older patients and intracellular water decreases, a decreased volume of distribution can occur and lead to a lower peak concentration and prolonged terminal half-life. Age-related changes also occur in renal and liver metabolism, which may require dose adjustments of treatment protocols (Lichtman, 2003; Sledge et al.).

Because many chemotherapy agents have pharmacokinetic data for the older adult, healthcare providers can use this information to help to guide practice in determining optimal protocols. Given the fact that older adults are underrepresented in clinical trials, more studies are needed regarding toxicities, drug metabolism, and drug effect. Future studies are needed that help to determine the effect of comorbidity, functional status, performance status, and geriatric assessment on desired outcomes.

State of Geriatric Nursing Research

According to Whall (2004), "Gerontologic nursing research currently is recognized across disciplines, published widely in non-nursing journals, and recognized for its important contribution to healthcare science" (p. 5). Excellent benchmark studies have produced scientific knowledge that has changed the face of health care. Whall further noted that, "because theory is the basis for and outcome of all research, the accelerated speed of gerontologic nursing theory development is due, in large part, to this successful research trajectory" (p. 5).

Early gerontologic nurse researchers reached out to other disciplines and created strong cross-disciplinary efforts (Whall, 2004). Nursing's past research trajectory has addressed important issues with the older adult population that other disciplines had not focused on, specifically issues revolving around functional status, independence and maintaining activities of daily living, nursing home concerns, quality of life, and impact on caregivers.

Nurse Competence in Aging

A new initiative, Nurse Competence in Aging (NCA), specifically focuses on the 400,000 practicing nurses who belong to specialty nursing associations (Scholder, Kagan, & Schumann, 2004). Scholder et al. provide an excellent and critical overview of the goal of NCA, which is to improve the quality of health care to older adults by enhancing the geriatric competence—the knowledge, skills, and attitudes of nurses who are identified as members of approximately 60–80 national specialty nursing associations.

NCA relies on the strength and experience of the American Nurses Association (ANA), American Nurses Credentialing Center (ANCC), and the John A. Hartford Foundation Institute for Geriatric Nursing (Hartford Institute) in working with specialty nurses and with specialty nursing associations. ANA represents the nation's entire RN population and is at the forefront of policy initiatives pertaining to health-care reform. ANCC is the credentialing branch of ANA, and its mission is to promote excellence in nursing and health care globally through credentialing programs and related services (Scholder et al., 2004). The Hartford Institute identifies and promotes best practices in nursing care of older adults. These authors reinforce the goal of NCA, which is to underscore the need of specialty nurses for a dual professionalism of their specialty and geriatrics when caring for their patients. "Specifically, NCA addresses the knowledge and skills of oncology nurses to address the complexity of care of geriatric health issues, including cancer issues. It also has a component to identify opportunities to promote the development of interdisciplinary geriatric competence that would address physicians, pharmacists, social workers, and other healthcare workers" (Scholder et al., p. 431).

Older adults still are underrepresented in most research clinical trials, especially pharmaceutical trials. Although studies investigating symptom management and individual responses to treatment such as chemotherapy, radiation therapy, and surgery have included older adult patients, studies specific to older adult patients with cancer typically have not been conducted. Exceptions to this pervading thought include studies looking at metastatic breast cancer (O'Brien et al., 2004; O'Shaughnessy et al., 2002; O'Shaughnessy, Twelves, & Aapro, 2002; Sledge et al., 2003), lymphomas, which demonstrate a decreased duration of complete response (National Comprehensive Cancer Network [NCCN], 2005), and acute myeloid leukemia (AML), which shows that AML appears to act differently in older patients (Mayer et al., 1994; Rees, Gray, Swirsky, & Hayhoe, 1986; Stone, 2004). An equally important concern is that minimal attention has been given to what outcomes are considered important in the care of older adults, including older adult patients with cancer. In response to an increasing awareness of the importance of developing ways to look at geriatric oncology outcomes and eventual improvements, NCCN and the ONS/Geriatric Oncology Consortium have developed position papers on cancer care in older adults. These papers address outcomes such as comorbidity, function, quality of life, and guidelines to begin to establish standards of care for outcomes in this highly vulnerable patient population (ONS, 2004).

According to Scholder et al. (2004), "Nursing traditionally views care of elders as a specialty set apart from disease-based subspecialties such as oncology, rheumatology, critical care, or perioperative care even though older adults are the largest group of healthcare users cared for by nurses in most subspecialties" (p. 429). These authors contend that as the size of the older adult population continues to increase, nursing and other healthcare providers cannot afford to maintain the perspective that geriatrics is only a subspecialty. Rather, older adults are the specialty. As an example of research studying a problem targeting an older population, Champion et al. (2003) conducted a comparison study of tailored interventions to increase mammography screening in nonadherent older women. More studies addressing the care needs of older adults are needed. The unique and complex needs of older adults are significant issues relevant to all practicing nurses.

The field of nursing research continues to address topics focused on improving the quality of care for cancer survivors (Ferrell, Virani, Smith, & Juarez, 2003). This is especially important considering the fact that a large number of cancer survivors are older adults with cancer. In addition to clinical practice and education, ONS has been a leading force in oncology nursing research, including initial efforts in cancer survivorship. The National Institute of Nursing Research (NINR) is the main source of funding for nursing research in the United States. NINR also collaborates with the National Institute on Aging and the National Cancer Institute (NCI) in supporting various research endeavors relevant to the older adult with cancer. Prominent oncology nurse researchers have provided eight specific recommendations to the National Cancer Policy Board and the Institute of Medicine that address the role of oncology nurses to ensure quality of care for cancer survivors, many of whom are older adults (Ferrell et al., 2003).

At this point, however, little nursing research exists that has been conducted in older patients with cancer. As with any discussion of research or evidence-based research guiding practice, it is important to provide an explanation of what rating system was used in describing levels of research. Most research generally is viewed according to the following levels of evidence: (a) evidence obtained from at least one properly designed randomized controlled trial, (b) evidence obtained from well-designed controlled trials without randomization (evidence obtained from well-designed cohort or case-controlled analytic studies, preferably from more than one center or research group, and evidence obtained from multiple time series with or without the intervention), and (c) opinions of respected authorities based on clinical experience, descriptive studies, or reports of expert communities. A summary of select EBP rating systems is provided in Figure 2-1.

A search of the literature was conducted through Ovid's MEDLINE and CINAHL using the following search terms: *aged* (65–79 years and 80 and older) and *research, nursing,* and *cancer.* MEDLINE produced 11 citations, and CINAHL generated 25 sources. A separate literature search also was conducted through PubMed using the terms *aged* (65+ years) and *cancer nursing research,* which produced an additional 11 citations. After reviewing the content of the articles generated (several of which were not nursing related or did not address older adults with cancer), 43 references total were considered nursing articles on older adults with a cancer diagnosis. These citations provide an overview of nursing research contributions concerning cancer and older adults (see Table 2-2). Although other articles were identified through a review of references cited in current articles dealing with older adults with cancer and nursing research, they were not captured from the literature search using Ovid, CINAHL, MEDLINE, or PubMed; thus, the table is not all inclusive. This is a potential problem that oncology nurse researchers need to be aware of when selecting key terms in articles for publication and when conducting literature searches. It is important to become familiar with what search terms to use (different search engines use different terms) and include specific age limits to capture nursing research on older adults with cancer.

It is imperative that there is an understanding from a holistic view regarding the physiologic and psychological differences that exist between different age groups, such as between young and older adults. Although common threads are apparent in the care, expected outcomes, and treatment modalities provided for different age groups of people with cancer, great differences also exist in practice and standards of care provided among pediatric, adult, and older adult populations. Unfortunately, more information is needed to know exactly what differences exist between adult patients with cancer and older adult patients with cancer. It is suspected, although with scant EBP, that differences exist in the biology of tumors, mechanisms of treatment protocols, responses to treatments, functional status, and quality of life between the adult and the older adult populations with cancer. The most recent clinical practice guidelines (NCCN, 2005) provide a brief summary of disease-specific issues related to age and include common clinical problems.

Type of Evidence (Agency for Healthcare Research and Quality [AHRQ], 2001; American Pain Society [APS], 1999)
- Meta-analysis of multiple well-designed studies
- At least one well-designed experimental study
- Well-designed quasi-experimental studies, such as a nonrandomized, controlled, single-group pre-test or post-test, cohort, time series, or matched-case controlled studies
- Well-designed nonexperimental studies, such as comparative and correlational descriptive and case studies
- Case reports and clinical examples

Strength and Consistency of Evidence (AHRQ, 2001; APS, 1999)
- Evidence of type I or consistent findings from multiple studies of types II, III, or IV
- Evidence of types II, III, or IV; findings are generally consistent.
- Evidence of types II, III, or IV; findings are inconsistent.
- Little or no evidence, or there is type V evidence only.

Quality of Evidence (Rosswurm & Larrabee, 1999)
- Meta-analysis of randomized controlled trials
  - One randomized controlled trial
- One well-designed controlled study without randomization
  - One other type of a well-designed quasi-experimental study
- Comparative, correlational, and other descriptive studies
- Evidence from expert committee reports and expert opinions

Strength and Consistency of Grading the Evidence (Gerontological Nursing Interventions Research Center, 1999)
- Evidence from a well-designed meta-analysis
- Evidence from well-designed controlled trials, both randomized and nonrandomized, with results that consistently support a specific action (e.g., assessment), intervention, or treatment
- Evidence from observational studies (e.g., correlational, descriptive studies) or controlled trials with inconsistent results
- Evidence from expert opinion or multiple case reports

Strength of Evidence (Stetler, Brunell, et al., 1998; Stetler, Morsi, et al., 1998)
- Meta-analysis of multiple controlled studies
- Individual experimental study
- Quasi-experimental study, such as a nonrandomized, controlled, single-group pretest or post-test, time series, or matched case-controlled studies
- Nonexperimental study, such as correlational descriptive research and qualitative or case studies
- Case report or systematically obtained, verifiable quality, or program evaluation data
- Opinions of respected authorities or the opinions of an expert committee, including their interpretation of non-research-based information

Figure 2-1. Examples of Evidence-Based Practice Rating Systems

Note. From "Use of Research in Practice" (5th ed., p. 164), by M. Titler in G. LoBiondo-Wood and J. Haber (Eds.), *Nursing Research: Methods, Critical Appraisal, and Utilization*, 2002, St. Louis, MO: Mosby. Copyright 2002 by Mosby. Adapted with permission.

These disease-specific issues occur, in part, because of the different behavior of the disease in older versus younger patients and because of the decreased tolerance of treatment by older patients (NCCN). Clearly, more research is needed in all areas of symptom management and in how individuals respond to treatments specific to age and anticipated nurse-sensitive outcomes. Disparities in health care exist despite efforts to include all cultural, ethnic, racial, and minority groups. Yet many clinicians and researchers forget that older adults are a minority group. Older adults, specifically older patients with cancer, are vulnerable, understudied, and

Table 2-2. Sources of Geriatric Oncology Nursing Research

Author(s)/ Date	Purpose	Design	Sample/ Population	Results
Bailey, 2001	Develop an understanding of research determinants of involvement in decision making.	Qualitative	337 patients age 58–95 with adenocarcinoma of the colon and rectum	The analysis suggests that patients often lack a sense of agency in the face of disease and treatment-related events, and many do not believe they possess the relevant knowledge or authority to act positively in these circumstances.
Bailey et al., 2003	Investigate role of age and multidimensional functional status in treatment decisions in older people with adenocarcinoma of the colon and rectum.	Exploratory; descriptive	337 patients age 58–95 with adenocarcinoma of the colon and rectum	Care should be taken to ensure that patients are not excluded from treatment because of age, and the question of providing social support during adjuvant chemotherapy should be reexamined.
Ballantyne, 2004	Describe the social context and outcomes of aging patients with breast cancer.	Integrative essay; literature search; non-research	Older adults with breast cancer	Concludes with the suggestion that clinical practitioners need to be aware of the resources and limitations facing the older patient with breast cancer
Boyle, 1994	Review relevant literature pertaining to nursing care of older adults facing cancer.	Literature review; non-research	Not applicable	Six realities to guide cancer nursing planning were identified that address key issues in the older adult continuum.
Boyle, 2003	Propose topics for nursing investigation relative to prevention and early detection, response to disease and treatment, and psychosocial responses in the older adult at risk for or having cancer.	Commentary; non-research	Not applicable	Topics for future investigations by nurse researchers were identified.

(Continued on next page)

Table 2-2. Sources of Geriatric Oncology Nursing Research *(Continued)*

Author(s)/ Date	Purpose	Design	Sample/ Population	Results
Boyle & Engelking, 1993	Discuss a potential framework to meet the cancer-specific needs of the older adult.	Commentary; non-research	Not applicable	European oncology nurses should be establishing a framework to meet the cancer-specific needs of the older adult.
Cameron & Horsburgh, 1998	Explore issues facing younger and older women with breast cancer.	Non-research; essay	Younger and older women with breast cancer	Although similarities exist, differences are noted between younger and older women with breast cancer.
Carter, 2001	Identify older female cancer caregivers' need for information.	Qualitative	22 older female caregivers of people with advanced-stage cancer	Healthcare providers need to evaluate their caregivers' individual needs for information and to provide this information in a sensitive and factually accurate manner.
Clotfelter, 1999	Determine if an educational intervention decreases pain intensity in older patients with cancer.	Quasi-experimental; pretest, post-test design	36 subjects age 65 and older with a cancer diagnosis	Statistical difference in pain intensity exists between the control group and experimental group.
Coker & Sitzes, 1996	Describe the need for a community-based cancer education and screening program for older women.	Content analysis; non-research	Not applicable	Older women have different needs than younger women in regard to education and screening.
Coleman et al., 2003	Evaluate a multi-method intervention targeting rural healthcare providers to increase breast cancer screening among rural minority and older women.	Intervention; pre-test and post-test design	224 healthcare providers in 27 counties in the Arkansas Delta	Healthcare providers significantly improved in breast cancer screening practices after the intervention.
Cope, 2001	Present news briefs related to medical care of older adult patients with cancer in the United States.	Non-research; commentary	Not applicable	Decline in the number of patients receiving hospice care for lymphedema

(Continued on next page)

Table 2-2. Sources of Geriatric Oncology Nursing Research *(Continued)*

Author(s)/ Date	Purpose	Design	Sample/ Population	Results
Crooks, 2001	Describe contributions of using grounded theory research to gain new understandings of the cancer experience in the study of older women with breast cancer.	Qualitative; grounded theory	146 women age 61 or older	Grounded theory provides greater understanding of the cancer experience for older women.
Ferrell, 1999	Examine pain and quality of life of older adults.	Interview by Ann Schmidt Luggen	Not applicable	Pain and quality of life of older adults has not been adequately addressed.
Ferrell, Juarez, et al., 1999	Describe current use of routine analgesics in home care and the treatment of breakthrough pain.	Descriptive; companion study	Convenience sample, 369 patients with various types and stages of cancer. Older adults were targeted for accrual (82% older than 55 years); mean age was 65 years.	A discrepancy was found between recommended pain management in clinical practice guidelines and the actual practice of pain management at home. Deficiencies were found in medications prescribed as well as in actual use by patients.
Fitch et al., 2001	Describe perspectives of older women regarding their experience with ovarian cancer.	Descriptive; survey	161 older women (61 and older) diagnosed with ovarian cancer	Ovarian cancer has a significant impact on older women, and many perceive that they are not receiving adequate assistance for problems they experience.
Gift et al., 2004	Identify the number, type, and combination of symptoms experienced by patients with lung cancer.	Secondary data analysis; correlational; factor analysis	220 patients newly diagnosed with lung cancer, age 65–89	Factor analysis determined that symptoms of fatigue, nausea, weakness, appetite loss, weight loss, altered taste, and vomiting form a cluster.
Gil et al., 2004	Examine sources of uncertainty in older African American and Caucasian long-term survivors of breast cancer.	Randomized controlled intervention study	244 older women with a history of breast cancer with a mean age of 64 years	Illness uncertainty persisted long after cancer diagnosis and treatment. Most women experienced multiple triggers of uncertainty about recurrence and a range of symptoms.

(Continued on next page)

Table 2-2. Sources of Geriatric Oncology Nursing Research *(Continued)*

Author(s)/ Date	Purpose	Design	Sample/ Population	Results
Given & Given, 1989	Describe cancer nursing and identify a target for research.	Review	Not applicable	Areas lacking research and suggestions for proposed nursing research were identified.
Given & Keilman, 1990	Describe cancer in the older adult and identify research issues.	Review	Older adults with cancer	Research areas pertinent to the older adult with cancer were identified.
Goodwin et al., 2003	Evaluate the effect of nurse case management on the treatment of older women with breast cancer.	Randomized prospective trial	335 women age 65 and older newly diagnosed with breast cancer (166 control group and 169 intervention group)	Greater percentages of women in the case management group received adjuvant radiation and breast reconstruction. Women with indicators of poor social support were more likely to benefit from nurse case management.
Hodgson, 2002	Explore epidemiologic trends of cancer in older adults.	Descriptive	Older adults with cancer	The study cited the need for clarification of the multiple factors affecting the heterogeneous response of cancer to develop effective cancer treatment and control strategies for older adults.
Hodgson & Given, 2004	Examine the psychosocial and disease-specific factors that influence functional recovery in older adults newly diagnosed with cancer and treated with surgery.	Correlational; multivariate logistic regression	Community-residing adults older than 65 years of age (N = 172)	Psychological well-being was a significant factor influencing functional recovery when age, comorbidities, site of disease, and symptom severity were controlled; findings suggest a need for psychological support following cancer surgery.

(Continued on next page)

Table 2-2. Sources of Geriatric Oncology Nursing Research *(Continued)*

Author(s)/ Date	Purpose	Design	Sample/ Population	Results
Howell et al., 1998	Promote nurses' attitudes toward cancer prevention and screening.	Program evaluation; program pretest, post-test, and at six month follow-up	60 nurses in Colorado rural settings	Significant differences in pre- and post-training attitude scores and family high-level confidence ratings suggest that nurses will continue to use their cancer prevention and detection skills in practice.
Kagan, 2004	Analyze the development of gero-oncology research through critical review.	Data synthesis	Not applicable	Shifting perspectives on research in aging and cancer are necessary to meet the needs of aging society.
Kurtz et al., 2001	Identify factors to assess which older adults are experiencing problems with function in association with cancer.	Correlational	420 patients 65–98 years of age, with a cancer diagnosis	Prediagnosis physical functioning, symptom severity, and days since surgery were significant predictors of physical functioning.
Lee, 2001	Provide a synthesis of existing research on sleep and fatigue.	Comprehensive review	Not applicable	Further research is needed to understand relationships between nonrestorative sleep, fatigue, and symptoms related to poor quality of life. Nonpharmacologic interventions may be useful.
Ludwick et al., 1994	Examine information on breast cancer explaining the degree of risk and special needs of older women.	Content analysis	Reviewed 113 articles for content on breast cancer relevant to older women	Authors in the professional nursing literature and the popular media have inadequately addressed the degree of risk and the special needs of the older woman.
McCorkle et al., 1998	Determine effectiveness of nursing interventions provided by advanced practice nurses in oncology to newly diagnosed older patients with cancer who are facing terminal illness.	Secondary data analysis from a longitudinal randomized clinical trial; descriptive	Sample of 37 adults age 60 years or older, discharged from the hospital having undergone surgical treatment of cancer with a prognosis of greater than six months	Nurses were responding to complex patient problems and needs. Findings show that these patients needed help to make the transition from a crisis state to a terminal phase in their illness trajectory.

(Continued on next page)

Table 2-2. Sources of Geriatric Oncology Nursing Research *(Continued)*

Author(s)/ Date	Purpose	Design	Sample/ Population	Results
McCorkle et al., 2000	Determine factors that influence outcomes, including the survival of older patients with cancer after surgery. Compare the length of survival of older patients with cancer post-surgery who received a homecare intervention by advanced practice nurses with usual follow-up care in an ambulatory setting.	Randomized controlled intervention study	375 newly diagnosed patients with solid tumors, age 60–92 years	This is the first study of postsurgical patients with cancer to link a specialized homecare intervention by advanced practice nurses with improved survival.
Narsavage & Romeo, 2003	Examine the use, satisfaction with, and need for cancer education and support services.	Program evaluation	243 younger adult cancer survivors compared to 295 older cancer survivors	Education and support programs should be targeted toward the age of people being served, as well as incidence, prevalence, expected trajectory, and prognosis of cancer types in the service area.
Neumark et al., 2001	Determine if subject or research design factors predicted who was less likely to participate in panel surveys of older families with cancer.	Multivariate model explored simultaneous effects of subject or research design on nonparticipation.	748 nonconsenters, 208 consenters who dropped out prior to data collection, and 992 consenters who participated. Age range not specified.	Findings suggest that both subject and research design characteristics affect the likelihood of nonparticipation in a panel of older patients with cancer and family caregivers.
Powe & Weinrich, 1999	Determine the effectiveness of a video intervention to decrease fatalism in patients with cancer.	Repeated measures; pre- and post-test intervention	70 rural older adults who attended senior centers (42 intervention group and 28 control group); mean age 73 years	People who viewed the intervention video had a greater decrease in fatalism scores and a greater increase in knowledge of colorectal scores than the control group.

(Continued on next page)

Table 2-2. Sources of Geriatric Oncology Nursing Research *(Continued)*

Author(s)/ Date	Purpose	Design	Sample/ Population	Results
Robinson et al., 1999	Describe the nursing care of postsurgical men with prostate cancer.	Retrospective chart review	32 homecare records; age not specified	Findings suggest that at the end of one month of home care, patients had not yet shifted from the crisis to the chronic phase of their illness.
Sammarco, 2003	Investigate relations among perceived social support, uncertainty, and quality of life.	Survey	103 breast cancer survivors older than 50	Social support decreased illness uncertainty and increased quality of life.
Schechterly, 2000	Investigate knowledge about the physical and behavioral aspects of aging and attitudes toward older adults.	Survey; dissertation	247 oncology RNs (Oncology Nursing Society members)	Results suggest a need for nurses to receive geriatric content in schools of nursing and a need to develop a positive philosophy contrary to the negative one held by society toward aging, particularly with a cancer diagnosis.
Sloman et al., 2001	Investigate nurses' knowledge of pain and pain management with respect to older adults.	Survey	RNs at several general hospitals and nursing homes	Findings suggest a knowledge deficit in RNs regarding pain management in the older adult, and differences were found between general hospital nurses and those working in nursing homes. Conclusions were that nurses need more education about pain management of older adults.
Tang et al., 2001	Examine factors associated with fecal occult blood test and sigmoid screening in Chinese American women.	Descriptive	100 Chinese American women from senior centers, age 60 and older	Older Chinese American women underuse fecal occult blood test and sigmoidoscopy screening as recommended by the American Cancer Society; cultural factors may influence screening practices of these women.

(Continued on next page)

Table 2-2. Sources of Geriatric Oncology Nursing Research *(Continued)*

Author(s)/ Date	Purpose	Design	Sample/ Population	Results
Thome et al., 2003	Investigate the experience of older people living with cancer and how it affects activities of daily life.	Qualitative	41 subjects age 75 and older, mean age 83 years old	Main role for health-care professionals is to empower older adults to make choices for themselves. It is important that health-care professionals support older people in their choices.
Utley, 1999	Explore the meaning of life for long-term survivors of breast cancer.	Qualitative	A sample of eight women using network sampling; age not specified	Group learned the meaning of cancer after surviving the disease and treatment centered around positive, insightful experiences.
Wallace, 2003	Explore uncertainty, anxiety, and personal manner in which uncertainty is understood; explain quality of life.	Descriptive	21 men diagnosed with prostate cancer; mean age 76 years old	Significant relationships were found among uncertainty, anxiety, and the perception of danger (a dimension of quality of life).
Wood et al., 2002	Test whether age- and race-sensitive, self-monitored video breast health kits increase knowledge about breast cancer risk and screening and breast self-examination proficiency.	Quasi-experimental; pre- and posteducational intervention	328 patients age 60 and older (206 received intervention, 122 control subjects did not receive the intervention)	The intervention group displayed increased knowledge about breast cancer risk and screening and breast self-examination.
Yarbrough, 2004	Perform a systematic review to (a) describe current research regarding screening practices and outcomes among older women; (b) describe factors associated with mortality or quality-of-life outcomes related to screening in older women; and (c) compare the strength of evidence supporting or refuting screening recommendations in older women.	Research synthesis	15 reports provided data for this review that focused on women older than age 65 (and also included women older than age 74 in sampling)	The data indicate that older women tolerate screening and treatment as well as younger women. Findings suggest that screening practices among older women and life expectancy or quality-of-life outcomes are equivocal and further research is needed. Decisions for screening recommendations in older women should be based on individual needs.

underserved. However, it is estimated that by 2030, 60%–70% of all cancers may occur in this population (Yancik & Ries, 2000).

There is a pressing need for geriatric oncology nurse researchers to determine what gero-oncology practice involves and how care differs from young adult to older adult populations. This includes the need to determine the standards of care for this population and to examine nurse-sensitive outcomes. The model depicted in Figure 2-2 can be useful in guiding research efforts to build a theory applicable to geriatric oncology practice and research.

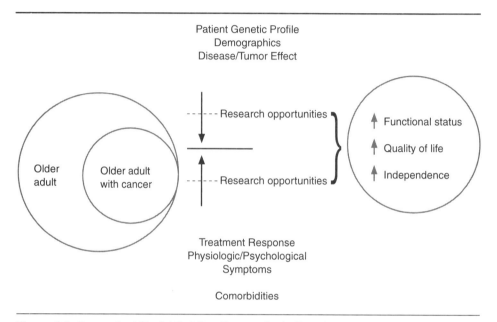

Figure 2-2. Conceptual Model Guiding Gerontologic Oncology Research

Assessment of the Older Adult Patient With Cancer

Conditions such as disabilities, comorbidity, and functional status in concert with tumor type and stage influence the evaluation and treatment of older patients with cancer. According to Rae, Seo, and Cohen (2004) and Bernabei et al. (1998), a comprehensive geriatric assessment (CGA), which can help to guide therapy and affect prognosis and quality of life, can identify these conditions and other geriatric syndromes. Bernabei et al. also suggested that using CGA facilitates better management and more efficient care of older adults with cancer. Geriatric assessment is a multidisciplinary and multidimensional process, which identifies medical, functional, and psychosocial problems, that is used to develop a comprehensive management and care plan (Rae et al.). The main domains of CGA are functional status, gait, balance, risk for falls, cognitive status, affective status, nutritional status, pain, and social function. The guidelines for senior adult oncology (NCCN, 2005) present a comprehensive overview of issues related to the management of cancer in older patients, including geriatric assessment, frailty, disease-specific issues related to age, and life expectancy for men and women at selected ages. Additionally, a detailed outline of the procedure for functional assessment screening is included in these guidelines. This guideline is evidence-based according to NCCN categories of consensus on levels of evidence (also included in the guidelines).

Research Focused on Treatment Modalities and Responses

Surgery

Surgery remains the most important treatment modality for patients with solid tumors regardless of age. Because healthcare clinicians often underestimate the life expectancy of older patients, cancer frequently is undertreated (Kemeny, 2004). Care involving pre- and postoperative procedures is similar across the life span. However, research is needed to determine differences in symptom management across age groups. For example, pain management in older adults is different than with adolescents or adults. Minimal research has been conducted to compare older adult noncancer groups with older adult cancer groups. Based on clinical observations, the healing process is different in older patients than in younger, yet no research exists in this important area of care.

Chemotherapy

Chemotherapy is a common treatment for many types of cancer, including hemato-logic and in combination with surgery for solid tumors. According to Lichtman (2004), cancer chemotherapy needs to be tailored to the individual, and oncologists should take into consideration aspects of aging, such as functional status and comorbidity.

Most adverse side effects and adverse events that occur during and following treat-ment are a result of specific pharmacokinetics attributable to individual pharmaceuti-cal agents rather than the type of cancer. For example, neutropenia causing bone marrow suppression is a frequently mentioned side effect in the older adult patient receiving chemotherapy and is an area that has received considerable investigation (Lichtman, 2004). Because limited data are available from prospective randomized phase III trials regarding adjuvant chemotherapy for breast cancer in older women, the choice of an adjuvant chemotherapy regimen is somewhat limited and random (Kimmick & Muss, 2004). More studies are needed in the areas of toxicity, drug metabolism, and drug effect, as well as research and educational initiatives targeted to this population (Lichtman, 2004).

Issues in Palliative Care Research

According to Reb (2003), as the number of older people living with chronic condi-tions increases, the need for palliative and supportive services throughout the illness continuum and at end of life also will be greater. Older people with cancer frequently experience unique challenges that younger people may not encounter (Matulonis,

2004). NINR and NCI, both housed within the National Institutes of Health (NIH), have established a strong leadership presence on palliative and end-of-life research issues. In concert with these federal funding agencies, the oncology nursing profession has played a key role in advancing improvements in palliative care through its leadership in educational, quality improvement, research, and legislative initiatives (Ferrell, Grant, & Virani, 1999; Ferrell, Virani, & Grant, 1998; Reb).

Other challenges relevant to older adults with advanced cancer include the presence of comorbid conditions that may increase the risk of severe toxicity from usual and standard treatments, such as surgery, antineoplastic medications, and other treatment modalities. In addition, these older adults may have unique social situations, such as residing in a nursing home or the need for a dedicated caregiver to assist in the home. The complexity of care involving older adults with cancer can contribute to a wide array of symptoms that may overlap and require geriatric knowledge as well as oncology training. Matulonis (2004) noted that "early initiation of advance directives is also important to specify levels of care at the end of life" (p. 274).

Advance Directives and Legal Considerations

An advance directive is a legal document recognized under state law that provides guidance to the family and healthcare providers as to the subject's wishes for health care in the event that he or she is unable to articulate those wishes. Three main types of documents are used to provide advance directives: a living will, a durable power of attorney for health care, and a durable power of attorney for financial concerns (Birke, 2004). It is important for physicians and nurses involved in recruitment for clinical trial research to have a clear understanding of the patient's wishes. These documents do not prevent a patient from participating in research; however, as with all patient care, providers need to be clear on the wishes of their older patients. Advance directives and palliative care are critical components of health care. Because cancer is the second major cause of death in the United States, these issues are of great concern for patient safety, quality of life, and an integral good death.

Long-Term Care, Home Care, and Oncology Issues

Minimal research on oncology issues in long-term care and home care has been conducted. Yet, these healthcare arenas are the fastest growing institutions in the United States and are especially important to the rapidly growing older adult patient populations. Nurses unfamiliar with oncology standards of care need evidence-based protocols readily available to help them to assess, plan, and implement quality cancer care to this burgeoning population. Patients with cancer receiving long-term care and home care often are not included in national statistics; thus, their numbers and care needs usually are absent from benchmark institution numbers and quality indicators. The older adult patient with cancer frequently is not included in cancer care trends and typically shows up only as a geriatric long-term care or homecare patient, with actual care and quality EBP "hidden" from reported data.

Caregivers of Older Adults With Cancer

The number of older adults with cancer is growing, and with the shift from inpatient to outpatient care, the significance and need for informal caregiving continues to increase (Ferrell et al., 2003; Reb, 2003). Most caregivers of patients with cancer are family members who may be unprepared for or lack the resources and energy to meet the needs of the patient.

Examples of agencies and professional organizations focusing on the need for research in the areas of palliative care, long-term and home care, and related caregiving demands on family members include the following: NIH, the Institute of Medicine, and ONS. For example, NINR has prioritized research themes, including interventions to address caregiver needs and support for older adult and rural caregivers.

Models of Evidence-Based Care and Existing Evidence-Based Protocols

Few clinical practice guidelines exist regarding the care of older patients, especially for older adult patients with cancer. Although EBP increasingly is being integrated into clinical nursing practice, minimal research exists on EBP specific to older patients in the geriatric research literature. In the EBP that exists in geriatric literature, none was identified specific to geriatric research, including people with cancer.

Several existing models of EBP in nursing have developed from earlier research utilization models (Goode, 1995; Horsley, Crane, & Bingle, 1978; Stetler, 1994; Tang & Titler, 2003; Titler et al., 1999, 2001). The first published research utilization model was the "Conduct and Utilization of Research in Nursing" (CURN) model (Haller, Reynolds, & Horsley, 1979; Horsley et al., 1978; Horsley, Crane, Crabtree, & Wood, 1983) developed at the University of Michigan. The CURN Project was designed to develop and test a model for using research-based knowledge in clinical practice settings. This project viewed research utilization as an organizational process, and planned change was integrated throughout the research utilization process. A necessary component of this model is that a systems change is essential to establishing research-based practice on a large scale.

The Iowa Model of EBP incorporated some components from the CURN project as an organizational, collaborative model developed by the University of Iowa Hospital and Clinics and the University of Iowa College of Nursing. In this environment, research utilization also is viewed as an organizational process. The Iowa Model infuses research into practice to improve the quality of care (Goode, 1995; Goode & Titler, 1996; Titler et al., 1994, 1999, 2001; Titler & Mentes, 1999) and accomplishes this by using planned change principles to integrate evidence-based healthcare research and practice with a multidisciplinary team approach. The University of Iowa College of Nursing Geriatric Nursing Intervention Research Center created a Research Dissemination Core in 1999 with the purposes of distributing scientific information to the professional nursing community and to consumers, as well as promoting the adoption of evidence-based interventions to improve the care of older adults. Currently, colleagues from the University of Iowa have developed 30 evidence-based nursing practice protocols designed for the older adult population. Although these EBP protocols are not specific to geriatric oncology or for disease-specific populations, they are evidence-based specific to the older adult population. Select examples common to and inclusive of older adult patients with cancer include acute pain management, falls prevention, management of constipation, detection of depression in the cognitively intact older adult, advance directives, and clinical trials. The author currently is developing an evidence-based protocol for clinical trials and the older adult.

The Stetler Model of Research Utilization applies research findings at the individual practitioner level (Stetler, 1983, 1985, 1994; Stetler & Marram, 1976). This model has six phases: (a) preparation, (b) validation, (c) comparative evaluation, (d) decision making, (e) translation and application, and (f) evaluation. A cornerstone of this model is the role of the advanced practice nurse to employ a mentoring process to accomplish organizational changes and outcomes. Critical thinking and decision making are emphasized in this model. This model has considerable "buy in" from staff because the focus is at the individual practitioner level, and implementing changes occurs at the clinical level.

Closely related to the previously referenced EBP models are rigorous and innovative efforts aimed at developing practice process guidelines (Hogan & Logan, 2004; Logan & Graham, 1998; Mezey & Zwicker, 2003). The Ottawa Model of Research Use (Hogan & Logan; Logan & Graham) evolved out of a clinical problem identified by a clinical nurse specialist who determined that usual neonatal transport was not based on evidence nor was it conducive to viewing the family as client. This organization concluded that use of a family assessment tool is an effective way of appraising families and addressing suffering. The Ottawa Model of Research Use provided a framework for implementing the clinical innovation (Hogan & Logan).

Mezey, Fulmer, and Abraham (2003) have developed geriatric nursing protocols to ensure quality care for older adults. Although not specifically evidence-based or specific to older adults with cancer, they are written with at least one level of evidence and provide guidance in the care of older adults. According to Lucas and Fulmer (2003), "clinical practice guidelines are statements derived from the best available evidence for making decisions about the care of specific patient populations" (p. 2).

In an effort to improve the care of older adults in hospitals, albeit not specific to oncology, the John A. Hartford Foundation Institute for Geriatric Nursing at New York University started the Nurses Improving Care for Health System Elders (NICHE), a comprehensive program that implements best practice models for geriatric care (Boltz, Harrington, & Kluger, 2005; Mezey et al., 2003). Components of the NICHE program include four practice models to enhance the knowledge of staff nurses: the Geriatric Resource Nurse model, the Geriatric Syndrome Management model, the Acute Care of the Elderly Nursing Unit model, and the Quality Cost Model of Transitional Care (Boltz et al.).

Although the previously described models have established innovative ways to ensure "best" practice in the care of patients and in the delivery of health care, it is equally important to find ways to ensure that EBP is continued and constantly kept current. This task is not easy, as there are inherent challenges in conducting research to determine levels of evidence. Excellent resources are available to find the best geriatric practices, including www.medicine.uiowa.edu.igec, www.nursing.upenn.edu/centers/hcgne/default.htm, www.hartfordign.org, www.americangeriatrics.org/products/gnr_syllabus.shtml, www.merck.com/pubs/mm_geriatrics/contents.htm, www.nia.nih.gov/healthInformation, and www.hartfordign.org/resources/policy/coalition.html.

Research Challenges Encountered With Older Adult Populations

Barriers to Older Adult Participation in Clinical Trials

Important barriers to recruitment, enrollment, and retention of older adults for clinical trials are fear, distrust, or misunderstanding of the clinical trial process; the perception that appropriate trials are not available; and the inconvenience of protocol requirements and perhaps extra visits for data collection (Connolly, Schneider, & Hill, 2004; Payne, 2003; Schilsky, 2004). These barriers are listed in Table 2-1. According to federal agencies such as NIH, NCI, and the Institute of Medicine, professional organizations such as ONS, and other organizations such as the Geriatric Oncology Consortium, older adults with cancer frequently are underserved with regard to prevention and screening measures and are less likely to be treated with curative therapy intent. Barriers to access and enrollment in clinical trials vary among different organizations, healthcare providers, and patient populations. However, evidence suggests that these barriers can be assembled into three categories: system barriers, healthcare provider barriers, and patient barriers. Changing attitudes, changing perceptions, and increasing awareness about clinical trials among these groups are paramount to overcoming many of the current barriers (Payne, 2003).

Changing the Mindset

Specific communication and education strategies may help potential subjects to overcome the fears, suspicions, and misconceptions that keep older adults with cancer from participating in clinical trials. It has been suggested that healthcare providers need to develop a new attitude about recruitment as well as change the community's mindset of what clinical trials are about to dispel some of the apprehensions that older people feel (Payne, 2003). Clinicians need to take time to explain the purpose of the research, the meaning of randomization, and the benefits that patients derive from research. These benefits include access to the newest and most innovative treatment and best-quality follow-up care. It also should be stressed that the research center is a "special" place with a team that is personally committed to helping to facilitate the patient's care at every stage of the trial (Payne, 2003). Communication skills can help to build trust and must be honed to accommodate the older adult, some of whom may be hard of hearing or have poor vision.

Strategies to Increase Enrollment

Research nurses are in a unique position to provide strategies that address recruitment as well as affect the attitudes of patients, physicians, and the greater community. Several factors have been identified that negatively influence whether potential individuals agree to study participation, including the belief that compensation is not adequate; the potential need for hospitalization; the possibility of receiving a placebo rather than the treatment; travel expenses; inconvenient location; risk of side effects; and reluctance of healthcare providers to offer clinical trials to the older adult. Strategies to overcome these factors include increasing public awareness, honing communication skills appropriate to the older patient, and increasing education efforts. These efforts include informing patients and communities about the availability of clinical trials, providing education about research trials, and explaining the potential benefits of participation, such as innovative state-of-the-art treatment as well as careful follow-up care.

Efforts to increase awareness of cancer clinical trials are ongoing. For example, NCI developed the Cancer Clinical Trials Education Program (CCTEP) in the 1990s to provide tools for healthcare professionals to educate the public about clinical trials. CCTEP recently was updated to include various educational materials in the new Clinical Trials Education Series (Michaels, Denicoff, Bright, Abrams, & Robinson, 2002). Another recent demonstration project was based on a national level partnership designed to increase knowledge about clinical trials among older adults in the community (Ehrenberger, Breeden, & Donovan, 2003). This project represents a successful grassroots effort in increasing awareness of clinical trials among older adults.

New Recruitment Techniques

Traditional recruitment strategies focus on a clinician or designated research personnel approaching a potential individual with prepared informational materials about the disease and treatment. A patient consent form also is usually presented at this initial meeting, and discussion occurs between the individual and clinician. Other traditional examples include posters with a research number and tear-off information and printed material displayed on sign-in counters and in elevators. New strategies include CD-ROM and more interactive visual materials for the older adult to share with his or her family and caregivers. Call centers also are being offered to decrease the time-consuming and clinical burdens that recruitment traditionally has required of clinicians. However, recruitment of older adults to clinical trials requires an additional time commitment from both the institution and the healthcare provider. Community outreach efforts to increase awareness of available clinical trials, being available to listen to stories and answer questions, and preparing age-appropriate teaching materials need to be performed. The time is well spent in an effort to include older adults in research studies.

Caregiver Issues

When approached by healthcare clinicians regarding participation in a clinical trial, older patients frequently say that they have to rely on a caregiver to drive them to and from doctor appointments, treatments, and follow-up surveillance. Many older adults hesitate to ask for any help and feel uncomfortable asking for transportation required for multiple follow-up visits. The general population also holds the perception that all cancer diagnoses and treatment modalities cause severe side effects. Resultant fears may include older adults facing the possibility that they may be left alone at home to deal with symptom management issues.

Informed Consent

Research facilitates a strong role in the development of treatment plans, standards of care, and policies in health care. Thus, participants of all ages and gender need to be included in research projects. Obtaining informed consent is a critical and necessary process. It is not a single event as much as a system of giving and processing information with the desired outcome being the subjects' understanding of the purpose and aims of the study, procedures involved, time commitment, and any risks or benefits. It is always optimal to explain the study and then provide a written copy to the patient and family to take home and read, make notes of any questions, and come back to sign the consent form for actual enrollment. This enables the patient to have time to read documents thoroughly and discuss any concerns with family or friends. Informed consent is an important component of the research process and can involve complicated language and terminology, complex procedures with numerous data collection points, clarification of patients' responsibilities and rights, and expected risks and benefits.

Nursing Roles and Contributions

The role of nursing is vital to successful clinical trials and especially for trials involving minority and older adult populations. Whether nurses are functioning as a research assistant, project director, or an individual principal investigator, understanding the research process is absolutely critical to the success of patient-focused clinical research trials. The nurse often is the first one to initiate a bond between the patient and the healthcare system and establish the beginning of a trusting long-term relationship. Based on the literature and clinical observation, this initial step of trust has to be present to successfully engage older adults into clinical trials (Payne, 2003). Nurses play a key role as educator in the research team. However, equally important is their role in the initial and ongoing assessment and symptom management of the older adult patient during and following study procedures.

Recommendations for Future Directions

Cooperation among gerontologic and oncology researchers must be developed and sustained if a theory is to be developed on which to base programs of research. Theory is the basis for and outcome of most research. Well-designed research studies will guide the development of practice standards and EBP guidelines in the emerging field of older adult oncology. Research implications and specific recommendations include

1. Encourage new oncology investigators to build a program of research. Mentoring junior investigators to think in terms of focusing research efforts on a topic or patient population will help them to develop skills and credibility in an area.
2. Provide evidence-based symptom management for this growing population. Older adult oncology nurse researchers and advanced practice nurses are optimally prepared for this role. In the high-technology–driven healthcare environment, symptom management (an area where oncology nurses are experts) is an area that is critical to patients' functional status and overall quality of life. A paucity of research exists that specifically targets older adults with cancer, and this presents a variety of opportunities for nurse researchers to make a difference and contribute to the science of care for this population.
3. Determine age not as an influencing variable but as the focus of the investigation. For example, how does the frail older adult respond to surgical treatment, and what nursing interventions work best for this age population?

4. Conduct large, multisite, and collaborative cooperative studies to get good data on which to build a research base.
5. Most importantly, develop well-designed studies with validated and age-appropriate measures. An excellent beginning foundation for examining the care of older adults with a cancer diagnosis has been established. However, challenges remain to create better-designed studies focusing on the priorities of national and professional organizations, including the study of older adults with cancer. This population needs to be studied in relation to care issues as an entity rather than viewing age as one variable.
6. Prioritize research oriented toward establishing nurse-sensitive oncology outcomes for this vulnerable and understudied population. Other research priorities include obtaining large data sets of treatment trends, costs, and the impact of healthcare policy on patient care.
7. Prioritize research, including longitudinal studies investigating comorbidity and survival data.
8. Conduct research aimed at affecting healthcare policy to secure and maintain ongoing quality health care for older adults with cancer.
9. Finally, design educational curricula to increase the knowledge base and awareness of students to the growing need for more research focused on older adults with cancer.

References

Agency for Healthcare Research and Quality. (2001). *Management of cancer pain*. Rockville, MD: Author.

American Pain Society. (1999). *Principles of analgesic use in the treatment of acute pain and cancer pain* (4th ed.). Glenview, IL: Author.

Bailey, C. (2001). Older patients' experiences of pre-treatment discussions: An analysis of qualitative data from a study of colorectal cancer. *NT Research, 6,* 736–746.

Bailey, C., Corner, J., Addington-Hall, J., Kumar, D., Nelson, M., & Haviland, J. (2003). Treatment decisions in older patients with colorectal cancer: The role of age and multidimensional function. *European Journal of Cancer Care, 12,* 257–262.

Balducci, L. (2003). New paradigms for treating elderly patients with cancer: The comprehensive geriatric assessment and guidelines for supportive care. *Journal of Supportive Oncology, 1*(4), 30–37.

Ballantyne, P.J. (2004). Social context and outcomes for the ageing breast cancer patient: Considerations for clinical practitioners. *Journal of Clinical Nursing, 13*(3a), 11–21.

Beers, M.H., & Berkow, R. (Eds.). (2000–2005). *Merck manual of geriatrics*. Retrieved February 18, 2005, from http://www.merck.com/pubs/mm_geriatrics/contents.htm

Bernabei, R., Gambassi, G., Lapane, K., Landi, F., Gatsonis, C., Dunlop, R., et al. (1998). Management of pain in elderly patients with cancer. *JAMA, 279,* 1877–1882.

Birke, M. (2004). Elder law, Medicare, and legal issues in older patients. *Seminars in Oncology, 31,* 282–292.

Boltz, M., Harrington, C., & Kluger, M. (2005). Nursing counts: Nurses Improving Care for Health System Elders (NICHE). *American Journal of Nursing, 105*(5), 101–102.

Boyle, D. (1994). Realities to guide novel and necessary nursing care in geriatric oncology. *Cancer Nursing, 17,* 125–136.

Boyle, D. (2003). Establishing a nursing research agenda in gero-oncology [Review]. *Critical Reviews in Oncology/Hematology, 48*(2), 103–111.

Boyle, D.M., & Engelking, C. (1993). Cancer in the elderly: The forgotten priority. *European Journal of Cancer Care, 2*(3), 101–107.

Cameron, S., & Horsburgh, M.E. (1998). Comparing issues faced by younger and older women with breast cancer. *Canadian Oncology Nursing Journal, 8,* 40–44.

Carter, P. (2001). A not-so-silent cry for help: Older female cancer caregivers' need for information. *Journal of Holistic Nursing, 19,* 271–284.

Champion, V., Maraj, M., Hui, S., Perkins, A.J., Tierney, W., & Menon, U. (2003). Comparison of tailored interventions to increase mammography screening in nonadherent older women. *Preventive Medicine, 36,* 150–158.

Clotfelter, C.E. (1999). The effect of an education intervention on decreasing pain intensity in elderly people with cancer. *Oncology Nursing Forum, 26,* 27–33.

Coker, M.A., & Sitzes, C. (1996). The need for more information: A Community-based breast cancer education and screening program for elderly women. *Geriatric Nursing, 17,* 154–155.

Coleman, E.A., Lord, J., Heard, J., Coon, S., Cantrell, M., Mohrmann, C., et al. (2003). The Delta project: Increasing breast cancer screening among rural minority and older women by targeting rural healthcare providers. *Oncology Nursing Forum, 30,* 669–677.

Connolly, N.B., Schneider, D., & Hill, A.M. (2004). Improving enrollment in clinical trials. *Oncology Nursing Forum, 31,* 610–614.

Cope, D. (2001). News briefs. *Clinical Journal of Oncology Nursing, 5,* 54.

Crooks, D.L. (2001). Older women with breast cancer: New understanding through grounded theory research. *Health Care for Women International, 22,* 99–114.

Denduluri, N., & Ershler, W.B. (2004). Aging biology and cancer. *Seminars in Oncology, 31,* 137–148.

Ehrenberger, H.E., Breeden, J.R., & Donovan, M.E. (2003). A demonstration project to increase the awareness of cancer clinical trials among community-dwelling seniors [Online exclusive]. *Oncology Nursing Forum, 30,* E80–E83.

Estabrooks, C.A. (1998). Will evidence-based nursing practice make practice perfect? *Canadian Journal of Nursing Research, 30*(1), 15–36.

Ferrell, B., Grant, M., & Virani, R. (1999). Strengthening nursing education to improve end-of-life care. *Nursing Outlook, 47,* 252–256.

Ferrell, B., Juarez, G., & Borneman, T. (1999). Use of routine and breakthrough analgesia in home care. *Oncology Nursing Forum, 26,* 1655–1661.

Ferrell, B., Virani, R., & Grant, M. (1998). HOPE: Home Care Outreach for Palliative Care Education. *Cancer Practice, 6,* 79–85.

Ferrell, B., Virani, R., Smith, S., & Juarez, G. (2003). The role of oncology nursing to ensure quality care for cancer survivors: A report commissioned by the National Cancer Policy Board and Institute of Medicine [Online exclusive]. *Oncology Nursing Forum, 30,* E1–E11.

Ferrell, B.R. (1999). Pain and quality of life of older adults: Betty R. Ferrell, PhD, FAAN. Interview by Ann Schmidt Luggen. *Geriatric Nursing, 20,* 273–274.

Fitch, M.I., Gray, R.E., & Franssen, E. (2001). Perspectives on living with ovarian cancer: Older women's views. *Oncology Nursing Forum, 28,* 1433–1442.

Gerontological Nursing Interventions Research Center. (1999). *Guidelines for writing evidence-based protocols.* Iowa City, IA: Gerontological Nursing Interventions Research Center, Research Dissemination Core, University of Iowa.

Gift, A.G., Jablonski, A., Stommel, M., & Given, C.W. (2004). Symptom clusters in elderly patients with lung cancer. *Oncology Nursing Forum, 31,* 203–212.

Gil, K.M., Mishel, M.H., Belyea, M., Germino, B., Germino, L.S., Porter, L., et al. (2004). Triggers of uncertainty about recurrence and long-term treatment side effects in older African American and Caucasian breast cancer survivors. *Oncology Nursing Forum, 31,* 633–639.

Given, B., & Given, C.W. (1989). Cancer nursing for the elderly: A target for research. *Cancer Nursing, 12,* 71–77.

Given, B., & Keilman, L. (1990). Cancer in the elderly population: Research issues. *Oncology Nursing Forum, 17,* 121–123.

Goode, C.J. (1995). Evaluation of research-based nursing practice. *Nursing Clinics of North America, 30,* 421–427.

Goode, C.J., & Titler, M.G. (1996). Moving research-based practice throughout the health care system. *Medsurg Nursing, 5,* 380–382.

Goodwin, J., Satish, S., Anderson, E., Nattinger, A., & Freeman, J. (2003). Effect of nurse case management on the treatment of older women with breast cancer. *Journal of the American Geriatrics Society, 51,* 1252–1259.

Haller, K.B., Reynolds, M.A., & Horsley, J.A. (1979). Developing research-based innovation protocols: Process, criteria and issues. *Research in Nursing and Health, 2,* 45–51.

Hodgson, N.A. (2002). Epidemiological trends of cancer in older adults: Implications for gerontological nursing practice and research. *Journal of Gerontological Nursing, 28,* 52–53.

Hodgson, N., & Given, C.W. (2004). Determinants of functional recovery in older adults surgically treated for cancer. *Cancer Nursing, 27,* 10–16.

Hogan, D., & Logan, J. (2004). The Ottawa model of research use: A guide to clinical innovation in the NICU. *Clinical Nurse Specialist, 18,* 255–261.

Horsley, J.A., Crane, J., & Bingle, J.D. (1978). Research utilization as an organizational process. *Journal of Nursing Administration, 8*(7), 4–6.

Horsley, J.A., Crane, J., Crabtree, M.K., & Wood, D.J. (1983). *Using research to improve practice.* Orlando, FL: Grune & Stratton.

Howell, S.L., Nelson-Marten, P., Krebs, L.U., Kaszyk, L., & Wold, R. (1998). Promoting nurses' positive attitudes toward cancer prevention/screening. *Journal of Cancer Education, 13,* 76–84.

Kagan, S. (2004). Shifting perspectives: Gero-oncology nursing research. *Oncology Nursing Forum, 31,* 293–299.

Kemeny, M.M. (2004). Surgery in older patients. *Seminars in Oncology, 31,* 174–184.

Kimmick, G., & Muss, H. (2004). Breast cancer in older adults. *Seminars in Oncology, 31,* 234–248.

Kurtz, M.E., Kurtz, J.C., Stommel, M., Given, C.W., & Given, B. (2001). Physical functioning and depression among older persons with cancer. *Cancer Practice, 9*(1), 11–18.

Lee, K.A. (2001). Sleep and fatigue. *Annual Review of Nursing Research, 19,* 249–273.

Lichtman, S. (2003). Guidelines for the treatment of elderly cancer patients. *Cancer Control, 10,* 445–453.

Lichtman, S. (2004). Chemotherapy in the elderly. *Seminars in Oncology, 31,* 160–174.

LoBiondo-Wood, G., & Haber, J. (2002). *Nursing research: Methods, critical appraisal, and utilization* (5th ed.). St. Louis, MO: Mosby.

Logan, J., & Graham, I. (1998). Toward a comprehensive interdisciplinary model of health care research use. *Scientific Communication, 20,* 227–246.

Lucas, J., & Fulmer, T. (2003). Evaluating clinical practice guideline: A best practice. In M. Mezey, T. Fulmer, & I. Abraham (Eds.), *Geriatric nursing protocols for best practice* (2nd ed., pp. 1–14). New York: Springer.

Ludwick, R., Rushing, B., & Biordi, D.L. (1994). Breast cancer and the older woman: Information and images. *Health Care for Women International, 15,* 235–242.

Matulonis, U. (2004). End of life issues in older patients. *Seminars in Oncology, 31,* 274–281.

Mayer, R.J., Davis, R.B., Schiffer, C.A., Berg, D.T., Powell, B.L., Schulman, P., et al. (1994). Intensive postremission chemotherapy in adults with acute myeloid leukemia. Cancer and Leukemia Group B. *New England Journal of Medicine, 331,* 896–903.

McCorkle, R., Hughes, L., Robinson, L., Levine, B., & Nuamah, I. (1998). Nursing interventions for newly diagnosed older cancer patients facing terminal illness. *Journal of Palliative Care, 14,* 39–45.

McCorkle, R., Strumpf, N.E., Nuamah, I.F., Adler, D.C., Cooley, M.E., Jepson, C., et al. (2000). A specialized home care intervention improves survival among older post-surgical cancer patients. *Journal of the American Geriatrics Society, 48,* 1707–1713.

Mezey, M., Fulmer, T., & Abraham, I. (Eds.). (2003). *Geriatric nursing protocols for best practice* (2nd ed.). New York: Springer.

Mezey, M., & Zwicker, D. (2003). Introduction. In M. Mezey, T. Fulmer, & I. Abraham (Eds.), *Geriatric nursing protocols for best practice* (2nd ed., p. xix). New York: Springer.

Michaels, M., Denicoff, A.M., Bright, M.A., Abrams, J., & Robinson, D. (2002). Current initiatives at the National Cancer Institute. *Oncology Issues, 17,* 33–35.

Morrow, G., Hickok, J., & Burish, T. (1994). Behavioral aspects of clinical trials. An integrated framework from behavior theory. *Cancer, 74*(Suppl. 9), 2676–2682.

Murthy, V., Krumholz, H., & Gross, C. (2004). Participation in cancer clinical trials. *JAMA, 291,* 2720–2726.

Muss, H.B., Cohen, H.J., & Lichtman, S.M. (2000). Clinical research in the older cancer patient. *Hematology/Oncology Clinics of North America, 14,* 283–291.

Narsavage, G., & Romeo, E. (2003). Education and support needs of young and older cancer survivors. *Applied Nursing Research, 16,* 103–109.

National Comprehensive Cancer Network. (2005). *Clinical practice guidelines in oncology: Senior adult oncology.* Jenkintown, PA: Author.

Neumark, D.E., Stomel, M., Given, C.W., & Given, B.A. (2001). Brief report. Research design and subject characteristics predicting nonparticipation in a panel survey of older families with cancer. *Nursing Research, 50,* 363–368.

O'Brien, M.E.R., Wigler, N., Inbar, M., Rosso, R., Grischke, E., Santoro, A., et al. (2004). Reduced cardiotoxicity and comparable efficacy in a phase III trial of pegylated liposomal doxorubicin HCL. *Annals of Oncology, 15,* 440–449.

Oncology Nursing Society. (2004). *Oncology Nursing Society and Geriatric Oncology Consortium joint position on cancer care in the older adult.* Retrieved February 23, 2005, from http://www.ons. org/publications/positions/Geriatric.shtml

O'Shaughnessy, J., Miles, D., Vukelja, S., Moiseyenko, V., Ayoub, J., Cervantes, G., et al. (2002). Superior survival with capecitabine plus docetaxel combination therapy in anthracycline-pretreated patients with advanced breast cancer: Phase III trial results. *Journal of Clinical Oncology, 20,* 2812–2823.

O'Shaughnessy, J., Twelves, C., & Aapro, M. (2002). Treatment for anthracycline-pretreated metastatic breast cancer. *Oncologist, 7,* 4–12.

Payne, J. (2002). An integrated model of evidence-based nursing practice [Abstract]. *Oncology Nursing Forum, 29,* 1–3.

Payne, J. (2003, September 18–19). *Enrolling elderly cancer patients in clinical trials: Changing the mindset.* Abstract presented at the Geriatric Oncology Consortium, Washington, DC.

Powe, B.D., & Weinrich, R. (1999). An intervention to decrease cancer fatalism among rural elders. *Oncology Nursing Forum, 26,* 583–588.

Rae, A., Seo, P., & Cohen, H. (2004). Geriatric assessment and comorbidity. *Seminars in Oncology, 31,* 149–159.

Reb, A. (2003). Palliative and end-of-life care: Policy analysis. *Oncology Nursing Forum, 30,* 35–50.

Rees, J.K., Gray, R.G., Swirsky, D., & Hayhoe, F.G. (1986). Principal results of the Medical Research Council's 8th acute myeloid leukaemia trial. *Lancet, 29,* 1236–1241.

Robinson, L., Hughes, L.C., Adler, D.C., Strumpf, N., Grobe, S.J., & McCorkle, R. (1999). Describing the work of nursing: The case of postsurgical nursing interventions for men with prostate cancer. *Research in Nursing and Health, 22,* 321–328.

Rosswurm, M.A., & Larrabee, J.H. (1999). A model for change to evidence-based practice. *Image: The Journal of Nursing Scholarship, 31,* 317–322.

Rutledge, D.N., & Grant, M. (2002). Evidence-based practice in cancer nursing. Introduction. *Seminars in Oncology Nursing, 18,* 121–126.

Sammarco, A. (2003). Quality of life among older survivors of breast cancer. *Cancer Nursing, 26,* 431–438.

Schechterly, G.J. (2000). *Oncology registered nurses' knowledge about and attitudes toward the elderly.* Unpublished doctoral dissertation, Pennsylvania State University, State College.

Schilsky, R. (2004, September 11). *Opportunities and pitfalls of clinical trials in older patients.* Abstract presented at the Geriatric Oncology Consortium, Washington, DC.

Scholder, J., Kagan, S., & Jean Schumann, M. (2004). Nurse competence in aging overview. *Nursing Clinics of North America, 39,* 429–442.

Sledge, G., Neuberg, D., Bernardo, P., Ingle, J., Martino, S., Rowinsky, E., et al. (2003). Phase III trial of doxorubicin, paclitaxel, and the combination of doxorubicin and paclitaxel as front-line chemotherapy for metastatic breast cancer: An intergroup trial (E1193). *Journal of Clinical Oncology, 21,* 588–592.

Sloman, R., Ahern, M., Wright, A., & Brown, L. (2001). Nurses' knowledge of pain in the elderly. *Journal of Pain and Symptom Management, 21,* 317–322.

Stetler, C.B. (1983). Nurses and research responsibility and involvement. *National Intravenous Therapy Association, 6,* 207–212.

Stetler, C.B. (1985). Research utilization: Defining the concept. *Image: The Journal of Nursing Scholarship, 17,* 42.

Stetler, C.B. (1994). Refinement of the Stetler/Marram model for application of research findings to practice. *Nursing Outlook, 42,* 15–25.

Stetler, C.B., Brunell, M., Giuliano, K., Morsi, D., Prince, L., & Newell-Stokes, V. (1998). Evidence-based practice and the role of nursing leadership. *Journal of Nursing Administration, 28*(7–8), 45–53.

Stetler, C.B., & Marram, G. (1976). Evaluating research findings for applicability in practice. *Nursing Outlook, 24,* 559–563.

Stetler, C.B., Morsi, D., Rucki, S., Broughton, S., Corrigan, B., Fitzgerald, J., et al. (1998). Utilization-focused integrative reviews in a nursing service. *Applied Nursing Research, 11,* 195–206.

Stone, R.M. (2004). *Challenges in the management of cancer in older patients—A delicate balance.* Symposium proceeding presented at the annual meeting of the American Society of Clinical Oncology, New Orleans, LA.

Tang, J.H.C., & Titler, M. (2003). Evidence-based practice: Residency program in gerontological nursing. *Journal of Gerontological Nursing, 29*(11), 9–14.

Tang, T.S., Solomon, L.J., & McCracken, L.M. (2001). Barriers to fecal occult blood testing and sigmoidoscopy among older Chinese-American women. *Cancer Practice, 9,* 277–282.

Thome, B., Dykes, A., Gunnars, B., & Hallberg, I.R. (2003). The experiences of older people living with cancer. *Cancer Nursing, 26,* 85–96.

Titler, M., Kleiber, C., Steelman, V., Goode, C., Rakel, B., Barry-Walker, J., et al. (1994). Infusing research into practice to promote quality care. *Nursing Research, 43,* 307–313.

Titler, M., Kleiber, C., Steelman, V., Rakel, B.A., Budreau, G., Everett, L.Q., et al. (2001). The Iowa Model of Evidence-Based Practice to Promote Quality Care. *Critical Care Nursing Clinics of North America, 13,* 497–509.

Titler, M., & Mentes, J. (1999). Research utilization in gerontological nursing practice. *Journal of Gerontological Nursing, 25*(6), 6–9.

Titler, M., Mentes, J.C., Rakel, B., Abbott, L., & Baumler, S. (1999). From book to bedside: Putting evidence to use in the care of the elderly. *Joint Commission Journal on Quality Improvement, 25,* 545–556.

Utley, R. (1999). The evolving meaning of cancer for long-term survivors of breast cancer. *Oncology Nursing Forum, 26,* 1519–1523.

Wallace, M. (2003). Uncertainty and quality of life of older men who undergo watchful waiting for prostate cancer. *Oncology Nursing Forum, 30,* 303–309.

Whall, A. (2004). Looking past and looking forward to the preferred gerontologic nursing future: 2003 Doris Schwartz Award Presentation. *Journal of Gerontological Nursing, 30*(4), 4–6.

Wood, R.Y., Duffy, M.E., Morris, S.J., & Carnes, J.E. (2002). The effect of an educational intervention on promoting breast self-examination in older African American and Caucasian women. *Oncology Nursing Forum, 29,* 1081–1090.

Yancik, R., & Ries, L.A. (2000). Aging and cancer in America: Demographic and epidemiology perspectives. *Hematology/Oncology Clinics of North America, 14,* 17–23.

Yarbrough, S. (2004). Older women and breast cancer screening: Research synthesis [Online exclusive]. *Oncology Nursing Forum, 31,* E9–E15.

CHAPTER 3

Physiology of Aging

Anne M. Reb, MSN, NP

Introduction

Changes that result from aging are very individualized and poorly reflected in chronologic age (Balducci, 2003b; Repetto et al., 2003). Aging is associated with a reduction in functional reserves and progressive deterioration of physiologic systems (Balducci & Extermann, 2000; Masoro, 1998). Cross-sectional studies show that parameters such as weight, metabolism, renal clearance, and cardiovascular function decline with age in most people (Brink, 1999). However, a more recent evaluation of physiologic functions shows that certain previously described declines are no longer found when using more sensitive criteria for health. For example, earlier studies showing declines in cardiac output with age have not been consistently verified in more recent studies (see Duthie, 2004, for further discussion). Although most physiologic processes decline gradually over time, much variability exists in physiologic function in older adults. Further, aging is associated with a decreased ability to adapt to stress (Duthie).

The age-associated decline in functional reserve leads to increased susceptibility to disease (Ershler & Longo, 1997). Although age-associated disease is related to physiologic changes, there is some ambiguity in distinguishing disease and normal age-related physiologic deterioration. For example, the distinction between "normal" loss of bone mass from aging and extreme loss of bone mass from osteoporosis, a disease of aging, is not completely clear (Masoro, 1998). Heterogeneity also exists in age-related physiologic changes among individuals. For example, progressive declines in glomerular filtration rate (GFR) of the kidney are characteristic of aging. However, these changes show marked variation among older individuals of the same age as documented by the Baltimore Longitudinal Study of Aging (Lindeman, Tobin, & Shock, 1985). Other authors have documented that some older patients show significant decreases in creatinine clearance with age, whereas others show only small or no changes in this parameter (Duthie, 2004; Masoro). Although chronologic age often is considered in determining cancer treatment, it does not adequately predict the extent of physiologic changes (Lichtman, 2004). Therefore, measurement or estimation of pertinent parameters, such as renal and liver function, is important in tailoring treatment (Simpson & Rosenzweig, 2002). This chapter presents an overview of aging changes in certain organ systems and molecular changes associated with carcinogenesis.

Organ Systems

Diseases or stress can alter the balance between functional reserves and normal functioning in older adults. Changes in renal and hepatic function, lean body mass, and bone marrow reserves should be considered in determining the use of drugs in cancer treatment (Extermann & Aapro, 2000). In malnourished patients, serum albumin may be very low, which may result in increased free drug concentration and toxicity (Vestal, 1997). Renal and hepatic metabolism and elimination of chemotherapy drugs may be altered because of aging, the cancer itself, concurrent medications, or comorbidities (Skirvin, Vemulapalli, & Lichtman, 2001). In particular, changes in renal function always should be assessed because many drugs are excreted renally, and some decline in renal function is almost uniformly present in older adults.

Renal Function

Age-related physiologic changes in renal function usually are caused by a decrease in GFR because of the loss of functioning nephrons associated with aging. The physiologic declines in renal function may result in decreased clearance of drugs primarily or solely eliminated by the kidney (Bell & Schnitzer, 2001; Vestal, 1997). Many chemotherapy agents are primarily excreted by the renal system and thus require dosage adjustment (Lichtman, 1998). A few examples of drugs that are mainly excreted by the renal system are methotrexate, bleomycin, cyclophosphamide, and carboplatin. Therefore, renal function should be determined before administration of cancer therapy so that appropriate dosage adjustments can be made (Extermann & Aapro, 2000; Skirvin et al., 2001). Creatinine clearance is widely used to estimate GFR (DuFour, 2001) but requires a 24-hour urine collection. The GFR can be estimated by formulas such as the Cockcroft-Gault formula, based on serum creatinine, age, and weight: $Cl_{cr} = (140 - age) \times (wt\ [kg]) / (72) \times (serum\ creatinine\ [mg/dl])$. For women, the estimated value is multiplied by 0.85 (Balducci, 2001; Choudhury, Raj, & Levi, 2004; "Clinical Pharmacology," 2005). An important caution is that various measurements or estimates of creatinine clearance are less accurate in the older adult and in those with severe renal failure and decreased muscle mass (Balducci, 2001; Choudhury et al.). Therefore, standard chemotherapy doses may be too toxic, especially with the older adult, and dose adjustments should be considered (Lichtman, 2004; see also Duthie, 2004). Other factors to consider include cognitive function and hydration status. For example, older adults who have difficulty maintaining adequate hydration because of limited mobility or mental status changes may not be able to maintain their GFR at optimal levels and, therefore, may require additional dosage adjustments ("Drug Therapy," 2005). Older adults with severe comorbidities or who are dependent in activities of daily living also may require dose adjustments because they are at increased risk for chemotherapy-related toxicities (Balducci, Hardy, & Lyman, 2000; Lichtman, 2004).

Liver Function

Liver function may change with aging because of decreased hepatic blood flow, decreased liver mass, or decreased activity of drug-metabolizing enzymes (Balducci, 2001). Studies show a decreased metabolism of drugs by hepatic enzymes, particularly the cytochrome P450 enzymes in the older adult (Extermann & Aapro, 2000; Skirvin et al., 2001; Vestal, 1997). These changes result in a decreased clearance of drugs metabolized solely or partly by the liver. For example, the decreased clearance of cytochrome P450 1A2 may result in decreased first-pass metabolism of drugs such as morphine (Lichtman, 2004). Levels of such drugs also may be elevated because of liver dysfunction, which can increase hematologic toxicity and other morbidity associated with chemotherapy. For example, patients with decreased liver function have a reduction in taxane clearance and a higher rate of neutropenic sepsis, stomatitis, and major morbidity (Skirvin et al.).

Evaluation of liver function may be difficult in older patients with cancer, as decreases in plasma protein levels may be caused by malnutrition and wasting as well as or in addition to decreased liver function. Elevated liver enzymes should be used as indicators of ongoing liver damage. Patients also may have difficulty clearing hepatically metabolized drugs before their liver function is impaired to the extent of affecting coagulation parameters. In particular, drugs that interact at the level of the cytochrome P450 enzymes should be given with extreme caution to older patients with suspected hepatic dysfunction (Lichtman, 2004; Skirvin et al., 2001).

Hematologic Changes

Aging is associated with a decreased reserve of heme and stem cells and a decreased ability to tolerate hematopoietic stress (Balducci & Extermann, 2000; Balducci et al., 2000). This decline may occur as a result of aging or age-related comorbidities. The mechanism of this decline may involve a decline in pluripotent hematopoietic stem cells and an imbalance in cytokine levels (Balducci et al.). Although the evidence supporting a decline in the number of hematopoietic stem cells with aging is inconclusive, the functions and ability of stem cells to differentiate into different hematopoietic lines may be reduced (Balducci, 2003b). In healthy older adults, hematopoiesis is generally comparable to younger adults. On the other hand, older adults with chronic illnesses or underlying anemia may respond with decreased ability to increase hematopoiesis. For example, anemic older adults experience a defect in hematopoiesis during periods of stress or increased demand. Further, anemia is an independent risk factor for myelotoxicity associated with chemotherapy administration (Balducci, 2000, 2003b). In addition to these changes, regulatory signals that stimulate hematopoiesis may be disordered.

Evidence supports that aging is associated with cytokines that may compromise the response of stem cells to growth factors (Balducci, 2003a). Cytokines and other factors regulate the proliferation and differentiation of hematopoietic stem cells. Regulators of hematopoiesis include interleukin (IL)-1, IL-2, IL-6, granulocyte–colony-stimulating factor (G-CSF), and erythropoietin. Some studies show that the expression of certain cytokines or hematopoietic growth factors such as granulocyte macrophage–colony-stimulating factor (GM-CSF) is decreased in the older adult. Alternatively, inhibitory cytokines such as IL-6 and tumor necrosis factor increase with age (Balducci et al., 2000).

The normal neutrophil response also may diminish with age (Balducci, 2001). Although the decrease in hematopoietic reserve usually does not affect baseline granulocyte counts, it limits the response to stress that normally would result in rapid hematopoiesis (Balducci, 2001). Thus, older adults may be at increased risk for neutropenia associated with chemotherapy. For example, they may experience delayed recovery of neutrophil numbers after chemotherapy or severe infection. These changes may affect the ability of older people to tolerate chemotherapy (Baraldi-Junkins, Beck, & Rothstein, 2000; see also Balducci, 2003b).

Immune Changes

Although a decline in immune function occurs with advancing age, the consequences of this decline are not completely established (Denduluri & Ershler, 2004; Ershler, 2004a). Aging is associated with changes in the cellular and humoral response as well as defects in the function of macrophages and neutrophils. In secondary immune responses, older adults have a lower antibody response to vaccines compared to younger adults (Burns & Goodwin, 2004). Further, they are more susceptible to certain disorders such as herpes zoster and reactivation of tuberculosis (Denduluri & Ershler; Ershler & Longo, 1997). One role of the cellular immune response is thought to be protection from development of malignancy. However, direct links between the decline in immune response and cancer in older adults have not been shown (Burns & Goodwin), nor has the age-related decline in immune function fully explained the increase in cancer incidence and common types of cancers seen in older adults (Cohen, 1999; Denduluri & Ershler).

Cellular

Aging is associated with decreased immune response to viruses and tumor growth (Balducci, 2001). The cellular response is mediated by T lymphocytes, which regulate the immune system and kill intracellular organisms such as viruses and certain bacteria. Cellular immunity also is hypothesized to protect against tumor growth (Burns & Goodwin, 2004). Changes in T-cell function in the older adult include a decrease in T-cell response to antigen stimulation (Hazzard, 2000). For example, a decline in the number of reactive T cells and in their proliferative response to infectious agents occurs in older adults (Burns & Goodwin). Helper T cells also are required for full-blown antibody responses.

Humoral

The humoral immune system consists of antibodies produced by B cells (Burns & Goodwin, 2004). An immature B cell has a membrane-associated antibody that, when bound with antigen, initiates the activation and maturation of that B cell into an antibody-secreting plasma cell. Activated B cells also proliferate rapidly, increasing the number of antibody-producing plasma cells. The large amounts of antibody produced can bind to and neutralize the presenting antigen (Mavroukakis, Muehlbauer, White, & Schwartzentruber, 2001). The ability of B cells to respond to antigens decreases with aging (Burns & Goodwin). In addition, a decline occurs in the number of T-cell–dependent antibody-forming cells as well as in the amount of antibody produced in response to primary and secondary antigens (Burns & Goodwin; Kim et al., 1998).

Immunoregulatory

Other changes associated with aging include alterations in immunoregulatory functions. Certain T cells secrete cytokines or hormones, which cause T cells to interact with one another and with other lymphocytes (Mavroukakis et al., 2001). Cytokines such as IL-1, IL-2, and tumor necrosis factor regulate T and B lymphocytes (Brink, 1999). For example, "IL-1 and IL-2 are important in the activation, recruitment, and proliferation of T lymphocytes" (Burns & Goodwin, 2004, p. 163). The function of T cells may decrease because of their altered secretion of certain cytokines (Baraldi-Junkins et al., 2000; Burns & Goodwin; Denduluri & Ershler, 2004; Ershler & Longo, 1997; Hazzard, 2000). A decline in the proportion of helper T cells expressing IL-2 is one example. This cytokine provides the signal to induce activation of T cells, natural killer cells, and monocytes in response to antigen stimulation (Kim et al., 1998). Recombinant DNA technology can produce cytokines such as IL-2. For example, IL-2 is a biologic therapy used to enhance the body's cytotoxic immune response. The U.S. Food and Drug Administration approved IL-2 for use in metastatic renal cell cancer and metastatic melanoma, and clinical trials are ongoing in other cancers and HIV (Mavroukakis et al.). Some studies have shown that IL-2 is effective in generating anticancer cytotoxic cells in older patients. For example, brief exposures (1-hr pulse) of granulocytes to IL-2 stimulated cytotoxic lymphokine-activated killer cells in older patients with cancer (Provinciali, Di Stefano, Stronati, & Fabris, 1998). Another study evaluated the tolerability of two dosing schedules of IL-2 given immediately after chemotherapy in older patients with acute myeloid leukemia in first remission (Farag et al., 2002). The low-dose IL-2 was better tolerated with less severe hematologic and nonhematologic toxicities compared with the low-dose IL-2 with intermediate pulse doses.

Activated T cells also produce other cytokines, including IL-4 and IL-6. Increased levels of IL-6, an inflammatory cytokine, have been linked to age-associated diseases such as osteoporosis and cancer (Baraldi-Junkins et al., 2000; Ershler, 2004a; Ershler & Longo, 1997). Certain cytokines and other factors may play a role in regulating tumor growth (Burns & Goodwin, 2004). For example, some studies have found increased expression of IL-6 with certain cancers such as multiple myeloma, Hodgkin disease, chronic lymphocytic leukemia, and non-Hodgkin lymphomas (Baraldi-Junkins et al.; Repetto et al., 2003). In addition to changes in host defenses against tumor growth, other molecular changes occur that increase susceptibility to mutations and tumor development (Balducci, 2001).

Molecular Changes and Carcinogenesis

Both carcinogenesis and aging are associated with genomic alterations that may cause cancer (Anisimov, 2004). Tissue aging is associated with an increased susceptibility to mutations that can lead to cancer. Older cells may be more susceptible to environmental carcinogens, resulting in molecular changes and mutations (Repetto et al., 2003). Mutations are changes in DNA caused by carcinogens. The next section will present an overview of common causes of mutations and safeguards to prevent DNA damage. Mutations and genetic rearrangements of genes associated with cancer, including tumor suppressor (TS) genes and oncogenes, also are reviewed.

Intrinsic Factors

Mutations may result from many causes, including intrinsic and extrinsic factors. Intrinsic factors include a person's genetic constitution as well as essential processes that occur in living organisms. During normal aerobic metabolism, the generation of energy from nutrients is associated with the formation of reactive chemicals or free radicals such as superoxides, nitric oxide, and hydrogen peroxide. These compounds may damage membranes, proteins, and DNA (Brink, 1999; Fernandez-Pol, 2004; Kim et al., 1998; Masoro, 1998). According to the free radical theory of aging, aging is a result of DNA and protein damage by molecules containing free radicals (Denduluri & Ershler, 2004). The accumulation of oxidative damage to DNA may lead to genetic damage and disorders such as cancer. DNA damage may result in cross-links and changes in bases known as adduct formation. Other changes may include genetic instability, DNA hypomethylation, chromosomal translocation, and point mutations (Anisimov, 2004; Balducci & Extermann, 2000; Ershler, 1998). Reactive chemicals may attach to DNA bases and form DNA adducts. If a cell is proliferating, the wrong base may be incorporated into the new DNA strand at the site of the adduct, resulting in a permanent mutation. If the gene is mutated, the protein it codes for may be nonfunctional or have altered function. Oxidative damage to proteins and membranes also may lead to other disorders such as atherosclerosis and neurodegeneration (Kim et al.). Tissue aging is associated with molecular alterations that affect cell growth and development. These changes may make older tissues more susceptible to environmental carcinogens (Balducci & Extermann).

Extrinsic Factors

Environmental exposures, diet, and lifestyle factors may contribute to aging and susceptibility to disease (Brink, 1999; Masoro, 1998). Exposures to radiation, ultraviolet light, and chemical agents can cause DNA damage, as outlined earlier. Older people may have increased susceptibility to radiation-induced damage and decreased ability to repair such damage (Burns & Goodwin, 2004). People exposed to certain chemical or physical agents often have higher incidences of cancer, such as lung, scrotal, and skin cancers (Fernandez-Pol & Douglas, 2000). Many age-associated diseases are promoted by smoking, including chronic lung disease, cancer, and stroke (Masoro). These diseases are the direct result of tissue damage or DNA damage produced by components of cigarette smoke. Other chemical carcinogens include chromium, nickel, beryllium, copper, and iron. Although these metal ions are essential for biologic functions, high levels are toxic. For example, iron is involved in both cancer and aging by interfering with normal DNA binding functions and producing free radicals that damage DNA (Fernandez-Pol, 2004; Fernandez-Pol & Douglas). Although protective mechanisms or safeguards exist to help to prevent this damage, they may be less effective in older adults.

Safeguards

Mechanisms to prevent DNA damage or mutation include (a) neutralization of reactive chemicals, (b) DNA repair enzymes, (c) cell cycle checkpoints during proliferation, and (d) immune surveillance (McLeskey, 2003a). Protective mechanisms that neutralize reactive chemicals include both exogenous and endogenous factors. Exogenous factors include compounds that act as free radical scavengers such as vitamin C, ferritin, and antioxidants such as beta-carotene, vitamin A, homocysteine, and vitamin E (Brink, 1999; Fernandez-Pol, 2004; Fernandez-Pol & Douglas, 2000). Plant-derived chemicals such as flavonoids and phytoestrogens also have the ability to scavenge free radicals (Fernandez-Pol, 2004). Endogenous factors include enzymes within cells that degrade free radicals and enzymes that facilitate repair of damaged cells. Protective enzymes such as catalase, peroxidase, and superoxide dismutase remove or modify reactive free radicals, whereas other enzymes such as proteases or polymerases repair or restore damaged components (Brink). Although cells produce these protective enzymes, a small percent of the free radicals may escape the reparative process and cause molecular damage (Kim et al., 1998). DNA repair enzymes correct damage to DNA. These enzymes repair the damage before the cell divides so that the mutation does not become permanent. Other regulatory molecules monitor cell cycle checkpoints during mitosis to prevent progression through the cell cycle if DNA damage occurs. Disorders in growth regulatory genes such as DNA repair mechanisms may be altered with age and may lead to mutations.

Growth Regulatory Genes

Carcinogenesis is a multistage process involving alterations of cellular genes such as those involved in cell proliferation and programmed cell death (apoptosis) (Ershler, 2004b). Evidence suggests that sequential activation of several oncogenes and the inactivation of several TS genes are necessary for carcinogenesis (Park, 2002; Pierotti, Sozzi, & Croce, 2003; see also Oster, Penn, & Stambolic, 2005). This multistage process may explain why cancer incidence increases with age. One hypothesis is that the tissues of older people have sustained more damage or events leading to carcinogenesis. Another hypothesis is that the aging process itself involves genetic events similar to those in early carcinogenesis. The result is an increased number of cells susceptible to the effects of late-stage carcinogens (Denduluri & Ershler, 2004; Ershler, 2004b). Mutations in genes that control cell growth or DNA replication or repair are early steps in carcinogenesis. Genes that are commonly mutated in cancer include oncogenes and TS genes.

Oncogenes

Normally, cell growth and programmed cell death (apoptosis) are controlled and highly regulated processes. Both aging and cancer are associated with genetic changes that may result in unregulated cell growth. Age-related changes in DNA metabolism include genetic instability, DNA hypomethylation, and formation of DNA adducts. These changes may be associated with cancer development or growth. Genetic instability involves activation of genes that normally are suppressed such as oncogenes or inactivation of some TS genes (Anisimov, 2003). Oncogenes can be considered genes with structural or functional alterations that promote abnormal cell growth or cell survival. Any of the genes that code for molecules in the growth-signaling pathway may be oncogenes if they are mutated or overexpressed (see Figure 3-1). Oncogenes may be classified as (a) growth factors, (b) growth factor receptors, (c) cytoplasmic or intracellular effectors of the growth signal pathway

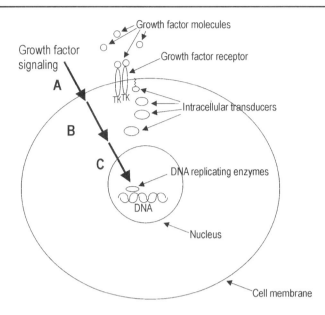

Figure 3-1. Growth Factor Signaling Pathway

Note. From "Biology of Lung Cancer With Implications for New Therapies," by M.F. Aberle and S.W. McLeskey, 2003, *Oncology Nursing Forum, 30,* p. 275. Copyright 2003 by the Oncology Nursing Society. Reprinted with permission.

(signal transducers), (d) transcription factors (located in the nucleus), and (e) others, including programmed cell death regulators (e.g., anti-apoptotic proteins or survival factors) (Pierotti et al., 2003; Ross, 1998). The protein products of oncogenes affect numerous biologic processes (Oster et al., 2005) and promote progression through the cell cycle to mitosis. Many tumors are associated with increased oncogene expression (see Table 3-1). When oncogenes are mutated or overexpressed, they can cause uncontrolled cell growth (Cohen, 1999). For example, mutations or overexpression leads to a growth signal that is "always on," producing unremitting growth (McLeskey, 2003b).

Growth Factor Receptors

Oncogenes do not have to be mutated to cause unremitting growth; they just may be expressed at very high levels. Chromosomal duplication of a growth factor receptor gene, such as *HER2/neu* or epidermal growth factor receptor, may yield multiple alleles resulting in overexpression of certain proteins. For example, the part of chromosome 17 that carries the *ErbB2* gene is duplicated in certain cancers, resulting in overexpression of the gene. The *ErbB2* protein is a growth factor receptor that transmits growth signals to the cytoplasm, thereby initiating the growth process. When this receptor is overexpressed, as in some breast, ovarian, lung, and other cancers, the growth signal is stronger and produces unremitting growth (McLeskey, 2003b). This oncogene is overexpressed in 20%–30% of breast cancers.

Table 3-1. Examples of Oncogenes and Associated Tumors

Oncogene	Tumor
Growth factors	
KS3	Kaposi sarcoma
v-sis	Glioma/fibrosarcoma
VEGF	Hematologic, colon and rectal, lung, breast, ovary, others
Growth factor receptors	
ErbB1 (EGFR)	Squamous cell carcinoma; glioblastoma; head and neck, colon; non-small cell lung cancer
ErbB2	Breast, ovarian
Signal transducers	
bcr-abl	Chronic myeloid leukemia
src	Colon
ras	Gastric, colorectal, thyroid; acute myeloid leukemia
Transcription factors	
fos	Osteosarcoma
jun	Sarcoma
myc	Breast, lung, colon, ovarian, head and neck; Burkitt lymphoma; leukemia; neuroblastoma
Anti-apoptotic proteins	
bcl-2	B-cell lymphomas; acute myeloid leukemia; multiple myeloma; breast, colon, lung, skin

Note. Based on information from Fernandez-Pol, 2004; Ferrara, 2004; Oster et al., 2005; Park, 2002; Perez-Soler, 2004; Pierotti et al., 2003.

Cytoplasmic Effectors of the Growth Signal Pathway

The Ras protein is associated within the membrane/cytoplasmic portion of the cell signaling pathway. It couples the growth signal received from the growth factor receptor to other proteins that transmit the signal to the nucleus. "Ras can be activated by a single point mutation, which leads to constitutive activation of growth promoting pathways" (Oster et al., 2005, p. 130). Abnormalities in this protein have been identified in many cancers, including lung, colon, and pancreas cancers and acute myeloid leukemia (Oster et al.; Ross, 1998).

Cytoplasmic kinases transmit the growth signal from the cell surface receptor through the cytoplasm to the nucleus. The *bcr-abl* oncogene, a cytoplasmic kinase, has a key role in tumorigenesis (Oster et al., 2005). This oncogene results from a translocation of the tips from chromosomes 9 and 22. The resultant "Philadelphia" chromosome is the hallmark of chronic myeloid leukemia (CML) and is present in other hematopoietic cancers, such as acute lymphoblastic leukemias (Oster et al.). The protein product of this gene may cause normal hematopoietic cells to undergo malignant transformation (Tennant, 2001). For example, the protein product can bind to various signaling molecules leading to the activation of kinase signaling pathways for cellular proliferation (Oster et al.).

Transcription Factors

The products of several genes located in the nucleus have a major role in the carcinogenesis process. Examples include steroid receptors in breast and prostate cancers and transcriptional factors (Oster et al., 2005). When the growth signal reaches the nucleus, genes are translated into proteins needed to complete the cell cycle. Certain transcription factors regulate the expression of these genes, and mutation of these factors is associated with certain types of cancers. Examples of transcription factors include *myc, fos,* and *jun.* Overexpression or mutation of *myc* is associated with Burkitt lymphoma, neuroblastomas, and colon and breast cancers (Fernandez-Pol, 1998). For example, the overexpression of the *c-myc* gene in Burkitt lymphoma directly contributes to this disease (Oster et al.).

Programmed Cell Death Regulators

"Normal tissues exhibit a regulated balance between cell proliferation and cell death" (Pierotti et al., 2003, p. 77). Programmed cell death is an important physiologic process needed to maintain cell number homeostasis. For example, normal development is characterized by the production of excess cells, which are removed by a genetically programmed process. Further, this same process is used to remove damaged cells such as virally infected cells (Zinkel & Korsmeyer, 2005). Studies have shown that the accumulation of excess cells because of excess proliferation or a decrease in programmed cell death can contribute to neoplasia and insensitivity to cancer treatments (Pierotti et al.; Zinkel & Korsmeyer) (see Figure 3-2).

The release of cytochrome c from the mitochondrial membrane triggers apoptosis, resulting in the activation of caspases that destroy the cell (Oster et al., 2005). The *bcl-2* oncogene is a regulator of apoptosis at the level of cytochrome c release. *Bcl-2* encodes proteins that interact with other proteins thought to be involved in the regulation of apoptosis (Pierotti et al., 2003). *Bcl-2* often is overexpressed in tumor cells, resulting in resistance to apoptosis, prolonged cell survival, and malignancy. For example, *bcl-2* overexpression is seen in follicular lymphomas, other leukemias such as acute myeloid leukemia and multiple myeloma, and various solid tumors (Oster et al.).

Research focused on oncogenes seeks to identify inducers of oncogenesis that are potential drug targets (Oster et al., 2005). For example, receptor tyrosine kinases are common drug targets because their location on the cell surface is readily accessible. Examples of drugs targeting these oncoproteins include trastuzumab (inhibits *HER2/ neu*) and erlotinib and gefitinib (inhibit epidermal growth factor receptor) (Oster et al.). The use of an anti–*bcr-abl* agent (imatinib mesylate) in the treatment of CML exemplifies one of the most successful applications of targeted therapy. This agent has shown significant efficacy against CML, especially in patients with early-stage disease (Oster et al.). *Bcl-2* and related anti-apoptosis proteins also are targets for therapeutic research. For example, antisense molecules such as G3139 have been used to inhibit *bcl-2* expression (Oster et al.). Initial studies of G3139 in xenograft lymphoma models were encouraging, and clinical trials are under way (Zinkel & Korsmeyer, 2005).

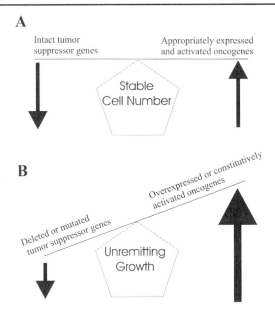

A. In organs and tissues, cell growth is tightly regulated by intact and appropriately expressed oncogenes, while intact, functional tumor suppressor genes regulate entry of defective cells into programmed cell death. The balance between growth and apoptosis maintains a stable cell number. **B.** In a neoplasm, mutated or overexpressed oncogenes provide a constitutive growth signal while deleted or mutated tumor suppressor genes fail to invoke apoptosis appropriately. The result is an unremitting growth signal.

Figure 3-2. Balance Between Cell Growth and Cell Death

Note. Figure courtesy of Dr. Sandra McLeskey. Used with permission.

Tumor Suppressor Genes

TS genes are associated with DNA repair or the suppression of malignant transformation through various regulatory functions. Some TS genes promote entry into apoptosis or prevent progression through the cell cycle if DNA damage is detected. Mutations in these genes may lead to accelerated carcinogenesis, with increased susceptibility of cells to carcinogens (Ershler, 2004b; Ershler & Longo, 1997) (see Table 3-2). TS genes commonly are involved in the development of familial as well as sporadic forms of cancer (Benchimol & Minden, 1998; Oster et al., 2005). Genetic predisposition to cancer may result from inborn errors in DNA repair or deficiencies in antioxidant mechanisms. Mutations of *BRCA1* and *BRCA2* account for a majority of familial breast cancers. Mutations in *BRCA1* also have been found in familial ovarian and prostate cancers, and mutations in *BRCA2* have been found in ovarian, prostate, pancreatic, and stomach cancers (Oster et al.). The *BRCA* genes code for proteins involved in repair of oxidative DNA damage. Cells with a defect in *BRCA1* are more sensitive to damage from radiation and superoxide ions (Fernandez-Pol & Douglas, 2000; Oster et al.). Loss of function of TS genes through mutation may lead to an

Table 3-2. Examples of Tumor Suppressor Genes and AssociatedTumors

Tumor Suppressor Gene	Tumor Type
p53	Li-Fraumeni, breast, brain, colon, lung, others
APC	Familial polyposis, sporadic colorectal tumors
BRCA1	Familial breast/ovarian
BRCA2	Familial breast, pancreatic cancer
RB1	Retinoblastoma, breast, prostate, bladder, others
hMSH2, hMLH1	Hereditary nonpolyposis colorectal, colon, gastric, endometrial
PTEN	Cowden syndrome, glioblastomas, prostate, breast, others

Note. Based on information from Fearon, 2002; Fernandez-Pol, 2004; Oster et al., 2005; Park & Vogelstein, 2003; Park, 2002.

inactive protein such that the cell cannot repair its DNA or cannot enter apoptosis when it is damaged beyond repair.

During normal growth, metabolic suppression of the action of TS genes that inhibit the cell cycle results in controlled cell proliferation. For example, gonadal hormones activate genes resulting in mitosis and growth of reproductive organs in a controlled fashion (Brink, 1999). Mutations in TS genes may increase the likelihood of tumors. Further, the loss of these genes is a common somatic mutation in human cancer. For example, deletions of *p53* and *RB* TS genes often are found in solid tumors (Brink; Cohen, 1999; Park & Vogelstein, 2003). The *p53* TS gene helps to regulate normal response to DNA damage and is associated with cell cycle arrest when DNA damage is detected (Oster et al., 2005). Mutations or deletions of *p53* are likely the most common genetic change in human cancer (Fisher, 2004; Park & Vogelstein). Deletion or mutation of *RB* removes its regulatory function at a cell cycle checkpoint during the process of mitosis (Oster et al.). Therefore, each of these mutations promotes inappropriate progression of the cell cycle and mitosis. Other TS genes include mismatch repair genes. For example, hereditary nonpolyposis colon cancer may be the result of mutations in mismatch repair genes. Inactivation of these genes increases the rate of mutations in all genes, including other TS genes and oncogenes.

Conclusion

Aging is associated with declines in functional reserves, including changes in renal, liver, and immune functions and hematologic reserves. However, physiologic changes are variable, and chronologic age alone does not necessarily predict the extent of these changes. Molecular changes associated with aging may result in increased susceptibility to genetic mutations and cancer. Because the development of cancer generally is a multistep, time-consuming process, the incidence of several cancers increases with age (Balducci, 2001; Ross, 1998). Intrinsic and extrinsic factors, such as chemicals, free radicals, radiation, or viruses, may cause DNA damage. If DNA repair is not successful, mutations may occur (Ross). Genes that are commonly mutated in cancer include oncogenes and TS genes. Oncogenes are associated with the cell cycle, and their protein products promote growth. The mutation or overexpression of oncogenes may disrupt the normal processes of the cell cycle and lead to unremitting growth and malignant transformation. TS genes are associated with DNA repair and cell cycle control. The loss of TS genes such as *p53* and *RB* often is related to solid tumors. Both oncogene activation and TS inactivation are thought to be necessary in the process leading to carcinogenesis.

The author acknowledges Sandra W. McLeskey, PhD, Associate Professor, University of Maryland School of Nursing, for her thoughtful comments on this chapter.

References

Anisimov, V.N. (2003). The relationship between aging and carcinogenesis: A critical appraisal. *Critical Reviews in Oncology/Hematology, 45,* 277–304.

Anisimov, V.N. (2004). Age as a risk factor in multistage carcinogenesis. In L. Balducci, G. Lyman, W.B. Ershler, & M.E. Extermann (Eds.), *Comprehensive geriatric oncology* (2nd ed., pp. 75–101). New York: Taylor & Francis.

Balducci, L. (2000). Evidence-based management of cancer in the elderly. *Cancer Control, 7,* 368–376.

Balducci, L. (2001). The geriatric cancer patient: Equal benefit from equal treatment. *Cancer Control, 8*(Suppl. 2), 1–25.

Balducci, L. (2003a). Anemia, cancer, and aging. *Cancer Control, 10,* 478–486.

Balducci, L. (2003b). Geriatric oncology. *Critical Reviews in Oncology/Hematology, 46,* 211–220.

Balducci, L., & Extermann, M. (2000). Cancer and aging. *Hematology/Oncology Clinics of North America, 14,* 1–16.

Balducci, L., Hardy, C.L., & Lyman, G.H. (2000). Hemopoietic reserve in the older cancer patient: Clinical and economic considerations. *Cancer Control, 7,* 539–547.

Baraldi-Junkins, C.A., Beck, A.C., & Rothstein, G. (2000). Hematopoiesis and cytokines: Relevance to cancer and aging. *Hematology/Oncology Clinics of North America, 14,* 45–61.

Bell, G.M., & Schnitzer, T.J. (2001). COX-2 inhibitors and other nonsteroidal anti-inflammatory drugs in the treatment of pain in the elderly. *Clinics in Geriatric Medicine, 17,* 489–502.

Benchimol, S., & Minden, M.D. (1998). Viruses, oncogenes, and tumor suppressor genes. In I.F. Tannock & R.P. Hill (Eds.), *The basic science of oncology* (3rd ed., pp. 79–105). New York: McGraw-Hill.

Brink, J.J. (1999). Cell biology and physiology of aging. In J.J. Gallo, J. Busby-Whitehead, P.V. Rabins, R.A. Silliman, J.B. Murphy, & W. Reichel (Eds.), *Reichel's care of the elderly: Clinical aspects of aging* (5th ed., pp. 631–636). Philadelphia: Lippincott Williams & Wilkins.

Burns, E.A., & Goodwin, J.A. (2004). Immunological changes of aging. In L. Balducci, G. Lyman, W.B. Ershler, & M.E. Extermann (Eds.), *Comprehensive geriatric oncology* (2nd ed., pp. 147, 158–170). New York: Taylor & Francis.

Choudhury, D., Raj, D.S.C., & Levi, M. (2004). Effect of aging on renal function and disease. In B.M. Brenner (Ed.), *Brenner & Rector's the kidney* (7th ed., pp. 2305–2344.). Philadelphia: Saunders.

Clinical pharmacology. (2005). In M.H. Beers & R. Berkow (Eds.), *The Merck manual of geriatrics.* Retrieved April 22, 2005, from http://www.merck.com/mrkshared/mm_geriatrics/sec1/ch6.jsp

Cohen, H.J. (1999). Oncology and aging: General principles of cancer in the elderly. In W.R. Hazzard, J.P. Blass, W.H. Ettinger, & J.G. Ouslander (Eds.), *Principles of geriatric medicine and gerontology* (pp. 117–130). New York: McGraw-Hill.

Denduluri, N., & Ershler, W.B. (2004). Aging biology and cancer. *Seminars in Oncology, 31,* 137–148.

Drug therapy in the elderly. (2005). In M.H. Beers & R. Berkow (Eds.), *The Merck manual of diagnosis and therapy.* Retrieved April 25, 2005, from http://www.merck.com/mrkshared/mmanual/section22/chapter304/304b.jsp

DuFour, D.R. (2001). Evaluation of renal function, water, electrolytes, acid-base balance, and blood gases. In J.B. Henry (Ed.), *Clinical diagnosis and management by laboratory methods* (20th ed., pp. 159–179). Philadelphia: Saunders.

Duthie, E.H. (2004). Physiology of aging: Relevance to symptoms, perceptions, and treatment tolerance. In L. Balducci, G. Lyman, W.B. Ershler, & M.E. Extermann (Eds.), *Comprehensive geriatric oncology* (2nd ed., pp. 207–222). New York: Taylor & Francis.

Ershler, W.B. (1998). Tumor-host interactions, aging and tumor growth. In L. Balducci, G. Lyman, & W.B. Ershler (Eds.), *Comprehensive geriatric oncology* (pp. 201–211). Amsterdam, The Netherlands: Harwood Academic.

Ershler, W.B. (2004a). Biology of aging and cancer. In L. Balducci, G. Lyman, W.B. Ershler, & M.E. Extermann (Eds.), *Comprehensive geriatric oncology* (2nd ed., pp. 67–74). New York: Taylor & Francis.

Ershler, W.B. (2004b). Tumor-host interactions, aging, and tumor growth. In L. Balducci, G. Lyman, W.B. Ershler, & M.E. Extermann (Eds.), *Comprehensive geriatric oncology* (2nd ed., pp. 147–157). New York: Taylor & Francis.

Ershler, W.B., & Longo, D.L. (1997). The biology of aging. *Cancer, 80,* 1284–1293.

Extermann, M., & Aapro, M. (2000). Assessment of the older cancer patient. *Hematology/Oncology Clinics of North America, 14,* 63–77.

Farag, S.S., George, S.L., Lee, E.J., Baer, M., Dodge, R.K., Becknell, B., et al. (2002). Postremission therapy with low-dose interleukin 2 with or without intermediate pulse dose interleukin 2 therapy is well-tolerated in elderly patients with acute myeloid leukemia: Cancer and Leukemia Group B study 9420. *Clinical Cancer Research, 8,* 2812–2819.

Fearon, E.R. (2002). Tumor-suppressor genes. In B. Vogelstein & K. Kinzler (Eds.), *The genetic basis of human cancer* (2nd ed., pp. 197–206). New York: McGraw-Hill.

Fernandez-Pol, J.A. (1998). Growth factors, oncogenes, and aging. In L. Balducci, G. Lyman, & W.B. Ershler (Eds.), *Comprehensive geriatric oncology* (pp. 179–196). Amsterdam, The Netherlands: Harwood Academic.

Fernandez-Pol, J.A. (2004). Growth factors, oncogenes, and aging. In L. Balducci, G. Lyman, W.B. Ershler, & M.E. Extermann (Eds.), *Comprehensive geriatric oncology* (2nd ed., pp. 102–126). New York: Taylor & Francis.

Fernandez-Pol, J.A., & Douglas, M.G. (2000). Molecular interactions of cancer and age. *Hematology/Oncology Clinics of North America, 14,* 25–44.

Ferrara, N. (2004). Vascular endothelial growth factor as a target for anticancer therapy. *Oncologist, 9*(Suppl. 1), 2–10.

Fisher, D.E. (2004). Apoptosis, chemotherapy, and aging. In L. Balducci, G. Lyman, W.B. Ershler, & M.E. Extermann (Eds.), *Comprehensive geriatric oncology* (2nd ed., pp. 128–146). New York: Taylor & Francis.

Hazzard, W.R. (2000). The clinical physiology of aging. *International Urology and Nephrology, 32,* 137–146.

Kim, S., Jiang, J.C., Kirchman, P.A., Rubelj, I., Helm, E.G., & Jazwinski, S.M. (1998). Cellular and molecular aging. In L. Balducci, G. Lyman, & W.B. Ershler (Eds.), *Comprehensive geriatric oncology* (pp. 123–155). Amsterdam, The Netherlands: Harwood Academic.

Lichtman, S.M. (1998). Recent developments in the pharmacology of anticancer drugs in the elderly. *Current Opinion in Oncology, 10,* 572–579.

Lichtman, S.M. (2004). Chemotherapy in the elderly. *Seminars in Oncology, 31,* 160–174.

Lindeman, R.D., Tobin, J.D., & Shock, N.W. (1985). Longitudinal studies on the rate of decline in renal function with age. *Journal of the American Geriatrics Society, 33,* 278–285.

Masoro, E.J. (1998). Physiology of aging. In R. Tallis, H. Fillit, & J.C. Brocklehurst (Eds.), *Brocklehurst's textbook of geriatric medicine and gerontology* (5th ed., pp. 85–95). New York: Harcourt Brace.

Mavroukakis, S.A., Muehlbauer, P.M., White, R.L., & Schwartzentruber, D.J. (2001). Clinical pathways for managing patients receiving interleukin 2. *Clinical Journal of Oncology Nursing, 5,* 207–216.

McLeskey, S.W. (2003a, February). *Genetic carcinogenesis.* Paper presented at the University of Maryland School of Nursing, Baltimore.

McLeskey, S.W. (2003b, February). *Oncogenes and proliferation.* Paper presented at the University of Maryland School of Nursing, Baltimore.

Oster, S., Penn, L., & Stambolic, V. (2005). Oncogenes and tumor suppressor genes. In I.F. Tannock, R.P. Hill, L. Harrington, & R.G. Bristow (Eds.), *Basic science of oncology* (4th ed., pp. 123–141). New York: McGraw-Hill.

Park, B.H., & Vogelstein, B. (2003). Tumor-suppressor genes. In D. Kufe, R. Pollock, R. Weichselbaum, R. Bast, Jr., T. Gansler, J. Holland, et al. (Eds.), *Cancer medicine* (6th ed., pp. 87–105). Hamilton, Ontario, Canada: BC Decker.

Park, M. (2002). Oncogenes. In B. Vogelstein & K. Kinzler (Eds.), *The genetic basis of human cancer* (2nd ed., pp. 177–196). New York: McGraw-Hill.

Perez-Soler, R. (2004). HER1/EGFR targeting: Refining the strategy. *Oncologist, 9,* 58–67.

Pierotti, M.A., Sozzi, G., & Croce, C.M. (2003). Oncogenes. In D. Kufe, R. Pollock, R. Weichselbaum, R. Bast, Jr., T. Gansler, J. Holland, et al. (Eds.), *Cancer medicine* (6th ed., pp. 73–85). Hamilton, Ontario, Canada: BC Decker.

Provinciali, M., Di Stefano, G., Stronati, S., & Fabris, N. (1998). Generation of human lymphokine-activated killer cells following an IL-2 pulse in elderly cancer patients. *Cytokine, 10*(2), 132–139.

Repetto, L., Venturino, A., Fratino, L., Serraino, D., Troisi, G., Gianni, W., et al. (2003). Geriatric oncology: A clinical approach to the older patient with cancer. *European Journal of Cancer, 39,* 870–880.

Ross, D.W. (1998). *Introduction to oncogenes and molecular cancer medicine.* New York: Springer-Verlag.

Simpson, J.K., & Rosenzweig, M.Q. (2002). Treatment considerations for the elderly person with cancer. *AACN Clinical Issues, 13*(1), 43–60.

Skirvin, J.A., Vemulapalli, S., & Lichtman, S.M. (2001). Pharmacology of antineoplastic agents in older cancer patients. *Oncology Spectrums, 2,* 404–413.

Tennant, L. (2001). Chronic myelogenous leukemia: An overview. *Clinical Journal of Oncology Nursing, 5,* 218–219.

Vestal, R.E. (1997). Aging and pharmacology. *Cancer, 80,* 1302–1310.

Zinkel, S.S., & Korsmeyer, S.J. (2005). Apoptosis. In V.T. DeVita, S. Hellman, & S. Rosenberg (Eds.), *Cancer: Principles and practice of oncology* (7th ed., pp. 95–103). Philadelphia: Lippincott Williams & Wilkins.

CHAPTER 4

Comprehensive Geriatric Assessment

Janine A. Overcash, PhD, ARNP, BC

Introduction

According to the National Center for Health Statistics (2003), the average human life expectancy in the United States has increased to more than 76 years of age, which is dramatically higher than the average 46 years of age in 1900. Increased life expectancy is a major factor in the importance of geriatric oncology as a specialty and the need to prioritize health care for older adults. An adequate knowledge base of assessment techniques specific to the older person is vital for healthcare providers. Cancer largely is a disease of the aged (Sahyoun, Lentzner, Hoyert, & Robinson, 2001), and the incidence of cancer is greater in the older adult population. The case study at the end of this chapter describes insensitivities that are all too common for many seniors seeking health care. Specialized cancer care of seniors is a necessary component of health care. This chapter will discuss some of the aspects of health care that differ with age and will define and describe the comprehensive geriatric assessment (CGA). The chapter also will discuss the role of the nurse in conducting the CGA, coordinating a multidisciplinary team, and facilitating necessary follow-up care. Limited research exists on the care of the older adult with cancer, showing the need for current information. Many studies that are available are considered "classic" and frequently are cited in the geriatric literature.

Aspects of Health Assessment

What makes assessing older adults different from assessing younger adults? One answer is comorbidities. Fried, Storer, King, and Lodder (1991) suggested that people 70 and older have 5.6 concurrent diagnoses. Healthcare providers must recognize, treat, and maintain many different types of ailments. Using clinical reasoning skills can help to determine whether a certain symptom is a consequence of many different diagnoses or a single diagnosis and is critical in providing adequate care for older adults (Repetto & Comandini, 2000). Moreover, clinical reasoning skills help to differentiate between whether a limitation is a consequence of older age or a potentially treatable problem (Izaks & Westendorp, 2003).

Another aspect of assessing the older adult is the use of assessment instruments to identify and monitor complex deficits in areas such as functional status, depression, and dementia (Overcash, 2003). Maintaining independence through proactive assessment is the axiom of geriatric assessment. Detecting health issues before they become limiting is crucial and requires a multidimensional assessment involving physical, functional, emotional, and cognitive abilities (Balducci & Beghe, 2000).

Functional Reserve

Functional reserve is an important consideration in the care of the older adult (Balducci & Yates, 2000). Functional reserve is the ability to maintain homeostasis when an insult is occurring to the body. For example, during extreme cold exposure, a healthy adult may tolerate the cold reasonably well for a limited amount of time. However, a baby or older person may not fare as well because of reduced subcutaneous fat and less vital support. Reduced functional reserve may contribute to some of the more global symptoms a seemingly minor diagnosis can inspire, such as a urinary tract infection causing confusion or dementia (Overcash, 2003). The issue of functional reserve is of importance when treating the older person with chemotherapy. For example, problems such as neutropenia may be more disabling or life threatening to an older person when compared to a younger person (Balducci & Repetto, 2004; Freyer et al., 2004).

Social Support

Not only are physical and emotional health important to assess, but social support systems and potential caregiver limitations also are important to evaluate (Overcash & Balducci, 2003). As older adults become more dependent, social support becomes a more important and challenging aspect of nursing care (Overcash, 2003). The gerontologic literature suggests that as people age, it is common to have a decrease in the available social support networks that provide assistance with such factors as transportation, instrumental tasks (bathing, dressing), and emotional support (Auslander & Litwin, 1990; Shaw & Janevic, 2004). Without the assistance of a support person, a patient may not be as able to tolerate or have access to adequate cancer therapy and, therefore, may experience a less positive treatment outcome (Balducci, 2003). Adequate social support networks have been linked with less depression, better adjustment to illness, less probability of nursing home placement, and even lower risk of mortality (Cohen & Syme, 1985; Funch & Marshall, 1983; Shaw & Janevic). Geriatric assessment deals with many of the same components as assessment of younger adults, with the addition of understanding multiple comorbidities, social support impairments, and geriatric syndromes such as falls, incontinence, and confusion. For further information, please refer to the National Comprehensive Cancer Network (NCCN) *Clinical Practice Guidelines in Oncology* (2004).

Definition of the Comprehensive Geriatric Assessment

For the older adult with cancer, a CGA can contribute to the identification of patients for whom treatment benefit may be most great and facilitate the formulation of an appropriate management plan, with ongoing monitoring of clinical outcomes (Bernabei, Venturiero, Tarsitani, & Gambassi, 2000; Overcash, 2003). General guidelines for the management of older people with cancer produced by the Senior Adult Care Task Force reported CGA to be a standard component of the assessment process (Balducci & Yates, 2000). The National Institutes of Health (NIH) released a consensus statement that included CGA as an accepted form of geriatric evaluation (Solomon, 1988). The American Geriatrics Society (AGS) adopted the NIH consensus statement in 1993 and recommended its integration into practice and educational curricula (AGS, 1993). A definition of the CGA developed in the NIH statement is as follows.

> A multidisciplinary evaluation in which the multiple problems of older persons are uncovered, described and explained if possible, and in which resources and strengths of the person are catalogued, need for services assessed and a coordinated care plan developed to focus interventions on the person's problems. (Solomon, 1988, p. 342)

CGA can be used and augmented depending on the environment and population served, such as outpatient ambulatory primary care, inpatient long-term care, or ambulatory oncology clinics (Overcash, 2003).

Components of the Comprehensive Geriatric Assessment

CGA generally assesses emotional, functional, and cognitive elements in addition to patient history and physical examination. Each element of the CGA is a distinct aspect of health. Generally, four basic instruments comprise the CGA: the Mini-Mental State Exam (MMSE) (see Figure 4-1) (Folstein, Folstein, & McHugh, 1975); Activities of Daily Living (ADL) (see Figure 4-2) (Katz, Downs, Cash, & Grotz, 1970); Instrumental Activities of Daily Living (IADL) (see Figure 4-3) (Lawton & Brody, 1969); and the Geriatric Depression Scale (GDS) (see Figure 4-4) (Yesavage et al., 1982–1983).

Comorbidities

Comorbid conditions can be simply defined as multiple diagnoses. For the purposes of this text, additional diagnoses are defined as other than the diagnosis of cancer. The most common comorbid conditions are hypertension, arthritis, and auditory impairment (Centers for Disease Control and Prevention, 2003) (see Table 4-1). As stated earlier in this chapter, the average number of comorbid conditions is 5.6 according to a classic study at Johns Hopkins by Fried et al. (1991). It is essential to assess for comorbidities and especially untreated comorbid conditions because of the potential for interaction with a cancer diagnosis and cancer treatment effects (Extermann, 2004; Rao, Seo, & Cohen, 2004). Comorbidity is a vital part of an

Orientation to Time
"What is the date?"

Registration
"Listen carefully. I am going to say three words. You say them back after I stop.
Ready? Here they are . . .
HOUSE (pause), CAR (pause), LAKE (pause). Now repeat those words back to me." [Repeat up to 5 times, but score only the first trial.]

Naming
"What is this?" [Point to a pencil or pen.]

Reading
"Please read this and do what it says." [Show examinee the words on the stimulus form.]
CLOSE YOUR EYES

Figure 4-1. Folstein Mini-Mental State Exam Sample Items

Note. Reproduced by special permission of the publisher, Psychological Assessment Resources, Inc., 16204 North Florida Ave., Lutz, FL 33549, from the Mini-Mental State Examination, by Marshal Folstein and Susan Folstein. Copyright 1975, 1998, 2001 by Mini Mental LLC, Inc. Published 2001 by Psychological Assessment Resources, Inc. Further reproduction is prohibited without permission of PAR, Inc. The MMSE can be purchased from PAR, Inc. by calling 800-331-8378 or 813-968-3003.

oncology assessment and can be a part of the decision to treat with more aggressive chemotherapy (AGS, 1993).

It is important to note that an older person may have multiple comorbid conditions; however, the individual may not have limitations in health and can be considered "healthy." This is because not all comorbidities have the same impact on health, and some patients may respond better to treatment than others (Extermann, 2000). It is important to define the comorbid condition while obtaining a patient health history and to understand the treatment history of each condition and the influence on general health. For example, a patient may have hypertension, osteopenia, and asthma and be well controlled and unlimited in functional status. Other patients may have the same diagnoses and be frail. Therefore, assessment of functional status is an important part of the evaluation. A study by Extermann, Overcash, Lyman, Parr, and Balducci (1998) found that issues such as comorbidity and functional status were not predictors of each other and required separate assessments for each construct.

Functional Status

Functional status looks at tasks that are required in everyday life that enable independence, such as bathing, dressing, ambulating, and toileting (Katz et al., 1970). For the older person with cancer, functional status may be related to the tolerance of chemotherapy, progression of cancer, and general health status (Balducci & Yates, 2000). The most common measures of functional status are ADL (Katz et al.) and IADL (Lawton & Brody, 1969). These instruments prompt the clinician to evaluate each task and determine whether a person is independent. If a person is dependent in any of the tasks, the healthcare provider generally explores decisions concerning assistance and rehabilitation. ADL is not necessarily score-based, as it is used to reveal a problem so that treatment and interventions can be made.

For each area of functioning listed below, check the description that applies. (The word "assistance" means supervision, direction, or personal assistance.)

BATHING—either sponge bath, tub bath, or shower

❐	❐	❐
Receives no assistance (gets in and out of tub by self, is usual means of bathing)	Receives assistance in bathing only one part of the body (such as back or a leg)	Receives assistance in bathing more than one part of the body (or not bathed)

DRESSING—gets clothes from closets and drawers, including underclothes and outer garments, and uses fasteners (including braces if worn)

❐	❐	❐
Gets clothes and gets completely dressed without assistance	Gets clothes and gets dressed without assistance except for assistance in tying shoe	Receives assistance in getting clothes or in getting dressed or stays partly or completely undressed

TOILETING—going to the "toilet room" for bowel and urine elimination; cleaning self after elimination and arranging clothes

❐	❐	❐
Goes to "toilet room," cleans self, and arranges clothes without assistance (may use object for support such as a cane, walker, or wheelchair and may manage night bedpan or commode, emptying same in morning)	Receives assistance in going to "toilet room" or in cleansing self or in arranging clothes after elimination or in use of night bedpan or commode	Does not go to room termed "toilet" for the elimination process

TRANSFER

❐	❐	❐
Moves in and out of bed as well as in and out of chair without assistance (may be using object for support such as cane or walker)	Moves in and out of bed or chair with assistance	Does not get out of bed

CONTINENCE

❐	❐	❐
Controls urination and bowel movement completely by self	Has occasional "accidents"	Supervision helps keep control; catheter is used, or is incontinent

FEEDING

❐	❐	❐
Feeds self without assistance	Feeds self except for cutting meat or buttering bread	Receives assistance in feeding or is fed partly or completely by using tubes or intravenous fluids

Figure 4-2. Evaluation of Activities of Daily Living

Note. From "Progress in the Development of the Index of ADL," by S. Katz, T.D. Downs, H.R. Cash, and R.C. Grotz, 1970, *Gerontologist, 10,* p. 21. Copyright 1970 by the Gerontological Society of America. Reprinted with permission.

Domains
- Using the telephone
- Getting to places beyond walking distance
- Grocery shopping
- Preparing meals
- Doing housework
- Doing handyman work
- Doing laundry
- Taking medications
- Managing money

Figure 4-3. Instrumental Activities of Daily Living

Note. Based on information from Lawton & Brody, 1969.

Choose the best answer for how you have felt over the past week.

1. Are you basically satisfied with your life? YES / NO
2. Have you dropped many of your activities and interests? YES / NO
3. Do you feel that your life is empty? YES / NO
4. Do you often get bored? YES / NO
5. Are you in good spirits most of the time? YES / NO
6. Are you afraid that something bad is going to happen to you? YES / NO
7. Do you feel happy most of the time? YES / NO
8. Do you often feel helpless? YES / NO
9. Do you prefer to stay at home, rather than going out and doing new things? YES / NO
10. Do you feel you have more problems with memory than most? YES / NO
11. Do you think it is wonderful to be alive now? YES / NO
12. Do you feel pretty worthless the way you are now? YES / NO
13. Do you feel full of energy? YES / NO
14. Do you feel that your situation is hopeless? YES / NO
15. Do you think that most people are better off than you are? YES / NO

Figure 4-4. Geriatric Depression Scale

Note. From "Development and Validation of a Geriatric Depression Screening Scale: A Preliminary Report," by J.A. Yesavage, T.L. Brink, T.L. Rose, O. Lum, M. V. Huang, M. Adey, et al., 1982–1983, *Journal of Psychiatric Research, 17*(1), p. 41. Copyright 1982 by Elsevier. Reprinted with permission.

IADL assesses more refined activities in nine domains (Lawton & Brody, 1969). Using the telephone, getting to places beyond walking distance, grocery shopping, cleaning and housekeeping activities, laundry, and managing money are examples of the domains assessed. For the items addressing housework and handyman work, it is important to ask the questions "If you had to, could you do housework; and if you had to, could you do handyman work?" IADL is scored such that the patient earns three points for being able to perform a task without assistance, two points for some assistance, and one point for completely being unable to perform the tasks (except for the medication domain). A best total score is 29, and anything less suggests some degree of dependence. It is important to assess whether patients have assistance for the activities in which they score in the latter two categories ("some assistance" or "completely unable"). For example, those who may require assistance and have a support person to provide help may be very different than an older adult living at home with activity deficits and no one to help. With ADL and IADL, each patient's score should be considered over time for assessment of general condition, response to interventions, or failing health.

Depression

Another common element of the CGA is the assessment for depression. One definition of depression is a clinical syndrome consisting of an inability to concentrate and feelings of sadness, loss, and grief (Kurlowicz, 1999). The incidence of depression increases with advanced age (Kurlowicz). Depression following a diagnosis of cancer is common and has been associated with a higher risk of mortality among patients with breast cancer (Hjerl et al., 2003). Depression also contributes to the decision not to undergo cancer treatment in older adults (Lyness et al., 1997). Moreover, when compared to anxiety in patients with cancer, depression seems to have a greater effect on quality of life (Skarstein, Aass, Fossa, Skovlund, & Dahl, 2000). For the general older population, mild depression may result in lower immunity and ability to fight off disease (McGuire, Kiecolt-Glaser, & Glaser, 2002). Despite these findings, researchers have done few studies on depression and the older patient with cancer (Charlson & Peterson, 2002). The GDS is a helpful instrument in screening for depression (see Figure 4-4).

The GDS is a valid and reliable screening tool for depression that consists of 15 "yes" or "no" items (Yesavage et al., 1982–1983). The GDS screening is positive if participants answer five or more questions positively for depression. A comparison

Table 4-1. Prevalence of Selected Conditions by Age and Sex: United States, 1984–1995 (NHIS) Other: Units (# of persons), sex (both sexes), age (65 and over)

Condition	Year					
	1990	**1991**	**1992**	**1993**	**1994**	**1995**
Diabetes	2,780,077	3,008,611	3,394,595	3,224,429	3,141,474	3,949,876
Hypertension	10,989,023	11,250,911	11,011,925	10,899,023	11,282,086	12,636,608
Cerebrovascular diseases	1,838,648	1,873,629	2,279,910	2,191,713	1,767,514	2,181,874
Diseases of heart	6,658,074	7,004,048	7,390,424	7,530,926	7,568,096	7,236,057
Asthma, bronchitis, emphysema	3,852,824	3,140,346	3,801,134	3,592,936	3,847,366	3,675,659
Arthritis	13,050,190	13,811,695	13,905,818	14,384,582	14,705,699	14,457,180
Blindness	2,175,546	2,397,511	2,680,126	2,991,407	2,550,643	2,390,079
Cataract	4,569,483	5,235,256	5,110,343	4,727,979	5,157,786	4,994,722
Deafness	9,583,358	9,710,108	9,866,464	9,821,561	8,885,645	8,933,011

Note. Based on information from Centers for Disease Control and Prevention, 2003.

with two well-known measures of depression, the Zung Self-Rating Scale for Depression (Zung, 1972) and the Hamilton Rating Scale for Depression (Hamilton, 1967), showed validation.

Cognition

The American Academy of Neurology (Petersen et al., 2001) recommended early screening for dementia, which can be caused by early Alzheimer disease, ischemic problems, and/or polypharmacy issues. They also recommended monitoring cognitive status for decline or improvement during the course of treatment for dementia. Older women with breast cancer who are on active chemotherapy should consider chemical-induced cognitive dysfunction when assessing the cause of the cognitive change (Barton & Loprinzi, 2002). One method of screening for dementia and also a common component of CGA is the MMSE (Folstein et al., 1975). Orientation, memory, language function, and praxis (translating an idea into practice) are the domains examined. Scores of less than 24 are indicative of dementia. Healthcare professionals can use the MMSE to screen for dementia in older adults who do not have overt cognitive loss, to assess dementia, and to evaluate the effectiveness of treatment. Researchers also commonly use the MMSE as a demonstration of cognition in research projects.

Little research exists in the area of dementia and older women with breast cancer. Questions dealing with the point at which cancer therapy outweighs the risk of treatment and other issues of screening in older women with dementia are germane to nursing clinical practice (Raik, Miller, & Fins, 2004). Motivating and participating in discussions on how to provide the best care to older women with breast cancer in order for further research to be developed is important.

Benefits of the Comprehensive Geriatric Assessment

Geriatric literature has demonstrated the benefits of the CGA since the 1980s (Boult et al., 2001; Burns, Nichols, Martindale-Adams, & Graney, 2000; Philp et al., 2001; Rubenstein et al., 1991; Trentini, Semeraro, & Motta, 2001; Williams, Williams, Zimer, Hall, & Podgorski, 1987). The CGA has been effective in a variety of settings and populations, including in-home assessments (Bula et al., 1999; Stuck et al., 2002), outpatient assessments, with community-dwelling older adults (Maly, Hirsch, & Reuben, 1997; Reuben, Fishman, McNabney, & Wolde-Tsadik, 1996; Wedding & Hoffen, 2003), and with inpatient hospitalized older adults (Rubenstein, Siu, & Wieland, 1989). As previously discussed, the issues of comorbidities and geriatric syndromes (e.g., falls, incontinence, dementia) are fundamental considerations when assessing older adults with cancer. Each of these diagnoses requires a critical understanding of the interrelatedness of the pathology and the treatment modalities specific to the older person. An older adult undergoing cancer treatment can be physiologically challenged. However, if further compromised by untreated multiple diagnoses, the older adult may experience additional health insult. By detecting comorbidities and geriatric syndromes and establishing a treatment plan, the older person may better tolerate chemotherapy (Maartense, Kluin-Nelcmans, & Noordijk, 2003; Overcash & Balducci, 2003; Winograd et al., 1991).

The CGA can detect problems that otherwise may go undetected until limitations arise or serious threats to independence occur (Burns et al., 2000; Rubenstein et al., 1989). The CGA can be the foundation of the patient treatment plan by establishing the functionality and emotional and physical well-being of an older person at the time of initial and repeated visits. Additionally, administration of the CGA with interventions delayed disability in activities such as bathing, dressing, and other basic ADL in a population of community-dwelling older adults (Bula et al., 1999).

Another benefit is that the CGA can detect problems in many older adults who appear very healthy and without overt problems. Specific screening measures address these problems (Balducci, 1994). For example, from 1995–1998, the administration of the CGA helped to detect dementia (20%) in an apparently highly functional population (Overcash, 1998). It is reasonable to assume that a percentage of this dementia may not have been detected without the generalized, systematic screening of the CGA. Other studies support that the CGA is an effective measure in assessing the older person with cancer (Balducci & Beghe, 2000; Overcash, Chen, Extermann, Cantor, & Balducci, 1998). In non-Hodgkin lymphoma, the CGA was used in the implementation of treatment modalities for people age 65 and older in the Netherlands (Maartense et al., 2003).

The CGA aids in understanding and identifying the extent of frailty and assessing treatment barriers such as caregiver problems, transportation problems, and coping concerns. Addressing problems discovered by the CGA may help to alleviate some of the barriers to cancer treatment (Balducci & Beghe, 2000; Repetto et al., 2003). An important premise of the use of the CGA in geriatric oncology is the detection of physical, social, and psychological barriers, which may hinder the effectiveness of cancer therapy (Repetto & Comandini, 2000). Healthcare professionals should address barriers such as transportation to the clinic and caregiver concerns. For example, the person with cancer also may be a caregiver to another and feel that he or she must delay or even forgo cancer treatment. These and other barriers may lead to dose reductions or treatment delays resulting from undetected problems or limitations, which may reduce the effectiveness of therapy (NCCN, 2004). Moreover, in a classic study in New Mexico of older adults with newly diagnosed cancer, those who had limited access to transportation along with impaired functional and cognitive status were less likely to receive radiation therapy but not surgical intervention. Radiation therapy often is a daily procedure, and surgical intervention usually is associated with limited visits (Goodwin, Hunt, & Samet, 1993).

One important consideration for a CGA is to focus on the type of patients who benefit from a thorough assessment. Older adults with comorbid conditions and/or geriatric syndromes such as frailty may be the most likely to benefit (Balducci, 2003). Inpatients or outpatients who have experienced falls, incontinence, and/or confusion and who have some type of functional limitation also benefit from a CGA (see Figure 4-5). Older adults who are most likely to *not* benefit from a CGA are those in need of acute hospitalization and those who have no health or functional limitations. One caveat is that many older adults seem as though they have no limitations, but, in fact, they have learned to compensate for their limitations (Overcash, 1998). Because it can be very difficult to determine who benefits from a CGA by cursory assessment, a CGA screening measure is necessary. Maly et al. (1997) found that the performance of rapidly administered standard screening

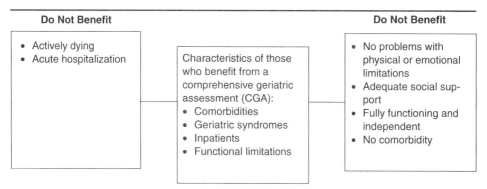

This figure illustrates each pole of the continuum of which older patients tend NOT to benefit from the CGA. Those seniors in between the boxes tend to benefit from the CGA.

Figure 4-5. Those Who Benefit and Do Not Benefit From the Comprehensive Geriatric Assessment

measures for geriatric syndromes in community-dwelling older adults helped to identify those who would most benefit from a CGA. In a more recent study, researchers used a mini-CGA to screen for older adults who require more complete assessment while undergoing treatment for prostate cancer (Terret, Albrand, & Droz, 2004).

Preliminary studies are being conducted to determine what items associated with MMSE (Folstein et al., 1975), ADL (Katz et al., 1970), IADL (Lawton & Brody, 1969), and GDS (Yesavage et al., 1982–1983) could be used as a screen for older adults with cancer who would benefit from the entire CGA (Overcash, Beckstead, & Cobb, 2004). Abbreviating the entire CGA would be a significant contribution to the care of the older person with cancer. Several of the CGA instruments have been abbreviated for use in the general older adult population. For example, researchers found the first five questions of the GDS to be as equally effective as the entire 15-item instrument (Hoyl, Valenzuela, & Marin, 2000). The first several questions of the MMSE also have been effective (Koenig, 1996). An abbreviated CGA performed by a nurse may help to focus on the groups of older adults who can benefit most from the entire CGA, thus reducing the costs associated with conducting an expensive, time-consuming, comprehensive examination.

Other options for expeditious CGA assessment are through self-reports (Ingram et al., 2002) and telephone questionnaires (Carrete et al., 2001). Both methods are reliable; however, with self-report, many older patients do not return the forms, and thus the assessment still has to take place during the clinic examination. Please refer to the NCCN *Clinical Practice Guidelines in Oncology* (2004) for more information on CGA screening measures.

Role of the Nurse in Coordination of the Comprehensive Geriatric Assessment and Follow-Up

One of the greatest indicators of CGA effectiveness is follow-up care (Burns et al., 2000; Waszynski, Murakami, & Lewis, 2000). Screening can be a complete waste of resources if the limitations detected are not referred for diagnostic evaluation and treatment. For many cancer treatment centers, follow-up is particularly difficult in that many people present to tertiary care clinics for a second opinion. If the CGA screening occurs in a tertiary care setting, then clinicians are obligated to follow up with primary care providers on elements of the exam that screen positive. Nurses play an important role in coordinating follow-up care.

Follow-up is a monumental task and principal role that often falls to the oncology nurse. Nurses who perform follow-up assessments to determine adherence to care management and evaluation of outcomes help to reduce overall healthcare costs by 33% (Waszynski et al., 2000). In a two-year randomized clinical trial of 128 veterans, ongoing care and evaluation of people age 65 and older resulted in fewer clinic visits, better IADL, improved social activity, improved depression scores, better general well-being, and better MMSE scores when compared to those who did not undergo continued care and medical support (Burns et al., 2000). Burns et al. also found that after initial CGA, long-term case management by a geriatric team resulted in enhanced scores on depression, dementia, and functional and life satisfaction screening instruments.

Little data exist on methods of follow-up. Recommendations from the CGA only are adhered to approximately 50%–70% of the time (Cefalu, Kaslow, Mims, & Simpson, 1995). Therefore, careful case management and follow-up are crucial and depend greatly on the population and the type of facility. If older adults are receiving some of their care at other clinics, communication between clinics should detail health assessment findings and recommendations. It also is helpful if the older adult receives a copy of the CGA medical report to take to any healthcare provider as a basis for the health history. If the geriatric team performs careful follow-up with patients, the nurse can help to schedule visits with the team when necessary and establish regular, ongoing multidisciplinary assessments. Case management and follow-up care are important nursing roles and are critical for many older adults to maintain some level of independence.

Geriatric care can be defined as the establishment of interventions for psychosocial support, caregiving, transportation needs, decreased mental status, impaired ADL, living arrangements, and financial concerns. Such care can be coordinated through a multidisciplinary team approach. Oncology nurses play an important role in coordination of the team. Many disciplines often administer the CGA. For example, social workers may perform the GDS and the MMSE; a dietitian may evaluate nutritional status; and a pharmacist may assess medications. Each of the disciplines should assimilate and communicate all of the data collected to the entire geriatric team for further interventions. The nurse often is responsible for compiling the recommended interventions to formulate a comprehensive plan of care (Evans, Yurkow, & Siegler, 1995).

Weekly team meetings, coordinated by nurses, typically facilitate dialogue among disciplines that deals with patient progress and any new interventions that should be added to the plan of care. The complete assessment and management of follow-up for older adults are useful in maintaining and even improving health (Overcash et al., 1998). In a nurse-led multidisciplinary program for delirium in older adults with a hip fracture, Milisen et al. (2001) showed that delirium was shorter in duration and less severe for those in the treatment group. Physical functioning also was enhanced in the treatment group. Moreover, in a retrospective study of patients age 70 and older with cancer, those who participated in a multidisciplinary approach to cancer care experienced a greater time to disease progression when compared to those who had not had a comprehensive team approach (Overcash et al., 1998).

Case Study

Carly opened the heavy door to the clinic. Cold air permeated her summer dress as she entered the office. The receptionist was speaking on the phone as she approached. "OK, sounds good. Oh . . . What are you wearing tonight? No . . . I'm wearing my black skirt . . . ." Carly stood patiently and wondered if she should sign in and sit in the waiting room. The young girl glanced up and mouthed something that Carly could not hear. Does she want me to sit down? Carly wondered. At that moment, the receptionist ended her phone conversation and harshly instructed Carly, "Sign your name and sit down." As Carly was situating herself in the waiting room, she began to think how breast cancer has changed her life. For 76 years, I have made my own decisions and have been very healthy and happy, and now I seem to be treated like a child, Carly thought. Carly began to flip through a magazine as a pretty, young woman in colorful scrubs erupted through the door to the exam room hallway and said, "Come on in, honey; it is time to see the doctor."

Carly was slow to rise from her chair in the waiting room. As she walked, the rattle of the medicine bottles in her bag accentuated her ataxic gait. The friendly nurse spoke softly as she commanded Carly to extend her arm for her blood pressure measurement. After the cuff was jerked off her arm, Carly gathered her possessions and went into the examination room. After a short wait, a young man gently opened the door and introduced himself as the nurse practitioner (NP) who was just hired. He said that he was going to ask some questions. Carly braced herself for the questions and listened to her medical records as the young man began to read her chart.

NP: . . . 76-year-old woman with stage II breast cancer. She is ER/PR+, *Her2/neu–*, 1/15 LN +, 2 cm tumor, moderately well differentiated. Path report showed infiltrating ductal carcinoma with a small component of intraductal carcinoma in situ. You underwent lumpectomy with axillary node dissection. Margins were found to be negative. Do you live alone?

Carly: Yes. I was widowed 15 years ago. I have four supportive children who all live out of state. I live in Florida year-round and have friends at church. The retirement community I live in has many activities and regular transportation to town and shopping.

NP: It looks like you have been diagnosed with diabetes mellitus (DM) and osteoporosis in addition to your breast cancer?

Carly: Yes.

NP: I see you have brought your medicine: vitamin E, vitamin A, multiple vitamin, Catapres® 0.1 mg po bid, Fosamax® 70 mg po q wk, and Glucophage® 850 mg po bid.

The following information completes Carly's medical history.

- Fractured elbow in 1995 from roller skating
- Remote history of migraines
- History of diabetes since 1984, controlled with diet and medication
  - Glucophage 850 mg po bid

- Benign cardiac arrhythmia; however, assessment and diagnostic workup revealed no pathology.
- Osteopenia; diagnosed with osteoporosis last year, treated with Fosamax (tolerating therapy well)
  - Fosamax 70 mg po q wk
- Surgical history
  - Internal reduction of left elbow in 1995
- Family medical history
  - Mother had breast cancer, which was resected 10 years before she died of cardiac issues.
- Comprehensive geriatric assessment
  - +4 on the GDS
  - 27 on the MMSE
  - No limitations on the ADL
  - Unable to do projects around the house and requires some help from her daughter to manage finances and IADL
- Assessment
  - Stage II breast cancer
  - DM type 2 controlled
  - Orthostatic hypotension
  - Osteoporosis controlled
  - Presbycusis
- Plan
  - Chemotherapy with CMF
    - o Cyclophosphamide 100 mg/m² po on days 1–14
    - o Methotrexate 40 mg/m² IV on days 1 and 8
    - o Fluorouracil 600 mg/m² on days 1 and 8
    - o Repeat cycle every 28 days for six cycles.
  - Hormonal therapy: Tamoxifen 10 mg bid following completion of chemotherapy and radiation therapy
  - Annual gynecologic exam and education to report any vaginal bleeding or gynecologic symptoms (Patient has not had a hysterectomy.)
  - Work with patient to arrange social support while undergoing cancer treatments.
  - Perform a gait inventory, and assess ataxia.
  - Continue to screen for falls.
  - Refer to audiologist for assessment and diagnosis.
  - Continue to follow the patient using the CGA as a baseline while receiving active chemotherapy by monitoring ADL and IADL, especially during chemotherapy. Also, continue to monitor MMSE because the patient's baseline score was 27. (Although not a positive screen, it suggests the need for ongoing assessment.)
  - Include caregiver in plan of care (either children or friends and neighbors at the retirement community). Develop a proactive plan of care with the patient concerning days when she does not feel well because of the cancer treatment.
  - Because of a history of breast cancer, teach the patient that daughters should be screened.
  - Send copy of dictation to primary care provider who is treating DM and osteoporosis.

Comprehensive Geriatric Assessment Summary

The CGA performed in this case study illustrates the importance of a thorough assessment for an older adult who has seemingly no or very few limitations. The CGA provided a baseline assessment of Carly's physical, functional, and emotional well-being. As Carly progresses through cancer treatment, continued assessment of functional, emotional, and physical health status is important. For example, episodic depression is common while undergoing cancer treatment. Regular screening with the GDS and close follow-up can detect depression before it becomes a life-limiting problem.

The breast cancer in this case is not the only consideration in managing Carly's care. Communication with the primary healthcare provider concerning the status of the CGA, the cancer, and the prescribed treatments also can help with the general patient management plan. Conversely, assessing the status of the DM and osteoporosis can be important in decision making regarding the cancer treatment plan. Additionally, any problems associated with the ataxia and altered gait should be diagnosed and treated. Carly also should be referred to audiology for hearing screening for sensory neuronal hearing loss.

Evaluation of social support and other resources is essential. Although Carly has friends in her retirement community, the support they offer may be limited to only very light tasks such as phone calls and occasional visits. If Carly's condition were to decline or if she were to experience complications from her cancer therapy and required more in-depth assistance, the available resources may not be adequate to meet her needs in the current situation. Proactive planning and assessment of resources are important to work out a reasonable plan should she require more assistance.

Conclusion

The CGA is a vital component of the care of the older adult with cancer. Nursing has a role in the forefront of geriatric oncology. The primary care nurse or advanced practice nurse must be familiar with current evidence-based practice guidelines and the principles of the CGA to help the older adult to maintain optimal function and quality of life during cancer diagnosis and treatment.

References

American Geriatrics Society. (1993). *Comprehensive geriatric assessment position statement.* New York: Author.

Auslander, G.K., & Litwin, H. (1990). Social support networks and formal help seeking: Differences between applicants to social services and a nonapplicant sample. *Journal of Gerontology, 45,* S112–S119.

Balducci, L. (1994). Do we need geriatric oncology? *Cancer Control, 1,* 91–93.

Balducci, L. (2003). New paradigms for treating elderly patients with cancer: The comprehensive geriatric assessment and guidelines for supportive care. *Journal of Supportive Oncology, 1,* 30–37.

Balducci, L., & Beghe, C. (2000). The application of the principles of geriatrics to the management of the older person with cancer. *Critical Reviews in Oncology/Hematology, 35,* 147–154.

Balducci, L., & Repetto, L. (2004). Increased risk of myelotoxicity in elderly patients with non-Hodgkin's lymphoma. *Cancer, 100,* 6–11.

Balducci, L., & Yates, J. (2000). General guidelines for the management of older patients with cancer. *Oncology (Huntington), 14*(11A), 221–224.

Barton, D., & Loprinzi, C. (2002). Novel approaches to preventing chemotherapy-induced cognitive dysfunction in breast cancer: The art of the possible. *Clinical Breast Cancer, 3*(Suppl. 3), S121–S127.

Bernabei, R., Venturiero, V., Tarsitani, P., & Gambassi, G. (2000). The comprehensive geriatric assessment: When, where, how. *Critical Reviews in Oncology/Hematology, 33,* 45–56.

Boult, C., Boult, L.B., Morishita, L., Dowd, B.M., Kane, R.L., & Urdangarin, C.F. (2001). A randomized clinical trial of outpatient geriatric evaluation and management. *Journal of the American Geriatrics Society, 49,* 351–359.

Bula, C.J., Berod, A.C., Stuck, A.E., Alessi, C.A., Aronow, H.U., Santos-Eggiman, B., et al. (1999). Effectiveness of preventive in-home geriatric assessment in well functioning, community-dwelling older people: Secondary analysis of a randomized trial. *Journal of the American Geriatrics Society, 47,* 389–395.

Burns, R., Nichols, L.O., Martindale-Adams, J., & Graney, M.J. (2000). Interdisciplinary geriatric primary care evaluation and management: Two-year outcomes. *Journal of the American Geriatrics Society, 48,* 8–13.

Carrete, P., Augustovski, F., Gimpel, N., Fernandez, S., Di Paolo, R., Schaffer, I., et al. (2001). Validation of a telephone-administered geriatric depression scale in a Hispanic elderly population. *Journal of General Internal Medicine, 16,* 446–450.

Cefalu, C.A., Kaslow, L.D., Mims, B., & Simpson, S. (1995). Follow-up of comprehensive geriatric assessment in a family medicine residency clinic. *Journal of the American Board of Family Practice, 8,* 337–340.

Centers for Disease Control and Prevention. (2003). *Summary health statistics for the U.S. population: National health interview survey, 2001.* Atlanta, GA: U.S. Department of Health and Human Services, National Center for Health Statistics.

Charlson, M., & Peterson, J.C. (2002). Medical comorbidity and late life depression: What is known and what are the unmet needs? *Society of Biological Psychiatry, 52,* 226–235.

Cohen, S., & Syme, A. (1985). *Social support and health.* New York: Academic Press.

Evans, L.K., Yurkow, J., & Siegler, E.L. (1995). The CARE Program: A nurse-managed collaborative outpatient program to improve function of frail older people. Collaboration Assessment and Rehabilitation for Elders. *Journal of the American Geriatrics Society, 43,* 1155–1160.

Extermann, M. (2000). Measurement and impact of comorbidity in older cancer patients. *Critical Reviews in Oncology/Hematology, 35,* 181–200.

Extermann, M. (2004). Management issues for elderly patients with breast cancer. *Current Treatment Options in Oncology, 5,* 161–169.

Extermann, M., Overcash, J.A., Lyman, G.H., Parr, J., & Balducci, L. (1998). Comorbidity and functional status are independent in older cancer patients. *Journal of Clinical Oncology, 16,* 1582–1587.

Folstein, M.F., Folstein, S.E., & McHugh, P.R. (1975). "Mini-mental state." A practical method for grading the cognitive state of patients for the clinician. *Journal of Psychiatric Research, 12,* 189–198.

Freyer, G., Lortholary, A., Delcambre, C., Delozier, T., Piot, G., Genin, F., et al. (2004). Unexpected toxicities in elderly patients treated with oral idarubicin in metastatic breast cancer: The GINECO experience. *Clinical Oncology, 16,* 17–23.

Fried, L., Storer, D., King, D.E., & Lodder, F. (1991). Diagnosis of illness presentation in the elderly. *Journal of the American Geriatrics Society, 39,* 117–123.

Funch, D., & Marshall, J. (1983). The role of stress, social support and age in survival from breast cancer. *Journal of Psychosomatic Research, 27,* 77–83.

Goodwin, J., Hunt, W., & Samet, J. (1993). A population-based study of functional status and social support networks of elderly patients newly diagnosed with cancer. *Archives of Internal Medicine, 151,* 366–370.

Hamilton, M. (1967). Development of a rating scale for primary depressive illness. *British Journal of Social Clinical Psychology, 6,* 278–296.

Hjerl, K., Andersen, E.W., Keiding, N., Mouridsen, H.T., Mortensen, P.B., & Jorgensen, T. (2003). Depression as a prognostic factor for breast cancer mortality. *Psychosomatics, 44,* 24–30.

Hoyl, T., Valenzuela, E., & Marin, P.P. (2000). Depression in the aged: Preliminary evaluation of the effectiveness, as a screening instrument, of the 5-item version of the Geriatric Depression Scale. *Revista Medica de Chile, 128,* 1199–1204.

Ingram, S.S., Seo, P.H., Martell, R.E., Clipp, E.C., Doyle, M.E., Montana, G.S., et al. (2002). Comprehensive assessment of the elderly cancer patient: The feasibility of self-report methodology. *Journal of Clinical Oncology, 20,* 770–775.

Izaks, G.J., & Westendorp, R.G. (2003). Ill or just old? Towards a conceptual framework of the relation between ageing and disease. *BioMed Central Geriatrics, 3,* 7.

Katz, S., Downs, T.D., Cash, H.R., & Grotz, R.C. (1970). Progress in the development of the Index of ADL. *Gerontologist, 10,* 20–30.

Koenig, H.G. (1996). An abbreviated Mini-Mental State Exam for medically ill older adults. *Journal of the American Geriatrics Society, 44,* 215–216.

Kurlowicz, L. (1999). *Try this: Best practices in nursing care to older adults.* New York: Hartford Institute for Geriatric Nursing.

Lawton, M.P., & Brody, E.M. (1969). Assessment of older people: Self-maintaining and instrumental activities of daily living. *Gerontologist, 9,* 179–186.

Lyness, J.M., Noel, T.K., Cox, C., King, D.A., Conwell, Y., & Caine, E.D. (1997). Screening for depression in elderly primary care patients: A comparison of the Center for Epidemiologic Studies Depression Scale and the Geriatric Depression Scale. *Archives of Internal Medicine, 157,* 449–454.

Maartense, R., Kluin-Nelemans, H.C., & Noordijk, E.M. (2003). Non-Hodgkin's lymphoma in the elderly. A review with emphasis on elderly patients, geriatric assessment and future perspectives. *Annals of Hematology, 82,* 661–670.

Maly, R.C., Hirsch, S.H., & Reuben, D.B. (1997). The performance of simple instruments in detecting geriatric conditions and selecting community-dwelling older people for geriatric assessment. *Age and Ageing, 26,* 223–231.

McGuire, L., Keicolt-Glaser, J., & Glaser, R. (2002). Depressive symptoms and lymphocyte proliferation in older adults. *Journal of Abnormal Psychology, 111,* 192–197.

Milisen, K., Foreman, M.D., Abaraham, I.L., DeGeest, S., Godderis, J., Vandermeulen, E., et al. (2001). A nurse-led interdisciplinary intervention program for delirium in elderly hip-fracture patients. *Journal of the American Geriatrics Society, 49,* 523–532.

National Center for Health Statistics. (2003). *Health, United States, 2003.* Atlanta, GA: Centers for Disease Control and Prevention.

National Comprehensive Cancer Network. (2004). *Clinical practice guidelines in oncology.* Jenkintown, PA: Author.

Overcash, J. (1998). Developing a senior adult oncology program. *Home Healthcare Consultant, 5,* 2–8.

Overcash, J. (2003). Assessing and caring for the older person with cancer: How comprehensive geriatric assessment and multidisciplinary teams can contribute to the caring for the older person with cancer. *Oncology Supportive Care Quarterly, 2*(1), 32–43.

Overcash, J., & Balducci, L. (2003). Social support and social networks of the older cancer patient. In J. Overcash & L. Balducci (Eds.), *The older cancer patient: A guide for nurses and related professionals* (pp. 223–241). New York: Springer.

Overcash, J., Beckstead, J., & Cobb, S. (2004, October). *A preliminary study of the abbreviated comprehensive geriatric assessment in the older person with cancer.* Abstract presented at the Sigma Theta Tau Conference, Augusta, GA.

Overcash, J., Chen, H., Extermann, M., Cantor, A., & Balducci, L. (1998, October). *Understanding the comprehensive geriatric assessment (CGA). Impact on survival and time to disease progression in older cancer patients.* Abstract presented at the IV International Conference on Geriatric Oncology, Rome, Italy.

Petersen, R.C., Stevens, J.C., Ganguli, M., Tangalos, E.G., Cummings, J.L., & DeKosky, S.T. (2001). Practice parameter: Early detection of dementia: Mild cognitive impairment (an evidence-based review). Report of the Quality Standards Subcommittee of the American Academy of Neurology. *Neurology, 56,* 1133–1142.

Philp, I., Newton, P., McKee, K.J., Dixon, S., Rowse, G., & Bath, P.A. (2001). Geriatric assessment in primary care: Formulating best practice. *British Journal of Community Nursing, 6,* 290–295.

Raik, B.L., Miller, F.G., & Fins, J.J. (2004). Screening and cognitive impairment: Ethics of forgoing mammography in older women. *Journal of the American Geriatrics Society, 52,* 440–444.

Rao, A.V., Seo, P.H., & Cohen, H.J. (2004). Geriatric assessment and comorbidity. *Seminars in Oncology, 31,* 149–159.

Repetto, L., & Comandini, D. (2000). Cancer in the elderly: Assessing patients for fitness. *Critical Reviews in Oncology/Hematology, 35,* 155–160.

Repetto, L., Venturino, A., Fratino, L., Serraino, D., Troisi, G., Gianni, W., et al. (2003). Geriatric oncology: A clinical approach to the older patient with cancer. *European Journal of Cancer, 39,* 870–880.

Reuben, D.B., Fishman, L.K., McNabney, M., & Wolde-Tsadik, G. (1996). Looking inside the black box of comprehensive geriatric assessment: A classification system for problems, recommendations, and implementation strategies. *Journal of the American Geriatrics Society, 44,* 835–838.

Rubenstein, L.Z., Goodwin, M., Hardley, E., Patten, S.K., Rempusheski, V.F., Reuben, D., et al. (1991). Targeting criteria for geriatric evaluation and management research. *Journal of the American Geriatrics Society, 39*(9 Pt. 2), 37S–41S.

Rubenstein, L.Z., Siu, A.L., & Wieland, D. (1989). Comprehensive geriatric assessment: Toward understanding its efficacy. *Aging, 1,* 87–98.

Sahyoun, N.R., Lentzner, H., Hoyert, D., & Robinson, K.N. (2001). *Trends in causes of death among the elderly.* Hyattsville, MD: National Center for Health Statistics.

Shaw, B.A., & Janevic, M. (2004). Associations between anticipated support, physical functioning, and education level among a nationally representative sample of older adults. *Journal of Aging and Health, 14,* 539–561.

Skarstein, J., Aass, N., Fossa, S.D., Skovlund, E., & Dahl, A.A. (2000). Anxiety and depression in cancer patients: Relation between the Hospital Anxiety and Depression Scale and the European Organization for Research and Treatment of Cancer Core Quality of Life Questionnaire. *Journal of Psychosomatic Research, 49,* 27–34.

Solomon, D. (1988). National Institutes of Health consensus development conference statement: Geriatric assessment methods for clinical decision-making. *Journal of the American Geriatrics Society, 36,* 342–347.

Stuck, A.E., Elkuch, P., Dapp, U., Anders, J., Iliffe, S., & Swift, C.G. (2002). Feasibility and yield of a self-administered questionnaire for health risk appraisal in older people in three European countries. *Age and Ageing, 31,* 463–467.

Terret, C., Albrand, G., & Droz, J.P. (2004). Geriatric assessment in elderly patient with prostate cancer. *Clinical Prostate Cancer, 2,* 236–240.

Trentini, M., Semeraro, S., & Motta, M. (2001). Effectiveness of geriatric evaluation and care. One-year results of a multicenter randomized clinical trial. *Aging, 13,* 395–405.

Waszynski, C.M., Murakami, W., & Lewis, M. (2000). Community care management. Advanced practice nurses as care managers. *Care Management, 2,* 148–152.

Wedding, U., & Hoffen, K. (2003). Care of breast cancer in the elderly woman—What does comprehensive geriatric assessment (CGA) help? *Supportive Care in Cancer, 11,* 769–774.

Williams, M.E., Williams, F., Zimer, J.G., Hall, W.Y., & Podgorski, C.A. (1987). How does the team approach to outpatient geriatric evaluation compare with traditional care: A report of a randomized controlled trial. *Journal of the American Geriatrics Society, 35,* 1071–1078.

Winograd, C.H., Gerety, M.B., Chung, M., Goldstein, M.K., Dominguez, F., & Vallone, R. (1991). Screening for frailty: Criteria and predictors of outcomes. *Journal of the American Geriatrics Society, 39,* 778–784.

Yesavage, J.A., Brink, T.L., Rose, T.L., Lum, O., Huang, V., Adey, M., et al. (1982–1983). Development and validation of a geriatric depression screening scale: A preliminary report. *Journal of Psychiatric Research, 17,* 37–49.

Zung, W.W. (1972). The depression status inventory: An adjunct to the self-rating depression scale. *Journal of Clinical Psychology, 28,* 539–543.

CHAPTER 5

Cancer Screening in the Older Adult

Anne M. Reb, MSN, NP

Introduction

Experts generally advocate population screening when studies demonstrate lower mortality from cancer in the screened versus the unscreened population (Champion, Rawl, & Menon, 2002). Cancer screening over the past 25 years has resulted in a decrease in mortality from most malignancies through early detection and more effective treatment (Heflin & Cohen, 2001). The evidence about the benefits of cancer screening in the older adult is limited because of a lack of randomized controlled trials in people older than 75 (Walter & Covinsky, 2001). In addition, barriers and controversial screening guidelines exist that hamper clinical judgment and screening decisions in the older adult. Barriers to adequate screening include factors such as finances, transportation, comorbidities, other physical factors, and attitudes of patients and healthcare providers. Lack of clinician support for screening is a strong variable that influences participation in screening (Balducci & Extermann, 2000). This factor may be especially problematic with the older adult population because current evidence about screening in this group is limited. Several organizations have created screening guidelines based primarily on age; however, conflicting recommendations exist. This chapter will discuss some of the benefits, limitations, and special considerations for cancer screening in the older adult. It also will review the evidence base for screening recommendations and present current screening guidelines from various agencies.

Screening Decisions

Various factors should be considered in screening decisions for the older adult, including the benefits, limitations, and potential harms of screening (see Figure 5-1).

- Risk of death from a particular cancer based on
  - Life expectancy and comorbidities
  - Age-specific mortality rate for that cancer
- Benefits of screening
  - Risk reduction associated with a screening test
  - Quality-of-life benefits associated with early detection
- Potential harms/limitations of screening
  - Treatment of cancer that may not become clinically significant in one's lifetime
  - Complications from additional diagnostic procedures in case of false-positive tests
  - Psychological distress associated with false-positive tests
  - Increased burden for older adults with multiple medical problems or short life expectancy
  - Lack of evidence supporting the benefit of certain screening tests on mortality reduction
- Patient values and preferences
  - Communicate benefits, risks, and potential for additional procedures for abnormal screening test.
  - Include older adults in decision-making process.
  - Individualize screening decisions rather than basing decisions on age alone.
- Need for increased participation and referrals of older adults to ongoing screening trials

Figure 5-1. Factors to Consider in Screening Decisions for the Older Adult

Note. Based on information from American Geriatrics Society, 2001; Champion et al., 2002; Walter & Covinsky, 2001.

The main benefit of screening is to reduce the risk of dying of a detectable cancer. The assumption is that screening and early detection/treatment will improve survival beyond what would be expected if the disease were not detected and treated (American Geriatrics Society [AGS], 2001). However, diagnosing an asymptomatic cancer is not beneficial when a person is likely to die of another cause such as heart failure or stroke (Saunders, 2001; Walter & Covinsky, 2001). One framework to guide screening decisions in the older adult considers the risk of dying of a screen-detectable cancer, the potential benefits and harms of screening, and patient preferences (Walter & Covinsky). The first step in this framework is based on the estimate of a person's risk of death because of a particular cancer. This estimate is derived from the person's life expectancy and the age-specific mortality rate of that cancer. Although variation exists in life expectancy at each age, healthcare professionals can calculate age-specific estimates based on the person's state of health, considering his or her comorbidities and functional impairments. Cancer screening is unlikely to be beneficial for those with life expectancies of less than five years because the survival benefits of screening are not immediate (AGS, 2001; Walter & Covinsky).

Benefits

One can calculate the absolute benefit of screening tests by determining the risk reduction associated with particular screening tests. This is referred to as the absolute risk reduction and can be quantified by calculating the number of people needed to screen (NNS) to prevent one cancer-specific death. These calculations have been approximated for various screening tests considering age and life expectancy. The NNS significantly increases as life expectancy decreases, meaning that many people need to be screened to prevent one death from a particular cancer. For further information regarding quantitative estimates of the benefits of screening, refer to Walter and Covinsky (2001).

Another consideration relates to the detection of rapidly progressive cancers. Screening that detects a rapidly progressive cancer is not likely to improve survival. Alternatively, detecting an aggressive cancer may improve quality of life by facilitating earlier initiation of palliative and supportive treatments. Some suggest that mortality benefits should not be the only consideration in screening decisions. Other factors such as quality of life and potential for less-invasive treatment with earlier detection also should be considered (Champion et al., 2002). In a comprehensive review of research regarding the benefits and burdens of breast cancer screening and treatment in older women, Yarbrough (2004) emphasized that quality of life should be an end point in research studies, especially when evaluating the costs and benefits of screening or treatment. The potential benefits of screening, such as improved survival and quality of life, should be considered in relation to possible burdens and harms from screening.

Potential Harms

Potential harms of screening include (a) complications from additional diagnostic procedures that may result from false-positive screening tests, (b) treatment of clinically insignificant cancers, and (c) psychological distress associated with a positive screening test (Walter & Covinsky, 2001). Further, older patients with multiple medical problems or short life expectancies may experience increased burdens from screening. For example, people with dementia or other conditions may be unwilling to undergo the discomfort associated with various screening tests such as colonoscopy or mammography (AGS, 2001). These harms may result in increased morbidity with no improvement in mortality because of early detection of disease (Silverman et al., 2000). For example, complications from colonoscopy performed after a positive fecal occult blood test (FOBT) may include perforation, bleeding, and cardiorespiratory events. Identifying and treating a cancer that would not become clinically significant represents a considerable potential harm of screening (Walter & Covinsky).

Patient Preferences

Patients' values and preferences should be incorporated in screening decisions. Prior to initiating screening, the healthcare provider should discuss risks and benefits as well as possible additional procedures in the event of an abnormal screening test (Walter & Covinsky, 2001). Screening decisions should be individualized, rather than determined by age alone, with consideration of the expected benefit of the screening test. Older adults should have access to screening tests for prognostic information, if desired, even if they do not plan to pursue active treatment if a cancer is discovered (AGS, 2001). The healthcare provider should consider life expectancy, comorbidities, benefits, and limitations of screening for particular types of cancers and patients' preferences in screening decisions. The following sections will address cancer screening guidelines for some of the common cancers in the older adult based upon government, private, and disease-related organization recommendations and evidence-based research. Table 5-1 includes screening guidelines for breast, prostate, and colorectal cancers because the guidelines for these cancers are more clearly defined. Screening considerations also will be discussed in the text for other common cancers for which the guidelines are less clearly defined at this time. Recommendations specific to the older adult will be highlighted, if available. Ongoing clinical screening trials relevant to the older adult also will be discussed (see Table 5-2).

Table 5-1. Cancer Screening Guidelines for People at Average Risk

Cancer	American Cancer Society	National Cancer Institute	National Comprehensive Cancer Network	U.S. Preventive Services Task Force	American College of Obstetricians and Gynecologists	American Urological Association	American Gastroenterological Association
Breast	Annual mammography starting at age 40	Annual or biennial mammography starting at age 40; annual or biennial mammography at age 50 and older	Annual mammography starting at age 40	Annual or biennial mammography at age 40 and older	Annual or biennial mammography starting at age 40; annual mammography starting at age 50	—	—
Prostate	Annual prostate-specific antigen (PSA) test and digital rectal exam (DRE) starting at age 50 for men who have at least a 10-year life expectancy	Insufficient evidence to determine whether screening with PSA or DRE reduces mortality	Baseline PSA at age 40; regular PSA screening starting at age 50	Insufficient evidence to recommend for or against routine screening using PSA or DRE	—	Annual PSA and DRE starting at age 50	—
Colorectal	Fecal occult blood test (FOBT) annually, flexible sigmoidoscopy every 5 years; or FOBT plus flexible sigmoidoscopy every 5 years; or double contrast barium enema (DCBE) every 5 years; or colonoscopy every 10 years starting at age 50	Annual FOBT testing; regular screening by sigmoidoscopy or colonoscopy beginning at age 50 for people at average risk	Annual FOBT and flexible sigmoidoscopy every 5 years; or DCBE every 5 years; or colonoscopy every 10 years starting at age 50	Periodic FOBT; sigmoidoscopy every 5 years; FOBT and sigmoidoscopy every 5 years; colonoscopy every 10 years; or DCBE every 5 years starting at age 50	—	—	FOBT annually, flexible sigmoidoscopy every 5 years; FOBT and sigmoidoscopy every 5 years, DCBE every 5 years; or colonoscopy every 10 years

Note. Based on information from American College of Obstetricians and Gynecologists, 2003; American Urological Association, 2000; National Cancer Institute, 2002b, 2005a, 2005b, 2005d; National Comprehensive Cancer Network, 2004, 2005a, 2005c; Smith et al., 2005; U.S. Preventive Services Task Force, 2002b, 2002c, 2002d; Winawer et al., 2003.

Table 5-2. Examples of Recent or Ongoing Screening Trials

Trial	Design	Purpose	Age at Enrollment
Prostate, Lung, Colorectal, and Ovarian (PLCO) Cancer Trial	Randomized controlled multicenter trial (Prorok et al., 2000)	To determine whether screening reduces mortality from prostate, lung, colorectal, and ovarian cancers Screening variables: – Digital rectal exam plus serum prostate-specific antigen test – Chest x-ray – Flexible sigmoidoscopy – CA-125 and transvaginal ultrasound	55–74 years
European Randomized Study of Screening for Prostate Cancer (ER-SPC)	Randomized controlled multicenter trial (De Koning et al., 2002)	To determine whether screening reduces prostate cancer mortality	Age varies by country between 55–74 years.
National Lung Cancer Screening Trial	Randomized controlled multicenter trial (Ford et al., 2003)	To determine if screening reduces lung cancer mortality in current and former heavy smokers Compares spiral computerized tomography scan and chest x-ray to determine which test is better in reducing deaths from lung cancer	55–74 years
The Digital Mammographic Imaging Screening Trial (DMIST)	Multicenter trial (Ford et al., 2003)	Compares accuracy of digital mammography versus screening mammography in women with no breast symptoms	No age limits; most women 40 or older
Randomized screening study of fecal occult blood test (FOBT) and multitarget DNA-based assay panel testing (MTAP) followed by colonoscopy in the detection of colorectal cancer	Randomized multicenter trial	Compares FOBT and MTAP applied to stools and plasma in identifying colorectal cancer	50–64 and 65–80 years
Study of computerized tomographic colonography (CTC) for screening healthy participants for colorectal cancer	Multicenter trial	Compares sensitivity of CTC versus colonoscopy for detecting large lesions in asymptomatic participants	50 and older
Randomized screening study of CA-125 and ultrasound in the detection of ovarian cancer in postmenopausal women	Randomized multicenter trial	Determines impact of screening for preclinical detection of ovarian cancer on ovarian cancer mortality in postmenopausal women	50–74 years

Note. Based on information from De Koning et al., 2002; Ford et al., 2003; National Cancer Institute, 2003, 2004a, 2004b; Prorok et al., 2000.

Breast Cancer

The purpose of screening for breast cancer is to detect cancer at earlier stages when treatment is more effective (Kimmick & Balducci, 2000). Breast cancer screening techniques include mammography, clinical breast exam (CBE), and breast self-exam (BSE), each with differing levels of evidence (Rimer, Schildkraut, & Hiatt, 2005). Randomized trials support the benefit of mammography screening in reducing mortality, with the strongest evidence seen in women ages 50–69 years (Iannuzzi-Sucich & Kenny, 2004; Rimer et al.). However, these trials have included inadequate numbers of women older than 70. Evidence of mammography effectiveness in older women is limited to two trials that included women older than age 65, the Malmo trial (45–69 years) and the Swedish Two-County Trial (40–74 years). Based on combined data from these trials, the U.S. Preventive Services Task Force (USPSTF) reported a breast cancer mortality reduction of 22% (summary relative risk = .78; CI, 0.62 to 0.99) in women ages 65–74 years (Humphrey, Helfand, Chan, & Woolf, 2002; Peek, 2003). One factor supporting mammography screening in the older adult is that the benefit in terms of absolute risk reduction increases with age, whereas the risk for false-positive results decreases. Randomized trials demonstrate that the sensitivity of mammography increases with increasing age because of decreased breast density. In addition, the positive predictive value of mammography screening increases because of the higher prevalence of breast cancer in older women (Smith, Saslow, et al., 2003).

Because many of the trials did not include women older than 75, the upper age limit for discontinuing screening is controversial (Kimmick & Muss, 2000; USPSTF, 2002b). One study used a decision analysis model to estimate the benefits of screening older women from different age, race, and health conditions. This study showed that screening saved lives of older adult women of all ages, but the magnitude of savings decreased with increasing age and comorbidities (Mandelblatt, 1992). A more recent systematic review of cost-effectiveness studies assessed the costs and benefits of screening women age 65 and older. The investigators concluded that "it remains cost-effective to screen older women for breast cancer every two years according to current medical spending" (Mandelblatt et al., 2003, p. 5). However, the costs and harms of screening may outweigh the benefits for women who have comorbidities that limit life expectancy (Mandelblatt et al., 2003). Research examining mammography in older women with chronic illnesses is limited because these women rarely are included in clinical trials. Silverman et al. (2000) found that women with breast cancer and two or more comorbidities were twice as likely to die from causes other than breast cancer in a three-year period, whereas Satariano and Ragland (1994) found that women with three comorbid conditions were 20 times more likely to die from other causes in a three-year period. Thus, women with significant comorbidities that limit their life expectancy are unlikely to benefit from screening (USPSTF, 2002b). Screening decisions should be individualized and consider the benefits and risks as well as the health status and life expectancy of older women (Smith, Cokkinides, & Eyre, 2003).

A consensus panel on breast cancer screening in older women, funded by the National Cancer Institute (NCI) and the National Institute on Aging, recommended monthly BSE, yearly CBE, and mammograms every two years for women 65–74 years of age. The recommendations were similar for women older than 75 with good life expectancies (Costanza, 1992). The American Cancer Society (Smith, Cokkinides, &

Eyre, 2005) and the National Comprehensive Cancer Network (NCCN, 2004) recommended annual CBE and mammography screening for all women older than 40 years of age as long as the patient is in good health. USPSTF (2002a, 2002b) recommended screening mammography with or without CBE annually or biennially from age 40 and older. The evidence is generalizable to women age 70 and older for those with a reasonable life expectancy. The American College of Obstetricians and Gynecologists (2003) recommended that all women have annual CBEs, mammography every one to two years starting at age 40, and annual mammography starting at age 50. NCI (2005a) noted that screening mammography, CBE, or both may decrease breast cancer mortality. For mammography, NCI (2002b) recommended screening every one to two years starting at age 40 for average-risk women. AGS (1999) recommended annual or biennial mammograms until age 75 and biennial mammograms or one at least every three years for women older than 75 with a life expectancy of at least four years. Screening guidelines for women at high risk of developing breast cancer are discussed in the NCCN (2005b) guidelines titled *Genetic/Familial High-Risk Assessment: Breast and Ovarian.*

Ovarian Cancer

The incidence of ovarian cancer increases with age. Screening tests may include pelvic examination, serum CA-125, and transvaginal ultrasound. However, these tests are not sufficiently accurate for general population screening (Karlan, Markman, & Eifel, 2005). CA-125 is a tumor marker used to monitor people with ovarian cancer and is elevated in the majority of women with advanced stage epithelial ovarian cancer (Karlan et al.; O'Rourke & Mahon, 2003). Although serum CA-125 correlates with progression or regression of the disease (Karlan et al.), this test does not have sufficient specificity for routine ovarian cancer screening when used as a sole test (Menon, 2004; Silverman et al., 2000). For example, other conditions such as endometriosis, fibroids, pancreatitis, cirrhosis, benign ovarian cysts, and other cancers also may be associated with elevations in CA-125 (Champion et al., 2002; Karlan et al.), thus leading to false-positive test results. Another important consideration affecting screening recommendations is that CA-125 is not elevated in 20%–50% of women diagnosed with early-stage disease (Karlan et al.).

Transvaginal ultrasound can detect small masses and frequently is used for diagnostic testing of pelvic masses. However, its use as a screening tool to detect malignant lesions is limited because of high rates of false-positive tests (Jacobs & Menon, 2004; Menon, 2004). For example, older women have a high prevalence of benign ovarian lesions contributing to false-positive tests (see Jacobs & Menon for further discussion). Therefore, women may face unnecessary surgery and anxiety when ultrasound alone is used for screening (Menon).

Screening to detect early-stage disease is particularly challenging because of the low prevalence rate of ovarian cancer as well as the need to identify a test or combination of tests with adequate sensitivity and specificity for detecting ovarian cancer (Jacobs & Menon, 2004). Another challenge is identifying the target population for screening because the majority of ovarian cancers are sporadic and occur in the general population (Jacobs & Menon). Current research does not conclusively demonstrate that screening will reduce mortality from ovarian cancer (Ferrini, 1997; NCI, 2005c; USPSTF, 2004). For example, a National Institutes of Health (1995) Consensus Development Panel concluded that evidence does not support the use of CA-125 and transvaginal ultrasound for widespread screening to reduce mortality. The Prostate, Lung, Colorectal, and Ovarian (PLCO) cancer trial is an ongoing randomized trial that will address this question. This study compares CA-125 and transvaginal ultrasound screening to routine care to assess the potential benefit of screening for ovarian cancer (Ferrini). Results of this trial should be available between 2005 and 2008 (Smith, Cokkinides, et al., 2003). Researchers are conducting another randomized multicenter trial (United Kingdom Collaborative Trial of Ovarian Cancer Screening, 2004) in the United Kingdom with postmenopausal women (ages 50–74) who are at average risk to assess the value of CA-125 testing and ultrasound in detecting ovarian cancer (NCI, 2003). Women are randomized to control, screening with ultrasound, or multimodal screening arm (annual screening with serum CA-125 as the primary test and CA-125 and ultrasound as the secondary test) groups (United Kingdom Collaborative Trial of Ovarian Cancer Screening). The primary end point is the impact of screening on ovarian cancer mortality (Jacobs & Menon). Other strategies that may help to reduce mortality include focusing on prevention and identifying high-risk populations (Barnes, Grizzle, Grubbs, & Partridge, 2002). Screening trials are ongoing to detect ovarian cancer in high-risk women. If ongoing trials show that screening has a beneficial effect on mortality, women at higher risk are likely to experience the most benefit (USPSTF, 2004). Older women should be encouraged to participate in clinical trials for early detection of ovarian cancer.

NCI (2005c) stated that insufficient evidence exists that screening for ovarian cancer will result in decreased mortality from the disease. The USPSTF (2004) recommended against routine screening for ovarian cancer. For women at high risk for developing ovarian cancer, see the NCCN guidelines (2005b).

Prostate Cancer

Screening for prostate cancer is controversial because it has not been shown to definitively reduce mortality (NCCN, 2005c; Silverman et al., 2000; Walter & Covinsky, 2001). However, early detection methods have been a factor contributing to diagnosis at earlier stages of disease (NCCN, 2005c). The most common screening methods include digital rectal exam (DRE) and serum prostate-specific antigen (PSA). Healthcare professionals may use imaging studies, such as transurethral ultrasonography, for further evaluation if screening tests are abnormal (Gambert, 2001; Silverman et al.). The DRE is a simple, inexpensive test that has a sensitivity of 55%–69%; however, in older males with high rates of prostatic hyperplasia, the test is less reliable (Heflin & Cohen, 2001). Additionally, the test is a poor predictor for cancers of the anterior prostate (Gambert; Silverman et al.). PSA is a sensitive tumor marker test that detects 90%–95% of prostate cancers while still localized (Gambert). However, the specificity of the PSA decreases in older males because of other factors that may cause elevations such as benign prostatic hypertrophy, prostatitis, prostate procedures, and medications (Heflin & Cohen; Raghavan & Skinner, 2004). Clinicians should inquire about the use of medications, such as finasteride, that may affect PSA levels. Clinicians also should inquire about the use of herbal supplements for lower urinary tract symptoms because several of these supplements, including saw palmetto, may affect PSA levels (NCCN, 2005c).

Data suggest that combining PSA and DRE improves the rate of cancer detection (American Urological Association [AUA], 2000). The U.S. Food and Drug Administration (2004) recently approved percent-free PSA for early detection in men with PSAs between 4 and 10 ng/ml. The percentage of free PSA is significantly lower in men with prostate cancer than in those without. This test has gained widespread approval, specifically for men with normal DREs who have had prior biopsies because of PSAs within the "gray zone" or for men with contraindications to biopsy (NCCN, 2005c).

Routine PSA screening for men older than age 75 generally is not recommended because early detection is unlikely to affect survival in that age group (Lu-Yao, Stukel, & Yao, 2003; NCCN, 2005c; Raghavan & Skinner, 2004). Clinicians should discuss the benefits and limitations of testing to facilitate informed decision making (Smith, Cokkinides, et al., 2003; Smith et al., 2005). Screening considerations should include life expectancy, comorbidities, quality of life, and patient priorities (Silverman et al., 2000). Two multicenter randomized trials of prostate cancer screening are ongoing: the NCI PLCO cancer trial and the European Randomized Study of Screening for Prostate Cancer. The PLCO trial is designed to determine whether screening with DRE plus PSA can reduce prostate cancer mortality in men ages 55–74 at entry (Prorok et al., 2000). Results from these trials should be available between 2005 and 2008 (Smith, Cokkinides, et al., 2003).

The American Cancer Society (ACS) and AUA recommended offering PSA and DRE testing annually starting at age 50 for men with a life expectancy of at least 10 years and earlier screening for men at high risk (AUA, 2000; Smith et al., 2005). NCCN (2005c) recommended a baseline PSA at age 40, with regular screening beginning at 50 years of age. NCI (2005d), USPSTF (2002d), and the American College of Physicians concluded that insufficient evidence is available to recommend for or against routine prostate cancer screening with DRE or PSA (USPSTF, 2002d).

Colorectal Cancer

Screening for colorectal cancer is cost effective and reduces mortality mainly because of early detection of cancer (Silverman et al., 2000; USPSTF, 2002c). The evidence for mortality reduction is based on three randomized trials for FOBTs and case-control studies for endoscopic exams (Enzinger & Mayer, 2004). Medicare currently provides reimbursement for FOBT plus sigmoidoscopy or barium enema or colonoscopy. Despite the evidence of benefit, however, only a small percentage of people in the United States undergo routine screening (Centers for Disease Control and Prevention, 2001).

Screening options for colorectal cancer include FOBT, flexible sigmoidoscopy, FOBT plus sigmoidoscopy, colonoscopy, and double-contrast barium enema (DCBE). The combination of FOBT and flexible sigmoidoscopy may detect more cases of cancer than either test alone. DCBE may be an alternative test to sigmoidoscopy in low-risk people. However, the sensitivity of this screening method for detecting large polyps and cancer is less than with colonoscopy (Winawer et al., 2003), and other screening tests are preferred when feasible (NCCN, 2005a). Patients with any positive screening test should undergo a colonoscopy (Silverman et al., 2000; USPSTF, 2002c). Colonoscopy is the most sensitive and specific test for detecting cancer. Colonoscopy is especially beneficial in older adults because of their higher incidence of proximal neoplasms, which are not visualized on sigmoidoscopy exams (Enzinger & Mayer, 2004). However, complications such as small risks of bleeding and perforation and risks associated with conscious sedation should be considered in screening decisions for older adults. Healthcare professionals do not know the upper age limit to discontinue colorectal screening because most screening studies have included patients younger than 80 (USPSTF, 2002c). However, because the risk of colorectal cancer is highest in older adults, clinicians should not discontinue screening arbitrarily without consideration of life expectancy, comorbidities, and functional status (Enzinger & Mayer; Stevens & Burke, 2003).

Ongoing studies are assessing the benefits of endoscopy in reducing colorectal cancer mortality. The PLCO is a randomized, controlled community trial that assesses whether screening with flexible sigmoidoscopy can reduce mortality from colorectal cancer in adults ages 55–74. The screening arm received sigmoidoscopy at entry and at three years, whereas the control arm received usual medical care. The screening interval was extended to five years in 1996 for consistency with current practice (Schoen et al., 2003). Results of the PLCO and other trials will increase knowledge about the benefits of screening on mortality and other variables such as incidence, stage, and biologic and prognostic characteristics of tumor tissues (Prorok et al., 2000).

ACS recommended offering FOBT or fecal immunochemical test (FIT) annually, flexible sigmoidoscopy or DCBE every 5 years, annual FOBT or FIT plus flexible sigmoidoscopy every 5 years, or colonoscopy every 10 years beginning at age 50 (Smith et al., 2005). NCCN (2005a) recommended offering FOBT and flexible sigmoidoscopy every 5 years, colonoscopy every 10 years, or DCBE every 5 years. NCI (2005b) recommended FOBT annually or biennially and regular screening by sigmoidoscopy beginning at age 50 for people at average risk. Although insufficient evidence is available to determine the optimal interval for repeat screening, data support a 5-year interval for sigmoidoscopy and a 10-year interval for colonoscopy (NCI, 2002a). USPSTF (2002c) recommended offering periodic FOBT, flexible sigmoidoscopy every 5 years, FOBT and flexible sigmoidoscopy every 5 years, colonoscopy every 10 years, or DCBE every 5 years starting at age 50. The American Gastroenterological Association (Winawer et al., 2003) recommended yearly FOBT or immunochemical test beginning at age 50, flexible sigmoidoscopy every 5 years, FOBT and sigmoidoscopy every 5 years, colonoscopy every 10 years, or DCBE every 5 years. ACS and other groups recommend more intensive surveillance for high-risk groups, such as people with a history of adenomatous polyps, colorectal cancer, or significant irritable bowel disease; a family history of colorectal cancer or adenomas in a first-degree relative before age 60; or the possibility of hereditary syndromes (Smith et al., 2005). However, the majority of hereditary syndromes, such as familial adenomatous polyposis and hereditary nonpolyposis colorectal cancer, is diagnosed before age 65 (Enzinger & Mayer, 2004). Clinicians should consider colonoscopy for people at increased risk because of a prior history of colorectal cancer, adenomatous polyps, or predisposing conditions, such as inflammatory bowel disease (Winawer et al.). For further information about screening for high-risk groups, see NCCN (2005a).

With regard to future trends, immunochemical FOBT techniques appear promising (Levin, Brooks, Smith, & Stone, 2003; NCCN, 2005a). Experts suggest that these techniques have advantages over guaiac-based testing in terms of improved specificity (Levin et al.). For example, the new tests will not react with vitamins, nonsteroidal anti-inflammatory drugs, or food sources. Large-scale investigations currently are under way in usual screening populations. Other new techniques under investigation include CT colonoscopy and molecular techniques for detecting DNA abnormalities in the stool (Levin et al.; NCCN, 2005a; Osborn & Ahlquist, 2005).

Lung Cancer

Lung cancer is the leading cause of cancer-related mortality in both men and women (Jemal et al., 2005), and most patients present with advanced disease (Bach, Niewoehner, Black, & American College of Chest Physicians, 2003). If lung cancer could be detected early through screening measures using new technology, many deaths could be prevented each year (Ford et al., 2003). Although chest x-rays and spiral CT scans have been used in the clinical setting to detect lung cancers in asymptomatic people, the evidence is inconclusive as to whether screening with either method will reduce lung cancer mortality (Ford et al.). Trials of chest x-ray screening have some limitations, and three randomized controlled trials did not show a mortality benefit (Bach et al.). However, the ongoing PLCO trial will obtain further data on the benefits of serial chest x-ray screening, which is designed to detect the effects of screening on lung cancer mortality. In this trial, smokers undergo a baseline chest x-ray at entry and an annual chest x-ray for three years, whereas nonsmokers undergo only two repeat annual chest x-rays.

The use of low-dose spiral computerized tomography (LDCT) is a focus of current research for the early detection of lung cancer. The LDCT obtains an image of the entire thorax using low-dose radiation. This technology is very sensitive in detecting small nodules and assessing growth patterns prior to invasive diagnostic tests (Bach et al., 2003). Observational studies suggest that LDCT detects more cancers and noncancerous nodules than chest x-ray, and the majority of cancers are detected at stage I. However, concerns exist about the high rate of false-positive results with LDCT and overdiagnosis that may result in unnecessary treatment (Bach et al.; Ford et al., 2003). Despite this concern, Henschke et al. (2001) found that false-positive screening tests in high-risk people were uncommon and usually manageable without biopsy based on diagnostic workups guided by the Early Lung Cancer Action Project's recommendations. Observational studies also suggested that serial LDCT may lessen the number of invasive procedures needed for people with an abnormal finding that is not cancer (Bach et al.). More definitive results will be available in the future based on ongoing observational and randomized studies.

The ongoing randomized National Lung Cancer Screening Trial compares LDCT and chest x-ray screening for detection of early lung cancer in current and former smokers (Ford et al., 2003). This trial seeks to evaluate risks and benefits of both tests and to compare mortality reduction. Several PLCO and American College of Radiology Imaging Network sites are conducting the trial, which should be complete in 2009. Some of these sites also are collecting specimens of tissue, blood, urine, and sputum for a repository for other studies evaluating biologic and genetic markers of lung cancer (Ford et al.). These and other ongoing trials should provide more definitive results to guide organizations issuing future screening guidelines (Smith, Cokkinides, & Eyre, 2004).

Based upon the current knowledge regarding lung cancer screening and the lack of evidence suggesting a decrease in lung cancer mortality, ACS, NCI, NCCN, and USPSTF do not recommend screening in asymptomatic people (Humphrey, Teutsch, Johnson, & USPSTF, 2004; Smith et al., 2005). For people without symptoms or history of cancer, the American College of Chest Physicians recommends against screening for lung cancer (Bach et al., 2003). However, screening should be considered on an individual basis for patients who are at high risk because of tobacco or occupational exposures. Further, people who wish to be tested should be informed of ongoing clinical studies using LDCT screening (Bach et al.) as well as the risks, benefits, and limitations of testing. Testing should occur at experienced centers linked to specialty groups for continuity of care (Smith et al., 2005). Findings from ongoing clinical trials will enhance the current evidence and provide more information regarding lung cancer screening technologies and mortality reduction.

Clinical Practice Implications

Screening decisions for the older adult should consider factors such as life expectancy, comorbidities, quality of life, risks/benefits, and patient preferences (Silverman et al., 2000; Walter & Covinsky, 2001). As a result of ongoing contact with patients, nurses are in a key role to perform a comprehensive geriatric assessment that will help to assess functional status, comorbidities, and other factors that impact screening decisions. Nurses also should be aware of current screening guidelines and keep abreast of new screening recommendations to provide patient education. In addition to patient education regarding screening recommendations, nurses should encourage prevention measures to reduce cancer risk, including smoking cessation and education about a healthy lifestyle such as diet and exercise.

Research Implications

Behavioral research addressing preventive behaviors and adherence to screening guidelines is needed, especially in at-risk older adult populations (Champion et al., 2002). Priorities include research to improve colorectal screening rates targeting older adults because this group has the highest risk of colorectal cancer. Testing interventions found to be successful in mammography screening may be useful in research focused on colorectal screening adherence (Champion et al.). Yarbrough (2004) discussed the need for further research targeting older women with breast cancer to describe the risks and benefits of screening, including research evaluating relationships among factors such as comorbidities, ability to tolerate screening or treatment, and the impact of screening or treatment on quality of life and mortality. Such research is needed before definitive public health recommendations can be made regarding screening in older women. Other priorities include research to address barriers to cancer screening such as patient, caregiver, and provider attitudes and strategies to increase access to screening services, especially in vulnerable and underserved populations. The National Institute of Nursing Research (2003) identified future research priorities, including the need for culturally sensitive interventions to reduce health disparities in access to care and incidence of disease in ethnic groups, the older adult, and other vulnerable populations. Interventions at the community level and research focusing on motivators for behavioral change are needed.

Healthcare providers should encourage older adults to participate in screening when appropriate, including discussion of benefits, risks, limitations of testing, and patient preferences. Healthcare providers also should encourage older adults to participate in clinical trials when eligible and should address barriers to screening to facilitate participation. In the future, the upper age limit for screening trials should be carefully considered because life expectancy is increasing, and many screening trials have not included patients older than 75. For example, approximately 25% of 75-year-old women will live more than 17 years, and 50% will live at least 11.9 years (Walter & Covinsky, 2001). Therefore, to set an arbitrary upper age limit for screening decisions or for participation in screening trials will unnecessarily exclude many older adults who are most likely to benefit from screening for certain cancers. Mandelblatt et al. (2000) addressed the question of whether an upper age limit should be set for breast cancer screening by using a framework that models the effects of physiologic rather than chronologic age on screening decisions. This approach considers broad questions that may be applicable for making public health decisions about breast cancer screening in older populations. For example, Mandelblatt et al. (2000) considered factors that may impact screening decisions, such as (a) whether a threshold exists where screening will not be beneficial (cost effectiveness), (b) whether estimating the probability of developing an aggressive versus an indolent tumor in a given population will change screening decisions or intervals (tumor characteristics), (c) whether cost-effective alternatives exist to mammography (e.g., CBEs by nurses), and (d) the boundaries of society's preferences for health for a given life expectancy (societal values). This framework may be applicable for decision making with regard to other types of common cancers in the older adult.

Conclusion

Various factors will have a direct impact on cancer screening considerations in research and clinical practice. The increased incidence of cancer in the older adult, the increase in life expectancy, and the projected increase in the number of individuals living past 65 years of age support the need for prioritizing research targeting older adults. Screening decisions should be individualized considering the expected benefits and burdens of screening while considering patients' values and preferences in decision making. Future research exploring cancer screening in the older adult will facilitate an evidence-based approach to cancer screening guidelines and clinical practice for this population.

The author acknowledges Diane G. Cope, PhD, ARNP, BC, AOCNP, for her thoughtful contributions to this chapter.

References

American College of Obstetricians and Gynecologists. (2003). *Breast cancer screening.* Retrieved May 6, 2005, from http://www.guideline.gov/summary/summary.aspx?doc_id=3990&nbr=3129&string=#s23

American Geriatrics Society. (1999). *Breast cancer screening in older women.* Retrieved October 13, 2004, from http://www.americangeriatrics.org/products/positionpapers/brstcncrPF.shtml

American Geriatrics Society. (2001). *Health screening decisions for older adults.* Retrieved October 15, 2004, from http://www.americangeriatrics.org/products/positionpapers/stopscreening.shtml

American Urological Association. (2000). *Prostate-specific antigen (PSA) best practice policy.* Retrieved November 2, 2004, from http://www.cancernetwork.com/journals/oncology/o0002e.htm

Bach, P.B., Niewoehner, D.E., Black, W.C., & American College of Chest Physicians. (2003). Screening for lung cancer: The guidelines. *Chest, 123*(Suppl. 1), 83S–88S.

Balducci, L., & Extermann, M. (2000). Cancer and aging. An evolving panorama. *Hematology/Oncology Clinics of North America, 14*(1), 1–16.

Barnes, M.N., Grizzle, W.E., Grubbs, C.J., & Partridge, E.E. (2002). Paradigms for primary prevention of ovarian cancer. *CA: A Cancer Journal for Clinicians, 52,* 216–225.

Centers for Disease Control and Prevention. (2001). Trends in screening for colorectal cancer—The United States, 1997 and 1999. *Morbidity and Mortality Weekly Report, 50,* 162–166.

Champion, V.L., Rawl, S.M., & Menon, U. (2002). Population-based cancer screening. *Oncology Nursing Forum, 29,* 853–861.

Costanza, M.E. (1992). Breast cancer screening in older women: Synopsis of a forum. *Cancer, 69*(Suppl. 7), 1925–1931.

De Koning, H.J., Auvinen, A., Berenguer Sanchez, A., Calais da Silva, F., Ciatto, S., Denis, L., et al. (2002). Large-scale randomized prostate cancer screening trials: Program performances in the European Randomised Screening for Prostate Cancer Trial and the Prostate, Lung, Colorectal and Ovary Cancer Trial. *International Journal of Cancer, 97,* 237–244.

Enzinger, P.C., & Mayer, R.J. (2004). Gastrointestinal cancer in older patients. *Seminars in Oncology, 31,* 206–219.

Ferrini, R. (1997). Screening asymptomatic women for ovarian cancer: American College of Preventive Medicine Practice Policy Statement. *American Journal of Preventive Medicine, 13,* 444–446.

Ford, L.G., Minasian, L.M., McCaskill-Stevens, W., Pisano, E.D., Sullivan, D., & Smith, R.A. (2003). Prevention and early detection clinical trials: Opportunities for primary care providers and their patients. *CA: A Cancer Journal for Clinicians, 53,* 82–101.

Gambert, S.R. (2001). Prostate cancer: When to offer screening in the primary care setting. *Geriatrics, 56*(1), 22–31.

Heflin, M.T., & Cohen, H.J. (2001). Cancer screening in the elderly. *Hospital Practice, 36,* 61–69.

Henschke, C.I., Naidich, D.P., Yankelevitz, D.F., McGuinness, G., McCauley, D.I., Smith, J.P., et al. (2001). Early lung cancer action project. *Cancer, 92,* 153–159.

Humphrey, L.L., Helfand, M., Chan, B.K.S., & Woolf, S.H. (2002). Breast cancer screening: A summary of the evidence for the U.S. Preventive Services Task Force. *Annals of Internal Medicine, 137,* 347–360.

Humphrey, L.L., Teutsch, S., Johnson, M., & U.S. Preventive Services Task Force. (2004). Lung cancer screening with sputum cytology examination, chest radiography, and computed tomography. *Annals of Internal Medicine, 140,* 740–753.

Iannuzzi-Sucich, M., & Kenny, A.M. (2004). Preventive medicine for older women: Gynecologic screening guidelines. *Family Practice Recertification, 26,* 53–59.

Jacobs, I.J., & Menon, U. (2004). Progress and challenges in screening for early detection of ovarian cancer. *Molecular and Cellular Proteomics, 3,* 355–366.

Jemal, A., Murray, T., Ward, E., Samuels, A., Tiwari, R., Ghafoor, A., et al. (2005). Cancer statistics, 2005. *CA: A Cancer Journal for Clinicians, 55,* 10–30.

Karlan, B.Y., Markman, M.A., & Eifel, P.J. (2005). Ovarian cancer, peritoneal carcinoma, and fallopian tube carcinoma. In V. DeVita, S. Hellman, & S. Rosenberg (Eds.), *Cancer: Principles and practice of oncology* (7th ed., pp. 1364–1397). Philadelphia: Lippincott Williams & Wilkins.

Kimmick, G.G., & Balducci, L. (2000). Breast cancer and aging. *Hematology/Oncology Clinics of North America, 14,* 213–234.

Kimmick, G.G., & Muss, H.B. (2000). Breast cancer in older women. In J. Harris, M. Lippman, M. Morrow, & C. Osborne (Eds.), *Diseases of the breast* (pp. 945–954). Philadelphia: Lippincott Williams & Wilkins.

Levin, B., Brooks, D., Smith, R.A., & Stone, A. (2003). Emerging technologies in screening for colorectal cancer. CT colonography, immunochemical fecal occult blood tests, and stool screening using molecular markers. *CA: A Cancer Journal for Clinicians, 53,* 44–55.

Lu-Yao, G., Stukel, T.A., & Yao, S.L. (2003). Prostate-specific antigen screening in elderly men. *Journal of the National Cancer Institute, 95,* 1792–1797.

Mandelblatt, J.S. (1992). Breast cancer screening for elderly women with and without comorbid conditions. *Annals of Internal Medicine, 116,* 722–730.

Mandelblatt, J., Saha, S., Teutsch, S., Hoerger, T., Siu, A.L., Atkins, D., et al. (2003). *The cost-effectiveness of screening mammography beyond age 65: A systematic review for the U.S. Preventive Services Task Force.* Retrieved May 2, 2005, from http://www.ahrq.gov/clinic/3rduspstf/breastcancer/brcancost.pdf

Mandelblatt, J., Yabroff, K.R., Lawrence, W., Yi, B., Orosz, G., Bloom, H.G., et al. (2000). Screening mammography in elderly women [Letter to editor]. *JAMA, 283,* 3202–3203.

Menon, U. (2004). Ovarian cancer screening. *Canadian Medical Association Journal, 171,* 323–324.

National Cancer Institute. (2002a). *National Cancer Institute trial yields new data on colon cancer screening test.* Retrieved May 6, 2005, from http://www.cancer.gov/newscenter/pressreleases/PLCO

National Cancer Institute. (2002b). *NCI statement on mammography screening.* Retrieved May 6, 2005, from http://www.cancer.gov/newscenter/mammstatement31jan02

National Cancer Institute. (2003). *Randomized screening study of CA 125 and ultrasound in the detection of ovarian cancer in postmenopausal women.* Retrieved November 27, 2004, from http://www.cancer.gov/clinicaltrials/UKCTOCS

National Cancer Institute. (2004a). *Randomized screening study of fecal occult blood testing and multitarget DNA-based assay panel testing followed by colonoscopy in the detection of colorectal cancer.* Retrieved April 13, 2005, from http://www.cancer.gov/search/ViewClinicalTrials.?cdrid=68783&protocolsearch id=1289455&version=healthprofessional

National Cancer Institute. (2004b). *Study of computed tomographic colonography for screening healthy participants for colorectal cancer.* Retrieved April 13, 2005, from http://www.cancer.gov/search/ViewClinicalTrials.aspx?cdrid=367101&protocolsearchid=1291650&version=healthprofessional #StudyIdInfo_CDR0000367101

National Cancer Institute. (2005a). *Breast cancer (PDQ®): Screening.* Retrieved May 6, 2005, from http://www.cancer.gov/cancertopics/pdq/screening/breast/healthprofessional

National Cancer Institute. (2005b). *Colorectal cancer (PDQ®): Screening.* Retrieved May 6, 2005, from http://www.cancer.gov/cancertopics/pdq/screening/colorectal/healthprofessional

National Cancer Institute. (2005c). *Ovarian cancer (PDQ®): Screening.* Retrieved April 26, 2005, from http://www.nci.nih.gov/cancertopics/pdq/screening/ovarian/healthprofessional

National Cancer Institute. (2005d). *Prostate cancer (PDQ®): Screening.* Retrieved May 6, 2005, from http://www.cancer.gov/cancertopics/pdq/screening/prostate/healthprofessional

National Comprehensive Cancer Network. (2004). *Breast cancer screening and diagnosis guidelines.* Retrieved November 2, 2004, from http://www.nccn.org/professionals/physician_gls/PDF/breast-screening.pdf

National Comprehensive Cancer Network. (2005a). *Colorectal screening.* Retrieved November 2, 2004, from http://www.nccn.org/professionals/physician_gls/PDF/colorectal_screening.pdf

National Comprehensive Cancer Network. (2005b). *Genetic/familial high-risk assessment: Breast and ovarian.* Retrieved April 26, 2005, from http://www.nccn.org/professionals/physician_gls/PDF/genetics_screening.pdf

National Comprehensive Cancer Network. (2005c). *Prostate cancer early detection.* Retrieved May 6, 2005, from http://www.nccn.org/professionals/physician_gls/PDF/prostate_detection.pdf

National Institute of Nursing Research. (2003). *Mission statement.* Retrieved November 28, 2004, from http://ninr.nih.gov/ninr/research/themes.doc

National Institutes of Health. (1995). Consensus development panel on ovarian cancer. Ovarian cancer screening, treatment, and follow-up. *JAMA, 273,* 491–497.

O'Rourke, J., & Mahon, S.M. (2003). A comprehensive look at the early detection of ovarian cancer. *Clinical Journal of Oncology Nursing, 7,* 41–47.

Osborn, N.K., & Ahlquist, D.A. (2005). Stool screening for colorectal cancer: Molecular approaches. *Gastroenterology, 128,* 192–206.

Peek, M.E. (2003). Screening mammography in the elderly: A review of the issues. *Journal of the American Medical Women's Association, 58,* 191–198.

Prorok, P.C., Andriole, G.L., Bresalier, R.S., Buys, S.S., Chia, D., Crawford, E.D., et al. (2000). Design of the Prostate, Lung, Colorectal and Ovarian (PLCO) cancer screening trial. *Controlled Clinical Trials, 21*(Suppl. 6), 273S–309S.

Raghavan, D., & Skinner, E. (2004). Genitourinary cancer in the elderly. *Seminars in Oncology, 31,* 249–263.

Rimer, B.K., Schildkraut, J.M., & Hiatt, R.A. (2005). Cancer screening. In V. DeVita, S. Hellman, & S. Rosenberg (Eds.), *Cancer: Principles and practice of oncology* (7th ed., pp. 567–579). Philadelphia: Lippincott Williams & Wilkins.

Satariano, W.A., & Ragland, D.R. (1994). The effect of comorbidity on 3-year survival of women with primary breast cancer. *Annals of Internal Medicine, 120,* 104–110.

Saunders, C.S. (2001). Cancer screening in older patients. *Patient Care for the Nurse Practitioner, 4*(11), 41–45.

Schoen, R.E., Pinsky, P.F., Weissfeld, J.L., Bresalier, R.S., Church, T., Prorok, P., et al. (2003). Results of repeat sigmoidoscopy 3 years after a negative examination. *JAMA, 290,* 41–48.

Silverman, M.A., Zaidi, U., Barnett, S., Robles, C., Khruana, V., Manten, H., et al. (2000). Cancer screening in the elderly population. *Hematology/Oncology Clinics of North America, 14,* 89–112.

Smith, R.A., Cokkinides, V., & Eyre, H.J. (2003). American Cancer Society guidelines for the early detection of cancer, 2003. *CA: A Cancer Journal for Clinicians, 53,* 27–43.

Smith, R.A., Cokkinides, V., & Eyre, H.J. (2004). American Cancer Society guidelines for the early detection of cancer, 2004. *CA: A Cancer Journal for Clinicians, 54,* 41–52.

Smith, R.A., Cokkinides, V., & Eyre, H.J. (2005). American Cancer Society guidelines for the early detection of cancer, 2005. *CA: A Cancer Journal for Clinicians, 55,* 31–44.

Smith, R.A., Saslow, D., Andrews Sawyer, K., Burke, W., Costanza, M.E., Evans, W.P., et al. (2003). American Cancer Society guidelines for breast cancer screening: Update 2003. *CA: A Cancer Journal for Clinicians, 53,* 141–169.

Stevens, T., & Burke, C.A. (2003). Colonoscopy screening in the elderly: When to stop? *American Journal of Gastroenterology, 98,* 1881–1885.

United Kingdom Collaborative Trial of Ovarian Cancer Screening. (2004). *GP information sheet.* Retrieved May 18, 2005, from http://www.ukctocs.org.uk/stats.htm

U.S. Food and Drug Administration. (2004). *AxSYM® Free PSA—P980007.* Retrieved April 26, 2005, from http://www.fda.gov/cdrh/pdf/p980007.html

U.S. Preventive Services Task Force. (2002a). *Screening for breast cancer.* Retrieved May 6, 2005, from http://www.ahrq.gov/clinic/3rduspstf/breastcancer/

U.S. Preventive Services Task Force. (2002b). Screening for breast cancer: Recommendations and rationale. *Annals of Internal Medicine, 137,* 344–346.

U.S. Preventive Services Task Force. (2002c). Screening for colorectal cancer: Recommendations and rationale. *Annals of Internal Medicine, 137,* 129–131.

U.S. Preventive Services Task Force. (2002d). *Screening for prostate cancer.* Retrieved May 6, 2005, from http://www.ahrq.gov/clinic/uspstf/uspsprca.htm

U.S. Preventive Services Task Force. (2004). *Screening for ovarian cancer.* Retrieved April 26, 2005, from http://www.ahrq.gov/clinic/uspstf/uspsovar.htm

Walter, L.C., & Covinsky, K.E. (2001). Cancer screening in elderly patients: A framework for individualized decision making. *JAMA, 285,* 2750–2756.

Winawer, S., Fletcher, R., Rex, D., Bond, J., Burt, R., Ferrucci, J., et al. (2003). Colorectal cancer screening and surveillance: Clinical guidelines and rationale—Update based on new evidence. *Gastroenterology, 124,* 544–560.

Yarbrough, S.S. (2004). Older women and breast cancer screening: Research synthesis [Online exclusive]. *Oncology Nursing Forum, 31,* E9–E15. Retrieved December 22, 2004, from http://journals.ons.org/ONF/2004/january/42.pdf

CHAPTER 6

Pharmacologic Issues

Rowena N. Schwartz, PharmD, BCOP

Introduction

As the population of the United States ages, interest increases in all issues associated with health care of the older adult. One of the most challenging healthcare issues to assess, predict, and manage in an older patient is the impact of aging on the use of medications. Older adults are the largest users of drugs, incurring 30% of total drug costs in the United States (Morris, Grossman, Barkdoll, Gordon, & Chun, 1987). A number of reviews described the potential pharmacologic changes of common anticancer agents in older adults (John, Mashru, & Lichtman, 2003; Lichtman, 2004; Lichtman, Skirvin, & Vemulapalli, 2003; Wildeiers, Highley, de Bruijn, & van Oosterom, 2003), but only recently has there been systematic evaluation of the pharmacokinetic and pharmacodynamic effects of single agents in the older adult with cancer. The use of combination chemotherapy regimens in the older adult with cancer, as well as other medications used in the management of cancer, is an area of increasing interest for oncology practitioners and clinical investigators. This chapter will review the aspects of drug therapy that should be considered for older patients with cancer, including the impact of aging on the pharmacokinetics and pharmacodynamics of drug therapy, issues with drug adherence, drug interactions, and adverse drug reactions in older patients with cancer. Healthcare practitioners should evaluate drug therapies for individual patients with these concepts in mind until more specific recommendations can be made for specific therapies through clinical trials.

Pharmacokinetics

Absorption

After the administration of most drugs, absorption of the medication into the blood stream often is required for pharmacologic effect. The absorption of oral medications may occur at different sites in the gastrointestinal tract. Therefore, the physiologic changes in the digestive system associated with aging may affect drug absorption after oral administration. Similarly, physiologic changes in the skin and/or fat that occur with aging may impact drug absorption after administration of certain medications applied to the skin (e.g., transdermal administration).

Absorption of a medication in the gastrointestinal tract requires a number of steps: disintegration and dissolution, absorption of the drug through the gut wall, gut wall metabolism for select products, and hepatic metabolism. These processes can be modified by the physiologic changes of aging and can impact the drug absorption process. These changes are listed in Figure 6-1. The overall surface of the intestinal epithelium decreases with age, which decreases the area for absorption of some medications. The age-related decrease in gastric motility may decrease absorption of some medications or increase absorption of other medications. The age-related decrease in the secretion of digestive enzymes and the decrease in gastric acid secretion may result in the decreased absorption of medications. The decrease in gastrointestinal blood flow (including splanchnic blood flow) seen in older individuals may also decrease absorption of some agents (Turnheim, 2003).

- Decrease in surface of intestinal epithelium
- Decrease in gastric motility
- Decrease in secretion of digestive enzymes
- Decrease in gastric acid secretion
- Decrease in gastrointestinal blood flow

Figure 6-1. Aging and Gastrointestinal Changes

The clinical impact of these changes associated with aging for patients with cancer should be considered for all medications used to treat cancer, manage cancer-related complications, and manage chronic and acute medical problems. For example, drugs that require an acid environment (e.g., ketoconazole used to manage fungal infections) may have decreased absorption in the older adult because of the age-related decrease in gastric acid secretion. Clinically, this could result in an inadequate concentration of these medications and, ultimately, decreased efficacy of the drug.

A practical concern with the absorption of drugs in the older adult is the impact of nutrition and drug absorption. Some drugs, such as capecitabine (Xeloda®, Roche Pharmaceuticals, Nutley, NJ), have decreased absorption with food. If an individual does not eat with each dose, an increase in the peak concentration of the drug and in exposure of the drug (or area under the curve) occurs, potentially leading to increased toxicity. Healthcare professionals should provide clear instructions to patients about oral administration of chemotherapy in relation to food.

As individuals age, changes in the skin occur, including a thinning of skin and an increase in subcutaneous fat. These changes may have significant consequences on the absorption of medications from the skin. Medications that are applied topically may be absorbed at a different rate or to a different extent in an older adult with these dermatologic changes.

When assessing the impact of physiologic changes of absorption that occur with aging, nurses should consider the potential physiologic changes at the site of absorption that may occur as an effect of cancer and/or cancer treatments. For example, chemotherapy-induced mucositis may significantly change the oral mucous membrane and increase absorption of certain oral medications. Nurses should assess individual patients for both age-related changes and other contributing changes at the site for drug absorption for all administered medications. The impact of the changes in absorption should be monitored to determine the real clinical significance of these changes on drug therapy outcomes.

Distribution

The volume of distribution (Vd) of a medication is the pharmacokinetic term that describes the degree that a drug partitions between body tissues and blood. The plasma concentration of a drug is inversely related to its Vd. Various factors influence the Vd of drugs, such as the binding of drugs to red blood cells and plasma proteins such as albumin, body composition (e.g., body fat), and fluid status. As individuals become older, age-related changes exist in most of these factors. Lean body mass, including skeletal muscle mass, declines with age. Total body water content declines with age, and total body fat increases with age. These changes in body composition impact how medications are distributed throughout the body.

As individuals age, they generally experience a decline in plasma proteins. Drugs that are highly protein bound, such as phenytoin (Dilantin®, Parke-Davis, New York, NY), will be less bound to proteins in an older adult who has decreased plasma protein. When a lesser amount of drug is bound to these plasma proteins, more drug is unbound and available to bind to receptors. Clinically, an increase in this unbound (or free) phenytoin means that higher levels of the active drug exist in the body. The total phenytoin level measured in the blood includes both bound (inactive) and unbound (active) phenytoin; the total phenytoin may appear to be within what is considered "normal" serum concentrations, even though more of the drug is free or active. Older adults with a decrease in albumin may have higher levels of unbound (active) phenytoin that can manifest as toxicities (e.g., nystagmus, ataxia, changes in mental status), even when their serum level is within or below the usual therapeutic range. In addition, if an older adult has cancer-related anorexia or cachexia, a greater than expected decline in plasma proteins may exist with age-related changes. Healthcare professionals should evaluate the patient's serum albumin plasma proteins in addition to the phenytoin level. They also should monitor the patient for clinical signs of phenytoin toxicity, even when the total phenytoin level appears normal.

Another example of the impact of changes in plasma protein on the pharmacologic effect of a chemotherapy drug is seen with ifosfamide (Ifex®, Bristol-Myers Squibb, Princeton, NJ). Hypoalbuminemia leads to an increased peak concentration of the active drug. This has been associated with an increased incidence of the neurotoxicity (encephalopathy) of the drug (Meanwell, Blake, & Kelly, 1986). In older patients with decreased plasma proteins, nurses should consider the potential of this change on the pharmacokinetics and pharmacology of ifosfamide and consider modification of treatment strategies based on assessment of patient-specific factors (e.g., lower doses infused over a longer time to decrease the peak concentration of the drug).

As individuals age, the amount of red blood cells present in their blood decreases. The Vd of drugs that are highly bound to red blood cells, such as taxanes (e.g., paclitaxel, [Taxol®, Bristol-Myers Squibb]), may be changed in patients with anemia related to age, cancer treatment, and/or cancer. The correction of anemia with blood and/or an erythropoietin product may change the Vd of these medications.

Older adults have an increase in body fat and a decrease of intracellular water. An increase in body fat results in an increase in the distribution of fat-soluble drugs (e.g., diazepam [Valium®, Roche Pharmaceuticals]). In older adults, an increase in body fat may cause a decrease in elimination of diazepam and result in a more prolonged effect of the drug. Total body fat increases to a greater extent in men than women, although women usually have a higher body fat percentage than men. Because the relative increase in fat content is greater in men, the volume of distribution of fat-soluble drugs may be more marked in men. These increases in body fat seen with aging may not persist in older individuals. The proportion of fat decreases in the frail older adult, and the Vd for lipophilic drugs also may decrease. Dosing of medications for the frail older adult should be considered in light of the individual's actual weight and assessment of body fat.

The decrease in total body water seen in older adults may result in a decrease in the expected volume of distribution of water-soluble drugs. Aminoglycoside antibiotics (e.g., tobramycin) are an example of water-soluble drugs. The clinical impact of the decrease in Vd for tobramycin is that an average dose may result in a higher plasma concentration and a higher incidence of toxicities such as ototoxicity. Again, evaluation of the fluid status of the older adult is important when determining appropriate dosing of water-soluble drugs.

Metabolism

Metabolism, the metabolic breakdown of a drug, occurs in a number of organs and tissues of the body (e.g., skin, liver, blood). The liver is one of the most common sites of drug metabolism. Age-related changes in the liver include a decrease in liver mass, hepatic enzyme activity, and hepatic blood flow. These changes result in an overall decrease in metabolic capacity of the liver in the older population. The impact of drug-induced changes in the liver is seen in the older population, who may be taking multiple drugs. Changes in the liver in older individuals may result in a change in both the rate and extent of metabolism of a medication to an inactive metabolite (e.g., longer exposure to an active drug results in an increase in therapeutic and adverse effects). Conversely, drugs that are converted to an active form in the liver may not be converted to the active form as quickly or as completely and, therefore, have a delayed onset of action and/or decrease in action.

Metabolism of medications in the liver occurs via phase I and II mechanisms. Phase I metabolism is the hydroxylation, epoxidation, and demethylation of substances via the cytochrome (CYP) P450 microsomal enzyme system. This system consists of a number of isoenzymes that appear to change with aging. The CYP P450 system constitutes a superfamily of heme proteins that are responsible for the biotransformation of substances, including medications. The human drug-metabolizing CYPs are concentrated in the smooth endoplasmic reticulum of liver hepatocytes, although lower levels of expression exist in the intestine, lungs, kidneys, and brain. The multiple CYP enzymes are classified into families, subfamilies, and isoforms. The major human drug-metabolizing CYPs belong to families 1, 2, and 3 with specific isoforms 1A1, 1A2, 2A6, 2B6, 2C8, 2C9, 2C19, 2D6, 2E1, 3A4, 2A5, 3A7. These enzymes are estimated to account for the biotransformation of approximately 60% of the commonly prescribed drugs in the United States (Venkatakrishnan, von Moltke, & Greenblatt, 2001).

In addition to age, other factors appear to impact the ability of the CYP P450 enzyme system to metabolize drugs in older adults. Genetic factors largely influence intersubject variability in metabolism, but environmental factors such as smoking, diet, and medications also may influence CYP enzyme activity (van der Weide & Steijns, 1999).

The impact of CYP P450 genetic polymorphisms on anticancer therapy has been recognized. The narrow therapeutic window between cancer drug therapeutic effect and drug toxicity means that interindividual variation in drug metabolism, because of individual variation in the CYP P450 enzymes, may complicate therapy among patients.

The potential of pharmacogenetic screening of an individual prior to treatment with cancer agents that are metabolized via the CYP P450 system has been suggested as a strategy to determine appropriate dosing modification(s) based on genetics (van Schaik, 2004). As the science and practicality of such strategies are evaluated in the general population, older adults may be of particular interest because of the multiple factors that may impact changes in drug metabolism in this population at risk for adverse drug reactions.

An increase or decrease in the synthesis of CYP protein may occur in the liver after exposure to select drugs or chemicals. Chemicals that may influence the synthesis of CYP proteins include nutritional supplements, herbs, and environmental exposures.

Induction of a CYP enzyme increases the rate of biotransformation of drugs metabolized by that protein and results in a decrease in the parent drug. Again, if a parent drug is biotransformed to an active agent via a CYP protein, the induction of the CYP protein may increase the amount of active drug in a patient. If a parent drug is metabolized to an inactive agent via a CYP protein, the induction of the CYP protein may increase the inactivation of the active parent drug.

Inhibition of a CYP enzyme decreases the rate of biotransformation of drugs metabolized by that protein and results in a prolonged exposure to the parent drug. If a parent drug is biotransformed to an active agent via a CYP protein, the inhibition of the CYP protein may decrease the amount of active drug in a patient. If a parent drug is metabolized to an inactive agent via a CYP protein, the inhibition of the CYP protein can result in the increase of the active drug in a patient.

Older adults often are taking multiple medications and are at an increased risk for one drug or substance interacting with the activation and/or inactivation of other drugs. These effects may result in a decrease in an active drug, an increase in a toxic substance, a shortened effect from medication, and/or a prolonged effect from medication.

The challenge of managing drug interactions in a patient is complex, as a single drug may have different effects on CYP enzymes. Drugs or substances may inhibit one or more of these isoforms, induce one or more of these isoforms, and/or be a substrate for one or more of these isoforms. A single drug may have different effects on a number of isoforms and therefore have different effects on the metabolism of different drugs. An example is aprepitant (Emend®, Merck & Co., West Point, PA), an antiemetic used for acute and delayed chemotherapy-induced nausea and vomiting. Aprepitant is a substrate, a moderate inhibitor, and an inducer of CYP3A4. Additionally, aprepitant is an inducer of CYP2C9. As an inhibitor of CYP3A4, aprepitant can increase plasma concentrations of medications that are metabolized through CYP3A4. As an inducer of CYP2C9, aprepitant can induce the metabolism of drugs that are metabolized through CYP2C9, such as warfarin. Because aprepitant usually is administered for a short course with chemotherapy (e.g., three days each month), these interactions with coadministered drugs change over the course of a month. Healthcare professionals should assess the impact of aprepitant on other medications prior to initiation of the medication and also assess the clinical impact of the drug during the course of therapy and after aprepitant is discontinued (Shadle et al., 2004).

Nutrition and/or diet may influence CYP enzyme activity. In the frail older adult, drug metabolism is decreased to a greater extent than in the older adult with normal body weight (Turnheim, 2003). An increasing interest exists in determining the cause(s) of this change in drug metabolism in the undernourished individual.

Researchers studied the impact of diet and nutrition on the metabolic rate of one isoform (CYP1A2) in the older adult in a small group of patients who were older than 80 years of age. The nutritional status of older patients did not appear to influence CYP1A2 activity (Hamon-Vilcot et al., 2004).

Phase II metabolism in the liver includes conjugation reactions that usually are unchanged in relation to age. It appears that the activities of glutathione transferase and glucuronyltransferase are not changed in the older adult.

The complexity of drug effects on the ability of the liver to metabolize drugs is of importance in older adults who often are taking multiple medications for both chronic and acute medical problems. The complexity of drug effects on the metabolism of chemotherapy, hormone, and biotherapy used in the management and treatment of cancer is also of significant interest in the older adult with cancer, as the potential of increasing or decreasing the therapeutic and toxic effects of the cancer therapy is of concern. Evaluation and ongoing monitoring of drug therapy with the initiation, change, or discontinuation of medication(s) is important.

Elimination

The therapeutic and adverse effects of a drug are related to the level of that drug within the body. Clearance is the measure of fractional loss of drug per unit time. Clearance also is the amount of blood flow completely extracted of drug per unit time. The major sites of drug clearance are the liver and the kidney, although other sites such as the lungs and the gastrointestinal tract may contribute to the clearance of certain medications. Total body clearance is the sum of the drug clearances by all organs. After drug distribution, the half-life of a drug is the time it takes for the drug concentration in plasma to decrease by 50% (Rowland & Tozer, 1995).

Many medications are eliminated from the body secondary to renal excretion. As individuals age, a number of changes occur to impact renal elimination of drugs. These changes include reduction in renal blood flow, decrease in renal tubular clearance, and reduction in creatinine clearance. Renal blood flow delivers medications and/or their metabolites to the kidney. Renal blood flow is reduced by approximately 1% per year after 50 years of age (Rowe, Andres, Tobin, Norris, & Shock, 1976) and may decrease the excretion of medications from the kidneys.

Changes in the kidney with age results in a decrease in renal clearance. Reduction in renal clearance often is measured clinically via creatinine clearance. Unfortunately, the true decline in creatinine clearance is difficult to estimate in certain populations, including the older adult. Most formulas used in clinical practice to estimate the creatinine clearance in a patient incorporate age, weight, and serum creatinine. Because serum creatinine formation is a function of muscle mass, older individuals with decreased muscle mass may have a low serum creatinine. Low serum creatinine in the older or cachectic patient does not always represent good kidney function and may lead to calculated creatinine clearances that are higher than the true (or measured) creatinine clearance.

Decreases in the clearance of a drug via the kidney may lead to increases in the serum half-life of medications that are routinely cleared by the kidneys. An example of a drug that should be used with extreme caution in older adults with decreased renal function is methotrexate. Methotrexate is one chemotherapeutic agent that is extensively cleared through renal excretion. Patients with decreased renal function have prolonged levels of methotrexate and increased toxicities from the drug such as myelosuppression and mucositis. Nurses should closely evaluate older adults for renal function prior to administration of methotrexate, and they should manage any evidence of prolonged effects from methotrexate following treatment. Subsequent courses of methotrexate should be modified based on changes that may occur with renal function over time.

Another medication that healthcare professionals should use with caution in the older adult patient with decreased renal function is morphine. Morphine is metabolized to a 6-glucoronide metabolite; the metabolite accumulates with renal dysfunction. Excessive sedation seen with morphine may be secondary to accumulation of this metabolite of the drug and may be a reason to change an older adult to another opiate for pain control (Portenoy et al., 1991).

Medications that are cleared by the kidney accumulate in patients with renal insufficiency and may result in increased parent drug and/or metabolites. Age-related change in renal function is one possible cause of renal insufficiency in the older patient with cancer. Side effects may occur secondary to accumulation of either the drug or metabolite(s).

Pharmacodynamic Changes

Many of the examples provided for the dose modifications of medications based on the pharmacokinetic changes seen in the older adult are based on the impact that the pharmacokinetic change has on the physiologic effects of the drug. In addition to the changes in the pharmacokinetics of drugs in the older adult, an alteration may exist in the pharmacologic response of the drug—the pharmacodynamics. The concentration of the drug at the site of action and the site of action of the drug influence the effects of a medication. A reason for a change in response to a medication in the older adult is the change in the biology of the target tissues of the drug therapy. In addition, with aging, a progressive reduction in homeostatic mechanisms occurs, and more time is required to regain the original steady state as counter regulatory measures have decreased.

An example of pharmacodynamic change seen with chemotherapy is the increased susceptibility of the bone marrow to the effect of myelosuppressive chemotherapeutic agents. The depth and duration of bone marrow suppression with chemotherapy may be greater in an older adult with cancer as compared to a younger individual. This difference could be, in part, secondary to pharmacokinetic changes of the specific agent but appears to be secondary also to bone marrow environment.

The pharmacodynamic changes seen with medication in the older adult have been well described in the older patient in the critical care setting (Moore & Blount, 2002). These changes are important for the older patient with cancer when critically ill.

Adherence

Adherence to medications is a major factor in the success of a drug therapy plan. *Compliance to medications* now is considered a dated term, suggesting that a patient is under the direction of the physician. *Adherence* is a term that suggests a relationship between the patient and the healthcare team, and adherence to medication(s) should be an important consideration in the development of a successful pharmacotherapy plan. Medication adherence is a challenge in the general population that has been well described in the literature. Studies have documented that many patients discontinue prescribed medications over time. At one year after the initial recommendation from a physician, only 10% of patients will follow advice on recommended lifestyle modifications. Only 50% of individuals will follow advice on drug treatment (McDonald, Garg, & Haynes, 2002). The problems associated with adherence include mismanagement of medical conditions, readmissions to the hospital, and adverse drug reactions. Although the older adult is not necessarily less adherent to medication regimens than younger individuals, the problems associated with nonadherence often are significant for the older adult. Problems associated with medication adherence in older patients have been shown to increase the number of medical problems and complications in the individual.

Medication mismanagement in older patients associated with adherence includes a number of issues with pharmacotherapy plans. Medication omissions involve patients not taking medications as prescribed. Commissions involve taking medications outside the prescribed medication regimen. Another common issue is scheduling nonadherence; this occurs when a patient does not take medications as scheduled. Scheduling nonadherence is an issue seen in older patients who are prescribed multiple drugs. Scheduling misconceptions also occur secondary to patients having problems understanding the prescribed drug regimen. All, or any, of these types of medication mismanagement in the older adult with cancer may lead to the inadequate treatment of the cancer, cancer-related complications, and cancer treatment–related complications. Understanding the reasons for problems with medication adherence and developing strategies for minimizing these problems are mechanisms for optimizing the pharmacotherapy in older patients with cancer.

The literature described and reviewed the reason(s) for problems with medication adherence (Banning, 2004). Issues include social, physical, and mental vulnerability and polypharmacy. A key factor in how patients will take their medication is the level of understanding patients and/or caregivers have about their medications and medication regimens. Studies evaluating knowledge of medication dosages and schedules show that older adults often have a poor understanding of their drug therapy (Spiers, Kutzik, & Lamar, 2004). Unfortunately, similar studies evaluating the understanding of medications have not been conducted in older adults with cancer or those who are undergoing cancer-related treatments.

An important factor in understanding the medication plan is receiving correct and consistent information from the healthcare team. Conflicting advice from the healthcare team contributes to patient confusion. In patients with multiple healthcare providers, generalist and specialist, frequent adaptations of medication regimens occur during and after cancer treatment. Healthcare professionals should ensure that communication to the patient from each of these team members is consistent. Additionally, other resources such as family or friends may impact both understanding and willingness to adhere to medication regimens. Healthcare professionals should assess older adults' support system and ensure that those involved in providing care are given appropriate information about medications.

Patients also alter their medication regimens based on how they feel, eliminating medications they feel have not helped a symptom or increasing medications they perceive as beneficial. Older adults with cancer must understand the importance of communicating any changes in medication to the healthcare team prior to making a change. Older adults may have handled past medical problems with over-the-counter medications, home remedies, or medications they have at home and may feel comfortable making decisions about using medications without talking to a healthcare professional. The healthcare team should reinforce the need for older patients to communicate what they may perceive as a simple decision, such as using an over-the-counter pain medication, to the healthcare team.

The cost and complexity of medication regimens also affect how a patient will adhere to drug therapy (Fick, Waller, & Maclean, 2001). Healthcare professionals should perform routine evaluations of the individuals' ability to afford medications and also should evaluate the ability to pay costs such as medication copayments and over-the-counter medications not covered by medication programs.

Understanding the many causes of nonadherence with drug therapy provides an opportunity for the healthcare team to work with older individuals to streamline drug therapy and to ensure patient understanding. Additionally, the healthcare team should develop individualized strategies for older patients with cancer to accurately assess how individuals are taking their prescribed (and nonprescribed) drugs.

In clinical trials, a variety of monitoring strategies have been used to assess patient compliance. Pharmacy records are one method to evaluate a patient's adherence, but this is a time-consuming strategy that may not be accurate if the patient uses multiple pharmacies. Nurses can perform pill counts at each patient visit, but because many patients do not keep their medications in the original containers, this often is not an effective method. One of the most effective strategies is direct questioning of the patient and/or the patient caregiver who "handles medications." Another method is to ask patients to bring their medications with them at each visit. Figure 6-2 outlines some questions that may be helpful in evaluating adherence. Figure 6-3 lists some predictors for medication nonadherence.

Cost of pharmacotherapy plays a significant role in adherence for some patients. These expenses include the costs of drug(s), side effects, prevention of side effects, management of side effects, and the costs associated with obtaining medications. When developing pharmacotherapy plans, healthcare providers should consider and discuss all aspects of cost of care with the patient. Weighed against the cost of treatment should be the consideration of the cost of untreated condition(s). An example is the cost of treating cancer-related pain. The expense of treatment includes the analgesic(s); medications to prevent side effects, such as constipation, from analgesic(s); medications to manage side effects, such as somnolence, from the treatment; and the availability of the medications for the patient. The cost of untreated pain is also significant in terms of quality of life, productivity, and impact on patient function and disease.

- Have any medications been added since your last visit?
- Have you started to use any new over-the-counter medications since your last visit?
- Have you changed your dose of any medications?
- At what times do you take medications?
- Do you have any concerns about your medications?
- What is the purpose of each of your medications?
- What problems could occur if you choose not to take your medication?
- What do you do if you forget to take your medications?
- How do you pay for your medications?

Figure 6-2. Questions for Assessing Medication Adherence

Education of patients and caregivers is one of the most obvious, yet difficult, strategies to help to optimize medication adherence in the older adult. Education should be provided at the initiation of all new medications and at every modification of a drug dose and/or schedule. Healthcare professionals should provide patient education through both verbal and written instructions. Development of patient

- Less frequent dosing
- Acute (versus chronic) illness
- Type of medications
- Severity of illness
- Symptoms score
- Older age of patient
- Female gender
- Patient belief in therapy
- Positive attitude of treating healthcare provider

Figure 6-3. Predictors for Medication Adherence

education materials is a helpful strategy to allow the older adult to review information. These educational efforts should be coordinated with the entire healthcare team. Effort should be made to keep general practitioners, all specialists, and members of the healthcare team informed about changes in all medications. The role of the entire healthcare team, including nursing and pharmacy, in the medication management for the older patient with cancer is important to the success of the pharmacotherapy plan (Bersten et al., 2001; Griffiths, Johnson, Piper, & Langdon, 2003).

Drug Interactions

The increased risk of drug interactions in the older adult has been attributed to the physiologic changes associated with aging and the multiple drug regimens commonly prescribed in these patients (Hussar, 1988). Drug interactions include drug-drug interactions, drug-food interactions, drug-laboratory interactions, and drug-disease interactions. The potential clinical impact of drug interactions should be evaluated in all patients but may be more complex in the older adult who is on multiple medications.

Healthcare providers should be aware of the potential for interactions even if no interaction has been described. This is especially important for over-the-counter medications, herbal preparations, nutritional supplements, and new medications. Often, these products have not been fully evaluated, and information from reliable sources may not reflect important interactions.

A number of strategies can help to minimize the clinical impact of drug interactions. Encourage older adults to coordinate medications through a single pharmacy to ensure that one pharmacist is aware of all medications. Additionally, suggest that patients develop a professional relationship with a pharmacist to ensure drug therapy is evaluated with each change in medication at their pharmacy. The same strategy should be used to coordinate prescribing of medication through a primary healthcare member, and one caregiver should be designated to coordinate administration of medications as a resource to the patient. Schedule a periodic review of all medications and a time for patients to bring in all medications, allowing time for discussion of drug therapy to ensure complete review for the patient and healthcare team. As with clinical trials, suggest that the patient report all side effects seen with therapy. Because it may be difficult for an older adult to recall side effects, healthcare providers may develop a tool for the patient to keep notes about drugs and drug effects (e.g., patient log). Instruct patients to inform all members of their healthcare team about new medications.

Adverse Drug Reactions

An adverse drug reaction (ADR) is a noxious or unwanted response that occurs with a dose of a drug that would be considered therapeutic. Older individuals are particularly susceptible to ADRs because of multimorbidity, a high number of medications used in this population, and age-associated changes in pharmacokinetic and pharmacodynamic properties. Adverse drug-related outcomes in older adults are related to poorer health outcomes such as lower health-related quality of life, higher utilization of healthcare resources, and higher costs (Okano, Malone, & Billups, 2001; Thomas & Brennan, 2000). Many of the adverse drug reactions are preventable. Preventable drug-related morbidities (PDRM) may be caused by the prescribing of potentially inappropriate medications (Zhan et al., 2001), under-use of technologies, and lack of ongoing patient monitoring. A review of the literature evaluated ADR with geriatric pharmacotherapy and identified risk factors for ADR: specific drug prescribed, qualities of the physician, qualities of the patients, and the healthcare system and practice (Tamblyn, 1996). A more recent retrospective review of an integrated healthcare database evaluated 52 newly developed clinical indicators of PDRM in older adults. Five risk factors were identified for approximately 47% of all PDRMs. The identified risk factors included four or more recorded diagnoses, four or more prescribers, six or more prescription medications, antihypertensive drug use, and male gender (Mackinnon & Hepler, 2003). Older adults with cancer are at high risk for developing ADRs. Some of the more appropriate strategies for this high-risk population may be streamlining care and careful monitoring.

One of the challenges for the healthcare team is to be aware of potentially important drug interactions that may occur in the older adult. A review of drug interactions in oncology (Lam & Ignoffo, 2003) is a good resource to assess drug interactions between cancer therapy and other medications. This review contains a table of drug-drug interactions that includes recommendations for management.

Conclusion

The importance of drug therapy for the management of older adults with cancer is well established. Drug therapy is a fundamental part of the care for older patients with cancer. Medications are needed to manage and treat the cancer, prevent and manage treatment-related toxicities, and manage cancer-related complications. Drug therapy is a fundamental aspect of care for older individuals to manage concomitant chronic and acute diseases. The success of these therapies, alone and together, is partially attributed to the appropriate use of each drug in individual patients. Future clinical trials will help to guide healthcare practices in the use of medications in older adults with cancer and increase understanding of the pharmacologic aspects of aging, which will help to provide some direction to evaluate and develop strategies for optimizing drug therapy.

References

Banning, M. (2004). Enhancing older people's concordance with taking their medications. *British Journal of Nursing, 13,* 669–674.

Bersten, C., Bjorkman, I., Caramona, M., Crealey, G., Frokeaer, B., & Grundberger, E. (2001). Improving the well-being of elderly patients via community pharmacy-based provision of pharmaceutical care. A multi centre study in seven European countries. *Drugs and Aging, 18,* 63–77.

Fick, D.M., Waller, J.L., & Maclean, J.R. (2001). Potentially inappropriate medication use in a Medicare managed care population: Association with higher costs and utilization. *Journal of Managed Care Pharmacy, 7,* 407–413.

Griffiths, R., Johnson, M., Piper, M., & Langdon, R. (2003). A nursing intervention for the quality use of medicines by elderly community clients. *International Journal of Nursing Practice, 10,* 166–176.

Hamon-Vilcot, B., Simon, T., Becquemont, L., Poirier, J.M., Piette, F., & Jaillon, P. (2004). Effects of malnutrition on cytochrome P450 1A2 activity in elderly patients. *Therapie, 59,* 247–251.

Hussar, D.A. (1988). Drug interactions in the older patient. *Geriatrics, 43*(Suppl.), 20–30.

John, V., Mashru, S., & Lichtman, S. (2003). Pharmacological factors influencing anticancer drug selection in the elderly. *Drugs and Aging, 20,* 737–759.

Lam, M.S.H., & Ignoffo, R.J. (2003). A guide to clinically relevant drug interactions in oncology. *Journal of Oncology Pharmacy Practice, 9,* 45–85.

Lichtman, S.M. (2004). Chemotherapy in the elderly. *Seminars in Oncology, 31,* 160–174.

Lichtman, S.M., Skirvin, J.A., & Vemulapalli, S. (2003). Pharmacology of antineoplastic agents in older cancer patients. *Critical Reviews in Oncology/Hematology, 46,* 101–114.

Mackinnon, N.J., & Hepler, C.D. (2003). Indicators of preventable drug-related morbidity in older adults. *Journal of Managed Care Pharmacy, 9,* 134–141.

McDonald, H.P., Garg, A.X., & Haynes, R.B. (2002). Interventions to enhance patient adherence to medication prescriptions: Scientific review. *JAMA, 288,* 2868–2879.

Meanwell, C.A., Blake, A.E., & Kelly, K.A. (1986). Prediction of ifosfamide/mesna associated encephalopathy. *European Journal of Cancer Clinical Oncology, 22,* 815–819.

Moore, L.A., & Blount, K.A. (2002). Medications and the elderly in the critical care setting. *Critical Care Nursing Clinics of North America, 14,* 111–119.

Morris, L.A., Grossman, R., Barkdoll, G., Gordon, E., & Chun, M.Y. (1987). Information search activities among elderly prescription drug users. *Journal of Health Care Marketing, 7*(4), 5–15.

Okano, G.J., Malone, D.C., & Billups, S.J. (2001). Reduced quality of life in veterans at risk for drug-related problems. *Pharmacotherapy, 21,* 1123–1129.

Portenoy, R.K., Foley, K.M., Stulman, J., Khan, E., Adelhardt, J., Layman, M., et al. (1991). Plasma morphine and morphine-6-glucuronide during chronic morphine therapy for cancer pain: Plasma profiles, steady-state concentrations and the consequences of renal failure. *Pain, 47,* 13–19.

Rowe, J.W., Andres, R., Tobin, J.D., Norris, A.H., & Shock, N.W. (1976). The effect of age on creatinine clearance in men: A cross-sectional and longitudinal study. *Journal of Gerontology, 31,* 155–163.

Rowland, M., & Tozer, T.N. (1995). *Clinical pharmacokinetics: Concepts and applications* (3rd ed.). Baltimore: Williams & Wilkins.

Shadle, C.R., Lee, Y., Majumdar, A.K., Petty, K.J., Gargano, C., Bradstreet, T.E., et al. (2004). Evaluation of potential inductive effects of aprepitant on cytochrome P450 3A4 and 2C9 activity. *Journal of Clinical Pharmacology, 44,* 215–223.

Spiers, M.V., Kutzik, D.M., & Lamar, M. (2004). Variation in medication understanding among the elderly. *American Journal of Health-System Pharmacy, 61,* 373–380.

Tamblyn, R.M. (1996). Medication use in seniors: Challenges and solutions. *Therapie, 51,* 269–282.

Thomas, E.J., & Brennan, T.A. (2000). Incidence and types of preventable adverse events in elderly patients: Population based review of medical records. *BMJ, 320,* 741–744.

Turnheim, K. (2003). When drug therapy gets old: Pharmacokinetics and pharmacodynamics in the elderly. *Experiential Gerontology, 8,* 842–853.

van der Weide, J., & Steijns, L.S. (1999). Cytochrome P450 enzyme system: Genetic polymorphisms and importance on clinical pharmacology. *Annals of Clinical Biochemistry, 36,* 722–729.

van Schaik, R.H.N. (2004). Implications of cytochrome P450 genetic polymorphisms on the toxicity of antitumor agents. *Therapeutic Drug Monitoring, 26,* 236–240.

Venkatakrishnan, K., von Moltke, L.L., & Greenblatt, D.J. (2001). Human drug metabolism and the cytochrome P450: Application and relevance of in vitro models. *Journal of Clinical Pharmacology, 41,* 1149–1179.

Wildeiers, H., Highley, M.D., de Bruijn, E.A., & van Oosterom, A.T. (2003). Pharmacology of anticancer drugs in the elderly population. *Clinical Pharmacokinetics, 41,* 1213–1242.

Zhan, C., Sangl, J., Bierman, A.S., Miller, M.R., Friedman, B., Wickizer, S.W., et al. (2001). Potentially inappropriate medication use in the community-dwelling elderly: Findings from the 1996 Medical Expenditure Panel Survey. *JAMA, 286,* 2823–2829.

CHAPTER 7

The Older Adult With Breast Cancer

Deborah A. Boyle, RN, MSN, AOCN®, FAAN

Introduction

The acknowledgment and focused investigation of experiences of older adults with cancer has been nonexistent (Oncology Nursing Society & Geriatric Oncology Consortium, 2004). Despite the fact that older Americans are diagnosed most frequently with, and die from, cancer, their recognition as a unique developmental subset has not transcended cancer care. Older adults' exclusion from clinical trials and the study of supportive therapies has resulted in a paucity of evidence on which to base scientifically sound treatment decision making. This aversion and bias seriously hamper the provision of optimum therapy. This is particularly relevant to the management of major solid tumors that represent malignancies most commonly diagnosed in the older adult: lung, prostate, colorectal, and breast cancer primaries. This chapter will address incidence, risk factors, screening issues, clinical presentation, and adjuvant treatment for newly diagnosed breast cancer in older women. The chapter will conclude with areas for future research and a case study exemplifying the many issues in caring for the older adult with, or at risk for, breast cancer.

In aging countries, breast cancer among older women is a significant public health concern (Jemal et al., 2005; Parkin, Pisani, & Ferlay, 1999; Sant et al., 2004). Yet, breast cancer's prominence in the older adult is in striking contrast to the degree of clinical inquiry it has received. The following facts illustrate the significance of older women's experience with breast cancer (Alberg & Singh, 2001; Balducci, Extermann, & Carreca, 2001; Edwards et al., 2002; Giordano, Cohen, Buzdar, Parkins, & Hortobagyi, 2004; Jemal et al.; Kimmick & Balducci, 2000; Kimmick & Muss, 2004; Peek, 2003; Sakorafas, 2003; Weir et al., 2003; Williams et al., 2003).

- Approximately one-half of women with breast cancer are age 65 or older at diagnosis, and one-third of these women are older than age 75.
- The mortality rate for women age 70 and older is more than twice that for women age 55.

- Breast cancer is the most common cause of death in American women older than age 65; this includes older Hispanic, African American, Asian/Pacific Islander (API), and American Indian/Alaska Native (AI/AN) women. However, death rates for API, AI/AN, and Hispanic women are lower than those for Caucasian and African American women.
- Male breast cancer is a rare disease; yet, similar to women, male breast cancer is a disease of older men. Incidence escalates with advancing age, with the median age at diagnosis being 67.
- Overrepresentation of older women in the cohort of women diagnosed with breast cancer is in stark contrast to participation rates in clinical trials; only 17% of women in breast cancer clinical trials are older adults.

Although the current state of awareness, knowledge, and clinical intervention is extremely problematic, the denial, aversion, and lack of quantitative findings related to breast cancer in older women assume overwhelming proportions as the future is pondered. Consider the following (Alberg & Singh, 2001; Balducci et al., 2001; Edwards et al., 2002; Howe et al., 2001; Kimmick & Muss, 2004; Merrill & Weed, 2001; President's Cancer Panel, 2004; Silliman, Balducci, Goodwin, Holmes, & Leventhal, 1993; Yancik & Ries, 2000).

- The projected number of cancer cases (based on current cancer incidence rates applied to U.S. Census population projections) by 2050 reveals an overwhelming increase when compared to 2005 data. Based on this estimation, both the age-specific prevalence and incidence rates of breast cancer in older women may increase by as much as 30% over the next decade if the growth of the older population continues at the current rate; this could result in two-thirds of women diagnosed with breast cancer being older than age 65 (see Figure 7-1).
- Both the absolute number of older women diagnosed with breast cancer and the age at which the diagnosis is made will increase exponentially in the future; as compared with incidence rates in 1998, by 2025, a 72% rise will occur in the number of older women diagnosed with breast cancer.
- The most rapid increase in breast cancer incidence will occur in the oldest old ($\geq$ 85 years).
- Of the 8.9 million cancer survivors in the United States, 61% are older than age 65, and 32% of these older adults are 75 years or older; nearly one quarter (22%) are survivors of breast cancer (see Figure 7-2).

The urgency of addressing and countering the negative stereotyping that fosters ageism is critical because today's knowledge will form the foundation of future care strategies that impact older women's encounter with breast cancer (Boyle, 2004; Kantor & Houldin, 1999). In the absence of rigorous study that supports evidence-based decision making, the care of older women with breast cancer will continue to be compromised. Hence, overall efforts to reduce cancer mortality will be jeopardized if this prominent malignancy in its most common age group remains ignored.

Risk Factors

Other than advancing age, approximately 85% of women who develop breast cancer have no identifiable risk factors (Blair, 1998). Hence, age is the single most important risk factor for breast cancer development (Holmes & Muss, 2003) (see Figure 7-3). One in 14 women between the ages of 60 and 79 are at risk for developing breast cancer.

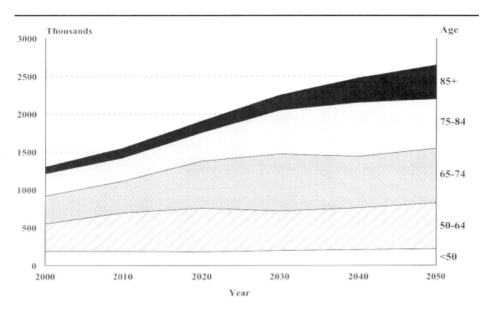

Projections based on projected census population estimates and age-specific cancer incidence rates, Surveillance, Epidemiology and End Results (SEER) Program and the National Program of Cancer Registries (NPCR) areas reported by the North American Association of Central Cancer Registries (NAACCR), 1995-1999. Projections based on current (1995-1999) age-specific incidence rates applied to projected census populations for 2000 to 2050. Population data from census populations 2000 - 2050. Cancer data from SEER and NPCR areas reported by NAACCR as meeting high data quality standards. The areas cover approximately 55% of the U.S. population: California (Los Angeles and Greater Bay area), Colorado, Connecticut, Delaware, Georgia (Atlanta area), Hawaii, Idaho, Illinois, Iowa, Kentucky, Louisiana, Michigan (Detroit area), Minnesota, Nebraska, New Jersey, New Mexico, New York, North Carolina, Pennsylvania, Rhode Island, Utah, Washington (Seattle area), West Virginia, Wisconsin, Wyoming.

Figure 7-1. Projected Number of Cancer Cases for 2000 Through 2050

Note. From "Annual Report to the Nation on the Status of Cancer, 1973–1999, Featuring Implications of Age and Aging on U.S. Cancer Burden," by B.K. Edwards, H.L. Howe, L.A.G. Ries, M.J. Thun, H.M. Rosenberg, R. Yancik, et al., 2002, *Cancer, 94*, p. 2786. Copyright 2002 by Wiley Interscience. Reprinted with permission.

This is in contrast to relative risks of 1 in 24 women ages 40–59 and 1 in 228 women age 39 and younger at risk for breast carcinoma (Singh, Hellman, & Heimann, 2004). Studies assessing the concurrence of other risk factors with age and their influence on risk have not been performed. These other risk factors include
• Hormone exposure (i.e., early menarche, late menopause, hormone replacement therapy, body mass index, alcohol intake)
• Positive family history
• Radiation exposure
• History of breast atypia (Hollingsworth et al., 2004).
    Additionally, although women ages 65 and older have a sixfold increased incidence for breast cancer, older women also have an eightfold higher risk for mortality compared with women younger than age 65 (Holmes & Muss, 2003).

Older African American Women as a Special Consideration

    Older adults and major minority populations bear a disproportionate share of the nation's cancer burden (Underwood, 2000). Thus, in terms of risk estimation, older

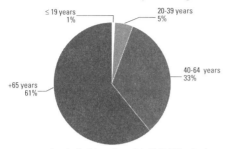

Estimated Percent of Persons Alive in the U.S. Diagnosed with Cancer in the Last 25 Years, By Current Age

≤ 19 years 1%
20-39 years 5%
40-64 years 33%
+65 years 61%

Invasive/1st Primary Cases Only, N=8.7 Million Survivors

Data Sources: November 2002 Submission. U.S. Estimated Prevalence counts were estimated by applying U.S. populations to SEER 9 Limited Duration Prevalence proportions. Populations from January 2000 were based on the average of the July 1999 and July 2000 population estimates from the U.S. Census Bureau

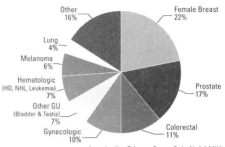

Estimated Percent of Persons Alive in the U.S. Diagnosed with Cancer, By Site

Other 16%
Female Breast 22%
Lung 4%
Melanoma 6%
Hematologic (HD, NHL, Leukemia) 7%
Other GU (Bladder & Testis) 7%
Gynecologic 10%
Colorectal 11%
Prostate 17%

Invasive/1st Primary Cases Only, N=9.6 Million

Prevalance proportions based on the standard SEER 9 registries. Complete Prevalence estimated using the completeness index method (Capocaccia, et al. 1997; Merrill, et al. 2000). U.S. prevalence counts estimated by applying SEER prevalence proportions to the U.S. populations. No attempt was made to adjust for demographic differences between the U.S. and SEER other than age.

Figure 7-2. Cancer Survivors in the United States by Age and Tumor Site

Note. Prepared by Suzanne H. Reuben for the President's Cancer Panel, May 2004. National Cancer Institute, National Institutes of Health, U.S. Department of Health and Human Services.

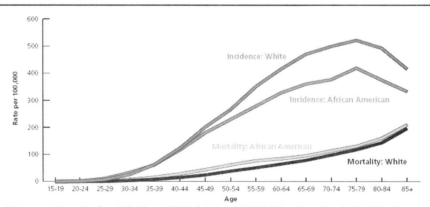

Data sources: *Incidence* – Surveillance, Epidemiology, and End Results Program, 1973-2002, Division of Cancer Control and Population Science, National Cancer Institute, 2005. *Deaths* – National Center for Health Statistics, Centers for Disease Control and Prevention, 2005.

American Cancer Society, Surveillance Research, 2005

Figure 7-3. Female Breast Cancer—Age-Specific Breast Cancer Incidence and Death by Race, United States, 1998–2002

Note. From *Breast Cancer Facts and Figures 2005–2006*, by the American Cancer Society, Atlanta, GA: Author. Copyright 2005 by the American Cancer Society. Reprinted with permission.

African American women can be characterized by double jeopardy. Breast cancer incidence rates are substantially higher in Caucasian women as compared with African American women (Chlebowski et al., 2005; Jemal et al., 2005). However, despite lower incidence rates, breast cancer causes death more frequently in African American women (Mandelblatt, Schecter, et al., 2004; Muss, 2001). In fact, at each stage of diagnosis, African American women have lower five-year survival rates than Caucasian women (Schairer, Mink, Carroll, & Devesa, 2004). This suggests possible disparity in access to and receipt of quality health care, differing prominence of comorbid conditions, and personal awareness of screening benefits. Figure 7-4 highlights racial discrepancies in mammogram ordering during physician office visits.

African American women generally are more likely to be diagnosed with advanced-stage disease (Chu, Lamar, & Freeman, 2003; Jemal et al., 2005). Even after accounting for stage at diagnosis, African American women are characterized by having poorer breast cancer survival rates (Schairer et al., 2004). Other racial differences to consider include lower receipt of radiation therapy following breast-conserving surgery, presence of more adverse prognostic factors, and cultural belief systems (Lannin et al., 1998; Magai, Consedine, Conway, Neugut, & Culver, 2004; Mandelblatt et al., 2002; Richardson, 2004; Shavers & Brown, 2002).

Despite common conjecture, when African American and Caucasian women receive comparable care, their treatment outcomes are similar (Bach et al., 2002; Newman, Theriault, Clendinnin, Jones, & Pierce, 2003). Hence, comparable care must be scrutinized when outcome by race is analyzed. This includes type of therapy, dose, schedule, delay, and toxicity profile. Because optimum care has been identified as a crucial issue in the outcome of older adults' experience with cancer, healthcare professionals must astutely address the older female African American population.

Tumor biology has been studied as an adverse prognostic factor in the African American patient cohort. These investigations have demonstrated a race-specific correlation between survival and unfavorable indices of cell proliferation (Chlebowski et al., 2005). Proportionately more aggressive tumors have been identified in African American women for each stage of disease and for each tumor size above 1.0 cm as revealed by the histologic grade (Henson, Chu, & Levine, 2003). Immunohistochemistry findings have revealed alterations in *p53* and c-*met* to be more common in African American women with breast tumors (Jones et al., 2004; Newman, 2004). Researchers have identified other genetic alterations such as mutations in *BRCA1* and *BRCA2* in African American families.

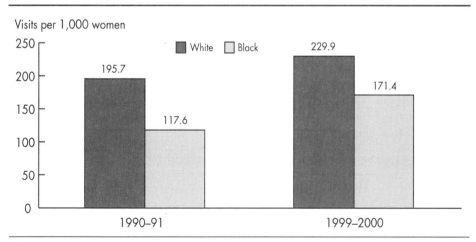

Figure 7-4. Physicians Visits With Mammograms Ordered or Provided for Women 45 Years of Age and Over, by Race: United States, 1990–2000

Note. From *Health Care in America: Trends in Utilization* (p. 73), by A.B. Bernstein, E. Hing, A.J. Moss, K.F. Allen, A.B. Siller, and R.B. Tiggle, 2003. Retrieved July 20, 2005, from http://www.cdc.gov/nchs/data/misc/healthcare.pdf.

However, because of a small study pool size, these findings require more investigation (Olopade et al., 2003). Negative status for both estrogen receptors and progesterone receptors also were more frequent in tumors of African American women. To date, no study or meta-analysis of prognostic factors and breast cancer treatment experience of older African American women has been compiled. However, data from those broad reviews can be extrapolated for more detailed investigation of the older woman's breast cancer trajectory.

Finally, belief systems are an important consideration in seeking, undergoing, and complying with breast cancer recommendations and care. The paucity of available materials integrating these perceptions into teaching and community education about breast cancer in older women precludes the delivery of cultural- and age-appropriate instruction (Watts, Merrell, Murphy, & Williams, 2004). Addressing race- and age-based perceptions about screening and breast cancer also require healthcare providers to be emotionally skilled in discussing the nature of these longstanding beliefs (Guidry, Matthews-Juarez, & Copeland, 2003).

Pathophysiology

Similar to young women, the most common type of breast cancer in older women is infiltrating ductal carcinoma (Holmes & Muss, 2003). Breast cancer in older women is considered to be more indolent in nature and has a more favorable biologic tumor profile (Gennari et al., 2004). Table 7-1 lists factors considered critical to this determination.

Table 7-1. Tumor Biology Indices Characteristic of Older Women's More Indolent Breast Cancer

Variable	Example
Cell proliferation	• Thymidine-3 labeling index lower • Higher frequency of diploid • Lower histologic grade
Genetic alterations	• More frequent normal *p53* • Higher incidence of epidermal growth factor receptor negativity • Absence of expression of c-*erbB2* • More frequent *HER2/neu* negativity
Hormone receptors	• Higher incidence of ER⁺/PR⁺ assays
Histology	• More frequent diagnoses of mucinous and papillary tumors

Note. Based on information from Holmes & Muss, 2003; Kimmick & Balducci, 2000; Kimmick & Muss, 2001.

Screening

Screening guidelines for women older than 40 generally have recommended mammography annually or semi-annually (Smith et al., 1999). No cutoff point has been identified for stopping routine screening. The majority of studies addressing the benefits of mammography have excluded women older than 70 (Kimmick & Muss, 2004); hence, this remains a controversial issue in the care of older women at risk for breast cancer.

An investigation of existing mammography rates for all age groups when available has documented the decreased use of mammography with advancing age (Alberg & Singh, 2001). Harrison et al. (2003) examined mammography use between 1993 and 1997 in a sample of 10,000 women 65 years of age and older. Results suggested that 43% had never undergone a mammogram, and 16% had undergone only one mammogram. This linear trend counters risk estimation. Ageism most likely plays a role in this finding.

The efficacy of mammography frequently is questioned as older women are considered being near the end of their life and would benefit little from having this procedure. The general medical impression that breast carcinoma in older women is less aggressive in nature reduces the likelihood of mammography being routinely ordered. Because physician recommendations for mammographic screening have been highly correlated with compliance with screening behaviors by older women, the absence of discussion about the importance of this test would most likely preclude the older woman's pursuit of this screening option (Alberg & Singh, 2001; Gulitz, Bustillo-Hernandez, & Kent, 1998; Mandelblatt & Yabroff, 2000). To date, no studies of nurse practitioner influence on mammography adherence exists. However, Coleman et al. (2003) published findings documenting that professional education by nurses targeting rural healthcare providers (e.g., physicians, nurses, mammography technicians) can influence the frequency of mammogram testing, clinical breast examination, and performance of breast self-examination. The patient sample in this two-year experimental study was low-income, African American, and older women. Figure 7-5 lists patient and provider barriers to breast cancer screening.

Provider barriers
- Inadequate knowledge of screening guidelines
- Lack of consensus or acceptance of guidelines
- Lack of knowledge of cancer treatment modalities for older adults
- Patient's age
- Gender of provider and patient
- Comorbidities associated with aging
- Time constraints
- Poor record keeping
- Failure to recognize social and cultural influences of patient population
- Lack of reimbursement for health promotion activities
- Assumption that older adults will not comply with recommendations
- Limited knowledge about the efficacy of screening tests

Patient barriers
- Assumption that it is "too late" for diagnosis or treatment
- Fear of cancer
- Fear of pain associated with diagnosis
- Perceived cancer susceptibility
- Fear of disfigurement
- Fear the treatment is worse than the disease
- Lack of accessibility to screening services
- Embarrassment associated with screening
- Lack of knowledge of screening guidelines
- Financial burden
- Limited knowledge about cancer risk
- Fatalism
- Failure of primary care provider to recommend or perform screening

---

Figure 7-5. Barriers to Cancer Screening

Note. Based on information from Blair, 1998.

Consideration of the older woman's current health status and estimation of her life expectancy should be the major influencing factors for the use of mammography screening (Alberg & Singh, 2001; Kimmick & Muss, 2004; Walter, Lindquist, & Covinsky, 2004). If the woman is highly functional with no serious comorbidities and could be a candidate for cancer treatment, then screening should occur (Holmes & Muss, 2003). On the contrary, if the woman has serious comorbidity with a limited life expectancy, mammography would not be indicated. A life expectancy of five to six years is necessary to confer survival benefit. Of note are life expectancy projections for older women. For example, a 65-year-old woman has a life expectancy of 17.5 years. Fifty percent of 75-year-olds will live 12 years, and 25% will live more than 17 years. Eighty-year-old women have a life expectancy of 8.6 years (Holmes & Muss; Walter & Covinsky, 2001). No rigid upper age limit should exist for the use of mammography in otherwise healthy older women (Kimmick & Balducci, 2000).

Results from a recent systematic review for the U.S. Preventive Services Taskforce proposed the recommendation that biennial breast cancer screening after age 65 reduces mortality at reasonable costs for women without clinically significant comorbid conditions (Mandelblatt et al., 2003). The American Geriatrics Society concurred with this recommendation (American Geriatrics Society Ethics Committee, 2003). Breast self-examination by older women is not recommended as a sole standard screening methodology (Saslow et al., 2004; Takahashi, Okhravi, Lim, & Kasten, 2004).

Clinical Presentation

Presenting symptoms of older women are not markedly different than those of younger women. A painless mass is the most common finding. However, in older women, a new lump is most likely a malignancy (Holmes & Muss, 2003; Kimmick & Muss, 2004; McDonald, Saslow, & Alciati, 2004). The majority of older women present with stage I or II disease except those older than 85 years of age, who most likely present with metastases (Holmes & Muss). Decreased breast density with age makes the clinical breast examination easier and enhances an accurate predictive value of an abnormal mammogram in women age older than 65 (Kimmick & Balducci, 2000). The sensitivity of mammography is estimated to be 63%–88% in women younger than age 65, but in women older than 65, the sensitivity increases to 90% (Takahashi et al., 2004). Healthcare providers should vigorously pursue breast pain, thickening, swelling, or nipple symptoms (e.g., discharge, retraction).

What is unique to the older woman at diagnosis is twofold. First, women older than 65 frequently will be diagnosed with breast cancer following earlier diagnoses of three to four chronic conditions. The most common intercurrent illnesses include hypertension, heart disease, arthritis, and gastrointestinal disturbances (Alberg & Singh, 2001). Comorbidity may compromise the early pursuit of a suspicious breast finding. Chronic conditions may limit manual dexterity, mobility, and physical access to various healthcare settings, endurance required for travel and appointment attendance, and individual financial resources. Any estimation of cost and expenses requires consideration of direct medical, direct nonmedical, time, and out-of-pocket costs (Hayman & Langa, 2003). Second, older women are characterized by their infrequent participation in breast cancer clinical trials, especially those targeting first-line therapy approaches. This limits the ability to develop evidence-based guidelines for treatment in this population.

Staging

The American Joint Committee on Cancer Staging System for Breast Cancer recently revised its defining criteria (Singletary et al., 2002). This revision was formally adopted for use in tumor registries in 2003. Major changes include size-based discrimination between micrometastases and isolated tumor cells; identifiers to indicate usage of innovative technical approaches; classification of lymph node status by number of involved axillary lymph nodes; and new classifications for metastasis to the infraclavicular, internal mammary, and supraclavicular lymph nodes. Figure 7-6 provides details of the most recent breast cancer staging framework. Diagnostic studies in older women are similar to those in younger women and consist of a breast biopsy to assess tumor size and a sentinel lymph node biopsy or lymph node dissection to assess lymph node involvement.

Comprehensive Geriatric Assessment

Healthcare providers have identified the use of a comprehensive geriatric assessment (CGA) in cancer care as a potential tool to demonstrate benefits in determining appropriate therapy, measuring response to treatment, and providing information on evaluative dimensions historically not ascertained at diagnosis. The CGA usually includes measurement of independent and instrumental activities of daily living, comorbidity, presence of geriatric syndromes, degree of polypharmacy, depression and cognition, social support, and nutritional status. In reviewing CGA prototypes used in general gerontology, however, no tool has emerged as the preferred choice for oncology settings (Holmes & Muss, 2003). Existing tools generally are too lengthy to administer, do not address symptom distress adequately, or fail to distinguish subtle change that may reflect progressive toxicity or recurrence. Yet, some version of this assessment framework could enhance the scope and depth of information retrieval germane to the older patient's cancer treatment experience. See Chapter 4 for further discussion of the CGA.

Treatment

Because of the historic absence of older women's inclusion in clinical trials, current treatment recommendations are based on study results of middle-aged and young women with breast cancer. This is problematic, as efficacy studies of young and middle-aged women cannot be extrapolated to older women because of the complicating nature of comorbidity, functional impairment, potential deficiencies in social support, variation in host physiology, and issues of adherence that may affect therapeutic outcomes (Silliman et al., 1993). The older adult population represents the only developmental subgroup in which cancer therapies are not determined based on the results of rigorous clinical trials. However, Web-based tools are available to assist in overall treatment planning. For example, the Mayo Clinic (www.mhs.mayo.edu/mhs/live/adjuvant) provides survival estimates with or without treatment based upon age, tumor size, lymph node involvement, and hormone receptor status (Kimmick & Muss, 2004).

Surgery and Radiation Therapy

One-half of older women with breast cancer are undertreated (Bouchardy et al., 2003). Older women are less likely to undergo breast-conserving surgery with axillary

TNM Definitions

Primary tumor (T)
- TX: Primary tumor cannot be assessed
- T0: No evidence of primary tumor
- Tis: Intraductal carcinoma, lobular carcinoma in situ, or Paget disease of the nipple with no associated invasion of normal breast tissue
  - Tis (DCIS): Ductal carcinoma in situ
  - Tis (LCIS): Lobular carcinoma in situ
  - Tis (Paget): Paget disease of the nipple with no tumor. [*Note:* Paget disease associated with a tumor is classified according to the size of the tumor.]
- T1: Tumor < 2.0 cm in greatest dimension
  - T1mic: Microinvasion < 0.1 cm in greatest dimension
  - T1a: Tumor > 0.1 cm but < 0.5 cm in greatest dimension
  - T1b: Tumor > 0.5 cm but < 1.0 cm in greatest dimension
  - T1c: Tumor > 1.0 cm but < 2.0 cm in greatest dimension
- T2: Tumor > 2.0 cm but < 5.0 cm in greatest dimension
- T3: Tumor > 5.0 cm in greatest dimension
- T4: Tumor of any size with direct extension to (a) chest wall or (b) skin, only as described below
  - T4a: Extension to chest wall, not including pectoralis muscle
  - T4b: Edema (including peau d'orange) or ulceration of the skin of the breast or satellite skin nodules confined to the same breast
  - T4c: Both T4a and T4b
  - T4d: Inflammatory carcinoma

Regional lymph nodes (N)
- NX: Regional lymph nodes cannot be assessed (e.g., previously removed)
- N0: No regional lymph node metastasis
- N1: Metastasis to movable ipsilateral axillary lymph node(s)
- N2: Metastasis to ipsilateral axillary lymph node(s) fixed or matted or in clinically apparent* ipsilateral internal mammary nodes in the absence of clinically evident lymph node metastasis
  - N2a: Metastasis in ipsilateral axillary lymph nodes fixed to one another (matted) or to other structures
  - N2b: Metastasis only in clinically apparent* ipsilateral internal mammary nodes and in the absence of clinically evident axillary lymph node metastasis
- N3: Metastasis in ipsilateral infraclavicular lymph node(s) with or without axillary lymph node involvement; in clinically apparent* ipsilateral internal mammary lymph node(s) and in the presence of clinically evident axillary lymph node metastasis; or metastasis in ipsilateral supraclavicular lymph node(s) with or without axillary or internal mammary lymph node involvement
  - N3a: Metastasis in ipsilateral infraclavicular lymph node(s)
  - N3b: Metastasis in ipsilateral internal mammary lymph node(s) and axillary lymph node(s)
  - N3c: Metastasis in ipsilateral supraclavicular lymph node(s)

* *Note: Clinically apparent* is defined as detected by imaging studies (excluding lymphoscintigraphy), by clinical examination, or grossly visible pathologically.

Pathologic classification (pN)
- pNX: Regional lymph nodes cannot be assessed (e.g., not removed for pathologic study or previously removed)
- pN0: No regional lymph node metastasis histologically, no additional examination for isolated tumor cells (ITC)
- pN0(I-): No regional lymph node metastasis histologically, negative IHC
- pN0(I+): No regional lymph node metastasis histologically, positive IHC, no IHC cluster > 0.2 mm
- pN0(mol-): No regional lymph node metastasis histologically, negative molecular findings (RT-PCR)*
- pN0(mol+): No regional lymph node metastasis histologically, positive molecular findings (RT-PCR)*

* *Note:* RT-PCR: reverse transcriptase/polymerase chain reaction
- pN1: Metastasis in 1 to 3 axillary lymph nodes and/or in internal mammary nodes with microscopic disease detected by sentinel lymph node dissection but not clinically apparent**
  - pN1mi: Micrometastasis (> 0.2 mm but < 2.0 mm)
  - pN1a: Metastasis in 1 to 3 axillary lymph nodes
  - pN1c: Metastasis in 1–3 axillary lymph nodes and in internal mammary lymph nodes with microscopic disease detected by sentinel lymph node dissection but not clinically apparent.** (If

Figure 7-6. Breast Cancer Staging *(Continued on next page)*

associated with > 3 positive axillary lymph nodes, the internal mammary nodes are classified as pN3b to reflect increased tumor burden.)
- pN2: Metastasis in 4–9 axillary lymph nodes or in clinically apparent* internal mammary lymph nodes in the absence of axillary lymph node metastasis to ipsilateral axillary lymph node(s) fixed to each other or to other structures
  - pN2a: Metastasis in 4–9 axillary lymph nodes (at least one tumor deposit > 2.0 mm)
  - pN2b: Metastasis in clinically apparent* internal mammary lymph nodes in the absence of axillary lymph node metastasis
- pN3: Metastasis in 10 or more axillary lymph nodes, in infraclavicular lymph nodes, or in clinically apparent* ipsilateral internal mammary lymph node(s) in the presence of 1 or more positive axillary lymph node(s); in more than 3 axillary lymph nodes with clinically negative microscopic metastasis in internal mammary lymph nodes; or in ipsilateral supraclavicular lymph nodes
  - pN3a: Metastasis in 10 or more axillary lymph nodes (at least 1 tumor deposit > 2.0 mm) or metastasis to the infraclavicular lymph nodes
  - pN3b: Metastasis in clinically apparent* ipsilateral internal mammary lymph nodes in the presence of 1 or more positive axillary lymph node(s); or in more than 3 axillary lymph nodes and in internal mammary lymph nodes with microscopic disease detected by sentinel lymph node dissection but not clinically apparent**
  - pN3c: Metastasis in ipsilateral supraclavicular lymph nodes

* *Note: Clinically apparent* is defined as detected by imaging studies (excluding lymphoscintigraphy) or by clinical examination.
** *Note: Not clinically apparent* is defined as not detected by imaging studies (excluding lymphoscintigraphy) or by clinical examination.

Distant metastasis (M)
- MX: Presence of distant metastasis cannot be assessed
- M0: No distant metastasis
- M1: Distant metastasis

American Joint Committee on Cancer stage groupings
Stage 0
- Tis, N0, M0
Stage I
- T1*, N0, M0
Stage IIA
- T0, N1, M0
- T1*, N1, M0
- T2, N0, M0
Stage IIB
- T2, N1, M0
- T3, N0, M0
Stage IIIA
- T0, N2, M0
- T1*, N2, M0
- T2, N2, M0
- T3, N1, M0
- T3, N2, M0
Stage IIIB
- T4, N0, M0
- T4, N1, M0
- T4, N2, M0
Stage IIIC**
- Any T, N3, M0
Stage IV
- Any T, any N, M1
* *Note:* T1 includes T1mic
** *Note:* Stage IIIC breast cancer includes patients with any T stage who have pN3 disease. Patients with pN3a and pN3b disease are considered operable. Patients with pN3c disease are considered inoperable.

Figure 7-6. Breast Cancer Staging *(Continued)*

Note. Data from *Breast Cancer Treatment,* by the National Cancer Institute, 2004. Retrieved July 8, 2004, from http//:www.cancer.gov/cancertopics/pdq/treatment/breast/HealthProfessional

dissection followed by radiation therapy postsurgery and receive adjuvant and systemic chemotherapy (Blackman, Lash, Fink, Ganz, & Silliman, 2002; DeMichele, Putt, Zhang, Glick, & Norman, 2003; Du & Goodwin, 2001b; Fyles et al., 2004; Kimmick & Muss, 2004; Repetto, Pietropalo, & Aapro, 2002; Woodard et al., 2003). Additionally, contrary to professional perception, many older women consider body image as an influencing factor in treatment decision making. A longitudinal study of 583 older women (age 67 or older) who were clinically eligible for breast conservation revealed that a third of this patient cohort used body image alteration as a factor in treatment choice (Figueiredo, Cullen, Hwang, Rowland, & Mandelblatt, 2004). These researchers also noted the positive impact on long-term mental health outcomes when shared decision making was practiced. Older women also appear to tolerate surgery and radiation therapy to the breast as well as younger women (Harris & Solin, 2000; Hughes et al., 2004; Samain, Schauvliege, Deval, & Marty, 2003; Wyatt & Friedman, 1998). Noted increased surgical risks in older adults, such as adverse reactions to anesthetics, deep vein thrombosis, delayed skin healing, and hypothermia, have not been identified with increased prominence in older women undergoing surgical resection (Dunn, 2004). Major desquamating skin reactions on the chest field site during radiation therapy also have lacked prominence in older women as compared to younger women (Zachariah et al., 1997). In evaluating the treatment course of older women undergoing radiation therapy, total dose, treatment interruptions, and treatment duration are comparable among younger and older women (Zachariah & Balducci, 2000). Hence, nonconventional fractionation in the form of higher dose accelerated treatment schedules generally is not required to reduce both toxicity and tolerance to breast field irradiation in older women (Olmi, Cefaro, Balzi, Becciolini, & Geinitz, 1997).

Chemotherapy

Factors that must be considered in choosing chemotherapy in older women with breast cancer include absorptive saturability limitations and pharmacokinetic and pharmacodynamic changes that occur with age (Green & Hacker, 2004; Lichtman, 2004). With the increasing trend of developing antineoplastics in oral formulation, healthcare providers must diligently address and assess methods to evaluate adherence to ensure optimum drug administration (Birner, 2003; Partridge, Avorn, Wang, & Winer, 2002). Additionally, the prescription of concomitant medications for the management of comorbid conditions increases the potential for altered pharmacokinetics through drug-drug absorption effects (Baker & Grochow, 1997). Changes that impact absorption may potentially result in altered toxicity and effectiveness of oral chemotherapy drugs (Lichtman, Skirvin, & Vemulapalli, 2003). Table 7-2 lists special considerations in the use of systemic chemotherapy in the older adult. Of particular concern are necessary dose adjustments required to minimize end organ dysfunction and toxicities in the setting of renal or hepatic dysfunction related to physiologic changes with age (Green & Hacker).

Age-related changes in the cytochrome (CYP) P450 microsomal system and the CYP 3A4 enzyme may alter metabolism of chemotherapy drugs by the liver. A 30% reduction in P450 capability results in decreased first-pass drug metabolism of medications that are highly extracted by the liver (Lichtman, 1998). In addition to age-related changes, a variety of commonly prescribed medications inhibit the CYP 3A4 enzyme, which is involved in the metabolism of cyclophosphamide, etoposide, teniposide, vincristine, the taxanes, and tamoxifen (Lichtman, 2004; Wildiers & Paridaens, 2004). Organ

Table 7-2. Selected Chemotherapeutic Agents Available for Breast Cancer Treatment and Special Considerations in the Older Population

Agent	Special Considerations
Anthracyclines (epirubicin and doxorubicin)	Limited cardiotoxicity in older patients. Avoid use of doxorubicin in patients with an ejection fraction < 50%. Significant alopecia, myelosuppression, nausea, and emesis potential. New liposomal doxorubicin preparation demonstrates improved side-effect profile. Epirubicin in metastatic breast cancer is associated with reduced cardiotoxicity, nausea, and myelosuppression more than doxorubicin.
Cyclophosphamide methotrexate	Elimination decreased in patients with impaired renal function. Excretion dependent on renal function, which decreases with age. Dose adjustments based on renal function in older women showed reduced toxicity. Patients with pleural effusions and ascites are at risk for prolonged drug elimination and toxicity.
Fluorouracil	No increased gastrointestinal toxicity noted in patients with breast cancer (as compared with patients with colorectal cancer). Fluorouracil-induced cardiac toxicity does not appear to increase with age. Oral 5-fluorouracil allows for home-based therapy. No trials to date in older patients.
Capecitabine	Minimal myelosuppression Hand-foot syndrome is frequently dose limiting, and diarrhea is possible. Age does not significantly affect pharmacology. Dose reduction suggested for renal impairment.
Vinca alkaloids (vincristine/ vinblastine)	Monitor carefully for neuropathy.
Vinorelbine	Pharmacokinetics comparable in older and younger women. Favorable toxicity profile seen in older patients.
Taxanes (paclitaxel/docetaxel)	Limited data available in older patients. Hepatic impairment increases toxicity. Sensory and motor neuropathy and fluid retention (docetaxel) side effects May cause mild to moderate myalgias and arthralgias
Gemcitabine*	Age-related differences in pharmacokinetics Favorable toxicity profile with mild myelosuppression as a single agent
Trastuzumab	Humanized monoclonal antibody approved for use in patients with *HER2/neu* overexpressing tumors. Early reports of cardiotoxicity may limit use in older women.

* Not FDA approved for use in breast cancer.

Note. From "Diagnosis and Treatment of Breast Cancer in the Elderly," by C.E. Holmes and H.B. Muss, 2003, *CA: A Cancer Journal for Clinicians, 53,* p. 241. Copyright 2003 by American Cancer Society. Reprinted with permission.

toxicities specific to each of these agents may be more pronounced. For example, liver dysfunction can increase hematologic toxicity and serious morbidity of therapy with taxanes (Lichtman, 2004). Because of a decline in glomerular filtration rates with age, estimation of creatinine clearance is especially required for antineoplastics primarily excreted by the kidneys (e.g., carboplatin, cisplatin, methotrexate). Standard doses of these agents may be too toxic, especially in the frail older adult (Lichtman, 2004).

Current investigation of chemotherapeutic agents for the older adult has many potential applications for future systemic therapy for older women with breast cancer. Agents that appear to have a beneficial therapeutic index, particularly in the older adult, include gemcitabine, vinorelbine, the taxanes, anthracyclines, platinum compounds, topoisomerase I and II inhibitors, and the oral fluoropyrimidines (Lichtman, 1998). Additionally, dose-intense regimens (such as Adriamycin® [Bedford Laboratories, Bedford, OH], cyclophosphamide, and its variations) given to women older than 70 are considered appropriate for first-cycle prophylaxis with human granulocyte–colony-stimulating factors to promote the delivery of planned dose-dense chemotherapy regimens on time (Frasci, 2002). Given the lack of data indicating older women in good health have poorer outcomes or increased toxicity after standard therapy, treatment recommendations should not be compromised based on age alone (Harris & Solin, 2000). Only limited life expectancy and serious comorbidities should influence the delivery of evidence-based care to older women.

Hormonal Therapy

Hormonal agents to manage breast cancer in the older woman in the adjuvant setting have been the focus of debate. Tamoxifen is the most established adjuvant hormonal treatment in pre- and postmenopausal women and is associated with a 50% reduction in recurrence and a 30% reduction in mortality (Kimmick & Muss, 2004). Anastrozole, an aromatase inhibitor, is another option for postmenopausal women with hormone receptor–positive breast cancer (Kimmick & Muss, 2004; National Comprehensive Cancer Network [NCCN], 2004). Recommendations for adjuvant therapy in women older than 70 are presented in Table 7-3. These emanate from expert consensus achieved at the St. Gallen Breast Cancer Conference and include the integration of recent information from large-scale adjuvant therapy clinical trials. Again, it must be noted that these guidelines for older women are based on extrapolation of evidence from trials of female participants aged 50–69 years (Kimmick & Muss, 2004). Older adult–specific breast cancer clinical trials that address the role of adjuvant therapy currently are ongoing. One of the first such studies, from the French Adjuvant Study Group, demonstrated significant efficacy of a weekly epirubicin-based chemotherapy plus tamoxifen regimen in disease-free survival in older women (age 65 or older) with node-positive operable breast cancer (Fargeot et al., 2004). This regimen, when compared with single-agent tamoxifen, also was characterized by efficacious hematologic, nonhematologic, and cardiac safety profiles (Fargeot et al.). Further detail concerning the use of antiestrogens and aromatase inhibitors in older women with breast cancer will enhance their application for older women with significant comorbidities and those who develop second breast cancers (Arora & Potter, 2004; Clemons, Danson, & Howell, 2002; Goss & Strasser, 2002). Additional information also is required on long-term sequelae of various hormonal therapies.

The evolving recognition of positive outcomes of older women treated comparatively with their younger counterparts has increased interest in the development of older adult–specific clinical trials (Muss, 2001). An increased use of chemotherapy in older

Table 7-3. Recommendations for Adjuvant Therapy in Women Older Than Age 70

Risk Category	Definition	Treatment
Node negative		
Minimal/low	≤ 1 cm, ER- and/or PR-positive, grade I	No treatment or hormonal therapy*
Moderate	> 1 cm and ≤ 2 cm, ER- and/or PR-positive, grade I or II	Hormonal therapy ± chemotherapy
High	> 2 cm, ER- and/or PR-negative, or grade II or III	Hormonal therapy; chemotherapy if ER/PR negative
Node positive		
ER-positive	Any	Hormonal therapy
ER-negative	Any	Chemotherapy

*Hormonal therapy consists of either tamoxifen for five years or anastrozole for five years.
ER—estrogen receptor; PR—progesterone receptor

Note. From "Breast Cancer in Older Patients," by G.G. Kimmick and H.B. Muss, 2004, *Seminars in Oncology, 31,* p. 242. Copyright 2004 by Elsevier. Reprinted with permission.

women with breast carcinoma occurred in the 1990s (Du & Goodwin, 2001a). Although still not adequate, this trend is promising, as perhaps firsthand accounts of treatment success has prompted provider revisiting of ageist-laden decision making.

Recurrent or Metastatic Disease

The overall goal of treatment for metastatic breast cancer in older women is palliation, improvement in quality of life, and prolongation of survival with minimal treatment side effects. The treatment of metastatic breast cancer in older women is not significantly different than treatment for other postmenopausal women (Kimmick & Muss, 2004). Older women with progressive disease always should be considered for clinical trial participation. In symptomatic older women with hormone receptor–positive tumors, sequential hormonal therapy is considered a reasonable option. Hormonal therapy agents include nonsteroidal aromatase inhibitors (anastrozole and letrozole); steroidal aromatase inhibitors (exemestane); pure antiestrogens (fulvestrant); progestins (megestrol acetate); and androgens (fluoxymesterone) (Kimmick & Muss, 2004; NCCN, 2004). Minimal toxicities and related impact on physical functioning associated with hormone therapies constitute an ideal profile for systemic therapy at this time. In symptomatic older women with hormone receptor–negative tumors, chemotherapy may be considered to palliate symptoms if functional status is not compromised. Chemotherapy agents may include taxanes, anthracyclines, vinorelbine, gemcitabine, or capecitabine (Kimmick & Muss, 2004; NCCN). In patients with HER2-positive tumors, trastuzumab may be given as single agent or in combination with chemotherapy. When serious comorbidities and significant functional decline is evident, palliative care rather than aggressive treatment should be continued with ongoing monitoring to minimize symptom distress.

Nursing Care Issues

Four major themes encompass critical issues of nursing care for older women facing breast cancer. These should be considered in devising guidelines for best practice and in planning comprehensive programs for older women with breast cancer along their illness trajectory.

Assessment, Monitoring, and Follow-Up

Ongoing surveillance of the health status of the older patient is required at the onset of treatment and throughout the survivor continuum. During treatment, phone contact optimizes assessment and offers patients an added sense of security that their response to therapy is being scrutinized in a continued fashion. Repeated efforts must be made to normalize the report of symptoms and other findings and to assure patients that disclosure is the norm, not the exception. The oncology nurse in ambulatory practice settings also must be skilled in advocating for the older patient when critical thinking results in the determination that symptom management is inadequate or comorbid conditions may be complicating care. The nurse must articulate the detailed problem analysis clearly, and the rationale for an alternate plan of care must be evidence-based.

By reiterating the need for continued follow-up and making an analogy to ongoing care requirements following a cardiac problem or other chronic illness, nurses can enhance compliance with post-therapy monitoring. Shortly after the cessation of therapy, decreased physical functioning may be the source of most concern and require creative problem solving (Ganz et al., 2004). Older patients with breast cancer are at risk for local recurrence (chest wall involvement or cancer in the contralateral breast) and systemic indices of recurrence (hepatic, lung, brain, or bone metastases, pathologic fracture, or spinal cord compression). Approximately 17% of breast cancer recurrences are diagnosed within five years of initial diagnosis (Mincey & Perez, 2004). Older women with a history of breast cancer also are at risk for the development of a second primary unrelated to the initial breast malignancy. The exact type and frequency of screening procedures in the older adult at risk for subsequent medical sequelae have not been determined (Boyle & Engelking, 2003). Yet, the goals for follow-up generally are to detect potentially curable local relapse and second primary tumors, manage the side effects of therapy, provide patients with psychosocial support, and provide care for patients who develop metastatic disease (Emens & Davidson, 2003). Continuity with nursing staff known to patients during treatment can facilitate data gathering with older adults following treatment cessation, as trust has been established and communication patterns solidified.

Comprehensive, Reinforced Education

Neurosensory compromise may deter the reception and assimilation of new information required for older patients to understand their treatment plan, carry out expectations for self-care, and be cognizant of signs and symptoms that warrant notification of staff. Determining reliance on hearing aids and glasses is imperative at initial contact and assessment. Any education offered must be duplicated and reinforced, as nurses should acknowledge that one attempt to teach is never enough. This also is true for the primary caregiver. The concerned and anxious spouse, sister, or son also needs repeated instruction and explanation of both routine and complex topics pertinent to the older woman's treatment experience. Information amount also should be assessed, as varying quantities of information complement individual coping. Caregivers who require high levels of information to enhance coping may paradoxically experience increased distress related to the nature of information garnered (Nikoletti, Kristjanson, Tataryn, McPhee, & Burt, 2003). Long-distance families (i.e., adult children geographically distant from their parents) may benefit from receiving copies of written materials given to the patient and audiotaped consultations detailing rationale for treatment and expectation of the patient for self-care. Navigation of the complex healthcare system can be particularly overwhelming to the older adult. Explicit directions in the form of visual pictures and maps drawn with large font size will aid transitioning through the maze of required consultations and appointments. Finally, communication style also must be considered paramount to teaching effectiveness. This factor has been documented to influence the receipt of information emanating from the patient-physician interaction (Maly, Leake, & Silliman, 2004). Demonstrating physical attentiveness (i.e., eye contact, facial expression, body posture), using optimum listening skills, and personalizing discussions are determinants of effective professional communication styles.

Coping and Caregiving

Although it is always an expectation that cancer be recognized as a family disease, it is of utmost importance when the patient/family unit is addressing older adult implications of cancer. Both the patient and the primary caregiver have their own unique needs, and in the absence of deliberative attention to both, any positive outcome of psychosocial support will be jeopardized (Boyle, 2003a).

Even in the older years, the threat of premature mortality may astound the patient and her family. Thinking of themselves as fit and having additional years in their future, older women may be shocked at the news of breast cancer. Other patients compromised by chronic illness may view themselves as vulnerable targets for cancer and may not be surprised by the diagnosis. Complicating the older adult's reaction to breast cancer may be cumulative grief. Juggling hope about a positive prognosis while concurrently mourning the loss of siblings and friends is indeed a difficult task. Although depression often is assumed to be a natural corollary of being old and having cancer, evidence has shown that younger patients may be more troubled by this symptom than older patients (Kurtz & Dufour, 2002). Older women with breast cancer may be the primary caregiver to an ill spouse, sibling, or grandchildren. Hence, they may experience guilt over their ongoing inability to provide care. Concerns about finances and perceptions of being a burden on their family may enhance remorse and interfere with asking for help when needed. Negative attitudes about sexuality in later life may preclude discussion about intimacy as an avenue of emotional comfort.

When family implications of cancer care are considered, caregiver burden must be anticipated (Ballantyne, 2004). Gender differences in coping distinguish male caregivers as having fewer confidantes in verbalizing psychological concerns and worries than female caregivers (Coristine, Crooks, Grunfeld, Stonebridge, & Christie, 2003). Male spouses may be "hidden patients," marginally functional with their own health problems. The thought of living on without one's spouse of four, five, or six decades may be too overwhelming to acknowledge. While dealing with recurrent breast cancer, the emotional well-being of family members may become compromised (Northouse et al., 2002). Reticent to ask for help or acknowledge profound sadness and anticipatory grief, family members' emotional endurance frequently deteriorates. Because of the mobility of Americans, middle-aged adult children may not be geographically available to provide support and care. For a number of reasons, some adult children may not be emotionally available to offer support to their parent(s). These factors negate the possibility of the older woman's ability to remain at home, particularly when end-of-life care is required (Gagnon, Mayo, Hanley, & MacDonald, 2004). Stress among children may evolve when a sibling does not handle his or her share of support in a time of need. The adult children, always perceiving their mother as "the Rock of Gibraltar," may experience disbelief over her vulnerability to breast cancer. Role reversal (i.e., "I am mother to my mother") may be particularly disheartening. Finally, grandchildren's reactions commonly are ignored, and they remain "unknown soldiers" in their own coping world. For many grandparents and grandchildren alike, these relationships are endearing and hold special significance. Yet, the acute and long-term ramifications of these dyads' encounters with loss remain virtually unexplored.

Managing Symptom Distress

As noted previously, the presence of comorbidity can complicate symptom recognition and the resolution of distress. Consideration of geriatric syndromes, conditions common to the older adult, must be taken into account when differentiating the nature of evolving problems. Table 7-4 identifies these syndromes and offers examples of potential etiologies specific to the breast cancer experience. Additionally, implications of polypharmacy (i.e., multiple drug therapies to manage chronic conditions) may be involved in the presentation of unusual symptoms or patterns of symptom distress. In the absence of one provider or group of office professionals overseeing all the older patients' medications, drugs may be prescribed that promote synergistic toxicity or render adverse effects when combined. Polypharmacy dilemmas, which include the use of over-the-counter and complementary supplements, often are not disclosed to the cancer care team. Although not considered problematic because of their ease in purchase, these drugs can precipitate symptom distress in the older patient with breast cancer undergoing treatment.

A model of gero-oncology nursing expertise incorporates awareness, knowledge, and skill in assessment, monitoring, and follow-up; provides education to the patient and family; enhances coping and seeks measures to reduce caregiving burden; and facilitates the optimum management of symptom distress. This expertise can be augmented by the integration of general gerontologic nursing scholarship with specialty cancer nursing competence. Cross training, peer clinical rounding, and formal collaborative instruction fosters this needed intradisciplinary proficiency.

Areas for Future Research

The volume and sophistication of research in cancer and aging within nursing and across disciplines are incongruent with the demographics of aging and the epidemiology of cancer (Kagan, 2004). A recent literature review on breast cancer outcomes, for example, identifies that less than 10% of study participants were non-Caucasian or older adults (Mandelblatt, Armetta, Yabroff, Liang, & Lawrence, 2004). Table 7-5 highlights studies by individual nurses or group researchers where older women with or at risk for

Table 7-4. SPPICEES Geriatric Assessment Model and Its Potential Application to the Older Patient With Breast Cancer

Common Problem	Cancer-Specific Examples/Issues
Skin integrity problems	Radiation-related skin compromise Wound healing postsurgery or postextravasation Vulnerability to skin breakdown during prolonged immobility in conjunction with fatigue Potential skin compromise promoting lymphedema
Problems with nutrition	Shortened periods of anorexia still may cause significant weight loss. Food tolerances and taste changes during episodes of symptom distress Difficulty with mastication without dentures during episodes of mucositis
Problems with pain	Dosing requirements of opioids, nonopioids, adjuvant medications Assessment issues with other comorbidities (e.g., arthritis, osteoporosis), potential treatment-related toxicities (e.g., arthralgias, myalgias, hand-foot syndrome), and/or symptoms of new or progressive recurrence (e.g., bone metastases) Assessment when cognitive impairment is an issue
Immobility	Infectious corollaries of immune compromise, access to young grandchildren Fall risk indicators during bone marrow depression with resultant deleterious outcomes (e.g., bleeding, fracture) Neurotoxicity related to chemotherapy
Confusional states	Identification of multiple risk factors and prodromal signs Nurse-friendly assessment tools to promote early recognition and objective documentation Memory prompters to foster adherence Optimum pharmacologic and behavioral management
Elimination problems	Prevalence and optimum management of constipation related to vinca alkaloids, taxanes, opioids, and inadequate fluid intake Prevalence and optimum management of diarrhea related to fluorouracil compounds or overuse of laxatives
Elder mistreatment	Identification of elder social support dilemmas Scope of pain mismanagement related to age bias Family withholding pain medications related to concerns about addiction Insurance/reimbursement issues
Sleep problems	Patterns during hospitalization Use and implications of over-the-counter sleep aids Implications of sleep deprivation on symptom intensity (e.g., pain, delirium)

Note. Based on information from Boyle, 2003a.

breast cancer were the target of investigation. Select findings from these studies may be extrapolated for consideration in the care of older women facing a breast malignancy.

Research issues of relevance to the older woman facing breast cancer can be categorized into those related to prevention and detection, responses to disease and treatment, psychosocial issues, long-term survivorship, and palliative end-of-life care (Boyle, 2003b). Some examples of research questions germane to this patient population include the following considerations.

Table 7-5. Nursing Research Targeting or Including Older Women With or at Risk for Breast Cancer

Author(s)	Study Title	Sample	Findings
McMillan, 1989	The relationship between age and intensity of cancer-related symptoms	25 outpatients being treated with cyclophosphamide, Adriamycin®, and fluorouracil (CAF) or cyclophosphamide, Adriamycin, and vincristine (CAV), evaluated for nausea/vomiting; 99 inpatients evaluated for pain; subsets in both groups compared by age	Older adults reported lower intensity of some physical symptoms than did younger individuals; however, relationship between age and symptom intensity was weak, suggesting individual responses (rather than age alone) should be the primary focus of assessment and interventions.
Morrison, 1996	Determining crucial correlates of breast self-examination [BSE] in older women with low incomes	204 women ages 40–86 self-referred or recruited from the community for free breast cancer screening; must be uninsured or underinsured and have income < 2.5 times the poverty level	Older subsets (≥ age 65) of participating women were not compared with younger participants; group analysis revealed 10 variables predictive of BSE behavior: confidence and confidence level, awareness of mammography, provider influence, desire for reconstruction, knowledge of parity risk factor, education, having been taught the correct time of month to perform BSE, adequate time devoted to BSE, and exposure to BSE messages from a clinician.
Blair, 1998	Cancer screening of older women	Retrospective chart review of 201 women age 60 years and older who were seen twice in one year in a Midwestern family practice residency program	Breast cancer screening was offered to approximately 70% of the sample; only one-third of the older women received mammography or clinical breast exam; recommendations for gynecologic screening given to 63% of older women; less than one-third received Pap smears; recommendations for digital rectal exam, fecal occult blood testing, and flexible sigmoidoscopy given to 58%, 59%, & 30%, respectively.
Wyatt & Friedman, 1998	Physical and psychosocial outcomes of midlife and older women following surgery and adjuvant therapy for breast cancer	46 patients with breast cancer age 55 or older	Two groups of women receiving surgery alone or surgery plus adjuvant therapy (either chemotherapy or radiation therapy) were compared; both groups did equally well with no differences in quality of life (QOL) or demands of illness; additionally, these scores did not change significantly over time following surgery.

(Continued on next page)

Table 7-5. Nursing Research Targeting or Including Older Women With or at Risk for Breast Cancer *(Continued)*

Author(s)	Study Title	Sample	Findings
Kurtz et al., 1999	The influence of symptoms, age, comorbidity and cancer site on physical functioning and mental health of geriatric women patients	299 women older than age 65 with breast (n = 183, 61.2%), colon (n = 58, 19.4%), or lung (n = 58, 19.4%) primaries	Higher symptom severity was more positively correlated with more comorbidity and more advanced age; greater symptom severity predicted worse mental health; older patients with lung cancer reported greater losses in physical functioning and higher average symptom severities than patients with either breast or colon cancer.
Hughes et al., 2000	Information needs of older post-surgical patients with cancer during the transition from hospital to home	Content analyses of 3,280 statements of teaching interventions with 148 patients surgically treated for a new diagnosis of prostate, breast, lung, head and neck, or gastrointestinal cancer	Information needs of older postsurgical patients with cancer during transition from hospital to home are extensive; teaching interventions ranged from giving concrete instructions about care of a surgical wound to interpreting complex information about options for cancer treatment.
McCorkle et al., 2000	A specialized homecare intervention improves survival among older post-surgical patients with cancer	375 newly diagnosed patients aged 60 or older with solid tumors treated surgically were randomized to an intervention group (n = 190) and a usual care group (n = 185); intervention consisted of protocols addressing standard assessment and management guidelines postsurgery, doses of instructional content, and schedules of contacts by an advanced practice nurse over four weeks that included three home visits and five phone contacts; patients and family members received assessments, monitoring, teaching and skills training.	Overall, the specialized homecare intervention group was found to have statistically increased survival; this is the first empirical study of postsurgical patients with cancer linked to a nurse-delivered homecare intervention that improves survival.

(Continued on next page)

Table 7-5. Nursing Research Targeting or Including Older Women With or at Risk for Breast Cancer *(Continued)*

Author(s)	Study Title	Sample	Findings
Given et al., 2001	Predictors of pain and fatigue in the year following diagnosis among older patients with cancer	839 patients aged 65 or older with newly diagnosed breast, colon, lung, or prostate malignancies were assessed at four time intervals (6–8 weeks, 12–16 weeks, 24–30 weeks, and 52 weeks); three questions related to the patient's pain and fatigue were posed.	Patients with three or more comorbid conditions had significantly more symptom distress (in addition to pain and fatigue); site and stage of disease had an independent effect on the number of other symptoms patients reported; a model proposed on the results of this research indicated a greater risk for reporting pain and fatigue if patients have three or more comorbid conditions, have lung cancer as compared to breast cancer, late-stage disease, or have had any treatment within the past 40 days; fatigue alone was reported by 30% of older patients with these solid tumors.
Cimprich et al., 2002	Age at diagnosis and QOL in breast cancer survivors	194 women at least five years postdiagnosis with no documented recurrence or other cancer diagnosis were stratified by age (< 45 years, ages 45–65, and > 65 years).	Long-term survivors of breast cancer diagnosed in older age (> 65 years) demonstrated worse QOL outcomes in the physical domain, whereas younger patients (ages 27–44 years) showed worse QOL outcomes in the social domain than other age groups; age at diagnosis and years of survival predicted QOL outcomes.
Hughes et al., 2002	Describing an episode of home nursing care for older postsurgical patients with cancer	Chart audits performed on 148 records of older postsurgical patients with cancer assigned to the intervention group in a randomized clinical trial to evaluate the effect of home care delivered by an advanced practice nurse on QOL and survival outcomes	The advanced practice nurses delivering the homecare intervention responded to numerous complex problems and used a variety of interventions to assist both older patients and their caregivers in the management of the illness experience; diversity in nursing care by cancer site was identified most prominently with patients with breast cancer; nursing intervention emphasis and dose intensity varied over time, suggesting care was customized along the illness trajectory.
Wood et al., 2002	The effect of an educational Intervention on promoting breast self-examination in older African American and Caucasian women	328 predominantly African American (77%) women aged 60 or older; 206 women were assigned to the intervention group (ethnically tailored breast health kits were used in teaching), and 122 women were assigned to the control group (generic educational pamphlets were used in teaching).	The intervention was effective in increasing knowledge about breast cancer risk and the proficiency of screening and BSE in older women; educational interventions designed specifically for age and race sensitivity may enhance cancer screening with vulnerable populations.

(Continued on next page)

Table 7-5. Nursing Research Targeting or Including Older Women With or at Risk for Breast Cancer *(Continued)*

Author(s)	Study Title	Sample	Findings
Jennings-Sanders & Anderson, 2003	Older women with breast cancer: Perceptions of the effectiveness of nurse case managers	106 older women (older than age 65) with newly diagnosed breast cancer	Community-based nurse case managers made a positive impact on older women with breast cancer by helping with the management of coexisting medical conditions, providing support and education, offering assistance with activities of daily living, and helping to navigate the healthcare system.
Sammarco, 2003	QOL among older survivors of breast cancer	103 breast cancer survivors older than 50 years	Increased age correlated with uncertainty that escalated in the presence of other diseases; positive correlations also were documented between support network size and the provision of social support; social support reduced illness uncertainty and improved QOL in older survivors of breast cancer.
Goodwin et al., 2003	Effect of nurse case management on the treatment of older women with breast cancer	335 newly diagnosed older (aged 65 or older) women with breast cancer were randomized to control (n = 166) and intervention groups (n = 169); the intervention consisted of receiving the services of a nurse case manager for 12 months following the diagnosis of breast cancer.	More women in the intervention group received breast-conserving therapy and radiation therapy and breast reconstruction surgery; more women with advanced breast cancer in the intervention group received chemotherapy; two months postsurgery, higher percentages in the intervention group had normal arm function and were more likely to state that they had a choice in their treatment decision making; women with inadequate social support were more likely to benefit from nurse case management.
Coleman et al., 2003	The Delta Project: Increasing breast cancer screening among rural minority and older women by targeting rural healthcare providers	224 nurses, physicians, and mammography technicians practicing in a primary healthcare provider's office in rural Arkansas	Healthcare provider instruction significantly increased breast cancer screening recommendations following the education intervention; performance competency in the clinical breast examination was higher for nurses as compared to physicians; mammogram frequency in those counties where staff received the education intervention was higher than in those counties where education was not provided to healthcare professionals.

(Continued on next page)

Table 7-5. Nursing Research Targeting or Including Older Women With or at Risk for Breast Cancer *(Continued)*

Author(s)	Study Title	Sample	Findings
Hodgson & Given, 2004	Determinants of functional recovery in older adults surgically treated for cancer	172 community-dwelling older adults (age 65 or older) recently diagnosed and surgically treated for lung, prostate, colorectal, or breast cancer	Sequential testing at 4–6 weeks and then again at 14–16 weeks revealed that prostatectomy patients were more likely to have recovered by the second survey period when compared to patients with lung, colorectal, or breast cancer; comorbidity and symptom severity were associated with decreased probability of recovery; for all groups, pain and fatigue were the most commonly reported symptoms.
Gil et al., 2004	Triggers of uncertainty about recurrence and long-term treatment side effects in older African American and Caucasian breast cancer survivors	244 older women (average age 64 years) between five to nine years post breast cancer diagnosis; 73 were African American and 171 were Caucasian.	The most frequent uncertainty triggers were hearing stories about another woman's breast cancer and the presence of new symptoms such as aches and pains; no ethnic differences existed in the symptom experience; Caucasian women were more likely to voice their fears of recurrence, triggered by hearing about another woman's cancer, environmental triggers (i.e., sights, sounds, and smells associated with the breast cancer experience), and the evolution of new information or controversy about breast cancer as discussed in the media; illness uncertainty manifested in the form of recurrence anxiety persisted long after treatment cessation, and most women experienced multiple triggers.
Yarbrough, 2004	Older women and breast cancer screening: Research synthesis	Medical and nursing databases were searched for research addressing women age 60 and older and their experience with breast cancer screening	Despite older women experiencing varied health problems and chronic illnesses, no empirical evidence indicated that they were less able than younger women to tolerate breast cancer screening or breast cancer treatment.
Overcash, 2004	Using narrative research to understand the quality of life of older women with breast cancer	12 women at least 70 years of age who were undergoing treatment for breast cancer (either radiation, chemotherapy, or hormonal therapy)	Following two to three one-hour interview encounters per participant, eight major themes evolved: importance of God, positive attitude, no alteration in lifestyle, physician trust, caregiver to others, importance of health, importance of family, and alteration in lifestyle; older women with breast cancer who serve as caregivers to other family members have unique role expectations despite their personal health limitations.

- What influence does the oncology advanced practice nurse provider have on compliance with older women's screening behaviors?
- Is toxicity incidence and severity increased in older women as compared with younger women? How dissimilar is treatment-related symptom distress in older women as compared with younger women, and within subsets of older adults (i.e., 65–74, 75–84, ≥ 85 years)?
- What is the prominence of cognitive changes (i.e., "chemo brain") in older women with breast cancer as compared with middle-aged and young women?
- How does polypharmacy affect medication adherence in women participating in chemoprevention clinical trials?
- How is caregiver burden characterized in varying "at-risk" social support scenarios (e.g., the patient as the primary caregiver to a chronically ill spouse, the patient and spouse have cancer concurrently, geographically removed middle-aged children attempting to coordinate their widowed mother's care from a distance)?
- Which older caregivers are most at risk for depression related to cumulative grief?
- How extensive are out-of-pocket costs for older adults receiving breast cancer treatment?
- Which symptoms during end-of-life care are most problematic for older women? Are they similar to younger patients during advanced stages of breast cancer?
- What cultural variables predict ongoing, routine screening and health surveillance following the completion of breast cancer therapy?
- What is the impact (i.e., degree of physiologic and emotional symptom distress, number of unscheduled office visits, hospital admissions, and emergency room visits) of a structured homecare support intervention by an oncology/homecare nurse team during the course of adjuvant chemotherapy for older women with breast cancer?

Instrument validation in the older population also is required (Di Maio & Perrone, 2003).

Targeting the older age group with breast cancer for research initiatives is imperative to enable the development of specific treatment guidelines, the employment of preventive and therapeutic symptom distress interventions, and the identification of psychosocial support therapies that work best with differing subsets of patients and families (Boyle, 2003b; Wyld & Reed, 2003).

Case Study

Mrs. S was a 79-year-old woman who resided in an assisted living residence for four years. Because of long-standing arthritis and diabetes that required daily glucose monitoring and oral hypoglycemics, she had sold her home and moved into this facility soon after her husband died. He had helped significantly with Mrs. S's medications and assumed responsibility for the housework, shopping, meal preparation, and transportation needs for both of them. Mrs. S had one adult daughter, Susan, who lived in a nearby suburb, and she visited frequently. With the assisted living staff now performing instrumental activities of daily living, Susan assumed primary responsibility for the general oversight of her mother's health, finances, and social activities.

Mrs. S visited the nurse weekly at the residential facility to discuss her glucose monitoring, nutrition, and self-care. Mrs. S confided to this nurse that she had felt a growth under her arm on the side of her breast. It had been there for about a month, but she thought it would go away, so she dismissed it. She remembered slightly losing her balance and bumping into her closet door one night when she went for her robe to go into the bathroom. She had considered this potential bruising the cause of the growth. But when no discoloration occurred in the area and the growth did not subside in size, she decided she should inform the nurse. Mrs. S stated, "If it's something bad, I don't want my daughter to know. She does enough for me already, and she has her own family, and I don't want to burden her any more than I have." The nurse spoke with Mrs. S about the need to get this assessed quickly. With prompt treatment, the nurse explained that Mrs. S's prognosis could be enhanced, and the overall requirements for physician visits and continued therapy could be minimized. Mrs. S then agreed to call her daughter about this finding and ask her to set up a doctor's appointment.

Susan chose to have her mother be seen by a surgeon who recently had performed breast biopsies on two of her friends. During this initial evaluation, Mrs. S confirmed that she had two mammograms since age 65, the last of which was performed at age 71. She said she had not had a mammogram since because no one told her she had to. She also assumed that because she had been menopausal for more than two decades, the test was not necessary.

Following workup and evaluation, Mrs. S was diagnosed with stage IIA (T1N0M0) infiltrating ductal carcinoma. When all the treatment options were initially discussed with her and her daughter, Mrs. S abruptly stated that she did not care if she lost her breast; she wanted to "get rid of the breast with the cancer." She also said that daily radiation treatments would be too much for her if she needed them and she preferred undergoing a simple mastectomy. This was subsequently scheduled.

Because she lived alone in an assisted living facility, the surgeon recommended an overnight stay following the mastectomy rather than performing the procedure in ambulatory surgery. Shortly after arrival to the inpatient unit, Mrs. S became increasingly agitated, pulling at her dressing, picking at the drains, and calling for Susan. The oncology clinical nurse specialist was asked to evaluate the patient. Along with the staff nurse caring for Mrs. S, they decided that a blood glucose level and pulse oximetry should be performed, that Susan be contacted, and that they needed to determine what recent medications had been given to Mrs. S in the postanesthesia care unit. Ultimately, several reversible etiologies of Mrs. S's acute confusion were identified and subsequently corrected. Her hyperglycemia was corrected by using hospital standing insulin orders; a short postoperative trial of oxygen by cannula improved her mild hypoxia. Susan quickly came to Mrs. S's bedside to decrease her disorientation, and postoperative orders for Demerol® (Sanofi Synthelabo, New York, NY) for pain were discontinued. Additionally, with Susan's assistance, it was determined that Mrs. S's hearing aid was not sent back from the operating room, and without this assistive device, Mrs. S was almost totally deaf. The operating room staff was called, and the hearing aid was found and brought to the unit. With these nursing interventions, Mrs. S's delirium totally subsided within two hours. She had no further cognitive compromise during the night and was discharged the next morning.

Conclusion

It is estimated that in 2005, nearly one-third (32%) of all cancers diagnosed in women will be breast malignancies (Jemal et al., 2005). As the geriatric population grows, the number of breast cancer cases will reach epidemic proportions (Kimmick & Balducci, 2000). The graying of society, the increasing incidence of cancer with age, the high prevalence of breast cancer as a major life-threatening disease, and lifespan projections concerning women outliving their male counterparts all coalesce to portend a novel future. The distinct patient cohort of vulnerable older women at risk for or who are diagnosed with breast cancer should become a priority focus of oncology nursing expertise.

References

Alberg, A.J., & Singh, S. (2001). Epidemiology of breast cancer in older women. *Drugs and Aging, 18,* 761–772.

American Geriatrics Society Ethics Committee. (2003). Health screening decisions for older adults: AGS position paper. *Journal of the American Geriatrics Society, 51,* 270–271.

Arora, A., & Potter, J.F. (2004). Aromatase inhibitors: Current indications and future prospects for treatment of postmenopausal breast cancer. *Journal of the American Geriatrics Society, 52,* 611–616.

Bach, P.B., Schrag, D., Brawley, O.W., Galaznik, A., Yakren, S., Begg, C.B., et al. (2002). Survival of blacks and whites after cancer diagnosis. *JAMA, 287,* 2106–2112.

Baker, S.D., & Grochow, L.B. (1997). Pharmacology of cancer chemotherapy in the older person. *Clinics of Geriatric Medicine, 13,* 169–183.

Balducci, L., Extermann, M., & Carreca, I. (2001). Management of breast cancer in the older woman. *Cancer Control, 8,* 431–441.

Ballantyne, P.J. (2004). Social context and outcomes for the aging breast cancer patient: Considerations for clinical practitioners. *Journal of Clinical Nursing, 13,* 11–21.

Birner, A. (2003). Safe administration of oral chemotherapy. *Clinical Journal of Oncology Nursing, 7,* 158–162.

Blackman, S.B., Lash, T.L., Fink, A.K., Ganz, P.A., & Silliman, R.A. (2002). Advanced age and adjuvant tamoxifen prescription in early-stage breast carcinoma patients. *Cancer, 95,* 2465–2472.

Blair, K.A. (1998). Cancer screening of older women: A primary care issue. *Cancer Practice, 6,* 217–222.

Bouchardy, C., Rapiti, E., Fioretta, G., Laissue, P., Neyroud-Caspar, I., Schafer, P., et al. (2003). Undertreatment strongly decreases prognosis of breast cancer in elderly women. *Journal of Clinical Oncology, 21,* 3580–3587.

Boyle, D.A. (2003a). Cancer in the elderly: Key facts. *Oncology Supportive Care Quarterly, 2*(1), 6–17.

Boyle, D.A. (2003b). Establishing a nursing research agenda in gero-oncology. *Critical Reviews in Oncology/Hematology, 48,* 103–111.

Boyle, D.A. (2004). Commentary on, "Effect of depression on diagnosis, treatment, and survival of older women with breast cancer." (Goodwin, J.S., Zhang, D.D., & Ostir, G.V. *Journal of the American Geriatrics Society, 52,* 106–111, 2004). *Breast Diseases: A Year Book Quarterly, 15,* 370–371.

Boyle, D.A., & Engelking, C. (2003). The evolution and future of breast cancer management. *Oncology Supportive Care Quarterly, 2*(2), 14–25.

Chlebowski, R.T., Chen, Z., Anderson, G.L., Rohan, T., Aragaki, A., Lane, D., et al. (2005). Ethnicity and breast cancer: Factors influencing difference in incidence and outcome. *Journal of the National Cancer Institute, 97,* 439–448.

Chu, K.C., Lamar, C.A., & Freeman, H.P. (2003). Racial disparities in breast carcinoma survival rates. *Cancer, 97,* 2853–2860.

Cimprich, B., Ronis, D.L., & Martinez-Ramos, G. (2002). Age at diagnosis and quality of life in breast cancer survivors. *Cancer Practice, 10,* 85–93.

Clemons, M., Danson, S., & Howell, A. (2002). Tamoxifen (Nolvadex®): A review. *Cancer Treatment Reviews, 28,* 165–180.

Coleman, E.A., Lord, J., Heard, J., Coon, S., Cantrell, M., Mohrmann, C., et al. (2003). The Delta Project: Increasing breast cancer screening among rural minority and older women by targeting rural healthcare providers. *Oncology Nursing Forum, 30,* 669–677.

Coristine, M., Crooks, D., Grunfeld, E., Stonebridge, C., & Christie, A. (2003). Caregiving for women with advanced breast cancer. *Psycho-Oncology, 12,* 709–719.

DeMichele, A., Putt, M., Zhang, Y., Glick, J.H., & Norman, S. (2003). Older age predicts a decline in adjuvant chemotherapy recommendations for patients with breast carcinoma. *Cancer, 97,* 2150–2159.

Di Maio, M., & Perrone, F. (2003). Quality of life in elderly patients with cancer. *Health and Quality of Life Outcomes, 1*(1), 44.

Du, X., & Goodwin, J.S. (2001a). Increase of chemotherapy use in older women with breast carcinoma from 1991 to 1996. *Cancer, 92,* 730–777.

Du, X., & Goodwin, J.S. (2001b). Patterns of use of chemotherapy for breast cancer in older women: Findings from Medicare claims data. *Journal of Clinical Oncology, 19,* 1455–1461.

Dunn, D. (2004). Preventing perioperative complications in an older adult. *Nursing, 34,* 36–41.

Edwards, B.K., Howe, H.L., Ries, L.A., Thun, M.J., Rosenberg, H.M., Yancik, R., et al. (2002). Annual report to the nation on the status of cancer, 1973–1999, featuring implications of age and aging on U.S. cancer burden. *Cancer, 94,* 2766–2792.

Emens, L.A., & Davidson, N.E. (2003). The follow-up of breast cancer. *Seminars in Oncology, 30,* 338–348.

Fargeot, P., Bonneterre, J., Roche, H., Lortholary, A., Campone, M., Van Praagh, I., et al. (2004). Disease-free survival advantage of weekly epirubicin plus tamoxifen versus tamoxifen alone as adjuvant treatment of operable, node-positive, elderly breast cancer patients: 6-year follow-up results of the French adjuvant study group 08 trial. *Journal of Clinical Oncology, 22,* 4622–4630.

Figueiredo, M.I., Cullen, J., Hwang, Y.T., Rowland, J.H., & Mandelblatt, J.S. (2004). Breast cancer treatment in older women: Does getting what you want improve your long-term body image and mental health? *Journal of Clinical Oncology, 22,* 4002–4009.

Frasci, G. (2002). Treatment of breast cancer with chemotherapy in combination with Filgrastim: Approaches to improving therapeutic outcomes. *Drugs, 62,* 17–31.

Fyles, A.W., McCready, D.R., Manchul, L.A., Trudeau, M.E., Merante, P., Pintilie, M., et al. (2004). Tamoxifen with or without breast irradiation in women 50 years of age or older with early breast cancer. *New England Journal of Medicine, 351,* 963–970.

Gagnon, B., Mayo, N.E., Hanley, J., & MacDonald, N. (2004). Pattern of care at the end of life: Does age make a difference in what happens to women with breast cancer? *Journal of Clinical Oncology, 22,* 3458–3465.

Ganz, P.A., Kwan, L., Stanton, A.L., Krupnick, J.L., Rowland, J.H., Meyerowitz, B.E., et al. (2004). Quality of life at the end of primary treatment of breast cancer: First results from the moving beyond cancer randomized trial. *Journal of the National Cancer Institute, 96,* 376–387.

Gennari, R., Curigliano, G., Rotmensz, N., Robertson, C., Colleoni, M., Zurrida, S., et al. (2004). Breast carcinoma in elderly women: Features of disease presentation, choice of local and systemic treatments compared with young postmenopausal patients. *Cancer, 101,* 1302–1310.

Gil, K.M., Mishel, M.H., Belyea, M., Germino, B., Porter, L.S., LaNey, I.C., et al. (2004). Triggers of uncertainty about recurrence and long-term side effects in older African American and Caucasian breast cancer survivors. *Oncology Nursing Forum, 31,* 633–639.

Giordano, S.H., Cohen, D.S., Buzdar, A.U., Parkins, G., & Hortobagyi, G.N. (2004). Breast carcinoma in men. *Cancer, 101,* 51–57.

Given, C.W., Given, B., Azzouz, F., Kozachik, S., & Stommel, M. (2001). Predictors of pain and fatigue in the year following diagnosis among elderly cancer patients. *Journal of Pain and Symptom Management, 21,* 456–466.

Goodwin, J.S., Satish, S., Anderson, E.T., Nattinger, A.B., & Freeman, J.L. (2003). Effect of nurse case management on the treatment of older women with breast cancer. *Journal of the American Geriatrics Society, 51,* 1252–1259.

Goss, P.E., & Strasser, K. (2002). Tamoxifen resistant and refractory breast cancer: The value of aromatase inhibitors. *Drugs, 62,* 957–966.

Green, J.M., & Hacker, E.D. (2004). Chemotherapy in the geriatric population. *Clinical Journal of Oncology Nursing, 8,* 591–597.

Guidry, J.J., Matthews-Juarez, P., & Copeland, V.A. (2003). Barriers to breast cancer control for African-American women: The interdependence of culture and psychosocial issues. *Cancer, 97,* 318–323.

Gulitz, F., Bustillo-Hernandez, M., & Kent, E.B. (1998). Missed screening opportunities among older women: A review. *Cancer Practice, 6,* 289–295.

Harris, E.E., & Solin, L.J. (2000). Treatment of early stage breast cancer in elderly women. *Medical and Pediatric Oncology, 34,* 48–52.

Harrison, R.V., Janz, N.K., Wolfe, R.A., Tedeschi, P.J., Huang, X., & McMahon, L.F. (2003). 5–year mammography rates and associated factors for older women. *Cancer, 97,* 1147–1155.

Hayman, J.A., & Langa, K.M. (2003). Estimating the costs of caring for the older breast cancer patient. *Critical Reviews in Oncology/Hematology, 46,* 255–260.

Henson, E.E., Chu, K.C., & Levine, P.H. (2003). Histologic grade, stage, and survival in breast carcinoma: Comparison of African American and Caucasian women. *Cancer, 98,* 908–917.

Hodgson, N.A., & Given, C.W. (2004). Determinants of functional recovery in older adults surgically treated for cancer. *Cancer Nursing, 27,* 10–16.

Hollingsworth, A.B., Singletary, S.E., Morrow, M., Francescatti, D.S., O'Shaughnessy, J.A., Hartman, A.R., et al. (2004). Current comprehensive assessment and management of women at increased risk for breast cancer. *American Journal of Surgery, 187,* 349–362.

Holmes, C.E., & Muss, H.B. (2003). Diagnosis and treatment of breast cancer in the elderly. *CA: A Cancer Journal for Clinicians, 53,* 227–244.

Howe, H.L., Wingo, P.A., Thun, M.J., Ries, L.A., Rosenberg, H.M., Feigal, E.G., et al. (2001). Annual report to the nation on the status of cancer (1973 through 1998), featuring cancers with recent increasing trends. *Journal of the National Cancer Institute, 93,* 824–842.

Hughes, K.S., Schnaper, L.A., Berry, D., Cirrincione, C., McCormick, B., Shank, B., et al. (2004). Lumpectomy plus Tamoxifen with or without irradiation in women 70 years of age or older with early breast cancer. *New England Journal of Medicine, 351,* 971–977.

Hughes, L.C., Hodgson, N.A., Muller, P., Robinson, L.A., & McCorkle, R. (2000). Information needs of elderly post-surgical cancer patients during the transition from hospital to home. *Journal of Nursing Scholarship, 32,* 25–30.

Hughes, L.C., Robinson, L.A., Cooley, M.E., Nuamah, I., Grobe, S.J., & McCorkle, R. (2002). Describing an episode of home nursing care for elderly post-surgical cancer patients. *Nursing Research, 51,* 110–118.

Jemal, A., Murray, T., Ward, E., Samuels, A., Tiwari, R., Ghafoor, A., et al. (2005). Cancer statistics, 2005. *CA: A Cancer Journal for Clinicians, 55,* 10–30.

Jennings-Sanders, A.J., & Anderson, E.T. (2003). Older women with breast cancer: Perceptions of the effectiveness of nurse case managers. *Nursing Outlook, 51,* 108–114.

Jones, B.A., Kasl, S.V., Howe, C.L., Lachman, M., Dubrown, R., Curnen, M., et al. (2004). African American/White differences in breast carcinoma: p53 alterations and other tumor characteristics. *Cancer, 101,* 1293–1301.

Kagan, S.H. (2004). Gero-oncology nursing research. *Oncology Nursing Forum, 31,* 293–299.

Kantor, D.E., & Houldin, A. (1999). Breast cancer in older women: Treatment, psychosocial effects, intervention and outcomes. *Journal of Gerontological Nursing, 25,* 19–25.

Kimmick, G.G., & Balducci, L. (2000). Breast cancer and aging. *Hematology/Oncology Clinics of North America, 14,* 213–234.

Kimmick, G.G., & Muss, H.B. (2001). Systemic therapy for older women with breast cancer. *Oncology, 15,* 280–292, 295.

Kimmick, G.G., & Muss, H.B. (2004). Breast cancer in older patients. *Seminars in Oncology, 31,* 234–248.

Kurtz, J.E., & Dufour, P. (2002). Strategies for improving quality of life in older patients with metastatic breast cancer. *Drugs and Aging, 19,* 605–622.

Kurtz, M.E., Kurtz, J.C., Stommel, M., Given, C.W., & Given, B. (1999). The influence of symptoms, age, comorbidity and cancer site on physical functioning and mental health of geriatric women patients. *Women and Health, 29,* 1–12.

Lannin, D.R., Matthews, H.F., Mitchell, J., Swanson, M.S., Swanson, F.H., & Edwards, M.S. (1998). Influence of socioeconomic and cultural factors on racial differences in late-stage presentation of breast cancer. *JAMA, 279,* 1801–1807.

Lichtman, S.M. (1998). Recent developments in the pharmacology of anticancer drugs in the elderly. *Current Opinion in Oncology, 10,* 572–579.

Lichtman, S.M. (2004). Chemotherapy in the elderly. *Seminars in Oncology, 31,* 160–174.

Litchtman, S.M., Skirvin, J.A., & Vemulapalli, S. (2003). Pharmacology of antineoplastic agents in older cancer patients. *Critical Reviews in Oncology/Hematology, 46,* 101–114.

Magai, C., Consedine, N., Conway, F., Neugut, A., & Culver, C. (2004). Diversity matters: Unique populations of women and breast cancer screening. *Cancer, 100,* 2300–2307.

Maly, R.C., Leake, B., & Silliman, R.A. (2004). Breast cancer treatment in older women: Impact of the patient-physician interaction. *Journal of the American Geriatrics Society, 52,* 1138–1145.

Mandelblatt, J., Armetta, C., Yabroff, K.R., Liang, W., & Lawrence, W. (2004). Descriptive review of the literature on breast cancer outcomes: 1990 through 2000. *Journal of the National Cancer Institute Monographs, 33,* 8–44.

Mandelblatt, J.S., Kerner, J.F., Hadley, J., Hwang, Y.T., Eggert, L., Johnson, L.E., et al. (2002). Variations in breast carcinoma treatment in older medicare beneficiaries: Is it black or white? *Cancer, 95,* 1401–1414.

Mandelblatt, J.S., Saha, S., Teutsch, S., Hoerger, T., Siu, A.L., Atkins, D., et al. (2003). The cost-effectiveness of screening mammography beyond age 65 years: A systematic review for the U.S. Preventive Services Task Force. *Annals of Internal Medicine, 139,* 835–842.

Mandelblatt, J.S., Schechter, C.B., Yabroff, R., Lawrence, W., Dignam, J., Muennig, P., et al. (2004). Benefits and costs of interventions to improve breast cancer outcomes in African American women. *Journal of Clinical Oncology, 22,* 2554–2566.

Mandelblatt, J.S., & Yabroff, K.R. (2000). Breast and cervical screening for older women: Recommendations and challenges for the 21st century. *Journal of the American Medical Women's Association, 55,* 210–215.

McCorkle, R., Strumpf, N.E., Nuamah, I.F., Adler, D., Cooley, M.E., Jepson, C., et al. (2000). A specialized home care intervention improves survival among older post-surgical cancer patients. *Journal of the American Geriatrics Society, 48,* 1707–1713.

McDonald, S., Saslow, D., & Alciati, M.H. (2004). Performance and reporting of clinical breast examination: A review of the literature. *CA: A Cancer Journal for Clinicians, 54,* 345–361.

McMillan, S.C. (1989). The relationship between age and intensity of cancer-related symptoms. *Oncology Nursing Forum, 16,* 237–241.

Merrill, R.M., & Weed, D.L. (2001). Measuring the public health burden of cancer in the United States through lifetime and age-conditional risk estimates. *Annals of Epidemiology, 11,* 547–553.

Mincey, B.A., & Perez, E.A. (2004). Advances in screening, diagnosis and treatment of breast cancer. *Mayo Clinic Proceedings, 79,* 810–816.

Morrison, C. (1996). Determining crucial correlates of breast self-examination in older women with low incomes. *Oncology Nursing Forum, 23,* 83–93.

Muss, H.B. (2001). Factors used to select adjuvant therapy of breast cancer in the United States: An overview of age, race and socioeconomic status. *Journal of the National Cancer Institute Monographs, 30,* 52–55.

National Comprehensive Cancer Network. (2004). *Breast cancer clinical practice guidelines in oncology.* Retrieved December 14, 2004, from http://www.nccn.com/professionals/physician_gls/PDF/breast.pdf

Newman, L.A. (2004). Breast carcinoma in African-American and White women: Application of molecular biology to understand outcome disparities [Editorial]. *Cancer, 101,* 1261–1263.

Newman, L.A., Theriault, L., Clendinnin, N., Jones, D., & Pierce, L. (2003). Treatment choices and response rates in African-American women with breast carcinoma. *Cancer, 97,* 246–252.

Nikoletti, S., Kristjanson, L.J., Tataryn, D., McPhee, I., & Burt, L. (2003). Information needs and coping styles of primary family caregivers of women following breast cancer surgery. *Oncology Nursing Forum, 30,* 987–996.

Northouse, L.L., Mood, D., Kershaw, T., Schafenacker, A., Mellon, S., Walker, J., et al. (2002). Quality of life of women with recurrent breast cancer and their family members. *Journal of Clinical Oncology, 20,* 4050–4064.

Olmi, P., Cefaro, G.A., Balzi, M., Becciolini, A., & Geinitz, H. (1997). Radiotherapy in the aged. *Clinics in Geriatric Medicine, 13,* 143–168.

Olopade, O.I., Fackenthal, J.D., Dunston, G., Tainsky, M.A., Collins, F., & Whitfield-Broome, C. (2003). Breast cancer genetics in African Americans. *Cancer, 97,* 236–245.

Oncology Nursing Society & Geriatric Oncology Consortium. (2004). *Oncology Nursing Society and Geriatric Oncology Consortium joint position on cancer care in the older adult.* Retrieved April 20, 2005, from http://www.ons.org/publications/positions/Geriatric.shtml

Overcash, J.A. (2004). Using narrative research to understand the quality of life of older women with breast cancer. *Oncology Nursing Forum, 31,* 1153–1159.

Parkin, D.M., Pisani, P., & Ferlay, J. (1999). Global cancer statistics. *CA: A Cancer Journal for Clinicians, 49,* 33–64.

Partridge, A.H., Avorn, J., Wang, P.S., & Winer, E.P. (2002). Adherence to therapy with oral antineoplastic agents. *Journal of the National Cancer Institute, 94,* 652–661.

Peek, M.E. (2003). Screening mammography in the elderly: A review of the issues. *Journal of the American Medical Women's Association, 58,* 191–198.

President's Cancer Panel. (2004). *Living beyond cancer: Finding a new balance* [2003–2004 annual report]. Bethesda, MD: U.S. Department of Health and Human Services, National Institutes of Health, National Cancer Institute.

Repetto, L., Pictropalo, M., & Aapro, M. (2002). Chemotherapy in the elderly with breast cancer. *Forum, 12,* 64–70.

Richardson, L.C. (2004). Treatment of breast cancer in medically underserved women: A review. *Breast Journal, 10,* 2–5.

Sakorafas, G.H. (2003). The management of women at high risk for the development of breast cancer: Risk estimation and preventative strategies. *Cancer Treatment Reviews, 29,* 79–89.

Samain, E., Schauvliege, F., Deval, B., & Marty, J. (2003). Anesthesia for breast cancer surgery in the elderly. *Critical Reviews in Oncology/Hematology, 46,* 115–120.

Sammarco, A. (2003). Quality of life among older survivors of breast cancer. *Cancer Nursing, 26,* 431–438.

Sant, M., Allemani, C., Berrino, F., Coleman, M.P., Aareleid, T., Chaplain, G., et al. (2004). Breast carcinoma survival in Europe and the United States: A population-based study. *Cancer, 100,* 715–722.

Saslow, D., Hannan, J., Osuch, J., Alciati, M.H., Baines, C., Barton, M., et al. (2004). Clinical breast examination: Practical recommendations for optimizing performance and reporting. *CA: A Cancer Journal for Clinicians, 54,* 327–344.

Schairer, C., Mink, P.J., Carroll, L., & Devesa, S.S. (2004). Probabilities of death from breast cancer and other causes among female breast cancer patients. *Journal of the National Cancer Institute, 96,* 1311–1321.

Shavers, V.L., & Brown, M.L. (2002). Racial and ethnic disparities in the receipt of cancer treatment. *Journal of the National Cancer Institute, 94,* 334–357.

Silliman, R.A., Balducci, L., Goodwin, J.S., Holmes, F.F., & Leventhal, E.A. (1993). Breast cancer in old age: What we know, don't know and do. *Journal of the National Cancer Institute, 85,* 190–199.

Singh, R., Hellman, S., & Heimann, R. (2004). The natural history of breast carcinoma in the elderly: Implications for screening and treatment. *Cancer, 100,* 1807–1813.

Singletary, S.E., Allred, C., Ashley, P., Bassett, L.W., Berry, D., Bland, K.I., et al. (2002). Revision of the American Joint Committee on Cancer Staging System for breast cancer. *Journal of Clinical Oncology, 20,* 3628–3636.

Smith, T.J., Davidson, N.E., Schapira, D.V., Grunfeld, E., Muss, H.B., Vogel, V.G., III, et al. (1999). ASCO 1998 update of recommended breast cancer surveillance guidelines. *Journal of Clinical Oncology, 17,* 1080–1082.

Takahashi, P.Y., Okhravi, H.R., Lim, L.S., & Kasten, M.J. (2004). Preventive health care in the elderly population: A guide for practicing physicians. *Mayo Clinic Proceedings, 79,* 416–427.

Underwood, S.M. (2000). Minorities, women, and clinical cancer research: The charge, promise and challenge. *Annals of Epidemiology, 10*(Suppl. 8), S3–S12.

Walter, L.C., & Covinsky, K.E. (2001). Cancer screening in elderly patients: A framework for individualized decision-making. *JAMA, 285,* 2750–2756.

Walter, L.C., Lindquist, K., & Covinsky, K.S. (2004). Relationship between health status and use of screening mammography and Papinicolaou smears among women older than 70 years of age. *Annals of Internal Medicine, 140,* 681–688.

Watts, T., Merrell, J., Murphy, F., & Williams, A. (2004). Breast health information needs of women from minority ethnic groups. *Journal of Advanced Nursing, 47,* 526–535.

Weir, H.K., Thun, M.J., Hankey, B.F., Ries, L.A., Howe, H.L., Wingo, P.A., et al. (2003). Annual report to the nation on the status of cancer, 1975–2000, featuring the uses of surveillance data for cancer prevention and control. *Journal of the National Cancer Institute, 95,* 1276–1299.

Wildiers, H., & Paridaens, R. (2004). Taxanes in elderly breast cancer patients. *Cancer Treatment Reviews, 30,* 333–342.

Williams, B.G., Iredale, R., Brain, K., France, E., Barrett-Lee, P., & Gray, J. (2003). Experiences of men with breast cancer: An exploratory focus group study. *British Journal of Cancer, 89,* 1834–1836.

Wood, R.Y., Duffy, M.E., Morris, S.J., & Carnes, J.E. (2002). The effect of an educational intervention on promoting breast self-examination in older African American and Caucasian women. *Oncology Nursing Forum, 29,* 1081–1090.

Woodard, S., Nadella, P.C., Kotur, L., Wilson, J., Burak, W.E., & Shapiro, C.L. (2003). Older women with breast carcinoma are less likely to receive adjuvant chemotherapy: Evidence of possible age bias. *Cancer, 98,* 1141–1149.

Wyatt, G.K., & Friedman, L.L. (1998). Physical and psychosocial outcomes of midlife and older women following surgery and adjuvant therapy for breast cancer. *Oncology Nursing Forum, 25,* 761–768.

Wyld, L., & Reed, M.W. (2003). The need for targeted research into breast cancer in the elderly. *British Journal of Surgery, 90,* 388–399.

Yancik, R., & Ries L.A. (2000). Aging and cancer in America: Demographic and epidemiologic perspectives. *Hematology/Oncology Clinics of North America, 14,* 213–234.

Yarbrough, S.S. (2004). Older women and breast cancer screening: Research synthesis [Online exclusive]. *Oncology Nursing Forum, 31,* E9–E15.

Zachariah, B., & Balducci, L. (2000). Radiation therapy of the older patient. *Hematology/Oncology Clinics of North America, 14,* 131–167.

Zachariah, B., Balducci, L., Venkattaramanabalaji, G.V., Casey, L., Greenberg, H.M., & Del Regato, J.A. (1997). Radiotherapy for cancer patients aged 80 and older: A study of effectiveness and side effects. *International Journal of Radiation Oncology, Biology, Physics, 39,* 1125–1129.

CHAPTER 8

The Older Adult With Colorectal Cancer

Deborah T. Berg, RN, BSN

Introduction

Colorectal cancer (CRC) is among the most common cancers in the United States. It is the third most common cancer in both men and women (after lung and prostate cancer and lung and breast cancer, respectively). According to American Cancer Society (ACS, 2005) estimates, 145,290 patients will be newly diagnosed, and 56,290 will die because of the disease in 2005. In the past few decades, the incidence initially declined, but the rate of decline recently has slowed or stabilized, whereas mortality rates have continued to decline since 1985 (Weir et al., 2003).

Disparities in outcomes exist when considering special populations such as the older adult or racial and ethnic groups. The trend in the United States is toward an aging population; subsequently, as the populace ages, the absolute number of cancer cases rises because many cancers are age-related diseases. CRC is an age-related disease with an average age at diagnosis of 72 years (National Cancer Institute [NCI], 2000c). More than two-thirds of the U.S. population with CRC is older than 65 (see Figure 8-1) (NCI, 2000a). For men aged 60–80, CRC is the second leading cause of death after lung cancer. In women aged 60–80, CRC is the third leading cause of death after breast and lung cancer. After the age of 80 in men, deaths from CRC drop to third after lung and prostate cancer; whereas in women age 80 or older, CRC becomes second only to lung cancer as the leading cause of death (Jemal et al., 2005). The highest mortality burden is in the group older than 85 years of age. In addition, the incidence and mortality vary considerably among racial groups, with African Americans carrying a disproportionate burden (see Figure 8-2). Although the trend in incidence is stable for men and women as a whole regardless of race, a greater improvement in mortality has been observed in Caucasian men and women than in African American men and women (NCI, 2003). Data also suggest that the

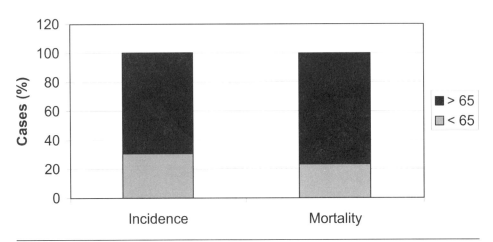

Figure 8-1. Proportion of Colon Cancer Incidence and Mortality, 1996–2000

Note. Based on information from the National Cancer Institute, 2000a.

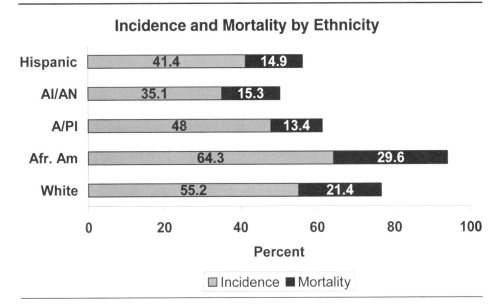

Figure 8-2. Incidence and Mortality by Ethnicity, 1975–2000

AI/AN—American Indian/Alaska Native; Afr. Am—African American; A/PI—Asian/Pacific Islander

Note. Based on information from Ward et al., 2004.

incidence is comparable in patients younger than 65 years versus those 65 years or older, regardless of race; however, mortality is greater in African Americans age 65 years or older, whereas it is comparable between the groups younger than 65, suggesting differences in diagnosis and treatment (Jemal et al., 2004) (see Figure 8-3).

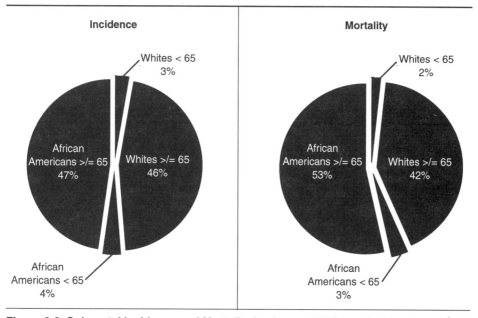

Figure 8-3. Colorectal Incidence and Mortality by Age and White and African American Race, 1975–2000

Note. Based on information from the National Cancer Institute, 2000b.

Risk Factors

The lifetime probability of developing CRC is approximately the same for both men and women at 6% (Jemal et al., 2005). The two major risk factors associated with the development of CRC are increasing age and personal or family history of predisposing diseases of the large intestine. The risk of developing CRC begins to increase after the age of 40 and rises sharply thereafter until it stabilizes around the age of 80 (see Figure 8-4). Personal history of predisposing diseases of the large intestine such as adenomatous polyps, previous history of CRC, inflammatory bowel disease, ulcerative colitis, and Crohn disease all are associated with a higher risk of CRC. Familial factors include a family history of CRC and polyposis syndromes. Hereditary nonpolyposis colorectal cancer (HNPCC), familial adenomatous polyposis (FAP), and the APC gene alteration—*APC I1307K* mutation—noted in Ashkenazi Jews of European descent are the common familial polyposis syndromes. Familial syndromes are rare and often are associated with diagnosis of CRC at a younger than expected age. For those with the genetic predisposition, the probability of developing CRC is high (70% risk in those with FAP, 100% risk in those with HNPCC, and 10%–20% risk in those with *APC I1307K*) (Berg, 2003). A family history of CRC without familial

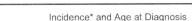

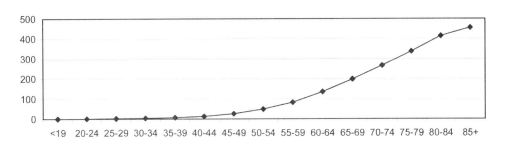

*Incidence rates are per 100,000 people

Figure 8-4. Incidence and Age at Diagnosis, 1975–2000

Note. Based on information from the National Cancer Institute, 2000b.

polyposis syndromes also increases an individual's risk of developing CRC (6% risk with one first-degree relative [parent, sibling, child] with CRC as compared to a 2% risk with a negative family history) (Fuchs et al., 1994).

Other risk factors are behavioral, nutritional, and environmental in nature. A high-fat, low-fiber, high-calorie diet; alcohol consumption; cigarette smoking; obesity, sedentary lifestyle; and anal intercourse and genital warts (for rectal cancer) all are implicated in the development of CRC (Byers et al., 2002). In the United States, the prevalence of these risk factors has increased, but the impact this trend will have on CRC incidence and mortality is unclear. Approximately 70% of cases of CRC are believed to be sporadic, 15%–25% are associated with a positive family history of CRC, and the remaining 5% are considered to be related to a familial mutation syndrome (Berg, 2003).

Pathophysiology

CRC is one cancer where a better understanding exists of the natural history, biologic features, and many of the genetic abnormalities. Normally, a balanced cycle of cellular division, proliferation, differentiation, and death of colonic epithelial cells occurs. Any disruption in this balance can result in overproliferation of cells or lack of cellular death, leading to the development of an adenomatous polyp. Polyps are prevalent in the general population; however, they are more common with increasing age, with those older than 50 at higher risk. People who eat a lot of fatty foods, smoke, drink alcohol, lack exercise, are overweight, and have a personal or family history of polyps also are more likely to produce polyps. Without intervention, the benign polyp continues to slowly enlarge, and genetic mutations accumulate over time. The benign cells may transform into cancerous cells and eventually begin to invade into the colonic wall and metastasize. Age is associated with cumulative damage to DNA and a decline in immune surveillance, making it easier for cells to become cancerous, proliferate, and survive. On average, this process takes approximately 10 years, which is why CRC is more prevalent in older adults because polyps have time to transform into cancerous tumors.

Histologic Types

Two main histologic types of CRC exist. Adenocarcinoma is the most common type, accounting for 90% of all tumors. Mucinous carcinomas are more common in younger patients and account for approximately 10% of all tumors. The remaining histologic types—signet-ring cell, squamous cell, small cell, carcinoid, adenosquamous, lymphoma, sarcoma, and melanoma—are infrequent. CRC can develop in any segment of the colon and rectum, with the majority of cases occurring in either the proximal or distal colon (Berg, 2003). Unique tumor characteristics exist depending on specific location of the tumor within the colon. Tumors in the right colon are more often ulcerative, necrotic, well differentiated, genetically stable, and carry a better prognosis (Curtas, 1999; DeVita, Hellman, & Rosenberg, 2001; Goldberg, 2000). DNA microsatellite instability (MSI) is primarily found in tumors in the right colon. MSI-positive tumors demonstrate a better response to adjuvant chemotherapy and a good prognosis (Prabhudesai & Kumar, 2002). Tumors in the left colon, especially in the distal colon and rectum, have similar molecular and clinical features (Prabhudesai & Kumar). These tumors tend to infiltrate the bowel wall, show more genetic instability, including *p53* mutations, and in general carry a poorer prognosis (Curtas; DeVita et al.; Goldberg; Prabhudesai & Kumar).

Tumors in the Older Adult

The older patient with CRC tends to have tumors that generally are well differentiated, are located in the proximal colon (especially in patients 85 years old or older), have a more indolent growth pattern with more frequent apoptosis, and are less aggressive (Kemppainen, Raiha, Rajala, & Sourander, 1993; Tanaka et al., 2002).

The patterns of metastasis and disease failure are distinct between colon and rectal cancers as a result of their anatomic location within the abdomen and their respective venous circulation. Colon tumors sit high in the abdomen, the circulation drains into the portal system, and the liver is the most common site of metastasis. Rectal tumors sit low in the pelvis, the circulation drains by way of the inferior vena cava, and the lungs are the most common site of distant metastasis. In addition, because of the same anatomic reasons, rectal tumors are more likely to recur in locoregional lymph nodes, whereas colon tumors often recur at a distant site. These differences in patterns of metastasis and disease failure dictate treatment strategies (Berg, 2004).

Clinical Presentation

CRC can be present without symptoms until the disease is well advanced, thereby causing disruption in the flow of stool or organ dysfunction from metastatic disease. General signs and symptoms commonly associated with CRC are blood in or on stool; bleeding from the rectum; stomach pains, cramps, or aches; change in bowel habits; weight loss; tenesmus; or anorexia and fatigue. Signs and symptoms vary depending on the location of the tumor within the colon and are similar in the older adult as compared with the patient population as a whole. Because the older adult often presents with a right-sided lesion, the most common presentation could include vague abdominal pain, palpable abdominal mass, melena, anemia, weight loss, anorexia, and potential bowel perforation and obstruction (Berg, 2003; Enzinger & Mayer, 2004).

Diagnostic Evaluation

Symptoms or suspicion of CRC will instigate a complete workup, including a medical history and physical examination with a focus on the abdominopelvic area. The tests used for CRC diagnosis are flexible sigmoidoscopy, colonoscopy, and double-contrast barium enema. Colonic examination with biopsy of suspicious lesions is necessary to determine if cancer is present and to determine the exact location of disease. Once the cancer diagnosis is confirmed, diagnostic imaging such as chest x-ray, computed tomography of the abdomen and pelvis, and transrectal ultrasound (for rectal tumors) is performed to determine the extent of disease; magnetic resonance imaging and positron emission tomography are optional. General blood tests identify anemia and liver dysfunction, if present. Carcinoembryonic antigen (CEA) and CA 19-9 levels often are elevated in CRC and may have prognostic value at diagnosis or disease recurrence, although they are not useful screening tools.

Staging

The stage of disease at the time of diagnosis is the most important prognostic factor and thus has implications for both therapeutic strategies and long-term outcome. CRC staging is based on three key elements: depth of tumor penetration through the bowel wall, lymph node involvement (including number of positive lymph nodes), and presence or absence of distant metastases. The Duke's and American Joint Committee on Cancer's (AJCC's) staging systems are well-known staging schemas; both describe the spread of the tumor through the bowel wall. The Duke's system was the original system and is based only on tumor penetration and lymph node involvement. The AJCC tumor-node-metastasis system is internationally accepted, provides the most prognostic detail, and therefore is the recommended staging system (see Figure 8-5). Additional factors that, along with staging, influence outcome are well or moderately differentiated tumor and MSI (both denoting good outcome), whereas poorly differentiated tumors, lymphatic or vascular invasion, regional lymph node metastasis, obstruction or perforation at diagnosis, and specific genetic abnormalities (e.g., *p53* mutations) predict a poor outcome. Age, gender, site of disease, perineural invasion, thymidylate synthetase expression, and preoperative CEA level have not yet impacted outcome but may be proved in the future to be associated either with prognosis or response to therapy independent of stage (Ellenhorn, Coia, Alberts, & Hoff, 2002; Goldberg, 2000; Greene et al., 2002).

The stage of disease at the time of diagnosis clearly has an impact on long-term outcome. Usually, the five-year survival rate for early localized disease, that which is confined only within the colon or rectum, is 90%; whereas if the disease is more advanced, the outcome is not as good. The survival rate is 67% for regional disease (tumor that has spread to regional lymph nodes) and 10% if metastatic disease is present at the time of diagnosis (Jemal et al., 2005). Unfortunately, 39% of individuals present with localized disease, 38% present with regional disease, 19% present with metastatic disease, and 5% are unstaged at diagnosis (Jemal et al., 2005; NCI, 2000b). All racial groups present with a similar stage of disease, except African Americans, who are more likely than any other group to present with metastatic disease (Ward et al., 2004). African Americans also are less likely to survive five years after diagnosis (55%), as compared to the population as a whole (63%) and

TNM Definitions

Primary tumor (T)
- TX: Primary tumor cannot be assessed
- T0: No evidence of primary tumor
- Tis: Carcinoma in situ: intraepithelial or invasion of the lamina propria*
- T1: Tumor invades submucosa
- T2: Tumor invades muscularis propria
- T3: Tumor invades through the muscularis propria into the subserosa or into nonperitonealized pericolic or perirectal tissues
- T4: Tumor directly invades other organs or structures, and/or perforates visceral peritoneum**,***

Regional lymph nodes (N)
- NX: Regional nodes cannot be assessed
- N0: No regional lymph node metastasis
- N1: Metastasis in 1 to 3 regional lymph nodes
- N2: Metastasis in 4 or more regional lymph nodes

Distant metastasis (M)
- MX: Distant metastasis cannot be assessed
- M0: No distant metastasis
- M1: Distant metastasis

American Joint Committee on Cancer stage groupings
Stage 0
- Tis, N0, M0
Stage I
- T1, N0, M0
- T2, N0, M0
Stage IIA
- T3, N0, M0
Stage IIB
- T4, N0, M0
Stage IIIA
- T1, N1, M0
- T2, N1, M0
Stage IIIB
- T3, N1, M0
- 4, N1, M0
Stage IIIC
- Any T, N2, M0
Stage IV
- Any T, any N, M1

Figure 8-5. Colon Cancer Staging

* *Note:* Tis includes cancer cells confined within the glandular basement membrane (intraepithelial) or lamina propria (intramucosal) with no extension through the muscularis mucosae into the submucosa.

** *Note:* Direct invasion in T4 includes invasion of other segments of the colorectum by way of the serosa, for example, invasion of the sigmoid colon by a carcinoma of the cecum.

*** *Note:* Tumor that is adherent macroscopically to other organs or structures is classified T4. If no tumor is present in the adhesion microscopically, however, the classification should be pT3. The V and L substaging should be used to identify the presence or absence of vascular or lymphatic invasion.

Note. Data from "Colon Cancer Treatment," by the National Cancer Institute, 2004. Retrieved July 8, 2004, from http://www.nci.nih.gov/cancertopics/pdq/treatment/colon/HealthProfessionals

Caucasians in particular (64%) (Jemal et al., 2005). Although conflicting data exist, CRC in the older adult tends to be more advanced at the time of diagnosis as compared to younger patients (Enzinger & Mayer, 2004; Kemeny, Busch-Devereaux, Merriam, & O'Hea, 2000; Kemppainen et al., 1993). The probability of living five years after diagnosis is generally similar when considering age; individuals younger than 65 have a 64% chance of living five years, whereas those 65 years and older have a 62% chance. However, a significant difference exists in five-year survival between the younger old (65–74 years) and the older old (75+ years) where the likelihood of survival is 64% versus 59%, respectively (NCI, 2000b). More advanced stage of disease and additional comorbid diseases most certainly contribute to the poorer outcome in the older adult.

Treatment

Prevention by Behavior Modification

The development of CRC may be reduced through surgical and behavioral interventions. For the last two decades, research has demonstrated that personal choices affect health outcomes even with such diseases as cancer. ACS supports behavior modification to decrease the likelihood of CRC development; eating a diet with plenty of fruits, vegetables, and whole grains and low in animal fat, drinking alcohol in moderation, quitting smoking, maintaining a healthy weight, and participating in 30 minutes of physical activity at least five times each week all are recommended (Byers et al., 2002). Research suggests that regular use of aspirin, nonsteroidal anti-inflammatory drugs (NSAIDs) (observational data), and the cyclooxygenase-inhibitor celecoxib (phase III randomized, double-blind, placebo-controlled clinical trial data) may reduce polyp formation and, consequently, the risk of CRC development (Enzinger & Mayer, 2004; Steinbeck et al., 2000). Other studies also support folic acid and calcium intake as beneficial in CRC prevention (Enzinger & Mayer). The benefit of these measures in the older adult is not known because the data are relatively recent, and such interventions likely need to be initiated early in life and maintained for many years. It can be theorized that for current older adults, the possible benefit may be derived only if they initiated these measures in their younger years. However, many adults now take aspirin to prevent coronary artery disease or NSAIDs to treat rheumatoid arthritis; therefore, older adults of the future may benefit from these interventions.

Several measures are either not effective or still controversial in CRC prevention. Increased fiber in the diet is not supported by current research, but this is still controversial (Ellenhorn, Cullinane, Coia, Alberts, & Alberts, 2004). The American Gastroenterological Association (2000) believes it is prudent to recommend high intake of dietary fiber even though sufficient scientific evidence is lacking. The antioxidants carotene, vitamin C, and vitamin E are not effective at protecting against CRC. Estrogen hormone replacement therapy in postmenopausal women may reduce the risk of CRC but carries increased risk for breast and uterine cancers, coronary artery disease, and stroke (Women's Health Initiative Investigators, 2002). State-of-the-art research is ongoing in an attempt to provide the public with evidence-based answers on how to prevent CRC (Berg, 2003).

Prevention by Surgical Excision

The natural history of CRC makes it conducive to prevention and early detection, which is crucial to improvement in survival, especially in the older adult. Preemptive excision of adenomatous polyps can reduce the likelihood of CRC development by eliminating the precursor lesion, thereby breaking the benign polyp to cancerous tumor transformation. Once the polyp is removed, CRC does not develop. Some special factors must be taken into account when caring for the older adult seeking early detection tests. Tumors in the older adult often are found in the proximal colon and therefore would be missed by a flexible sigmoidoscopy (Kemppainen et al., 1993). The patient's life expectancy also must be taken into consideration; hence, if the patient's life expectancy is at least another five to seven or more years, then it would be appropriate to test the patient for CRC, and the potential risks and benefits should be discussed.

The currently recognized schedule for CRC screening and early detection is based on risk and is outlined in Figure 8-6. The reader is referred to the National Comprehensive Cancer Network (NCCN) colorectal screening guidelines for further information (NCCN, 2005b). Medicare participants age 50 and older are eligible for CRC screening and early detection benefits, including colonoscopy screening for the average risk patient (Centers for Disease Control and Prevention [CDC], 2003a) (see Table 8-1 for Medicare benefit parameters). The increased acceptance of lower endoscopy, particularly colonoscopy, for CRC screening and early detection will greatly benefit the older adult who has a higher incidence of proximal lesions (see Figure 8-7) (CDC, 2003b, 2004a). Several initiatives are under way to improve the CRC screening and early detection rates, including the CDC funding of state screening projects and national education programs such as "Screen for Life" and "Call to Action: Prevention and Early Detection of CRC," which are for the public and healthcare providers, respectively (CDC, 2004b). In addition, the CDC has

---

Beginning at age 50, both men and women of average risk should undergo one or a combination of the following screening options.
- Annual home fecal occult blood test (FOBT)*
- Flexible sigmoidoscopy every five years*
- Annual FOBT plus flexible sigmoidoscopy every five years*‡
- Double-contrast barium enema every five years*
- Total colon examination by colonoscopy every 10 years

People with increased risk should begin colorectal cancer screening earlier and/or should undergo screening more often. Genetic counseling and testing also should be considered. People at increased risk include those with a
- Personal history of colorectal cancer or adenomatous polyps
- Strong family history of colorectal cancer or polyps
- Personal history of chronic inflammatory bowel disease, ulcerative colitis, or Crohn disease
- History of familial polyposis syndromes (familial adenomatous polyposis and hereditary nonpolyposis colorectal cancer).

Figure 8-6. Recommendations for Early Detection of Colorectal Cancer

---

*All positive results should be followed up with colonoscopy.
‡ American Cancer Society recommends this option.

Note. Based on information from the American Cancer Society, 2001.

Table 8-1. Colorectal Cancer Screening Tests and Medicare

Test	Medicare Coverage
Fecal occult blood test	• Yearly with no fee to patient
Flexible sigmoidoscopy	• Every four years • Patient pays 20% of approved amount after Part B deductible.*
Colonoscopy	• No age limit • Every 10 years if not at high risk but not within 4 years of a screening flexible sigmoidoscopy unless used as a follow-up test for abnormal finding. • Every two years if at high risk • Patient pays 20% of approved amount after Part B deductible.*
Double-contrast barium enema	• As a substitute for flexible sigmoidoscopy or colonoscopy • Every four years if patient is not at high risk • Every two years if patient is at high risk • Patient pays 20% of approved amount after Part B deductible.

* If flexible sigmoidoscopy or colonoscopy is performed in ambulatory surgical or hospital outpatient department, patient pays 25% of approved amount after Part B deductible.

Note. Based on information from Centers for Disease Control and Prevention, 2003a.

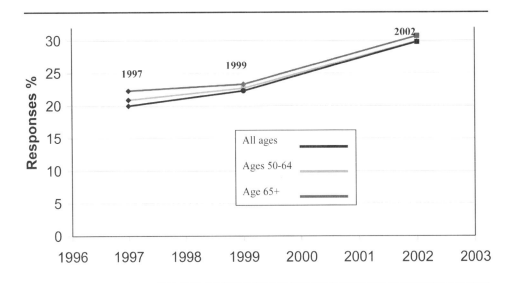

Figure 8-7. Prevalence of Sigmoidoscopy or Colonoscopy 1997–2002

Note. Based on information from Centers for Disease Control and Prevention, 2004a.

supported a new measure on the Health Plan Employer Data and Information Set that will assess whether adults aged 50–80 have been appropriately screened for CRC (CDC, 2004b).

Therapeutic Strategies

All patients with cancer, especially older adults, require individualized treatment strategies. The goals of treatment are highly personal, and the patients are extremely heterogeneous. For example, a big difference exists between an active, healthy 80-year-old and an inactive, chronically ill 70-year-old, although both would be labeled older or elderly. In the older adult, providers should not base treatment decisions solely on chronologic age because older adults have much more physiologic variability than younger patients, even when compared to those at the same chronologic age. The picture a provider has of what age 75 is like may not be reality in the patient sitting before him or her. Wide differences exist in organ function, types and number of comorbid illnesses, functional and cognitive status, and life expectancy.

Pattern of Undertreatment

In the United States, older adults often are undertreated either by receiving no treatment or by being offered less aggressive or inadequate treatment (Balducci, 2003). Clinicians often exclude treatment options because of a patient's age as a way to protect him or her from toxicity or by deciding the patient could not tolerate the treatment anyway. It is a myth that older patients cannot tolerate standard therapy. The reality is that outcomes are predicted by comorbidities and functional status, not age; efficacy is equal in the healthy older adult as compared with the younger adult; and healthy older patients tolerate therapy as well as younger patients, although attention and proactive supportive care may be required (Balducci, 2001). Therefore, healthcare providers should give older patients all the options, even if they ultimately choose not to participate or accept the treatment strategy. Provider bias based on chronologic age rather than physiologic age and the lack of clear treatment guidelines regarding benefits for older adults are problems. Limited research data are available to support recommendations because most trials historically included limited numbers of older adults, and those with comorbidities often were excluded. NCCN recommended using screening tests and established geriatric assessment tools to evaluate all patients ≥ 70 years in an effort to identify problems that may interfere with cancer treatment, hence increasing the delivery of optimal treatments and promoting a standard of care (see Table 8-2). See the NCCN senior adult oncology guidelines for more details (NCCN, 2005e). Consistent utilization of such tools, it is hoped, will assist in decision making about therapy and eradicate the fact that older patients are staged less and treated less aggressively or with substandard regimens.

Surgery

Initial Management

The initial treatment of choice for the primary management of CRC is surgery. The involved segment of the large intestine with disease-free margins (both radial

Table 8-2. Highlights of a Comprehensive Clinical Geriatric Assessment

Goals of Assessment	Three Stages of Aging
1. Discover problems that may compromise safety and efficacy of treatment; assess risk/benefit balance. 2. Identify potentially treatable conditions. 3. Determine functional reserve. 4. Estimate life expectancy. 5. Identify common language to classify older adults.	1. Functionally independent without comorbidity; candidates for standard therapy 2. Some dependence or comorbidity; candidates for dose reduction of therapy initially followed by later dose escalation based on tolerance 3. Frail; candidate for palliative therapy

Factor	Evaluating
Functional	Degree of independence; activity of daily living (Eastern Cooperative Oncology Group and Karnofsky performance scales have limited utility in elderly.)
Physical	Number and severity of chronic conditions; comorbidity (cardiovascular, respiratory, renal, and hepatic)
Mental	Memory; orientation; comprehension; logical thinking; ability to participate/comply
Emotional	Depression; reversibility with proper intervention
Polypharmacotherapy	Establish all medication usage—over-the-counter and prescription; number, appropriateness, and possible interactions
Socioeconomic	Caregiver adequacy; family support; insurance coverage; housing condition; transportation resources
Nutrition	Corrective problem?
Geriatric syndromes	Dementia; delirium; severe depression; frequent falls ($\geq$ 3 per month); neglect; abuse; spontaneous fractures; fecal incontinence; failure to thrive; frailty (subjective criteria by consensus versus formal definition)
Life expectancy	Gross estimate of typical longevity under prevailing or predicted circumstances

Note. Based on information from Balducci & Extermann, 2000; National Comprehensive Cancer Network, 2005e.

and distal), the surrounding mesentery, and the adjacent lymph nodes all are excised either by open or laparoscopic intestinal resection. An open colectomy is the standard technique because outcome results for the laparoscopic approach still are pending (NCCN, 2005a). The specific surgical procedure depends on whether the tumor is within the colon or rectum, because at premetastatic stages, colon and rectal cancers are very individual diseases and dictate different treatment approaches. Colon cancer has few surgical limitations with a low risk of local recurrence. The rectum is located low in the pelvis; therefore, important surgical limitations exist along with a high risk of local recurrence. The standard surgical procedure for colon cancer is a partial colectomy with an end-to-end anastomosis, with the exact segment excised varying depending on the specific location of the tumor within the colon and the clinical stage of disease (see Table 8-3). The standard procedure for rectal tumors is a low anterior resection with complete excision of the mesorectum, a 2 cm disease-free distal margin, and a coloanal anastomosis. Few permanent colostomies are required today, in part, because of new diagnostic technologies and improved sphincter-sparing surgical techniques. A temporary diverting colostomy still may be used to allow for healing of an intestinal segment. However, upon successful healing, this is reversed, allowing for normal bowel flow. The goal of surgical therapy may be for cure, disease control, or palliation. If the disease is localized at the time of diagnosis, surgery may be curative. If lymph node involvement or regional disease is present, surgery plus adjuvant therapy is required to increase the chance of cure. Finally, surgery may be performed for palliative intent (i.e., reduction of tumor burden, pain relief, and bleeding control).

Table 8-3. Colon and Rectal Cancer: Surgical Procedures

Tumor Location	Procedure
Cecum, ascending, hepatic flexure, or transverse colon	Right or extended right hemicolectomy
Middle or left transverse colon	Transverse or extended right colectomy
Splenic flexure or descending colon	Left hemicolectomy
Sigmoid	Low anterior resection
Middle or upper rectum	Low anterior resection with mesorectal excision
Middle or distal rectum	Low anterior resection with total mesorectal excision or sphincter-sparing approach
Lower/distal rectum	Abdominoperineal resection or sphincter-sparing approach

Note. Based on information from Ellis & Hubbard, 2000.

Research Studies

Assuming older adults are susceptible to postoperative complications, they may stay in the hospital longer and be at increased risk for loss of independence postoperatively. Stocchi, Nelson, Young-Fadok, Larson, and Ilstrup (2000) studied complication rates and benefits of laparoscopic-assisted patients versus patients with open colectomy in those older than age 75. Forty-four patients older than 75 were included in this study; 21 underwent laparoscopy, and 23 underwent open colectomy. The aim of the study was to determine rates of complications compared with the benefits of each approach in the older adult. The laparoscopic approach was associated with fewer postoperative complications, shorter hospitalization, reduced pain and narcotic use, earlier return of bowel function, earlier resumption of diet, quicker convalescence, and preservation of postoperative independence in the older adult when compared to open colectomy (Stocchi et al.). The short-term benefits and adequacy of laparoscopic colon resection are clear, but survival benefits and frequency of recurrence still must be established in the older adult. The Clinical Outcomes of Surgical Therapy Study Group (2004) recently reported that the rates of recurrence and overall survival at three years were very similar between those undergoing a laparoscopic colectomy and those undergoing a standard open colectomy. This study randomly assigned 872 patients with adenocarcinoma of the colon to either an open colectomy or a laparoscopically assisted surgical technique. The primary end point of this study was tumor recurrence. The results of this study suggest that the laparoscopic approach is an acceptable alternative to the standard surgical technique (Clinical Outcomes of Surgical Therapy Study Group).

Morbidity and Mortality

Advanced chronologic age is not a sole contraindication to surgery. Mortality does not increase dramatically with age, even up to age 100 for elective surgery (Balducci, 2000). However, mortality is greater in the older adult undergoing emergency surgery. This factor can be a concern because the older adult with CRC has a greater likelihood of an acute presentation secondary to obstruction or perforation (Balducci, 2000; Enzinger & Mayer, 2004). The decision as to whether a patient is a surgical candidate is made based upon the patient's health status using the American Society of Anesthesiology's (ASA's) physical status score and the known extent of tumor burden. ASA's physical status score is used to stratify operative patients by risk, prompting clinicians to consider comorbid conditions, functional abilities, and risks of the surgical procedure. In this score, advanced age is considered a minor clinical predictor, whereas physical functional status is given more weight, signifying that chronologic age is less important than the type, severity, and number of comorbid medical problems (see Figure 8-8 for a listing of common comorbid conditions and Figure 8-9 for an outline of preoperative assessments and postoperative complications). Many older patients who are deemed surgical candidates are not referred to oncologists for postoperative therapy because of the belief that they are too old to tolerate it, yet they were healthy enough to undergo surgery (Schrag, Cramer, Bach, & Begg, 2001).

- Chronic pulmonary disease (obstructive or restrictive)
- Diabetes mellitus
- Renal insufficiency
- Hepatic insufficiency
- Depression
- Peripheral neuropathy
- Cardiovascular disease (atherosclerotic heart disease, congestive heart failure, valvular heart disease, cerebrovascular disease)
- Hypertension
- Benign prostatic hypertrophy
- Immune suppression
- Arthritis
- Coexisting malignancies

Figure 8-8. Common Comorbid Conditions

Note. Based on information from Repetto, 2003.

Preoperative Assessments
- History, physical, medical chart review
- Laboratory testing (dictated by comorbid conditions and specific surgical procedure)
- Cognitive assessment
- Cardiovascular evaluation
- Pulmonary assessment
- Functional capacity
- Prior surgery (complications)
- Understand medication usage.
- Miscellaneous (e.g., anorexic, dehydrated, frail)
- Education related to safety of anesthesia

Possible Postoperative Complications
- Infection: wound, intra-abdominal abscess, urinary, pulmonary
- Pain
- Fluid and electrolyte imbalance
- Anastomotic leak
- Poor wound healing
- Abdominal distention
- Impaired bowel function/paralytic ileus
- Bleeding or clotting disorders
- Urinary retention/neurogenic bladder
- Impotence/sexual dysfunction
- Cognitive decline (e.g., acute delirium, persistent cognitive decline)

Figure 8-9. Preoperative Assessments and Possible Postoperative Complications

Radiation Therapy

Rectal Cancer

Because of the high risk of local recurrence and the low risk of distant metastasis, radiation therapy (RT) is an important therapeutic modality in the treatment of rectal cancers. RT may be given either pre- or postoperatively, alone or in combination with chemotherapy. Preoperative RT often is administered to shrink tumors, allowing for a better surgical outcome. Postoperative RT given along with chemotherapy decreases the frequency of disease recurrence and improves survival better than RT or surgery alone. Ongoing clinical trials are trying to answer which chemotherapy combination is best and what is the best sequence of RT plus chemotherapy. Currently, RT at doses of 45–55 gray (Gy) plus 5-fluorouracil (5-FU)-based chemotherapy given as a continuous infusion is recommended. Clinical trials are investigating replacing the continuous-infusion 5-FU with capecitabine (Xeloda®, Roche Laboratories, Nutley, NJ), as well as adding novel agents such as oxaliplatin (Eloxatin®, Sanofi-Synthelabo, New York, NY), irinotecan (Camptosar®, Pfizer, New York, NY), and bevacizumab (Avastin®, Genentech, Inc., South San Francisco, CA) to the chemotherapy regimen.

Colon Cancer

In colon cancer, RT has limited value because of possible damage to adjacent organs and the small intestine. However, postoperative chemotherapy with radiation may benefit patients with T3 tumors with localized perforation or positive margins or patients with T4, N0 colon cancer (NCCN, 2005a). Researchers have documented that older adults tolerate standard RT as well as younger patients, although they may have more radiation enteritis. The safety and efficacy of hyperfractionation radiation techniques have not yet been demonstrated (Balducci, 2000; Enzinger & Mayer, 2004) (see Table 8-4 for RT side effects). Unfortunately, older adults are referred to oncologists less often for postoperative adjuvant therapy (Enzinger & Mayer). In all patients, including the older adult, RT also has palliative benefits as a means to control pain, treat bowel obstruction, control bleeding, and preserve organ function, which may avert ostomy placement.

Table 8-4. Radiation Therapy Side Effects

Side Effect	Acute Presentation	Chronic Toxicity
Skin reactions	Local reactions: erythema, desquamation (dry or moist), hyperpigmentation	Hyper- or hypopigmentation changes, fibrosis, telangiectasias, scrotal tenderness and irritation
Diarrhea	With or without cramping, urgency, incontinence, mucous or bloody discharge, tenesmus	Incontinence, small bowel obstruction, fibrosis, adhesions, fistulas
Myelosuppression	Anemia, thrombocytopenia, leukopenia	Hypoplasia
Proctitis	Frequent or continuous sensation to have a bowel movement, constipation, a feeling of rectal fullness, left-sided abdominal pain, passage of mucus through the rectum, rectal bleeding, and anorectal pain may occur.	–
Fibrosis	–	Colonic, rectum, vagina
Atrophy	–	Bladder, vagina
Cystitis	Frequency, dysuria, urgency, urinary tract infection	Rare, bladder ulceration and bleeding
Fatigue	Begins second to third week of treatment, peaks near completion	–
Organ or sexual dysfunction	Vaginal dryness, vaginitis, hot flashes	Impotence, vaginal stenosis

Note. Based on information from Gosselin, 2001.

Chemotherapy and Biotherapy

Chemotherapy for the treatment of CRC is an area of active investigation. For years, the only active agent was 5-FU, but now several new chemotherapy agents and novel molecularly targeted agents are available that have demonstrated clinical advances in efficacy. The recommendations in this chapter are based on the regimens approved by the U.S. Food and Drug Administration (FDA) and guidelines published by NCCN (2005a) (see Table 8-5).

Table 8-5. U.S. Food and Drug Administration's and National Comprehensive Cancer Network's Recommended Regimens for Metastatic Colorectal Cancer (CRC)

Chemotherapy Regimen	Recommended First-Line Metastatic CRC	Recommended Second-Line Metastatic CRC
5-FU and leucovorin (bolus)	National Comprehensive Cancer Network (NCCN) recommended if patient cannot tolerate intensive therapy and has received no adjuvant therapy or relapsed for more than six months after adjuvant therapy	–
5-FU and leucovorin (infusional)	NCCN recommended if patient cannot tolerate intensive therapy and has received no adjuvant therapy or relapsed for more than six months after adjuvant therapy	–
Irinotecan + bolus 5-FU and leucovorin (IFL)	U.S. Food and Drug Administration (FDA) approved	–
Irinotecan + infusional 5-FU and leucovorin (FOLFIRI)	FDA approved NCCN recommended	NCCN option for patients who failed bevacizumab +/–5-FU/ leucovorin or FOLFOX
Oxaliplatin + infusional 5-FU and leucovorin (FOLFOX)	FDA approved NCCN recommended	FDA approved NCCN option for patients who failed FOLFIRI
Bevacizumab + IV 5-FU–based chemotherapy	FDA approved NCCN recommended	–
Capecitabine	FDA approved for patients in whom 5-FU therapy alone is preferred NCCN recommended if patient cannot tolerate intensive therapy; combination therapy not recommended pending phase III data	–
Cetuximab alone or with irinotecan	–	FDA approved NCCN recommended alone if intolerant to irinotecan or with irinotecan if refractory to irinotecan-based chemotherapy and FOLFOX
Irinotecan	–	FDA approved NCCN option if patient failed 5-FU/leucovorin or FOLFOX +/–bevacizumab

Note. Based on information from Genentech, Inc., 2004; Imclone Systems Inc. & Bristol-Myers Squibb, 2004; National Comprehensive Cancer Network, 2005a; Pfizer Inc., 2005; Roche Pharmaceuticals, 2003; Sanofi-Synthelabo Inc., 2005.

Chemotherapy and Biologics: Adjuvant

Stage II Colon Cancer

Adjuvant chemotherapy is not standard for stage II disease because, to date, it has not demonstrated a survival advantage compared to surgery alone. In spite of this, patients with lesions that are nonmetastatic but have invaded through the muscle into the subserosa (T3) and have other factors suggesting a high risk for systemic recurrence, such as poorly or undifferentiated lesions, lymphatic or vascular invasion, or bowel obstruction, may be considered for adjuvant therapy (NCCN, 2005a). Healthcare providers also may consider adjuvant chemotherapy plus RT for patients with T3 lesions with localized perforation or close or positive surgical margins or tumors that have directly invaded adjacent organs (T4) without positive lymph nodes (NCCN, 2005a). Researchers have investigated biologic therapies but with poor results thus far in stage II colon cancer. A new approach is to design clinical trials that will prospectively evaluate molecular genetic markers (e.g., MSI that may help to target specific patients for whom the treatment will work) (Berg, 2003).

Stage III Colon Cancer

Adjuvant chemotherapy given after surgery has been recommended for stage III colon cancer since the 1990s. 5-FU plus leucovorin is the standard regimen. However, a new combination of 5-FU, leucovorin, and oxaliplatin (FOLFOX) has been shown to delay disease recurrence better than 5-FU plus leucovorin alone, but its effect on overall survival is unknown (Hickish et al., 2004; Sanofi-Synthelabo, 2005). The combination of bolus irinotecan, 5-FU, and leucovorin (IFL) should not be used in the adjuvant setting. Data are pending on the use of adjuvant infusional 5-FU, leucovorin, and irinotecan (FOLFIRI) (NCCN, 2005a). Additional clinical research with other chemotherapy combinations has completed accrual and is awaiting analysis. The new National Surgical Adjuvant Breast and Bowel Project Adjuvant Colon Cancer trial is investigating biologic therapy. The trial will consist of FOLFOX administered alone or with the antiangiogenesis agent bevacizumab.

Rectal Cancer

In rectal cancer, regimens include both concomitant chemoradiation therapy and adjuvant chemotherapy as standard care. The concomitant chemoradiation therapy may be given either pre- or postoperatively and can consist of bolus 5-FU plus RT or continuous infusional 5-FU plus RT. The adjuvant chemotherapy is 5-FU and leucovorin given either weekly for six out of eight weeks or daily for five days once a month (NCCN, 2005c). FOLFOX also is being used adjuvantly in rectal cancer (NCCN, 2005c).

Research in Older Adults

Several analyses from retrospective data regarding the older adult and adjuvant therapy have been reported in the literature. These analyses consistently show that older adults experience the same benefits from adjuvant therapy compared with adults younger than 65 years of age (Sargent et al., 2001; Sundararajan et al., 2002). Most studies suggest that older adults generally tolerate the chemotherapy as well as younger patients, with an occasional slight increase in leukopenia or stomatitis (Enzinger & Mayer, 2004; Sargent et al.). Unfortunately, the use of adjuvant chemotherapy in the older adult declines sharply with advancing age (see Table 8-6) (Schrag et al., 2001; Sundararajan et al.). It is unclear from these retrospective reviews of data in the Surveillance, Epidemiology, and End Results (SEER)/Medicare-linked database if the older adults refused therapy or if they did not get the therapy as advised by their clinician. Given the reasonable life expectancy of adults in their sixth, seventh, and eighth decades of life and the clear benefit of adjuvant therapy, the older adult with stage III colon cancer should be informed of all treatment options (Sargent et al.; Schrag et al.; Sundararajan et al.).

Table 8-6. Surveillance, Epidemiology, and End Results (SEER)/Medicare-Linked Database 1991–1996 Age and Adjuvant Chemotherapy Use for Stage III Colon Cancer

Age	% Older Adults Receiving Adjuvant 5-FU Therapy
Overall—Age ≥ 65 years	52%–55%
Age 65–69 years	77%–78%
Age 70–74 years	72%–74%
Age 75–79 years	58%
Age 80–84 years	32%–34%
Age 85–89 years	10%–11%
Age ≥ 90 years	2%

Note. Based on information from Schrag et al., 2001; Sundararajan et al., 2002.

Chemotherapy and Biotherapy: Metastatic Disease—Colon and Rectal Primaries

In the metastatic setting, tumors originating in the colon or rectum are treated in the same manner with similar chemotherapy regimens. Some issues that must be considered early are what is the timing from prior adjuvant therapy; are the metastatic lesions isolated and operable; and what is the goal of the therapy? In a few cases, metastatic disease may present as isolated lesions in the liver or lungs. In this situation, if the tumors are resectable, a standard colectomy involving the primary tumor and resection of the isolated metastasis is recommended (NCCN, 2005a).

Research Studies

Studies have shown that appropriately selected older adults can tolerate liver or lung resections for metastatic CRC with acceptable morbidity and mortality (Enzinger & Mayer, 2004). For patients with resected liver metastasis, adjuvant hepatic artery infusion chemotherapy plus systemic chemotherapy has been shown to be better than systemic chemotherapy alone (NCCN, 2005c). If a limited number of liver lesions exist, intralesion therapy with selective internal RT, ethanol injections, radiofrequency ablation, chemoembolization, and cryotherapy are additional treatment options. All of these methods use a local approach to destroy the cancer cells and are beneficial in select patients with small, discreet tumors isolated to the liver. Radiofrequency ablation uses heat; ethanol injections use absolute ethanol; chemoembolization uses a foreign substance "soaked" with chemotherapy; and cryosurgery directly freezes the lesion to kill the cancerous cells. The only intralesion option that is FDA approved is selective internal RT. This technique selectively delivers high doses of RT in small, biocompatible microspheres to liver tumors. However, it has not demonstrated an improvement in overall survival when compared with systemic chemotherapy (Gray et al., 2002). For patients with resectable lung metastasis, systemic therapy with 5-FU/leucovorin (bolus or continuous infusion), IFL, or observation is suggested postoperatively (NCCN, 2005a). If the metastatic lesions are not resectable because of location or number, standard systemic chemotherapy should be considered.

New Agents

In the past five years, five new agents have been FDA approved as part of the systemic treatment of metastatic CRC: irinotecan, capecitabine, oxaliplatin, bevacizumab, and cetuximab (Erbitux®, Imclone Systems, Princeton, NJ). The FDA and NCCN recognize the importance of several of these in combination owing to the significant impact on overall survival in patients with newly diagnosed metastatic disease (see Tables 8-5 and 8-7). In addition to combination regimens, use of some of these agents alone also can be beneficial. The following is a summary of the indications for the available agents and regimens.

- Bevacizumab (a monoclonal antibody that inhibits vascular endothelial growth factor and therefore angiogenesis) was FDA approved in February 2004 in combination with IV 5-FU-based chemotherapy for the first-line treatment of metastatic CRC. A phase III trial demonstrated an improvement in tumor shrinkage, a significantly longer duration before disease recurrence, and a statistically significant and clinically meaningful increase in overall survival as compared to bolus IFL. In addition, a third arm of the phase III trial and data from a phase II trial support the use of bevacizumab with IV 5-FU and leucovorin (Genentech, Inc., 2004).
- Infusional FOLFOX4 was FDA approved January 2004 for the first-line treatment of metastatic CRC. In a phase III trial (N9741), FOLFOX was shown to be statistically better in overall response rate, time to tumor progression, and survival than bolus IFL (Sanofi-Synthelabo Inc., 2005). According to NCCN (2005a), the survival advantage in this trial is not definitive because of several complexities in the trial (e.g., one regimen used infusional 5-FU, whereas the other used bolus 5-FU; and an inequality in crossover existed to a second-line regimen.
- Irinotecan plus either bolus or infusional 5-FU and leucovorin were recognized and approved by the FDA in 2000 as regimens that statistically improved survival as compared with the previous standard 5-FU and leucovorin (Pfizer Inc., 2005). NCCN (2005a) cautions clinicians about the possible increased toxicities of the bolus IFL regimen.
- Capecitabine, an oral agent, was FDA approved in 2001 and is recommended for patients in whom clinicians typically would recommend 5-FU alone. It has not demonstrated a survival benefit (Roche Pharmaceuticals, 2003).
- Options also are available for patients who have been previously treated for metastatic CRC.
  - Single-agent cetuximab or cetuximab in combination with irinotecan was approved in February 2004 for the treatment of epidermal growth factor receptor (EGFR) expressing metastatic CRC in patients that is refractory or intolerant

Table 8-7. Highlights of Chemotherapy Regimen Efficacy, Toxicity, and Other Issues

Regimen	Overall Efficacy	Older Adult Efficacy	Overall Toxicity	Older Adult Toxicity	Miscellaneous
Oxaliplatin with infusional 5-FU/leucovorin (LV)	First line: improved survival 19.4 months Second line: improved RR and TTP over 5-FU/LV	First line: same efficacy	Most common: Peripheral sensory neuropathy; fatigue; neutropenia; nausea, vomiting, and diarrhea	Adverse events are similar; older adults are more susceptible to diarrhea, dehydration, hypokalemia, leukopenia, fatigue, and syncope.	• Age has no effect on platinum clearance. • No starting dose adjustment is required in patients age ≥ 65. • Coadministration of nephrotoxic agents may decrease clearance via the kidneys. • No data are available for patients with renal impairment; use with caution if preexisting conditions.
Irinotecan	First line: survival benefit with both bolus irinotecan, 5-FU, and LV (IFL) (14.8 months) and adjuvant infusional 5-FU, LV, and irinotecan (FOLFIRI) (17.4 months) Second-line single agent: survival benefit 9.2 and 10.8 months, respectively	First line: improvement in RR and TTP similar Second line: similar RR	Most clinically significant toxicities: diarrhea (early and late), nausea, vomiting, neutropenia, and alopecia	• Patients > age 65 are at greater risk for late diarrhea. • No difference seen in severe neutropenia by age. • Healthcare providers should monitor older adult patients closely.	• Reduce starting dose to 100 mg/m^2 weekly and 300 mg/m^2 every three weeks for patients age ≥ 65, PS 2. • Patients with PS 2 have higher rates of hospitalization, neutropenic fever, thromboembolism, first cycle discontinuation, and early deaths with IFL. • Hold diuretics and laxatives during dosing to decrease exacerbation of dehydration and diarrhea. • Hyperglycemia is seen in patients with a history of diabetes or intolerance to glucose.

(Continued on next page)

Table 8-7. Highlights of Chemotherapy Regimen Efficacy, Toxicity, and Other Issues *(Continued)*

Regimen	Overall Efficacy	Older Adult Efficacy	Overall Toxicity	Older Adult Toxicity	Miscellaneous
Bevacizumab with IV 5-FU–based chemotherapy	First line: improved survival (20.3 months)	First line: effect on survival is similar in older patients.	In metastatic colorectal cancer: hypertension, epistaxis, proteinuria, gastrointestinal perforation, wound healing complications, deep vein thrombosis	Limited data are available; toxicities higher ($\geq$ 2%) in older adult subset: fatigue, sepsis, deep vein thrombosis, hypertension, hypotension, myocardial infarction, stroke, congestive heart failure, diarrhea, constipation, anorexia, leukopenia, anemia, dehydration, hypokalemia, hyponatremia	• No recommended dose adjustments or reductions based on age • Discontinue bevacizumab for gastrointestinal perforations, wound dehiscence requiring medical intervention, serious bleeding, nephritic syndrome, or hypertensive crisis. • Temporarily suspend bevacizumab for moderate to severe proteinuria and uncontrolled severe hypertension. • No data are available regarding use of bevacizumab in patients with renal or hepatic impairment.
Capecitabine	First line: superior to 5-FU/LV in RR but similar TTP and survival	No data	Common toxicities: diarrhea, hand-foot syndrome, nausea, vomiting, hyperbilirubinemia, myelosuppression	• Patients aged $\geq$ 80 are vulnerable to greater frequency of severe adverse events. • Healthcare providers should monitor older adult patients closely. • Compliance concerns exist regarding oral drug administration.	• Age has no significant influence on pharmacokinetics. • Insufficient data are available on dosage recommendations in older adult patients. • The effect of hepatic dysfunction on capecitabine is not known. • A dose reduction of 25% is recommended for patients with moderate renal dysfunction. • Healthcare providers may need to reduce doses of concomitant phenytoin or coumarin-derived anticoagulants. • Concomitant intake of aluminum- or magnesium-containing antacids may increase bioavailability.

(Continued on next page)

Table 8-7. Highlights of Chemotherapy Regimen Efficacy, Toxicity, and Other Issues *(Continued)*

Regimen	Overall Efficacy	Older Adult Efficacy	Overall Toxicity	Older Adult Toxicity	Miscellaneous
					• Contraindicated in patients with known dihydropyrimidine dehydrogenase deficiency or hypersensitivity to 5-FU • Cardiotoxicity is more common in patients with a prior history of coronary artery disease.
5-FU plus LV	Improved RR and TTP	Similar efficacy	Common toxicities (vary depending on dose and schedule): mucositis, diarrhea, myelosuppression, skin reactions	Older adult patients are at higher risk for mucositis and diarrhea.	• Contraindicated in patients with poor nutritional status, active ischemic heart disease, or a history of myocardial infarction
Cetuximab +/– irinotecan	Second line: improved RR	No differences in efficacy	Most common: acneform rash, fatigue, diarrhea, nausea, abdominal pain, vomiting. Most serious: acneform rash, severe infusion reactions, diarrhea, dehydration, fever, and, rarely, interstitial lung disease, sepsis, kidney failure, pulmonary embolus	Researchers observed no differences in toxicity.	• Age has no significant influence on pharmacokinetics. • Interstitial lung disease is rare, but if acute or worsening pulmonary symptoms appear, discontinue cetuximab. • Sunlight can exacerbate skin reactions; instruct patients to wear sunscreen and hats and to limit sun exposure. • No drug-drug interaction data are available, except for irinotecan.

5-FU—5-fluorouracil; PS—performance status; RR—response rate; TTP—time to tumor progression

Note. Based on information from Enzinger & Mayer, 2004; Genentech, Inc., 2004; Imclone Systems Inc. & Bristol-Myers Squibb, 2004; Pfizer Inc., 2005; Roche Pharmaceuticals, 2003; Sanofi-Synthelabo Inc., 2005.

to irinotecan-based chemotherapy. This monoclonal antibody, specific for the EGFR, has demonstrated improvements in tumor shrinkage but not overall survival (Imclone Systems Inc. & Bristol-Myers Squibb, 2004).

– Irinotecan monotherapy also is a treatment option, having demonstrated a significant improvement in survival as compared with infusional 5-FU and best supportive care (Pfizer Inc., 2005).

Therapy with 5-FU and leucovorin as either a bolus or continuous infusion remains a standard option for patients with previously treated metastatic disease. NCCN guidelines do not specify a sequence recommendation favoring 5-FU and leucovorin plus either irinotecan or oxaliplatin. Tournigand et al. (2004) conducted a small randomized trial looking at the sequence of FOLFOX or FOLFIRI in the treatment of chemotherapy-naïve metastatic CRC. The results demonstrated that the sequence of which combination was given first and which was second was not as important as the fact that patients received all the agents. Grothey, Sargent, Goldberg, and Schmoll (2004) conducted a review of seven recent phase III trials in metastatic CRC that confirmed these results. Therefore, if the patient received one of the combinations first line, the other combination could be considered second line if the patient was still an appropriate candidate for chemotherapy (NCCN, 2005a).

Individualized Treatment

In the setting of metastatic disease, all patients with cancer, especially older adults, require individualized treatment strategies. Many therapeutic options are available, and although these regimens should be given in sequence, the exact sequence has not yet been defined. The therapeutic benefit of these combination therapies in the older adult has been demonstrated in numerous trials consistently revealing that response to chemotherapy, survival benefit, and toxicity are similar in younger and older patients (Best et al., 2005; Enzinger & Mayer, 2004; Popescu, Norman, Ross, Parikh, & Cunningham, 1999). However, only a small percentage of older adults participated in these clinical trials, and those who did had a high functional score. Therefore, little evidence exists on which to base therapeutic decisions in old or frail older adults (i.e., those with multiple comorbidities and poor function). A complete assessment of the patient's wishes, comorbidities, life expectancy, goals for therapy, functional status, type and timing of prior therapy, and toxicity profiles must be taken into consideration. For older adults, this is an especially optimal time to use a comprehensive geriatric assessment to assist in decision making and to offer patients the best treatment options based on the available evidence and not on chronologic age bias. As has been discussed previously, chronologic age is an imprecise predictor of physiologic age and functional status.

Nursing Care and Considerations With the Older Adult

Symptom Management

Healthy older adults tolerate elective surgery, standard RT, and chemotherapy as well as younger adults; however, older adults may need attention and proactive supportive care (Balducci, 2000). Two important patient-dependent factors include comorbid diseases and the individual's overall functional status. These factors may have an influence on older adults' tolerance of standard therapies, whereas age itself is not a predictor of tolerability. The potential types of side effects secondary to surgery, standard RT, and chemotherapy are the same in older adults as reported by younger patients. However, older adults treated for CRC may have decreased tolerance of fluorinated pyrimidines (NCCN, 2005e). Older adults also may be at increased risk for diarrhea and mucositis when treated for CRC. The focus of symptom management is on the patient's physical and metabolic needs, preventing complications, reinforcing self-care strategies, and providing emotional support. Standard measures to control the side effects of therapy are warranted while considering issues of polypharmacy, drug interactions, and patient compliance. The measures used to prevent and treat toxicity from chemotherapy and RT are the same in younger and older adults. Although proactive symptom management is important for all patients with cancer, healthcare professionals must provide older adults with the best chance for a positive outcome. The reader is referred to other references for an extensive review of symptom management in patients with CRC (Berg, 2003; NCCN, 2005d; Yarbro, Frogge, & Goodman, 2004). The nurse frequently must evaluate the impact of the disease and treatment on patients, their functional status, and their significant others, and then make adjustments in the plan of care as appropriate.

Follow-Up Care and Recommendations

Postoperative surveillance is important to identify additional tumors early. The American Society of Clinical Oncology (ASCO, 2001) recommended a physical examination every three to six months for three years, then yearly; colonoscopy within one year after diagnosis, then every three to five years based on the results; and CEA determinations every two to three months for two years, then at the healthcare provider's discretion. Additional guidelines for surveillance, especially in patients with previous adenomas, inflammatory bowel disease, and genetic syndromes, can be found in NCCN's guidelines for colorectal screening (NCCN, 2005b). The greatest risk for recurrence is within the first five years. Unfortunately, retrospective data analysis suggests that younger patients are more likely to undergo postoperative surveillance than are older patients (Enzinger & Mayer, 2004). The fear of disease recurrence or progression can be overwhelming for all patients and requires counseling to put things into perspective. Financial issues can put a significant strain on patients and their families; although older adults often are covered by Medicare, co-payments and deductibles are the patient's responsibility and can be burdensome if not overwhelming. A collaborative approach to care is important to identify rehabilitation needs and appropriate social service referrals.

Areas for Future Research

Evidence-Based Literature Summary

- Median age at diagnosis for CRC is 72 years.
- More than two-thirds of people with CRC are older than 65 years of age.

- Major risk factors associated with development of CRC are increasing age and personal or family history of predisposing disease of the large intestine; other risk factors are behavioral, nutritional, and environmental in nature.
- Polyps are common, especially in people older than age 50.
- Older adults tend to have well-differentiated tumors located in the proximal colon, a more indolent growth pattern, and less aggressive tumors.
- The natural history of colon and rectal tumors differs.
  - Colon cancers recur at distant sites (i.e., liver).
  - Rectal cancers spread locally (i.e., locoregional lymph nodes).
- CRC signs and symptoms (blood in or on stool; bleeding from rectum; stomach pain, cramps, or aches; changes in bowel habits, weight loss, tenesmus, anorexia, and fatigue) are similar in all age groups.
- Colonic examination and histologic examination of the biopsy diagnose CRC, with further testing required to determine extent of disease.
- The AJCC (tumor-node-metastasis system) stages CRC with depth of penetration through the colon rather than size of the tumor as the important factor; staging is the most important prognostic factor.
- CRC may be prevented by behavior modifications and/or early detection with surgical excision.
- Surgery is the primary therapeutic option.
  - Standard procedures
    o Colon: partial open colectomy, lymph node dissection, with end-to-end anastomosis.
    o Rectum: lower anterior resection with complete excision of the mesorectum, disease-free margin, and coloanal anastomosis.
  - Laparoscopic colectomy may be an acceptable alternative to open colectomy in patients overall but still is investigational in the older adult.
- Concomitant chemoradiation plus adjuvant chemotherapy is the standard of care in early-stage rectal cancer.
  - RT (45-55 Gy) given either pre- or postoperative, alone or in combination with bolus or infusional 5-FU–based chemotherapy
- Adjuvant chemotherapy is not the standard of care for stage II colon cancer but may be considered in patients at high risk for systemic recurrence.
- Adjuvant 5-FU and leucovorin (low-dose or high-dose) chemotherapy for six months is the standard of care for stage III colon cancer. The use of a new regimen, continuous FOLFOX, is supported by improved three-year disease-free survival (data from phase III randomized trial).
  - Older adults experience the same benefits from adjuvant therapy as do patients younger than 65 years of age (retrospective data reviews).
- Chemotherapy for metastatic CRC is an important therapeutic option, with some regimens extending survival.
  - FDA approved and NCCN recommended first-line treatment options
    o Bevacizumab plus IV 5-FU–based chemotherapy increases survival (phase III randomized trial compared with IFL).
    o Infusional FOLFOX increases survival (phase III randomized trial compared with IFL).
    o Infusional FOLFIRI and bolus 5-FU, leucovorin, and irinotecan (IFL) increase survival (phase III randomized trial compared with 5-FU and leucovorin).

 o Capecitabine recommended in patients who typically would be treated with single-agent 5-FU increases response rate but has no survival benefit (phase III randomized trial compared with 5-FU and leucovorin).

 – FDA approved and NCCN recommended second-line treatment options

  o Single-agent cetuximab or cetuximab plus irinotecan increases response rate but has no survival benefit (phase II and phase III randomized trials).

  o Irinotecan monotherapy increases survival (phase III randomized trials compared with 5-FU and leucovorin and best supportive care).

  o 5-FU and leucovorin

- NCCN guidelines recommend using the available agents in a sequential manner but do not specify the exact sequence (supported by retrospective data and a phase II trial).

Research With Older Adults

The decisions about what regimen to use and when are more complicated in older adults, as little evidence-based data are available. Few clinical trials look specifically at the treatment of older adults with carcinoma of the colon or rectum; in fact, most trials include a small number of older adults in the entire group and usually only those who are functionally fit. If older adults are included in the trial, the results for these patients are seldom reported separately. In addition, inconsistent definitions of "older" exist, leading to incompatible methods of reporting data (e.g., some report results for patients $\geq$ 65 years of age, whereas others report data in patients $\geq$ 70 years of age). Randomized trials are needed to evaluate novel drug regimens in the older adult to facilitate an understanding of the risks and benefits of such treatments. Response rates and progression-free survival may be the most meaningful outcomes in the older adult, as comorbidities and geriatric issues may negatively impact overall survival. In addition, research needs to look at the toxicity of treatment, drug metabolism, drug effect, and quality of life of specific regimens in the older adult to reduce the bias of treating this population and improve the understanding of drug-related adverse reactions.

Case Study

A 77-year-old man was treated with adjuvant 5-FU and leucovorin for stage III colon cancer. Two years later, his CEA was noted to be 200 ng/ml (upper limit of normal 5 ng/ml). Follow-up computed tomography showed metastatic disease with five new liver lesions. He is basically asymptomatic and lives in a senior citizen housing complex with his wife, who is 75 years old with multiple comorbid conditions. Several members of his extended family live within a 20-mile radius. He is an active golfer (was a professional player); his performance status is 0 (Eastern Cooperative Oncology Group scale); and his hypertension is controlled with a diuretic. What are the next treatment steps for this patient?

The first step is to complete a basic comprehensive geriatric assessment and determine the patient's goals for therapy. The results of the assessment highlight his overall excellent health status, but social concerns arise should he experience complications (e.g., his wife may be too ill with her own comorbidities). However, he has some family members who are reasonably nearby. This gentleman has some comorbidity but is quite independent and, along with his family, is interested in receiving standard therapy. Surgery is not an option because of the location of the liver metastases, and RT also is not an option. The most appropriate chemotherapy options for this patient include FOLFOX, FOLFIRI, bevacizumab plus 5-FU–containing regimens (5-FU/leucovorin, FOLFOX, FOLFIRI, IFL), and participation in a clinical trial (NCCN, 2005a). Issues to be considered when obtaining informed consent include diuretic use (dehydration) and diarrhea with irinotecan; controlled hypertension and arterial thrombosis with bevacizumab; and cumulative neurotoxicity with oxaliplatin that may interfere with his love for golf. Other side effects from these therapies could include stomatitis, myelosuppression, hair loss (irinotecan), and nausea with or without vomiting. The patient agrees to treatment with bevacizumab and FOLFIRI because of concern of neurotoxicity from the oxaliplatin interfering with his golf game. However, all of the strategies noted are feasible in selected older adults (Aparicio et al., 2003; Comella et al., 2003; Genentech, Inc., 2004).

Conclusion

CRC presents many challenges along the continuum of prevention, early detection, and treatment. Promotion of ACS's recommendations for healthy lifestyle choices and the benefits and value of screening and early detection can decrease the incidence of this disease while increasing survival. Operative procedures, standard RT, and chemotherapy all are safe and effective in the appropriately selected older adult. Therapeutic clinical trials offer the hope for new treatment regimens and are extremely needed in the older adult, especially those older than 75 years, where a balance must exist between efficacy and toxicity. As noted by Lerner (1996) "At every turn there are bewildering arrays of choices, and often there is no adequate external guidance that you can count on. So when all the information is before you, consider turning inward to discover from as deep a source as possible what makes sense to you" (p. 25). In the future, older adults should not hope the clinician looked into as deep a source as possible to find the appropriate therapeutic recommendations but rather looked to evidence on which to base the therapeutic strategy.

The opinions and ideas expressed in this chapter are those of the author and are not intended to be construed as the opinions or recommendations of Genentech, Inc.

References

American Cancer Society. (2001). American Cancer Society guidelines on screening and surveillance for the early detection of adenomatous polyps and colorectal cancer—Update 2001. *CA: A Cancer Journal for Clinicians, 51,* 44–54.

American Cancer Society. (2005). *Colorectal cancer facts and figures.* Atlanta, GA: Author.

American Gastroenterological Association. (2000). American Gastroenterological Association medical position statement: Impact of dietary fiber on colon cancer occurrence. *Gastroenterology, 118,* 1233–1234.

American Society of Clinical Oncology. (2001). *A patient's guide: Follow-up care for colorectal cancer.* Alexandria, VA: Author.

Aparicio, T., Desrame, J., Lecomte, T., Mitry, E., Belloc, J., Etienney, I., et al. (2003). Oxaliplatin- or irinotecan-based chemotherapy for metastatic colorectal cancer in the elderly. *British Journal of Cancer, 89,* 1439–1444.

Balducci, L. (2000). Prevention and treatment of cancer in the elderly. *Oncology Issues, 51,* 26–28.

Balducci, L. (2001). The geriatric cancer patient: Equal benefit from equal treatment. *Cancer Control, 8*(Suppl. 2), 1–25.

Balducci, L. (2003). New paradigms for treating elderly patients with cancer. *Journal of Supportive Oncology, 1,* 30–37.

Balducci, L., & Extermann, M. (2000). Management of cancer in the older person: A practical approach. *Oncologist, 5,* 224–237.

Berg, D.T. (2003). *Pocket guide to colorectal cancer.* Sudbury, MA: Jones and Bartlett.

Berg, D.T. (2004). Colorectal cancer. In C.G. Varricchio (Ed.), *A cancer source book for nurses* (8th ed., pp. 187–200). Sudbury, MA: Jones and Bartlett.

Best, L., Simmonds, P., Baughan, C., Buchanan, R., Davis, C., Fentiman, I., et al. (2005). Palliative chemotherapy for advanced or metastatic colorectal cancer (Cochrane Review). *Cochrane Library, 2.* Chichester, United Kingdom: Wiley.

Byers, T., Nestle, M., McTiernan, A., Doyle, C., Currie-Williams, A., Gansler, T., et al. (2002). American Cancer Society guidelines on nutrition and physical activity for cancer prevention: Reducing the risk of cancer with healthy food choices and physical activity. *CA: A Cancer Journal for Clinicians, 52,* 92–119.

Centers for Disease Control and Prevention. (2003a). *Colorectal cancer: Facts for people with Medicare.* Atlanta, GA: Author.

Centers for Disease Control and Prevention. (2003b, March 14). *Colorectal cancer test use among persons aged > 50 years—U.S., 2001.* Retrieved July 1, 2005, from http://www.cdc.gov/mmwr/pdf/wk/mm5210.pdf

Centers for Disease Control and Prevention. (2004a, February 26). *Behavioral risk factor surveillance system prevalence data: Colorectal cancer screening.* Retrieved April 2, 2004, from http://apps.nccd.cdc.gov/brfss/page.asp?yr=1997&state=US&cat=CC#CC

Centers for Disease Control and Prevention. (2004b, March 1). *Colorectal cancer prevention and control initiatives.* Retrieved April 2, 2004, from http://www.cdc.gov/cancer/colorctl/index.htm

Clinical Outcomes of Surgical Therapy Study Group. (2004). A comparison of laparoscopically assisted and open colectomy for colon cancer. *New England Journal of Medicine, 350,* 2050–2059.

Comella, P., Farris, A., Lorusso, V., Palmeri, S., Maiorino, L., De Lucia, L., et al. (2003). Irinotecan plus leucovorin-modulated 5-fluorouracil IV bolus every other week may be a suitable therapeutic option also for elderly patients with metastatic colorectal carcinoma. *British Journal of Cancer, 89,* 992–996.

Curtas, S. (1999). Diagnosing GI malignancies. *Seminars in Oncology Nursing, 15,* 10–16.

DeVita, V., Hellman, S., & Rosenberg, S. (Eds.). (2001). *Cancer: Principles and practices of oncology* (6th ed.). Philadelphia: Lippincott-Raven.

Ellenhorn, J.D.I., Coia, L.R., Alberts, S.R., & Hoff, P.M. (2002). Colorectal and anal cancers. In R. Pazdur, L.R. Coia, H.J. Hoskins, & L.D. Wagman (Eds.), *Cancer management: A multidisciplinary approach* (6th ed., pp. 295–318). Melville, NY: PRR, Inc.

Ellenhorn, J.D.I., Cullinane, C.A., Coia, L.R., Alberts, S.R., & Alberts, S.R. (2004). Colorectal and anal cancers. In R. Pazdur, L.R. Coia, W.J. Hoskins, & L.D. Wagman (Eds.), *Cancer management: A multidisciplinary approach* (8th ed., pp. 323–355). Melville, NY: PRR, Inc.

Ellis, C., & Hubbard, D.S. (2000). Colorectal cancer. In C.H. Yarbro, M.H. Frogge, M. Goodman, & S.L. Groenwald (Eds.), *Cancer nursing: Principles and practice* (5th ed., pp. 1117–1137). Sudbury, MA: Jones and Bartlett.

Enzinger, P.C., & Mayer, R.J. (2004). Gastrointestinal cancer in older patients. *Seminars in Oncology, 31,* 206–219.

Fuchs, C.S., Giovannucci, E.L., Colditz, G.A., Hunter, D.J., Speizer, F.E., & Willett, W.C. (1994). A prospective study of family history and the risk of colorectal cancer. *New England Journal of Medicine, 25,* 1669–1674.

Genentech, Inc. (2004). Avastin (bevacizumab) [Package insert]. South San Francisco, CA: Author.

Goldberg, R.M. (2000). Gastrointestinal cancers. In D.A. Casciato & B.B. Lowitz (Eds.), *Manual of clinical oncology* (4th ed., pp. 182–194). Philadelphia: Lippincott Williams & Wilkins.

Gosselin, T.K. (2001). Radiation therapy. In D.T. Berg (Ed.), *Contemporary issues in colorectal cancer: A nursing perspective* (pp. 135–156). Sudbury, MA: Jones and Bartlett.

Gray, B., van Hazel, G., Anderson, J., Price, D., Moroz, P., Bower, G., et al. (2002). Randomized phase II trial of SIR-Spheres plus fluorouracil/leucovorin chemotherapy versus fluorouracil/leucovorin chemotherapy alone on advanced colorectal hepatic metastases. *Proceedings of the American Society of Clinical Oncology,* Abstract 599.

Greene, F.L., Page, D.L., Fleming, I.D., Fritz, A., Balch, C.M., Haller, D.G., et al. (2002). *AJCC cancer staging manual.* New York: Springer.

Grothey, A., Sargent, D., Goldberg, R.M., & Schmoll, H.J. (2004). Survival of patients with advanced colorectal cancer improves with the availability of fluorouracil-leucovorin, irinotecan, and oxaliplatin in the course of treatment. *Journal of Clinical Oncology, 22,* 1209–1214.

Hickish, T., Boni, C., Tabernero, J., Clingan, P., Colucci, G., Nowacki, M., et al. (2004). Oxaliplatin/5-fluorouracil/leucovorin in stage II and III colon cancer: Updated results of the international randomized "MOSAIC" trial. *Proceedings of the American Society of Clinical Oncology,* Abstract 211.

Imclone Systems Inc. & Bristol-Myers Squibb. (2004). Erbitux (cetuximab) [Package insert]. Princeton, NJ: Authors.

Jemal, A., Murray, T., Ward, E., Samuels, A., Tiwari, R., Ghafoor, A., et al. (2005). Cancer statistics, 2005. *CA: A Cancer Journal for Clinicians, 55,* 10–30.

Jemal, A., Tiwari, R.C., Murray, T., Ghafoor, A., Samuels, A., Ward, E., et al. (2004). Cancer statistics, 2004. *CA: A Cancer Journal for Clinicians, 54,* 8–29.

Kemeny, M.M., Busch-Devereaux, E., Merriam, L., & O'Hea, B.J. (2000). Cancer surgery in the elderly. *Hematology/Oncology Clinics of North America, 14,* 169–192.

Kemppainen, M., Raiha, I., Rajala, T., & Sourander, L. (1993). Characteristics of colorectal cancer in elderly patients. *Gerontology, 39,* 222–227.

Lerner, M. (1996). *Choices in healing: Integrating the best of conventional and complementary approaches to cancer.* Cambridge, MA: MIT Press.

National Cancer Institute. (2000a). *Surveillance, Epidemiology, and End Results (SEER) cancer statistics review, 1975–2000: Age distribution at diagnosis and death.* Retrieved April 2, 2004, from http://www.seer.cancer.gov/csr/1975_2000/results_merged/topic_age_dist.pdf

National Cancer Institute. (2000b). *Surveillance, Epidemiology, and End Results (SEER) cancer statistics review, 1975–2000: Colon and rectum.* Retrieved April 2, 2004, from http://www.seer.cancer.gov/csr/1975_2000/results_merged/sect_06_colon_rectum.pdf

National Cancer Institute. (2000c). *Surveillance, Epidemiology, and End Results (SEER) cancer statistics review, 1975–2000: Median age of cancer patients at diagnosis.* Retrieved April 2, 2004, from http://www.seer.cancer.gov/csr/1975_2000/results_merged/topic_med_age.pdf

National Cancer Institute. (2003, September 2). *Quick facts: Annual report to the nation on the status of cancer 1975–2000, featuring the uses of surveillance data for cancer prevention and control.* Retrieved April 2, 2004, from http://www.cancer.gov/newscenter/pressreleases/ReportFactSheet

National Comprehensive Cancer Network. (2005a). *NCCN clinical practice guidelines in oncology: Colon cancer.* Retrieved September 20, 2005, from http://www.nccn.org/professionals/physician_gls/PDF/colon.pdf

National Comprehensive Cancer Network. (2005b). *Guidelines for prevention, detection, and risk reduction of cancer: Colorectal cancer screening.* Retrieved September 20, 2005, from http://www.nccn.org/professionals/physician_gls/PDF/colorectal_screening.pdf

National Comprehensive Cancer Network. (2005c). *NCCN clinical practice guidelines in oncology: Rectal cancer.* Retrieved September 20, 2005, from http://www.nccn.org/professionals/physician_gls/PDF/rectal.pdf

National Comprehensive Cancer Network. (2005d). *NCCN clinical practice guidelines in oncology: Guidelines for supportive care.* Retrieved September 20, 2005, from http://www.nccn.org/professionals/physician_gls/f_guidelines.asp#detection

National Comprehensive Cancer Network. (2005e). *NCCN clinical practice guidelines in oncology: Guidelines for supportive care—Senior adult oncology.* Retrieved September 20, 2005, from http://www.nccn.org/professionals/physician_gls/PDF/senior.pdf

Pfizer. (2005). Camptosar (irinotecan) [Package insert]. Kalamazoo, MI: Author.

Popescu, R.A., Norman, A., Ross, P.J., Parikh, B., & Cunningham, D. (1999). Adjuvant or palliative chemotherapy for colorectal cancer in patients 70 years or older. *Journal of Clinical Oncology, 17,* 2412–2418.

Prabhudesai, A.G., & Kumar, D. (2002). Adjuvant therapy of colorectal cancer: The next step forward. *Current Medical Research and Opinion, 18,* 249–257.

Repetto, L. (2003). Greater risks of chemotherapy toxicity in elderly patients with cancer. *Journal of Supportive Oncology, 4,* 18–24.

Roche Pharmaceuticals. (2003). Xeloda (capecitabine) [Package insert]. Nutley, NJ: Author.

Sanofi-Synthelabo Inc. (2005). Eloxatin (oxaliplatin) [Package insert]. New York: Author.

Sargent, D.J., Goldberg, R.M., Jacobson, S.D., MacDonald, J.S., Labianca, R., Haller, D.G., et al.

(2001). A pooled analysis of adjuvant chemotherapy for resected colon cancer in elderly patients. *New England Journal of Medicine, 345,* 1091–1097.

Schrag, D., Cramer, L.D., Bach, P.B., & Begg, C.B. (2001). Age and adjuvant chemotherapy use after surgery for stage III colon cancer. *Journal of the National Cancer Institute, 93,* 850–857.

Steinbeck, G., Lynch, P.M., Phillips, R.K.S., Wallace, M.H., Hawk, E., Gordon, G.B., et al. (2000). The effect of celecoxib, a cyclooxygenase-2 inhibitor, in familial adenomatous polyposis. *New England Journal of Medicine, 342,* 1946–1952.

Stocchi, L., Nelson, H., Young–Fadok, T.M., Larson, D.R., & Ilstrup, D.M. (2000). Safety and advantages of laparoscopic vs. open colectomy in the elderly: Matched-control study. *Diseases of the Colon and Rectum, 43,* 326–332.

Sundararajan, V., Mitra, N., Jacobson, J.S., Grann, V.R., Heltjan, D.F., & Neugut, A.I. (2002). Survival associated with 5-fluorouracil-based adjuvant chemotherapy among elderly patients with node-positive colon cancer. *Annals of Internal Medicine, 136,* 349–357.

Tanaka, K., Nagaoka, S., Takemura, T., Arai, T., Sawabe, M., Takubo, K., et al. (2002). Incidence of apoptosis increases with age in colorectal cancer. *Experimental Gerontology, 37,* 1467–1477.

Tournigand, C., Andre, T., Achille, E., Lledo, G., Flesh, M., Mery-Mignard, D., et al. (2004). FOLFIRI followed by FOLFOX6 or the reverse sequence in advanced colorectal cancer: A randomized GERCOR study. *Journal of Clinical Oncology, 22,* 229–237.

Ward, E., Jemal, A., Cokkinides, V., Singh, G.K., Cardinez, C., Ghafoor, A., et al. (2004). Cancer disparities by race/ethnicity and socioeconomic status. *CA: A Cancer Journal for Clinicians, 54,* 74–93.

Weir, H.K., Thun, M.J., Hankey, B.F., Ries, L.G., Howe, H.L., Wingo, P.A., et al. (2003). Annual report to the nation on the status of cancer, 1975–2000. Featuring the uses of surveillance data for cancer prevention and control. *Journal of the National Cancer Institute, 95,* 1276–1299.

Women's Health Initiative Investigators. (2002). Risks and benefits of estrogen and progesterone in healthy postmenopausal women. *JAMA, 288,* 321–333.

Yarbro, C.H., Frogge, M.H., & Goodman, M. (Eds.). (2004). *Cancer symptom management* (3rd ed.). Sudbury, MA: Jones and Bartlett.

CHAPTER 9

The Older Adult With Head and Neck Cancer

Sarah H. Kagan, PhD, RN, APRN, BC, AOCN®

Introduction

Providing evidence-based care to the older adult with head and neck cancers is a precarious process of knowing specific science, extrapolating available evidence from related errors, and employing critical clinical judgment (Kagan, 2004a). Although head and neck cancers disproportionately affect older adults, relatively little specific science has been conducted to address the unique needs of this group. Interestingly, the specialty of head and neck oncology has a small but cohesive body of age-focused research, dating from the 1990s, examining chronologic age effects (Kagan, 2004b). Newer science and clinical expert opinion focus on age-related issues such as comorbid disease and clinical outcomes for older adults with head and neck cancer (Kagan, 2004b). This science provides evidence specific to this population through reliance on retrospective clinical case series and clinical performance improvement reports. Despite inherent limitations and relative paucity, such evidence is useful in shaping practice when coupled with the earlier literature and clinical expert opinion.

This chapter offers a summary of evidence-based care of the older adult with head and neck cancer. It begins with an overview of head and neck cancer with attention to unique features in older adults. A discussion of the treatment trajectory follows with considerations of biologic age and comorbid disease, an area in which literature on head and neck cancer exceeds current standards for other diseases. Issues in nursing management and interdisciplinary collaboration are woven into the discussion. It concludes with a case study that integrates important concepts and management considerations.

Head and Neck Cancer, Aging, and Older Adults

Head and neck cancers, a group of relatively rare malignancies that are disproportionately prevalent among older adults, are among those cancers that clinically illustrate a clear association between advancing age and cancer (National Cancer Institute [NCI], 2004a, 2004b). The incidence of typical head and neck cancers, such as cancer of the larynx and oral cavity, has a pronounced curve beginning in the sixth decade of life (NCI, 2004a, 2004b). Recent basic and clinical science advances help to illuminate that gross connection, specifying elements of the relationship between head and neck cancer and advancing age.

Head and neck cancers account for approximately 7% of all cancers diagnosed in humans (Forastiere, Koch, Trotti, & Sidransky, 2001; Goepfert, 1998; Jemal et al., 2005). Although head and neck cancers are relatively uncommon in the United States, as a diagnostic group, they create disease- and treatment-related symptoms and side effects that are functionally disabling. These functional effects include changes in speaking and swallowing, xerostomia, chemosensory changes, chronic pain, depression, and spinal accessory and other syndromes related to anatomic nerve and musculoskeletal damage (Forastiere et al.). Managing these symptoms and side effects commonly entails complex intervention strategies combined with drug and rehabilitative therapies. An interdisciplinary team approach involving nursing, clinical nutrition, speech-language pathology, physical and occupational therapies, social work, specialty cancer services such as pain management and liaison psychiatry, and geriatric services must be routine in the care of the older adult with head and neck cancers. Dysfunction of this sort is paradigmatic of symptom clusters and functional loss and with interdisciplinary management and intensive health and social service use associated with cancer and other debilitating chronic illnesses in older adults. For this reason, older adults who have head and neck cancers often exemplify nursing and collaborative care needs illustrative of cancer in late life and of other geriatric chronic illnesses that create similar treatment burdens and symptom profiles (e.g., Parkinson disease, stroke, rheumatoid arthritis, heart failure) (Kagan, 2004a).

Incidence

Head and neck cancers are a set of cancer diagnoses grouped anatomically beginning with the oral cavity and moving through the pharynx and larynx (Forastiere et al., 2001) (see Figures 9-1 and 9-2). The group of anatomic sites generally includes the sinonasal passages and upper aerodigestive tract and select aspects of the skull base (Forastiere et al.). The sites that are identified as head and neck cancers include the oral cavity, with the lip, oral tongue, and palate as commonly involved subsites; the floor of the mouth, tonsil, and pharynx, which include the oropharynx, hypopharynx, nasopharynx, and pyriform sinus; and the larynx (Forastiere et al.). Most common sites of cancer in the older adult are the larynx, the oropharynx, and the oral cavity (Gillani & Grunberg, 2004). Head and neck cancers as an anatomic grouping most often exclude the thyroid, which is classified separately, and the esophagus, which is grouped with other gastrointestinal malignancies (Forastiere et al.). Skin cancer of the head and neck also often is included in the clinical practice of head and neck oncology. This is anatomically and clinically relevant, given exposure of this skin to ionizing solar radiation; however, accurate statistics on incidence, morbidity, and mortality are difficult to isolate. Nonetheless, perhaps the most striking element of the epidemiology of head and neck cancers in late life is the heterogeneity of disease patterns that makes assumptions without site-specific knowledge risky.

The public, for example, most commonly identifies cancer of the larynx with patients who have abused alcohol and tobacco and are made voiceless and disfigured

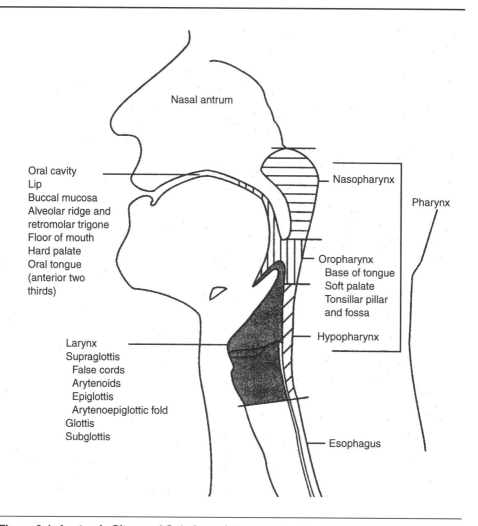

Figure 9-1. Anatomic Sites and Subsites of the Head and Neck

Note. From *Practice Guidelines in Oncology* (version 1.2005, p. 91), by the National Comprehensive Cancer Network, 2005, Jenkintown, PA: Author. Copyright 2005 by the National Comprehensive Cancer Network. Reprinted with permission.

by treatment. This image emerges for real epidemiologic reasons that are merged with stereotypic misapprehensions. Cancer of the larynx has the highest site-specific incidence in the United States and is among the highest for mortality rates (Jemal et al., 2005). The incidence of cancer of the larynx peaks, as seen in age-specific crude incidence rates, between 70 and 74 years of age and is highest for both African American and Caucasian men in that group. For women of both racial/ethnic groups, incidence peaks approximately five years earlier and is less than a fifth the peak rate for African American men, with 65 cases per 100,000 people during 1992–2000 (NCI, 2004a). Mortality is similarly patterned, with African American men experiencing the highest mortality at 70–74 years of age, with approximately 25–27 cases per

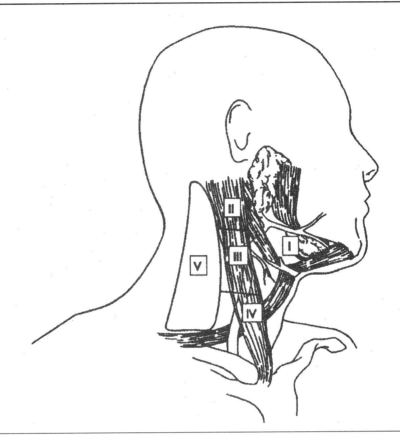

Figure 9-2. Level Designation for Cervical Lymphatics in the Right Neck

Note. From *Practice Guidelines in Oncology* (version 1.2005, p. 91), by the National Comprehensive Cancer Network, 2005, Jenkintown, PA: Author. Copyright 2005 by the National Comprehensive Cancer Network. Reprinted with permission.

100,000 (NCI, 2004c). Mortality for Caucasian men is considerably lower at its peak, with approximately 17 cases per 100,000 and a linear climb from a low of 2.5 cases at 50–54 years of age to a peak older than 85 years (NCI, 2004c). Women of both groups experience a low mortality of no more than 2.5 cases per 100,000 people, with rates peaking in the decade between 65 and 74 years (NCI, 2004c). Such differences provide evidence that understanding site-, gender-, and age-specific risk factors is critical to effective practice with older adults who have cancers of the larynx as well as cancers of other sites in the head and neck.

Risk Factors

The genesis of head and neck cancers and their connections to cellular senescence or the aging process is complex, especially given the number of discrete sites and variable histologies seen in this diagnostic group. Most commonly, cancers of the head and neck are squamous cell malignancies (Forastiere et al., 2001; Gillani & Grunberg, 2004). Head and neck cancers result from exposure to widely acknowledged carcinogens, such as tobacco and alcohol, for some site-specific diseases as well as the influence of less well-known viral and chemical carcinogens and oncogenes (Forastiere et al.; Goepfert, 1998). Exposure to known carcinogens offers an immediate link between head and neck cancers and aging, wherein cumulative exposure and possible expression of acquired mutations clearly takes place over time (Gibbs, 2003).

Evidence on the connection between cumulative exposure to carcinogens and acquired mutations in head and neck cancers for older adults is somewhat unclear, limited by the nature of the evidence available. Koch, Patel, Brennan, Boyle, and Sidransky (1995) offered a retrospective review of a cohort of two groups of individuals who were diagnosed with squamous cell cancer of the upper aerodigestive tract. The group of interest was composed of people who were diagnosed after age 75, and the comparison group was made up of younger individuals diagnosed between ages 40 and 70. Interestingly, although tobacco and alcohol exposure were significantly lower in the older cohort, the younger group showed greater expression of *p53* mutation compared with the older cohort (Koch et al.). The antecedents of this finding about the older cohort suggest that variability may exist in carcinogenesis and clinical presentation of cancer of the head and neck in late life and specifically in the "old-old." The findings reported by Koch et al. have yet to be pursued and replicated in subsequent literature.

Despite possible implications of the retrospective case control study reported by Koch et al. (1995), exposure to tobacco and alcohol as significant carcinogens and cocarcinogens in cancer of the head and neck generally is considered well established (Duffy et al., 2002; Forastiere et al., 2001). The relationships to advancing age and specific elements of senescence are less clear. Koch et al. are not alone in noting that the old-old appear to have a higher risk of multiple synchronous and metachronous cancers (Forastiere et al.; Goepfert, 1998). Tobacco and alcohol seem to create what is known as "field cancerization" that creates great risk for multiple malignancies in the upper aerodigestive tract or "field" (Forastiere et al.). Clinically, these synchronous or metachronous multiple primary cancers often appear in older adult males. Opportunities to prevent head and neck cancers linked to tobacco use and the cocarcinogenic effect of alcohol consumption then are tightly tied to public health initiatives to abolish or limit the consumption of both substances. Most public health campaigns seem to paradoxically ignore older adults in favor of younger populations and fail to recognize opportunities for symptom reduction and improved functional status even if primary prevention is not possible.

Prevention of malignancies where issues of carcinogenesis and the influence of aging are less understood is far more difficult. For example, Epstein-Barr virus (EBV) is strongly associated with certain types of nasopharyngeal cancers (NPCs), appearing in perhaps 100% of the World Health Organization NPC types 2 and 3 (Forastiere et al., 2001). Nonetheless, EBV infection alone, which is extraordinarily common across the world, does not account for the high incidence of NPC in some parts of the world, particularly South East Asia, implying again a complex process that likely involves more than one carcinogen and may rely on somatic genetic mutation or other genetic alterations. The influence of advancing age and especially the process of cellular senescence remains unclear. Similarly, human papillomavirus (HPV) is linked to approximately half of oropharyngeal cancers, especially those found in the tonsils and base of tongue (Forastiere et al.). Nonetheless, HPV infection is common, and the mismatch between benign or asymptomatic infection implies a more intricate equation that results in actual disease. What affects infection over time and the role senescence plays in development of oropharyngeal cancers are unexplored. Consequently, vigilance directed through knowledge of known carcinogens and avoidance of assumptions about the influence of aging must guide clinical practice.

Genetic evidence in the epidemiology of many head and neck site-specific cancers is growing rapidly (Cohen, Lingen, & Vokes, 2004; Forastiere et al., 2001; Gibbs, 2003). Much of the science reveals only mutations expressed in younger adulthood, unaffected by aging processes (Gibbs). Current evidence reveals a high prevalence of *p53* mutations in the squamous cell head and neck cancers of individuals who have smoked tobacco and drunk alcohol (Forastiere et al.; Koch et al., 1995). Other tumor suppressor genes, including *p16*, *PTEN*, and *Rb*, also are implicated in squamous cell cancer of the head and neck. Oncogenes (e.g., Cyclin D1, *p63*, epidermal growth factor receptor), which may alter the cell cycle or overall cell growth and proliferation, appear to be involved in head and neck cancers (Forastiere et al.). The specific effects of isolated elements of cellular senescence in expression of mutations associated with head and neck cancers have yet to be systematically explored. Emerging knowledge of the interplay among identified genetic factors, environmental carcinogen exposure, and the aging process will greatly aid in identifying the exact risk for site-specific malignancies. Research in this area will help to target public health and nursing efforts to prevent these malignancies within the aging population (Bourbonniere & Kagan, 2003).

Early Detection

Growing translational science in chemoprevention and photodynamic therapies may hold promise for treatment or reversal of dysplastic lesions or carcinoma in situ for younger and older adults (Cohen et al., 2004; Goepfert, 1998). However, early detection capacities remain very limited with no national guidelines or sensitive and specific technologies currently available beyond the annual cancer-related checkup after age 20 recommended by the American Cancer Society (Smith, Cokkinides, & Eyre, 2003). More broadly, public education efforts target the "Seven Warning Signs of Cancer," which include voice changes that may foretell laryngeal cancer and nonhealing lesions that may reveal nonmelanoma skin cancer of the head and neck. Early detection among older adults, however, often is confounded by difficulty distinguishing underlying cancer in the context of known comorbid illness and nonspecific complaints commonly associated with old age (e.g., dysphagia, voice changes) (Koch et al., 1995; Piccirillo, Lacy, Basu, & Spitznagel, 2002). Conversely, older adults may self-stereotype with regard to their complaints or have difficulty accessing health care, which may delay help seeking and appropriate management (Levy, 2003). Such behavioral and social issues make development of evidence-based practice through application of emerging science circuitous. No studies to date have begun to dissect behaviors connected to comorbidity and age-associated complaints in relation to screening and early detection of head and neck cancers.

Staging

Staging of head and neck cancers has changed little over time and is specific to subsites within the group of malignancies known as head and neck cancers. Laryngeal cancer is a clear example of the anatomic factors that are considered and the influence of lymph node involvement in the neck (see Figure 9-3). The tumor-node-metastasis and four-stage system is employed to frame treatment decisions and assess prognosis (Cohen et al., 2004). Advanced age and advanced stage at presentation are implicated in poor prognosis and five-year survival. Additionally, age effects are different among varying sites of disease. Davidson, Root, and Trock (2001) examined age and survival in cancer of the oral tongue and found a clear relationship. With a 10-year increase in age, risk of death rose 18%. Researchers have further outlined the association of comorbid disease to survival in site-specific disease and large samples of individuals with head and neck cancers (Chen, Matson, Roberts, & Goepfert, 2001; Piccirillo et al., 2002). Importantly, for nursing and comprehensive interdisciplinary care, the

---

TNM Definitions

Primary Tumor (T)
- TX: Primary tumor cannot be assessed
- T0: No evidence of primary tumor
- Tis: Carcinoma in situ

Supraglottis
- T1: Tumor limited to one subsite of supraglottis with normal vocal cord mobility
- T2: Tumor invades mucosa of more than one adjacent subsite of supraglottis or glottis or region outside the supraglottis without function of the larynx
- T3: Tumor limited to larynx with vocal cord fixation and/or invades any of the following: postcricoid area or pre-epiglottic tissues
- T4: Tumor invades through the thyroid cartilage and/or extends into soft tissues of the neck, thyroid, and/or esophagus

Glottis
- T1: Tumor limited to vocal cord(s) with normal mobility
- T2: Tumor extends to supraglottis and/or subglottis, and/or with impaired vocal cord mobility
- T3: Tumor limited to the larynx with vocal cord fixation
- T4: Tumor invades through the thyroid cartilage and/or to other tissues beyond the larynx

Subglottis
- T1: Tumor limited to the subglottis
- T2: Tumor extends to vocal cord(s) with normal or impaired mobility
- T3: Tumor limited to larynx with vocal cord fixation
- T4: Tumor invades through cricoid or thyroid cartilage and/or extends to other tissues beyond the larynx

Regional Lymph Nodes (N)
- NX: Regional lymph nodes cannot be assessed
- N0: No regional lymph node metastasis
- N1: Metastasis in a single ipsilateral lymph node, 3 cm or less in greatest dimension
- N2: Metastasis in a single ipsilateral lymph node, more than 3 cm but not more than 6 cm in greatest dimension, or in multiple ipsilateral lymph nodes, none more than 6 cm in greatest dimension or in bilateral or contralateral lymph nodes, none more than 6 cm in greatest dimension
  - N2a: Metastasis in a single ipsilateral lymph node more than 3 cm but not more than 6 cm in greatest dimension
  - N2b: Metastasis in multiple ipsilateral lymph nodes, none more than 6 cm in greatest dimension
  - N2c: Metastasis in bilateral or contralateral lymph nodes, none more than 6 cm in greatest dimension

---

Figure 9-3. Laryngeal Cancer Staging *(Continued on next page)*

Distant Metastasis (M)
- MX: Distant metastasis cannot be assessed
- M0: No distant metastasis
- M1: Distant metastasis

Stage 0
- Tis, N0, M0

Stage I
- T1, N0, M0

Stage II
- T2, N0, M0

Stage III
- T3, N0, M0
- T1, N1, M0
- T2, N1, M0
- T3, N1, M0

Stage IVA
- T4, N0, M0
- T4, N1, M0
- Any T, N2, M0

Stage IVB
- Any T, N3, M0

Stage IVC
- Any T, any N, M1

Figure 9-3. Laryngeal Cancer Staging *(Continued)*

Note. Data from "Laryngeal Cancer Treatment," by the National Cancer Institute, 2004. Retrieved July 8, 2004, from http://www.cancer.gov/cancertopics/pdq/treatment/laryngeal/HealthProfessional

effect of age on the experience of advanced disease, progression in single symptoms and symptom clusters, such as xerostomia, dysgeusia, and pain, and interaction of comorbid disease and symptoms on shortened survival time is unexplored (Hammerlid, Silander, Hornestam, & Sullivan, 2001).

Through an innovative program of research, Piccirillo et al. (2002) offered some of the most important investigations into head and neck cancer–specific comorbid disease. Piccirillo et al. developed an index of seven comorbid conditions significantly related to survival in head and neck cancers. These conditions (i.e., heart failure, cardiac arrhythmias, peripheral vascular disease, pulmonary disease, renal disease, and both controlled and uncontrolled other cancer diagnoses) were examined for their impact on survival (Piccirillo et al.). A large cohort of 1,153 individuals divided into three age groups, the oldest being composed of those 65 years of age and older at diagnosis, was followed for a five-year period. The diseases were weighted, and those weights were combined to develop a score (Piccirillo et al.). The scores for the samples showed a statistically significant association with five-year survival. Although this index still is under investigation and has yet to have clear clinical application in direct use, the larger implications for practice are important. Complete assessment of comorbid disease and a grasp of the differential influence of specific diseases are as essential in evidence-based care for older adults diagnosed with head and neck cancers as site-specific staging and prognosis.

Treatment

Once staged, individuals diagnosed with head and neck cancer will be offered a treatment plan that may include multiple modalities and a number of advances in single-modality therapies. Surgery and radiation therapy (RT) continue to be mainstays of treatment (Goepfert, 1998). Chemotherapy is increasingly offered, embedded in combined chemoradiation protocols (Cohen et al., 2004; Forastiere et al., 2001). Increasingly, literature on single- and multimodality treatment of head and neck cancers demonstrates a willingness to treat older adults (Kagan et al., 2002; McGuirt & Davis, 1995; Singh et al., 1999). Samples reported in retrospective case series or case-control studies often include individuals older than 75 years of age, and a growing number of papers specifically are focused on older adults' tolerance of treatment (Clayman, Eicher, Sicard, Razmpa, & Goepfert, 1998; Kagan et al.; McGuirt & Davis; Singh et al.). The single most important general finding stemming from this literature and literature that examines treatment tolerance across diagnostic categories is that older and younger adults benefit from the same treatment protocols (Kagan, 2004a; Piccirillo et al., 2002). However, older adults may experience greater use of resources such as hospital days and home caregiving, suggesting longer functional recovery times (Kagan et al.; McLane, Jones, Lydiatt, Lydiatt, & Richards, 2003). Conversely, older adults may not be at greater risk for treatment complications but rather protracted functional recovery. The evidence that suggests this conclusion, however, tends to emphasize surgical treatment protocols and emerges from studies with some variation in defining complications (Clayman et al.; Kagan et al.; McGuirt & Davis; Singh et al.). Caution then is required in considering the relevance of current evidence to RT, chemotherapy, and combined modalities.

Surgery

Several important surgical advances in treatment for head and neck cancers are influential in guiding care for the older adult. Organ conservation, using partial laryngectomy or chemoradiation for laryngeal cancers, allows less invasive treatment with optimal functional outcomes (Samlan & Webster, 2002). Movement away from radical neck dissection to modified and selective neck dissection involves removing only the lymph nodes that are likely to be involved with the primary site of disease. This modified procedure, used to control nodal spread, drastically has limited the incidence of scarring and severe neck deformity as well as upper extremity complications, such as spinal accessory nerve syndrome (Ferlito ct al., 2003). Technically advanced surgical reconstruction now is standard practice in comprehensive head and neck cancer care (Singh et al., 1999). Although advances in reconstruction do not offer opportunities for better control of cancers, these surgeries bolster quality of life and daily activities by improving appearance and function. These techniques include older rotation flaps and newer microvascular free flaps where skin, muscle, and often bone distant to the operative site are harvested and then implanted to reconstruct lost tissues. Postoperative care is made more technically complicated by monitoring flap perfusion and the secondary surgical incisions made during flap harvest. Rehabilitation more commonly requires intensive interdisciplinary care from speech-language pathology, clinical nutrition, and physical and occupational therapy.

Retrospective studies of older adults undergoing more complex microvascular reconstruction consistently show tolerance equal to that of younger adults, with no difference in complications or complication rates. Chen et al. (2001), McGuirt and Davis (1995), and Singh et al. (1999) uniformly emphasized the role of comorbid disease in prognosis and treatment complications. The evidence they reported implies the critical nature of assessing and managing comorbid conditions and in making decisions predicated on understanding differential influence of particular conditions given available evidence in the context of patients' capacity and desires (Piccirillo et al., 2002).

Radiation Therapy

Radiotherapeutics are advancing rapidly in head and neck cancer treatment. This progression makes RT a very prominent part of treatment for head and neck cancer and a primary treatment modality for older adults with radiosensitive tumors. New techniques for delivery of RT, protocols to better manage acute and chronic side effects, and related technologies such as photodynamic therapy all have a place in the treatment of head and neck cancers. Altered fractionation protocols and intensity modulated radiation therapy allow the radiation oncologist the opportunity to offer higher doses of therapy over shorter periods of time with better sparing of surrounding tissues, respectively (Lee et al., 2003). Use of radioprotective drugs such as amifostine offers the possibility of preserving the function of structures adjacent to the field, such as salivary glands, thereby reducing both acute and chronic side effects (Seikaly, 2003).

Advanced radiotherapeutic technologies logically benefit the older adult being treated with radiotherapy—protection of already senescent tissue, for example, seems obviously important—yet investigation into age-focused and age-related issues in radiotherapy for the older adult with head and neck cancer lags paradoxically. Treatment effects and experience at the patient level as well as management from the clinician perspective are poorly explored and leave important gaps in evidence-based practice. In clinical practice, concerns about functional mobility and ability to tolerate a full course of RT are discussed, but currently decisions are made without aid of evidence. Hence, in conjunction with prioritizing more sophisticated research agendas for the future, current practice must rely on comprehensive geriatric assessment for the frail older adult for whom treatment tolerance is at risk and optimal engagement of the patient in decision making is in practice.

Chemoradiation

Chemoradiation protocols are becoming established therapies for select site-specific cancers and likely will become a prevalent treatment option as new chemotherapeutic agents are developed (Cohen et al., 2004; Forastiere et al., 2001; Goepfert, 1998). Chemoradiation protocols use concurrent administration of the two modalities. Questions about preoperative and sequential use are being debated in clinical trials literature. The chemotherapeutic agents most commonly administered include carboplatin or cisplatin with or without fluorouracil, which may be given with leucovorin. Side effects and symptom clusters generally are more pronounced in combined protocols, but the extent and pattern of severity are unclear (Dodd, Miaskowski, & Paul, 2001). For example, radiation mucositis may be more severe with very thick, tenacious secretions necessitating enhanced self-care and enteral feeding support during and after therapy (Shih, Miaskowski, Dodd, Stotts, & MacPhail, 2002). Case series analyses that establish the nutritional outcomes of routine enteral feeding protocols do not, however, attend at all to issues of age or age-related concerns such as visual impairment, psychomotor slowing or dexterity loss, or cognitive impairment (Lee et al., 1998; Scolapio, Spangler, Romano, McLaughlin, & Salassa, 2001). Therefore, evidence that outlines any unique needs of older adults only can be derived from considering implications of such protocols in the context of findings for individual patients through comprehensive geriatric assessment, guidance from clinical nutrition, and an individualized plan of care.

Age and Treatment and the Risk of Ageism

Head and neck cancer treatment, as outlined by available literature, reveals an embedded understanding of the differences imparted by chronologic age, the age from one's birth, and biologic and functional age (Bourbonniere & Kagan, 2003; Levy, 2003). The attention to comorbidity in defining treatment effects, prognosis, and outcomes shifts study design and analysis away from gross measurement of chronologic age, which is clinically inefficient (Piccirillo et al., 2002). Delimiting clinical practices based on evidence that merely divides findings by age younger than and older than 65 years generally is not efficient in a busy cancer clinic. Emergence of work such as that reported by Piccirillo et al. is a fundamental advance in the level of evidence available for understanding biologic and functional age. Comorbidity can be viewed as a proxy variable that represents elements of biologic and functional age. Other proxy representations of biologic and functional age include variables such as functional status, performance status, and symptom profiles.

Although variables that go beyond comorbidity have yet to appear in the head and neck literature, work that addresses symptom clusters and long-term quality of life anticipates progress in this area and will yield more sophisticated understandings of age and treatment of head and neck cancers. Hammerlid et al. (2001) reported an examination of health-related quality of life among 232 patients who had a mean age of 61 years and were mostly men. Although they found few differences related to age, significant and persistent problems with xerostomia, chemosensory alterations, and dentition limited long-term quality of life. Conversely, Terrell, Fisher, and Wolf (1998) reported on long-term quality of life for 46 patients who participated in the Veterans Affairs study of surgery and radiotherapy versus chemoradiotherapy for cancer of the larynx. They found that although the subjects who received chemoradiotherapy were older than those who received surgery and radiotherapy (61.2 versus 55.7 years, p < .05), they reported significantly better quality of life. The data implied that better emotional well-being and less pain and depression contributed to better quality of life in the chemoradiotherapy group. Although their findings about age are not pronounced or congruent, these studies illustrate clinically important concerns that may vary specifically by age.

Data from Hammerlid et al. (2001) and Terrell et al. (1998) are sharply limited with respect to gender, setting for care, and self-report from health-related and disease-specific instruments that offer forced choice selection of intensity and impact. Nonetheless, the findings are provocative and suggest patterns to attend to in practice as well as direction for future research. Age-based patterns in treatment decisions, concerns about oral symptoms, attention to pain, and assessment and treatment of depression and associated phenomena such as tobacco, alcohol, and other substance use deserve attention in clinical practice (Bourbonniere & Kagan, 2003). Clinical decisions and management then are less likely to be based on assumptions about chronologic age if comprehensive assessment pursues individual characteristics and generalizations (Bourbonniere & Kagan, 2003). Most importantly, these studies outline critical topics to investigate in future research (Hammerlid et al.; Terrell et al.).

Nursing Care Issues

The association of depression with poor quality of life and connections to use of tobacco, alcohol, and possibly other drugs is particularly consequential for the older adult with head and neck cancer (Duffy et al., 2002). Nursing care is critical to successful assessment and intervention in these complex problems. Nursing attention to tobacco and alcohol cessation efforts among older adults at risk for or diagnosed with head and neck cancer should be heightened. The tendency to take a "you can't teach old dogs new tricks" or a "what use would it be?" stance to preventive health behaviors with older adults is inherently ageist and ignores opportunities to reduce disease risk and to improve symptoms exacerbated by poor health habits in late life (Bourbonniere & Kagan, 2003; Duffy et al.). Areas for future research include explicating the unique aspects of emotional and psychological responses and comorbid psychiatric disease for the older adult with head and neck cancer. Although further research is required in these areas, detailed assessment, avoidance of ageist assumptions, and adherence to standards of care for community-dwelling older adults offer tremendous initial opportunities to improve nursing and interdisciplinary practice.

The impact of the head and neck cancer experience for the older family encompasses a broad range of psychosocial concerns from depression to caregiving stress to potential for abuse and neglect. The implications of head and neck cancer and its treatment combine with age-related functional decline to impair communication and increase the need for functional assistance. This additive effect may influence the older adult with head and neck cancer, family members directly involved in daily care, and other family and social support network members.

McLane et al. (2003) reported the grounded theory that illustrates the complex interactions, needs, and impact that the head and neck cancer caregiving experience imparts. In part, the complexity seen in caregiving is a direct result of the sophisticated technologies such as enteral feeding tubes, tracheotomy tubes, and surgical dressings necessitated by current care practices. McLane et al. investigated the specific process of cooperative care, interviewing seven patients, only one of whom was younger than 65 years of age, and their "carepartners" or family caregivers, illustrating the typical age of individuals with head and neck cancers. Twelve themes emerged, ranging from preservation of autonomy to education for self-care (McLane et al.). These themes, although not specific to older adults, addressed salient concerns for the interdisciplinary team led by nursing and social work and suggested the breadth and depth needed in future investigation.

Areas for Future Research

Surviving head and neck cancer while facing the possibility of metachronous primary cancers, recurrence, and often frightening symptoms at the end of life add further complexity to psychosocial care for the older adult with head and neck cancer and for his or her family and friends. The absence of specific evidence to guide practice in these areas underscores the need for individualized interdisciplinary care that attends to the older adult's voice (Bourbonniere & Kagan, 2004; Happ, Williams, Strumpf, & Burger, 1996). Individualized care begins with knowing the individual at all levels and clearly framing those areas of behavioral and psychosocial care that remain unaddressed in current science (Happ et al.). Attending to the older adult's narrative, developing a trusting relationship, and probing with focused questions as indicated by accumulated data provide optimal data for intervention (Happ et al.). Conducting well-designed, prospective studies with precisely framed methods and analyses is a challenge set with obstacles to sampling, statistical power, and instrumentation.

Case Study

Ms. W is an 82-year-old retired journalist who has just been diagnosed with stage III laryngeal cancer. Ms. W has smoked one pack of unfiltered cigarettes per day since the age of 15 when she was a "copy girl" for her hometown newspaper. Since her retirement nine years ago, she has volunteered about 20 hours per week in church-run English literacy programs for immigrants from Hispaniola, as she speaks French, Haitian Creole, Spanish, and English. Ms. W tells you that she has always had a harsh voice and sought health care only after friends commented for approximately one year that her voice had changed.

On clinical examination, Ms. W is found to have a supraglottic exophytic lesion that is expanding outward and is beginning to compress her airway. Her vocal cords are fixed. She has one pathologic ipsilateral lymph node determined by imaging criteria. Her medical history is significant for continued tobacco use with complaints of a non-productive nocturnal cough that was evaluated with a negative chest radiograph and computed tomography scan during the diagnostic evaluation; mild hypertension, which is controlled with a diuretic; arthritis of both hands; and a 10-pound weight loss in the past year. Notably, Ms. W is edentulous and reports losing the last of her teeth about 25 years ago from gingivitis. She wears full dentures. Ms. W's functional status is unimpaired in activities of daily living. She is five feet tall and weighs 95 pounds. A friend accompanies her to diagnostic visits.

In a tumor conference, the interdisciplinary team reviews Ms. W's clinical data and decides to recommend definitive RT with the option of surgical salvage should she not respond completely to the RT. The team feels that Ms. W is at high risk for treatment toxicity, specifically mucositis, further weight loss, and poor tumor response with continued tobacco use. The plan is created to include dental, speech-language, nutrition, and social work evaluations before initiation of treatment, with coordination of the overall plan by the head and neck cancer advanced practice nurse (APN). A primary goal to maximize treatment success is enrollment in a smoking cessation program prior to treatment initiation. Additionally, a percutaneous gastrostomy (PEG) tube will be placed before RT begins. The APN and the surgeon review the plan and the role of salvage surgery, as well as the need for close follow-up after treatment, given the relatively higher risk of recurrence in the first two to three years. She seems amenable to both treatment and planned follow-up.

In the two weeks before RT begins, Ms. W's evaluations go well, her PEG tube is placed, and she begins the smoking cessation program. She appears on time for all of her appointments and takes copious notes. Ms. W seems particularly happy with the nutritionist and the speech-language pathologist. Her nutritional assessment shows stable weight with borderline transport proteins (albumin = 3.0 g/dl, prealbumin = 12.0 mg/dl). The nutritionist counsels Ms. W on management of common side effects of RT and continues to teach her to use her PEG tube, building on what was begun during her ambulatory surgery preparation for its placement.

The behavioral counselor from the smoking cessation program notifies the APN that Ms. W scored 18 on the long-form Geriatric Depression Scale, indicating the high end of the range for mild depression. The behavioral counselor thinks a psychiatric evaluation is indicated for further assessment and possible use of bupropion for treatment of depression and nicotine withdrawal. The APN coordinates a referral even though Ms. W resists. The APN acknowledges her concerns and encourages Ms. W to rely on her ability to collect information, as she has in her job as a journalist, before drawing conclusions. Ms. W appears to enjoy the opportunity to use her prior life experience.

In the week before treatment begins, the radiation oncologist approaches the APN and the surgeon, voicing concerns after having seen Ms. W for the first time. The radiation oncologist is concerned that Ms. W is chronologically old, thin, and a long-time smoker and asks for confirmation that the APN and surgeon feel she can complete treatment or if the dose should be altered. The APN and surgeon refocus discussion on her intact functional status, openness to the treatment team's suggestions, and social support network. The radiation oncologist seems unconvinced but agrees to begin treatment on schedule at full dose.

Ms. W and her friend are both learning to use the PEG tube in the days leading to the start of RT. Both the APN and the nutritionist begin to receive several calls each day from the patient, who asks the same questions of them about the PEG tube. In conferring with each other, the APN and the nutritionist express concern that the patient is showing signs of cognitive impairment. The APN calls the psychiatrist who works with the smoking cessation program, who reports that Ms. W scored 30 out of 30 on the Mini-Mental Status Exam and has been successful in achieving the goals of the cessation program to date. The psychiatrist feels that the escalating number of calls from Ms. W more likely represents anxiety about treatment and encourages the APN to gently confront the patient about her behavior to elicit underlying anxiety. The APN asks Ms. W to come into clinic and review PEG tube use with her. During this interview, the APN reflects that many people may find RT frightening because of negative ideas associated with it. Ms. W starts to cry. The APN and the radiation oncology nurse make arrangements to explore her concerns and address the fears that she has about RT. The APN suggests Ms. W attend a local meeting of the support group Support for People with Oral and Head and Neck Cancers.

The social worker meets with Ms. W as radiation begins. On further exploration, the social worker determines that Ms. W is requesting increasing amounts of personal assistance from her friend. The social worker assesses Ms. W's other social and financial resources as well as her needs in activities of daily living in collaboration with the physical and occupational therapists on the team. Ms. W currently needs assistance with bathing and errands. She became essentially housebound during the beginning of RT and complains of fatigue that increases over the course of the day. The social worker investigates opportunities for support and funding from the county's Area Agency on Aging, which can provide a homemaker to help with activities of daily living and light housekeeping and assistance with errands. The American Cancer

Society can provide transportation to RT. Services are arranged, and the social worker communicates these findings to the APN, the nutritionist, the radiation oncology nurse, and the physicians.

Radiotherapy continues over the following weeks. In the last two weeks of treatment, Ms. W sees the radiation nurse most frequently of all team members. The radiation nurse monitors for toxicities and notices the onset of patchy wet desquamation. The radiation nurse initiated oral and skin care teaching at the beginning of treatment. The radiation nurse confirms that Ms. W is no longer smoking and escalates the frequency of oral and skin care for Ms. W, emphasizing salt and soda oral rinses every two hours while awake and use of Domeboro® (Bayer, Morristown, NJ) soaks and a hydrophilic ointment four times each day. After speaking with Ms. W about more help at home, the radiation nurse contacts the social worker to arrange for home nursing visits and a personal care assistant to help Ms. W to complete her self-care activities each day. The social worker is able to obtain precertification for two nursing visits per week and four assistant visits per week for the last two weeks of radiotherapy and the first week following therapy.

At Ms. W's final radiotherapy appointment, the nutritionist reviews her weekly weight and transport protein levels and notes a weight loss of 1.5 pounds with stable transport protein levels. The nutritionist reinforces Ms. W's success in maintaining her nutrition and emphasizes the use of enteral feeding until her mucositis resolves and she has a follow-up appointment with the speech-language pathologist. The APN and the radiation nurse assess Ms. W's skin reaction and reinforce continued use of the skin care routine established to treat the wet desquamation. Ms. W is given her post-treatment follow-up schedule and future imaging appointments to evaluate the tumor response in the coming year.

Conclusion

Head and neck cancers are a group of relatively rare malignancies that predominantly affect older adults. Complex problems can exist for the older adult with head and neck cancer and can include xerostomia; changes in speech, swallowing, and nutritional intake; pain; and depression. As a result of these potential problems, an interdisciplinary team approach with astute nursing assessment and care is critical. Future research is needed to explore treatment tolerance, side effects, symptom management, and caregiver issues relevant to the older adult with head and neck cancer.

References

Bourbonniere, M.E., & Kagan, S.H. (2003). Ageism can affect how older adults receive care when cancer is the diagnosis. *Advance for Nurses On-line Editions, 5*(19), 32.

Bourbonniere, M.E., & Kagan, S.H. (2004). Nursing intervention and older adults who have cancer: Specific science and evidence based practice. *Nursing Clinics of North America, 39,* 529–543.

Chen, A.Y., Matson, L.K., Roberts, D., & Goepfert, H. (2001). The significance of comorbidity in advanced laryngeal cancer. *Head and Neck, 23,* 566–572.

Clayman, G.L., Eicher, S.A., Sicard, M.W., Razmpa, E., & Goepfert, H. (1998). Surgical outcomes in head and neck cancer patients 80 years of age and older. *Head and Neck, 20,* 216–223.

Cohen, E.E.W., Lingen, M.W., & Vokes, E.E. (2004). The expanding role of systemic therapy in head and neck cancer. *Journal of Clinical Oncology, 22,* 1743–1749.

Davidson, B.J., Root, W.A., & Trock, B.J. (2001). Age and survival from squamous cell carcinoma of the oral tongue. *Head and Neck, 23,* 273–279.

Dodd, M.J., Miaskowski, C., & Paul, S.M. (2001). Symptom clusters and their effect on the functional status of patients with cancer. *Oncology Nursing Forum, 28,* 465–470.

Duffy, S.A., Terrell, J.E., Valenstein, M., Ronis, D.L., Copeland, L.A., & Connors, M. (2002). Effect of smoking, alcohol, and depression on the quality of life of head and neck cancer patients. *General Hospital Psychiatry, 24,* 140–147.

Ferlito, A., Rinaldo, A., Robbins, K.T., Leemans, C.R., Shah, J.P., Shaha, A.R., et al. (2003). Changing concepts in the surgical management of the cervical node metastasis. *Oral Oncology, 39,* 429–435.

Forastiere, A., Koch, W., Trotti, A., & Sidransky, D. (2001). Medical progress: Head and neck cancer. *New England Journal of Medicine, 345,* 1890–1900.

Gibbs, W.W. (2003). Untangling the roots of cancer. *Scientific American, 289*(1), 56–65.

Gillani, A.A., & Grunberg, S.M. (2004). Aerorespiratory tract cancer in older patients. *Seminars in Oncology, 31,* 220–233.

Goepfert, H. (1998). Squamous cell carcinoma of the head and neck: Past progress and future promise. *CA: A Cancer Journal for Clinicians, 48,* 195–198.

Hammerlid, E., Silander, E., Hornestam, L., & Sullivan, M. (2001). Health-related quality of life three years after diagnosis of head and neck cancer—A longitudinal study. *Head and Neck, 23,* 113–125.

Happ, M.B., Williams, C.C., Strumpf, N.E., & Burger, S.G. (1996). Individualized care for frail elders: Theory and practice. *Journal of Gerontological Nursing, 22,* 6–14.

Jemal, A., Murray, T., Ward, E., Samuels, A., Tiwari, R., Ghafoor, A., et al. (2005). Cancer statistics, 2005. *CA: A Cancer Journal for Clinicians, 55,* 10–30.

Kagan, S.H. (2004a). The advanced practice nurse in an aging society. *Sourcebook for Advanced Practice Nurses, 12,* 4–16.

Kagan, S.H. (2004b). Shifting perspectives: Gero-oncology nursing research. *Oncology Nursing Forum, 31,* 293–299.

Kagan, S.H., Chalian, A.A., Goldberg, A.N., Rontal, M.L., Weinstein, G.S., Prior, B., et al. (2002). Impact of age on clinical care pathway length of stay after complex head and neck resection. *Head and Neck, 24,* 545–548.

Koch, W.M., Patel, H., Brennan, J., Boyle, J.O., & Sidransky, D. (1995). Squamous cell carcinoma of the head and neck in the elderly. *Archives of Otolaryngology—Head and Neck Surgery, 121,* 262–265.

Lee, J.H., Machtay, M., Unger, L.D., Weinstein, G.S., Weber, R.S., Chalian, A.A., et al. (1998). Prophylactic gastrostomy tubes in patients undergoing intensive irradiation for cancer of the head and neck. *Archives of Otolaryngology—Head and Neck Surgery, 124,* 871–875.

Lee, N., Xia, P., Fischbein, N.J., Akazawa, P., Akazawa, C., & Quivey, J.M. (2003). Intensity-modulated radiation therapy for head-and-neck cancer: The UCSF experience focusing on target volume delineation. *International Journal of Radiation Oncology, Biology, Physics, 57,* 49–60.

Levy, B.R. (2003). Mind matters: Cognitive and physical effects of aging self-stereotypes. *Journals of Gerontology. Series B, Psychological Sciences and Social Sciences, 58,* P203–P211.

McGuirt, W.F., & Davis, S.P. (1995). Demographic portrayal and outcome analysis of head and neck cancer surgery in the elderly. *Archives of Otolaryngology—Head and Neck Surgery, 121,* 150–154.

McLane, L., Jones, K., Lydiatt, W., Lydiatt, D., & Richards, A. (2003). Taking away the fear: A grounded theory study of cooperative care in the treatment of head and neck cancer. *Psycho-Oncology, 12,* 474–490.

National Cancer Institute. (2004a). *SEER incidence, larynx—Crude rates for additional races/registries, 1992–2001.* Retrieved June 2, 2004, from http://canques.seer.cancer.gov/cgi-bin/cq_submit?dir= seer2001&db=4&rpt=LINE&sel=1^0^1^0^^^&x=Age%20at%20diagnosis^1,2,3,4,5,6,7,8,9,10,11 ,12,13,14,15,16,17,18&y=Race/ethnicity^1,2,3,4,5^Sex^1,2&dec=4

National Cancer Institute. (2004b). *SEER incidence, oral cavity/pharynx—Crude rates for additional races/registries, 1992–2001.* Retrieved June 2, 2004, from http://canques.seer.cancer.gov/cgi-bin/ cq_submit?dir=seer2001&db=4&rpt=LINE&sel=1^0^42^0^^^&x=Age%20at%20diagnosis^1,2,3, 4,5,6,7,8,9,10,11,12,13,14,15,16,17,18&y=Race/ethnicity^1,2,3,4,5^Sex^1,2&dec=4

National Cancer Institute. (2004c). *U.S. mortality (total U.S.), larynx—Crude rates for additional races, 1990–2001.* Retrieved June 2, 2004, from http://canques.seer.cancer.gov/cgi-bin/cq_submit? dir=seer2001&db=10&rpt=LINE&sel=1^32^2^^^&x=Age%20at%20death^1,2,3,4,5,6,7,8,9,10,1 1,12,13,14,15,16,17,18&y=Race/ethnicity^1,2,3,4,5^Sex^1,2&dec=4

Piccirillo, J.F., Lacy, P.D., Basu, A., & Spitznagel, E.L. (2002). Development of a new head and neck cancer-specific comorbidity index. *Archives of Otolaryngology—Head and Neck Surgery, 128,* 1172–1179.

Samlan, R.A., & Webster, K.T. (2002). Swallowing and speech therapy after definitive treatment for laryngeal cancer. *Otolaryngologic Clinics of North America, 35,* 1115–1133.

Scolapio, J., Spangler, P.R., Romano, M.M., McLaughlin, M.P., & Salassa, J.R. (2001). Prophylactic placement of gastrostomy feeding tubes before radiotherapy in patients with head and neck cancer: Is it worthwhile? *Journal of Clinical Gastroenterology, 33,* 215–217.

Seikaly, H. (2003). Xerostomia prevention after head and neck cancer treatment. *Archives of Otolaryngology—Head and Neck Surgery, 129,* 250–251.

Shih, A., Miaskowski, C., Dodd, M.J., Stotts, N.A., & MacPhail, L. (2002). A research review of the current treatments for radiation-induced oral mucositis in patients with head and neck cancer. *Oncology Nursing Forum, 29,* 1063–1080.

Singh, B., Cordeiro, P.G., Santamaria, E., Shaha, A.R., Pfister, D.G., & Shah, J.P. (1999). Factors associated with complications in microvascular reconstruction of head and neck defects. *Plastic and Reconstructive Surgery, 103,* 403–411.

Smith, R.A., Cokkinides, V., & Eyre, H.J. (2003). American Cancer Society guidelines for the early detection of cancer, 2003. *CA: A Cancer Journal for Clinicians, 53,* 27–43.

Terrell, J.E., Fisher, S.G., & Wolf, G.T. (1998). Long-term quality of life after treatment of laryngeal cancer. The Veterans Affairs Laryngeal Cancer Study Group. *Archives of Otolaryngology—Head and Neck Surgery, 124,* 964–971.

CHAPTER 10

The Older Adult With Lung Cancer

Marie Aberle, MS, APRN-BC, BNSc, RN, AOCN®, and
Sandra W. McLeskey, PhD, RN

Introduction

This chapter will outline the incidence, diagnosis, and treatment of the two main types of lung cancer in the older adult. Pathophysiology of lung cancer with rationale and impact of new, targeted biologic therapies will be discussed.

Incidence

The American Cancer Society (ACS) (2005) estimated 172,570 new cases of lung cancer in 2005, which accounts for approximately 13% of all cancer diagnoses. The incidence rate has declined drastically in men from a peak of 102.1 per 100,000 in 1991 to 79.8 per 100,000 in 2000 (ACS, 2004a). African American men are 40% more likely to develop lung cancer than Caucasian men. In women, the incidence rate decreased from 52.8 per 100,000 in 1998 to 49.1 in 2001 (ACS, 2005). African American women have the highest incidence of lung cancer followed by Caucasian, Asian Pacific Islander, Hispanic, and Native American or Alaska Native women. Although the prevalence of smoking has decreased over the past two decades, lung cancer cases still reach epidemic numbers. This results from the prolonged lag time between smoking exposure and the development of cancer. Even if all smokers stopped today, a significant number of lung cancer cases would still exist for many years (ACS, 2004a).

Lung cancer can be described as a disease of the older adult because the vast majority of patients with lung cancer are older than age 65. The National Cancer Institute (NCI) Surveillance, Epidemiology, and End Results (SEER) program reported age-adjusted incidence rates for 1997–2001 at 23.4 per 100,000 for individuals younger than age 65 and up to 350.7 per 100,000 for those older than 65 (Ries et al., 2004). Sixty percent of newly diagnosed patients with lung cancer are older than 65, and 30% are older than 70. The prevalence of lung cancer is expected to increase dramatically over the next 10 years because of the aging population (Syrigos & Dionellis, 2003).

Mortality

Cancer accounts for nearly one-fourth of deaths in the United States, surpassed only by heart disease (ACS, 2005). Lung cancer causes 32% of cancer-related deaths for men and 25% for women. ACS (2005) estimated 163,510 deaths from lung cancer in the United States for 2005. Death rates for lung cancer for men have declined significantly since 1991 at a rate of approximately 1.9% per year. However, female lung cancer deaths have increased in both Caucasians and African Americans, although the rate of increase has slowed since the early 1990s in both groups. In 1987, lung cancer overtook breast cancer as the leading cause of cancer death in women. This is because of a large increase in the lung cancer death rate in women coupled with a somewhat smaller decline in the breast cancer death rate (ACS, 2004b).

Clinical Presentation

A typical patient with lung cancer presents between ages 50–70, with fewer than 5% of patients younger than age 40. A minority of asymptomatic patients has incidental findings of a lesion on a chest x-ray (CXR). Unfortunately, most patients present with advanced disease and exhibit symptoms that are directly related to their primary tumor or to metastasis. Presenting symptoms depend on the histologic type and stage of lung cancer, systemic effects of the disease, and location and effects of metastasis, if present (Aberle & McLeskey, 2003; Knop, 2005).

Approximately 2% of patients with lung cancer present with a paraneoplastic syndrome. Examples of paraneoplastic syndromes in lung cancer include syndrome of inappropriate antidiuretic hormone, clubbing, hypertrophic pulmonary osteoarthropathy, hypercalcemia, and hypercoagulable states (Van Houtte, McDonald, Chang, & Salazar, 2001).

Presenting symptoms of lung cancer can differ depending on the location of the tumor and its proximity to other structures that are compressed or compromised by the tumor (see Table 10-1). Practitioners should be suspicious of lung cancer with

Table 10-1. Symptoms Produced by Lung Tumors in Various Locations

Tumor Location	Symptoms
Central or endobronchial	Bronchial obstruction (cough, unilateral wheezing, or stridor), hemoptysis, sputum production, pneumonitis, dysphagia because of esophageal obstruction
Right-sided apical or peripheral	Superior vena cava syndrome
Apical, either side	Hoarseness because of compression of the recurrent laryngeal nerve, arm weakness or shoulder pain because of compression of the brachial plexus
Invasion of pleura or pericardium	Pleuritic pain, dyspnea, chest pain

any unexplained symptoms referable to the chest, particularly in smokers (Aberle & McLeskey, 2003; Knop, 2005).

Lung cancer has a propensity to spread to the bone, liver, or brain. In such cases, presenting symptoms from bony metastases can include bone pain or pathologic fracture. Central nervous system metastasis can cause seizures, altered mental status, and/or motor and sensory defects. Liver metastasis may cause right hypochondrial pain as well as icterus and altered mentation. Patients with advanced disease may have fatigue or weight loss, possibly from humoral factors elaborated by the tumor (Aberle & McLeskey, 2003; Knop, 2005).

Lung Cancer in the Older Adult

Until recently, many older adult patients with lung cancer were excluded from therapy and clinical trials based solely on their chronologic age. Recently published studies show that advanced age is not a barrier for aggressive lung cancer therapy for patients at any stage of disease (Gridelli, 2002a; Gridelli, De Vivo, & Monfardini, 2002; Langer, 2002). Older adults have been shown to tolerate treatment and enjoy responses much like their younger counterparts. Therefore, treatment should be based on physiologic age, which is reflected in functional status. Specific considerations should be made when treating older individuals with lung cancer because of their risk for comorbid conditions and multiple medications, as well as financial and physical limitations (Gridelli, 2002a; Gridelli et al., 2002; Langer).

Changes of Aging

Metabolic changes that occur with aging can include an approximately 30% decrease in the capacity of the cytochrome P450 enzyme system, the most important system in hepatic metabolism of drugs (Hennessy, Hanrahan, & Breathnach, 2003). This may prolong metabolism of some drugs, resulting in higher plasma levels and prolonged half-lives. Additionally, older patients have a loss of lean body mass with a proportional increase in fat and decrease in intracellular water. This means that hydrophilic drugs will have a lower volume of distribution and variability in peak plasma concentrations, which could cause unpredictable toxicities (Hennessy et al.).

Unpredictable myelotoxicities have been seen in older patients receiving chemotherapy agents, even with dose adjustments. A contributing factor may be the decrease in glomerular filtration rate by approximately 1 ml/minute per year beginning at age 40. For instance, cisplatin is considered the standard of care chemotherapy for lung cancer but is renally toxic and can be poorly tolerated by older adults. Some newer agents, including gemcitabine, vinorelbine, docetaxel, paclitaxel, and oral fluoropyrimidines, have better therapeutic indexes with demonstrated activity in older patients. Regimens with carboplatin, which is widely used in lung cancer, are adjusted according to area under the curve, allowing the clinician to take age and renal function into consideration for safer delivery (Curran & Plosker, 2002; Hennessy et al., 2003; Matsui et al., 2001).

Several physiologic changes affect the ability of older patients to tolerate surgery or thoracic radiation. First, the older adult is at risk for pulmonary infections, partly because of a loss of ciliary function in the respiratory tract. This loss is greatly exacerbated in smokers, who are overrepresented in lung cancer populations. Loss of elastic recoil of thoracic structures with aging can result in a decrease in chest wall compliance, with a consequent decrease in negative intrapleural pressure with air trapping and inadequate ventilation. Vital capacity progressively drops, and respiratory centers become less responsive along with a general slowing of reflexes. However, these changes usually do not compromise the patient's ability to receive therapy unless the patient suffers from other comorbid conditions (Jaklitsch, Mery, & Audisio, 2003).

Risk Factors

Smoking

Smoking remains the greatest contributor to the development of lung cancer and is thought to contribute to 87% of all lung cancer cases. Lung cancer mortality rates are 22 times higher for current male smokers and 12 times higher for current female smokers compared with nonsmokers. Decreasing lung cancer incidence and mortality rates correlate with a decreased incidence of smoking over the past 30 years. Cigarette smoking rates among adults aged 18 and older declined 20% between 1965 and 2000, from 42% to 22% (ACS, 2004a). Unfortunately, the Centers for Disease Control and Prevention's (CDC's) (2003) latest report in 2001 estimated that 46.2 million U.S. adults were current smokers. This represents 22.8% of all adults (20.7% women, 25.2% men). Lung cancer is considered one of the most preventable diseases because smoking abstinence and cessation would drastically reduce its incidence (ACS, 2004a).

At least 43 carcinogens are found in tobacco smoke, including formaldehyde, arsenic, and cyanide. The Environmental Protection Agency (EPA) has identified secondhand smoke as a human carcinogen (Knop, 2005). Secondhand smoke, also known as "side stream" smoke, is released from the smoldering part of the cigarette. It carries up to 100 times the concentration of some of the chemicals that are inhaled by smokers because of the effect of cigarette filters and unburned tobacco on ingredients of inhaled cigarette smoke. Smoke-filled rooms have up to six times the air pollution of a busy highway, and it takes hours to weeks to clear the air (ACS, 2004a). Smoking prevention should be stressed in older patients with lung cancer as well as younger ones, and healthcare providers should advise patients that they are more likely to respond to their treatment if they stop smoking (ACS, 2004b).

Incidence of lung cancer increases with age; however, the risk of getting lung cancer is proportional to smoke exposure, not advancing age. Interestingly, former smokers' risk does not increase with age; their risk remains at the same level that it was at the point they stopped smoking (Syrigos & Dionellis, 2003).

The connection between marijuana smoking and lung cancer has been hard to demonstrate because marijuana is an illegal substance, and smokers often smoke both cigarettes and marijuana. However, marijuana contains some of the same carcinogens as tobacco smoke. Furthermore, it is deeply inhaled and held in and is smoked to the end of the cigarette where the tar is the highest. Because it is illegal, no surveillance is taken of pesticide, fungus, or other chemical content (Jemal, Chu, & Tarone, 2001).

Occupational Risk Factors

Table 10-2 presents occupational exposures that may result in lung cancer.

Table 10-2. Occupation-Related Exposures to Carcinogens

Occupational Setting	Carcinogen	Tumor
Roofing, insulation installation and manufacture, remodeling	Asbestos	Mesothelioma, lung
Mining	Radon from the ground, radiation from ores such as uranium, nickel, coal	Many, including lung
Plastics manufacture	Vinyl chloride	Liver, lung
Traffic or petroleum exposure	Aromatic hydrocarbons in gasoline and diesel fuels and exhaust	Lung

Asbestos

Asbestos workers have a seven times increased risk for developing lung cancer, and asbestos is linked to 2%–4% of lung cancer cases. For those who have both smoked cigarettes and worked with asbestos, the risk for mesothelioma (a cancer of the pleura) is 50–90 times greater than the general population. Asbestos use now is prohibited in commercial and industrial products. However, asbestos still is present in many homes and commercial buildings and is harmful if released into the air through demolition or renovation (ACS, 2004b).

Radon

The EPA (2003) reported annual lung cancer deaths from radon exposure at approximately 21,000. Radon-related lung cancers usually develop 5–25 years after exposure, and smokers are at a higher risk for developing radon-related lung cancer.

Other

Tuberculosis and some types of pneumonia are thought to increase the risk of adenocarcinomas because of prolonged inflammation (ACS, 2004b).

Screening

The purpose of screening is to prevent or delay the development of cancer by means of early detection of cancer or of premalignant states. The main reason to screen populations for diseases is to improve the quality of health care and reduce healthcare costs. Lung cancer is an appropriate target, with more than one million attributable deaths worldwide in 2000. However, randomized controlled trials have not been able to demonstrate a decrease in lung cancer mortality through the use of screening with CXR and/or sputum cytology (Marcus et al., 2000; NCI, 2004). False-positive results are a risk and can lead to percutaneous needle biopsy or thoracotomy. Overdiagnosis can occur, which is the diagnosis of a tumor that would not have become clinically significant had it not been detected by screening. ACS (2004b) currently does not recommend screening tests for lung cancer, even for people at high risk. The National Comprehensive Cancer Network (NCCN, 2005a) recommended that people at high risk for non-small cell lung cancer (NSCLC) participate in prospective trials evaluating spiral computed tomography (CT) (Bach, Niewoehner, & Black, 2003).

Although CXR is not officially recommended, many physicians believe that smokers, especially those age 50 or older, should undergo one annually. Recently, a screening procedure known as helical or spiral CT of the chest has attracted considerable attention. The Early Lung Cancer Action Project enrolled 1,000 symptom-free healthy individuals aged 60 or older with at least a 10 pack–year history of smoking who had no previous evidence of cancer (Henschke et al., 1999). Subjects received both low-dose spiral CT and CXR. Spiral CT identified 233 (23%) noncalcified nodules compared with 68 (7%) shown by CXR. Of the positive findings from CT, 2.7% (27 patients) were found to have malignant disease, with 23 of the 27 patients having stage I disease. Of the 27 with malignancy, 26 were able to undergo a complete resection with a goal of cure. The authors reported that the cost of the low-dose CT scanning was only slightly higher than standard CXR. This trial indicated that high-resolution, rapid, low-dose-intensity CT scanning can improve the likelihood of detection of small noncalcified nodules and possibly detect lung cancer at an earlier stage than CXR, when it is potentially curable (Henschke et al., 1999). NCI is conducting a much larger randomized controlled trial, the National Lung Screening Trial, to evaluate whether screening asymptomatic individuals at high risk for lung cancer with spiral CT or standard CXR can reduce the number of lung cancer deaths (ACS, 2004b). Enrollment and follow-up data will be analyzed for eight years as of February 2004.

In the future, better screening tests for lung cancer may be developed. The scientists of the Human Genome Project, together with NCI, are undertaking a project to identify the genetic events that are involved in the process of carcinogenesis. Genetic markers could be used to screen individuals for genetic mutations and predict malignant potential, allowing identification, reversal, or treatment of preneoplastic lesions (Lea, Calzone, Masny, & Bush, 2002).

It is noteworthy that enrollment of smokers in the Early Lung Cancer Action Project trial was limited to those 60 years of age or older (Henschke et al., 1999). In the past, many screening trials have not included older individuals because it was felt that the benefits of screening would not be evident in patients with a limited life span. Because lung cancer is largely a disease of older adults and most patients with lung cancer currently have a very limited life span after diagnosis, this concern may not be valid for lung cancer. However, the National Lung Screening Trial recruited patients between the ages of 55 and 74 (ACS, 2004b), implying that the designers of the study felt that including subjects older than 74 might prevent the demonstration of benefit in younger subjects. Nonetheless, exclusion of adults 75 and older eliminates the opportunity to gain any useful information on the value of screening in these subjects.

Chemoprevention in Lung Cancer

Chemoprevention involves the use of a substance, including vitamins, mineral supplements, or medications, to prevent the development of cancer. Many compounds, such as retinoids, carotenoids, soy isoflavones, nonsteroidal anti-inflammatory drugs, green tea polyphenols, and antioxidants, are suggested to be chemopreventive based on epidemiologic data in lung cancer or data from other cancers. However, only a few of these have survived studies in cell culture or animals and advanced to randomized clinical intervention trials.

These primary prevention trials recruit subjects likely to develop lung cancer (smokers or previous smokers). Various retinoids were studied in such trials and found to be without effect in preventing the development of metaplasia, a preneoplastic change (Cohen & Khuri, 2003). Surprisingly, beta-carotene was found to increase incidence of premalignant atypical pulmonary epithelial cells in sputum of active smokers, implying that it was increasing the risk of lung cancer (Cohen & Khuri). Six-year follow-up is available from this study and showed that the adverse effects of beta-carotene had persisted throughout the interval (Goodman et al., 2004).

Tertiary chemoprevention studies in subjects who had developed a first lung cancer with the end point of second primary tumor development have shown equivocal results with retinyl palmitate and no overall benefit with retinoic acid, N-acetyl-cysteine, or beta-carotene (Cohen & Khuri, 2003). In a study with beta-carotene and isotretinoin, multivariate analysis showed a possible increase in lung cancer with current smokers and possible benefit with former smokers (Cohen & Khuri). Some of these studies still are ongoing and may provide more definitive results at some future time. At this time, sufficient evidence is unavailable to support the use of any agent alone or in combination for the primary, secondary, or tertiary prevention of lung cancer outside of a clinical trial (Dragnev, Stover, & Dmitrovsky, 2003). However, patient education is an important primary prevention strategy, because experts estimate that nearly one-third of all cancers could be prevented by lifestyle changes, primarily smoking cessation in the case of lung cancer (Henschke, McCarthy, & Wernick, 2002).

Types of Lung Cancer in Older Adults

The median age at diagnosis of lung cancer is 70 (Edwards et al., 2002), which dictates that more than half of patients with lung cancer are older than 65. Characterization of types of lung cancers and their distribution in the population is inherently biased toward the types of disease found in older adults; however, no evidence suggests that lung cancer is more aggressive in older adults. Comorbidities in this population may dictate alternative approaches to potentially curative surgery or palliative but aggressive approaches to widespread disease. This suboptimal therapy may result in poorer outcomes in older adults with lung cancer.

Lung (bronchiogenic) cancer is divided into two subgroups, NSCLC and small cell lung cancer (SCLC), which was formerly known as oat cell carcinoma. Differentiating between the two main types of lung cancer is crucial because SCLC and NSCLC are treated differently. Each type of lung cancer has unique biologic characteristics resulting in different responses to different therapies. Evidence shows that current methods of tissue diagnosis in lung cancer are accurate, and the chance for error in diagnosing an SCLC that is actually an NSCLC averages 0.09%, and the chance of diagnosing an NSCLC that is actually an SCLC is 0.02% (Minna, Dekido, Fong, & Gazdar, 2001). Currently, more than 80% of diagnosed lung cancers are NSCLC, and less than 20% are SCLC (Hurria & Kris, 2003).

NSCLC is further classified based on histology into adenocarcinoma, bronchoalveolar cell carcinoma (a variant of adenocarcinoma), large cell carcinoma, and squamous cell carcinoma. Each of these subtypes has its own characteristics and might be treated differently, although the differences between types of NSCLC are not as marked as those between NSCLC and SCLC.

The percentage of patients diagnosed with SCLC decreased from 17.4% in 1986 to 13.8% in 1998. Nearly one-fourth of patients diagnosed with SCLC are at least 70 years of age. SCLC differs from NSCLC by its rapid doubling time, early spread, and high growth fraction (Minna et al., 2001).

Diagnostic Evaluation

Diagnosis of lung cancer most often is relatively simple, given that the advanced disease that most patients present with can easily be visualized on a routine CXR. However, for treatment considerations, it is imperative that the type of lung cancer be determined and careful estimation of the extent of disease be made to provide aggressive treatment to those most likely to benefit while offering palliative treatment to those whose disease has little likelihood of cure. Determination of the extent of disease enables patients to be categorized according to staging criteria (see Figure 10-1), to which are attached specific treatment recommendations. Various imaging or biopsy modalities are used in diagnosis and/or staging in lung cancer (Minna et al., 2001).

Imaging

The CXR is the primary tool for diagnosing lung cancer and can reveal an abnormal mass or nodule $\geq$ 1 cm in size, effusions, atelectasis, and tumors in the peripheral parenchyma (Van Houtte et al., 2001). SCLC presents with a mass in or adjacent to the hilum and/or massive hilar lymphadenopathy, with direct mediastinal invasion in as many as 78% of cases (Rivera, Detterbeck, Mehta, & the American College of Chest Physicians [ACCP], 2003). However, CXR is poor at differentiating structures, determining precise locations, or identifying small lymph nodes, all of which are necessary in staging lung cancer. Magnetic resonance imaging (MRI) is not routinely used but may offer some advantage when evaluating for metastasis to the brain or spine. CT scans of the lungs and the upper abdomen, liver, and adrenal glands can help to define the location of lesions or lymphadenopathy and the presence of liver or adrenal gland metastasis. These should be performed at baseline and routinely following therapy to evaluate response and/or monitor for recurrence (Knop, 2005). CT scans have a sensitivity of 75% and a specificity of 66% but are limited in their ability to identify subtleties in the mediastinum or chest wall (Van Houtte et al.).

Positron emission tomography (PET) is a newer form of nuclear medicine scanning that involves the acquisition of physiologic images based on the detection of [18]-fluoro-deoxy-glucose (FDG), which localizes in metabolically active cells such as cancer cells. PET scans are more useful than CT scanning or MRI in identifying local spread to mediastinal and hilar lymph nodes. Whole body PET scanning can be useful in detecting metastatic disease at distant sites. PET scanning has a sensitivity of 95% and an 85% specificity and can eliminate the need for biopsies in some settings. However, PET scan does not provide measurable images, whereas CT scans allow for the measurement of tumors. The Health Care Foundation Association for reimbursement by Medicare has approved PET scans for NSCLC for diagnosis, staging, and restaging (Centers for

TNM definitions

Primary tumor (T)
- TX: Primary tumor cannot be assessed or tumor is proven by the presence of malignant cells in sputum or bronchial washings but is not visualized by imaging or bronchoscopy
- T0: No evidence of primary tumor
- Tis: Carcinoma in situ
- T1: A tumor that is < 3 cm in greatest dimension is surrounded by lung or visceral pleura and is without bronchoscopic evidence of invasion more proximal than the lobar
- T2: A tumor with any of the following features of size or extent:
  - > 3 cm in greatest dimension
  - Involves the main bronchus and is < 2 cm distal to the carina
  - Invades the visceral pleura
  - Associated with atelectasis or obstructive pneumonitis that extends to the hilar region but does not involve the entire lung
- T3: A tumor of any size that directly invades any of the following: chest wall (including superior sulcus tumors), diaphragm, mediastinal pleura, parietal pericardium; tumor in the main bronchus < 2 cm distal to the carina but without involvement of the carina; or associated atelectasis or obstructive pneumonitis of the entire lung
- T4: A tumor of any size that invades any of the following: mediastinum, heart, great vessels, trachea, esophagus, vertebral body, carina; separate tumor nodules in the same lobe; or tumor with a malignant pleural effusion

Regional lymph nodes (N)
- NX: Regional lymph nodes cannot be assessed
- N0: No regional lymph node metastasis
- N1: Metastasis to ipsilateral peribronchial and/or ipsilateral hilar lymph nodes, and intrapulmonary nodes including involvement by direct extension of the primary tumor
- N2: Metastasis to ipsilateral mediastinal and/or subcarinal lymph node(s)
- N3: Metastasis to contralateral mediastinal, contralateral hilar, ipsilateral or contralateral scalene, or supraclavicular lymph node(s)

Distant metastasis (M)
- MX: Distant metastasis cannot be assessed
- M0: No distant metastasis
- M1: Distant metastasis present

American Joint Committee on Cancer stage groupings
Occult carcinoma
- TX, N0, M0

Stage 0
- Tis, N0, M0

Stage IA
- T1, N0, M0

Stage IB
- T2, N0, M0

Stage IIA
- T1, N1, M0

Stage IIB
- T2, N1, M0
- T3, N0, M0

Stage IIIA
- T1, N2, M0
- T2, N2, M0
- T3, N1, M0
- T3, N2, M0

Stage IIIB
- Any T, N3, M0
- T4, any N, M0

Stage IV
- Any T, any N, M1

Figure 10-1. Lung Cancer Staging

Note. Data from "Lung Cancer Treatment," by the National Cancer Institute, 2004. Retrieved July 8, 2004, from http://www.nci.nih.gov/cancertopics/pdq/treatment/non-small-cell-lung/HealthProfessionals

Medicare and Medicaid Services, 2004). Studies in SCLC have shown that PET scanning will be useful in staging disease, but further prospective trials are necessary before it is adopted as the standard of care (Simon, Wagner, & ACCP, 2003).

Tissue Diagnostic Procedures

As with any cancer, lung cancer only can be definitively diagnosed by a biopsy or cytologic examination, which involves looking at tissue or cells under a microscope (Knop, 2005). Guidelines for biopsies and cytologies have been established, with specific recommendations on the diagnosis of lung cancer. A multidisciplinary team should make the decision regarding a particular technique with input from the patient, pulmonologist, chest radiologist, and thoracic specialist. The presumed type and stage of the lung cancer and the location and size of the tumor will determine the appropriate diagnostic procedure (Rivera et al., 2003). Tissue diagnostic methods are compared in Table 10-3.

Table 10-3. Tissue Diagnostic Modalities in Lung Cancer

Modality	Advantages	Disadvantages
Sputum cytology	Easily obtained, noninvasive, inexpensive, sensitivity increased with serial sputum collections, no complications	Low sensitivity for a single specimen, high false-negative rate, central tumors give better results
Bronchoscopy	High specificity, subcarinal lymph nodes are accessible, autofluorescence techniques improve sensitivity	Invasive, requires sedation, limited to large bronchi, only moderate sensitivity, high false-positive rate with autofluorescence, major complications (rare)
Mediastinoscopy	High specificity and sensitivity, reaches otherwise inaccessible lymph nodes and other mediastinal structures	Invasive, requires general anesthesia, major complications, including those of anesthesia (rare)
Transthoracic needle biopsy	Minimally invasive, high specificity and sensitivity, reaches peripheral tumors not accessible by other means	Analgesia required, serious complications possible but rare, air leaks may persist
Video thoracoscopy and thoracentesis	Increased sensitivity, high specificity, pleural fluid examination possible	Invasive, requires anesthesia and incision, complications possible, including persistent air leaks

Sputum Cytology

Sputum cytology can be a cost-effective means of obtaining a pathologic diagnosis when collected properly. Sputum specimens should be collected with deep coughing early in the morning for three to five days. With repeated examinations, positive results can be found in as many as 75% of lung carcinomas (Van Houtte et al., 2001). Central tumors can yield a positive result in approximately 80% of cases, but the accuracy drops to 20% if the tumors are smaller and located in the periphery (Ingle, 2000). Therefore, sputum cytology is a reasonable approach in patients with central lesions, but the accuracy will depend on the rigorous collection, processing, and interpretation of the specimens (Rivera et al., 2003).

Bronchoscopy

Fiberoptic bronchoscopy is a primary method for diagnosing lung cancer and allows direct visualization of the upper and lower respiratory tract for the additional diagnosis of a spectrum of infectious, inflammatory, and malignant diseases of the chest. During bronchoscopy, tissue specimens can be retrieved with a bronchial brush, forceps, or needle. Cell washings via bronchial lavage allows for removal of abnormal tissues. Suspicious subcarinal lymph nodes may be biopsied using transbronchial fine-needle aspiration during bronchoscopy (Fretz & Peterson, 2004).

Autofluorescence bronchoscopy involves examining the bronchi with illumination from an ultraviolet light source. Normal cells fluoresce red, but abnormal cells appear brown. These abnormal-appearing areas are removed with a bronchial brush or forceps and evaluated for malignancy. This technique is particularly useful in patients with positive sputum cytology and normal CXR. Similar to bronchoscopy without fluorescence, its use is limited in bronchi not large enough to pass the bronchoscope, and it cannot detect peripheral tumors. A high false-positive rate engenders unnecessary biopsies (Kennedy, Lam, & Hirsch, 2001).

For centrally located tumors, bronchoscopy offers high sensitivity. However, if lesions are located peripherally, transthoracic needle aspiration will have a higher sensitivity than bronchoscopy. Major complications are rare (with a mortality rate of less than 0.1%) (see Table 10-3). Minor complications include minor bleeding (less than 50 cc), minor arrhythmias, and hypocalcemia, which occurs in less than 10% of patients (Fretz & Peterson, 2004).

Mediastinoscopy

The mediastinum is the membranous structure that contains the mediastinal lymph nodes, heart, thymus, esophagus, and trachea along with a variety of blood vessels, including the aorta and pulmonary artery and vein. X-rays or CT scans may identify enlarged mediastinal nodes that should be biopsied to determine whether they are malignant or benign. Ipsilateral lymph nodes (N2) involved with NSCLC indicate stage IIIa disease, and such patients are potential candidates for surgery after preoperative chemoradiation. Patients with positive contralateral mediastinal lymph nodes (N3) have stage IIIb disease and are not considered surgical candidates because complete surgical removal of the primary tumor and involved lymph nodes will not prevent recurrence of the cancer. Therefore, determining whether a patient has N2 or N3 disease is critical in managing patients with lung cancer (Van Houtte et al., 2001).

Mediastinoscopy is accomplished by insertion of an endoscope through a small incision at the superior border of the sternum, advancing the instrument throughout the chest, examining structures, and taking biopsies when necessary. General anesthesia with intubation is necessary (Ingle, 2000).

Transthoracic Needle Biopsy

A fine-needle aspiration can be performed on patients presenting with a solitary suspicious intrathoracic lesion. This procedure has a higher sensitivity than bronchoscopy (Rivera et al., 2003). With the help of fluoroscopic or CT guidance, transthoracic needle biopsy can access pulmonary lesions that are not accessible with bronchoscopy (Ingle, 2000). For patients who have extensive suspected tumor infiltration of the mediastinum as evidenced on plain CXR, either a transthoracic needle aspiration or endoscopic ultrasound-guided needle aspiration is the procedure of choice (Aelony, Bonnet, Colt, & Potkin, 2002; Detterbeck, DeCamp, Kohman, & Silvestri, 2003).

Video Thoracoscopy and Thoracentesis

Video thoracoscopy is accomplished through an incision between the ribs, which leads to partial collapse of the lung and allows the surgeon to pass an endoscope with a video camera to visualize the lung and perform biopsies. The lung will re-expand after the procedure (Koizumi et al., 2002; Rivera et al., 2003).

Approximately 10% of patients with lung cancer will have pleural effusions, and sampling this fluid by thoracentesis may allow for diagnosis and assist in staging. If a patient presents with an accessible pleural effusion, it should be sampled to determine whether it is because of cancer invading the pleura or lymphatic blockage, hypoproteinemia, or atelectasis. Malignant fluid indicates T4 disease. If the pleural fluid is cytologically negative after two separate attempts, pleural biopsy via thoracoscopy should be the next step, which improves the diagnostic sensitivity (Rivera et al., 2003). Thoracentesis also can be performed therapeutically to relieve dyspnea from malignant pleural effusions. Unfortunately, the relief is rarely long lasting, and more definitive treatment of the underlying disease or pleurodesis might be needed (Kvale, Simoff, & Prakash, 2003).

Staging

Accurate staging of both NSCLC and SCLC is critical because the prognosis and treatment options are different depending on the stage of the disease. As mentioned, most patients with lung cancer are older adults; therefore, conclusions about survival of various stages by definition are applicable to the older adult population.

Staging for NSCLC uses the TNM guidelines from the American Joint Committee on Cancer (AJCC) (Greene et al., 2002) based on three characteristics: T—size and location of tumor, N—extent of lymph node involvement, and M—presence or absence of metastases. These guidelines were last revised in 1997 and are due to be revised in 2007. In the interim, further research is being conducted to evaluate modifications that could give additional guidance on staging as well as new prognostic information (Ginsberg, 1998).

SCLC is classified as either extensive or limited. Limited-stage disease is confined to one hemithorax with ipsilateral regional lymph node involvement that can be included within a single radiotherapy port. Any disease beyond these limits is classified as extensive disease (Minna et al., 2001).

Evaluation of Metastasis

A thorough history and physical examination is the best predictor of metastatic disease. If the patient has stage I or II NSCLC and clinical evaluation of the chest and laboratory parameters are negative, published guidelines of the ACCP do not recommend further imaging studies of possible metastatic sites. However, if signs or symptoms are present, imaging of suspected sites should be performed. Tissue sampling should be performed if the radiographic findings are questionable as to whether they are malignant or benign (Silvestri, Tanoue, Margolis, Barker, & Detterbeck, 2003).

In addition to a CT of the chest and upper abdomen, patients with SCLC should have a bone scan and MRI of the brain to rule out metastasis because SCLC has a propensity to metastasize quickly to the bone and brain (Simon et al., 2003).

Preoperative Evaluation in Patients With Operable Tumors

Once staging is accomplished and potentially curative or palliative surgery is indicated, older adults should undergo a thorough preoperative evaluation. NCCN (2005b) recommended initial screening that includes assessment of the probability that the patient will die of the cancer compared with the likelihood that he or she will die of a comorbidity. If death from cancer is more likely, a thorough geriatric assessment should be performed to determine the patient's ability to tolerate cancer therapy (NCCN, 2005b). Particular attention should be paid to mental and functional status and nutritional, physical, social, and financial concerns, such as prescription coverage. Age alone should not prevent patients from undergoing surgical resection if indicated, because surgery remains the only treatment approach in lung cancer with the potential for cure (Beckles, Spiro, Colice, & Rudd, 2003). In fact, increasing age was a favorable prognostic factor for response to treatment (Borges et al., 1996) and did not predict outcomes from surgery in selected patient populations (Ishida, Yokoyama, Kaneko, Sugio, & Sugimachi, 1990; van Rens, de la Riviere, Elbers, & van Den Bosch, 2000). Tumor stage, performance status, and weight loss are the most accepted preoperative prognostic predictive factors for surgical morbidity and mortality (Beckles et al.).

Pulmonary Evaluation

Postoperative respiratory complications are the major cause of morbidity and mortality for the older adult. For that reason, preoperative pulmonary status should be evaluated with spirometry/pulmonary function tests, CXR, and arterial blood gas analysis. If the forced expiratory volume in one second (FEV1) is greater than 80% of the predicted norm (or > 2 L), the patient should be a candidate for surgery, including pneumonectomy. Patients may be considered for a lobectomy if the FEV1 is > 1.5 L. Additional testing should be done if the guidelines for FEV1 are not met. Diffusing capacity of the lung for carbon monoxide (DLCO), a measurement of carbon monoxide uptake from alveolar gas, should be determined if evidence of interstitial lung disease is present or if the patient is symptomatic, even if the FEV1 is adequate. Studies suggest that DLCO is a strong predictor of mortality (Jaklitsch et al., 2003).

Preoperative exercise has been found to better correlate with postoperative dyspnea than spirometry. Some authorities recommend the combination of exercise tolerance tests with stair climbing and walking for six minutes; spirometry; and DLCO as standard preoperative evaluation for all older adult patients with suspected lung cancer (Jaklitsch et al., 2003).

Patients with a FEV1 < 40% of the predicted norm are at high risk of perioperative death and cardiopulmonary complications. If the FEV1 is < 30%, patients should be counseled on nonsurgical options. If patients have any abnormal findings during their pulmonary workups, further tests such as perfusion scans should be obtained (Beckles et al., 2003; Jaklitsch et al., 2003).

Cardiac Evaluation

All older adult patients should have a detailed cardiac history and an electrocardiogram (ECG). Previous myocardial infarction (MI) and concurrent congestive heart failure (CHF) are two well-documented preoperative risk factors for cardiac morbidity after surgery. No further preoperative tests should be required if the older adult patient has no cardiac symptoms, a normal ECG, and no history of coronary artery disease (CAD), MI, or CHF. If the patient has a history of MI or CHF, an echocardiogram should be performed to evaluate ejection fraction. For patients with a history of CAD or previous coronary graft bypass, a stress test should be completed to evaluate cardiac function. High-risk patients can be treated preoperatively with anti-ischemic and antihypertensive medications and with intensive monitoring peri- and postoperatively (Jaklitsch et al., 2003).

Treatment of Non-Small Cell and Small Cell Lung Cancer

Treatment for lung cancer depends on the type of lung cancer (SCLC versus NSCLC), stage of the disease, performance status of the patient, and comorbidities. Some treatment modalities can be used at any stage of disease for palliative reasons. These would include bronchoscopy to relieve bronchial obstructing lesions, site-specific radiation for bone pain, or chemotherapy to relieve symptoms related to a paraneoplastic syndrome. However, treatment is largely dictated by the stage of the disease at diagnosis. Superimposed upon this are the patient's functional status and comorbidities because these will influence the patient's ability to tolerate treatment. Finally, the patient's wishes concerning treatment always should be respected, especially because lung cancer is quite often diagnosed at a late stage, and current treatment modalities of late-stage disease do not afford a cure (Bunn & Lilenbaum, 2003).

Non-Small Cell Lung Cancer Stages I and II

NSCLC can be considered a disease typical of advanced age, with more than 50% of patients with NSCLC older than age 65 and 30% older than age 70. Early findings showed that frequency of localized lung cancer is higher in patients older than 75 years of age when compared with patients younger than 54 years of age (O'Rourke, Feussner, Feigl, & Laszlo, 1987), and squamous NSCLC, which tends to be localized, is a more frequent diagnosis in older adults (North-Eastern Italian Oncology Group, 1990). However, these findings are countered by the fact that only 15%–20% of all patients, regardless of their age, present at an early stage or are able to undergo a complete resection (Gridelli, 2002b).

Surgery

Surgical resection with clear margins is the treatment of choice and the only curative approach available for early stage NSCLC (stages I and II). No difference exists in long-term survival for older adult patients who survive surgery compared with younger patients. However, older patients are less likely to be offered surgery. Resection rates range from 26%–32% for younger patients compared with 6% for older adult patients. As previously mentioned, age alone should not prevent a patient from undergoing surgery. The dilemma facing patients and their physicians is balancing the risk of surgery with improved long-term survival (Jaklitsch et al., 2003; Yamamoto et al., 2003).

In the past decade, thoracic surgery has been transformed by the development of minimally invasive surgeries. These procedures decrease operative risks, allowing older adult patients with comorbid conditions a greater opportunity to undergo curative surgery (Conti, Brega Massone, Lequaglie, Magnani, & Cataldo, 2002; Jaklitsch et al., 2003).

A trained surgeon who is board certified or board eligible in thoracic surgery should perform the surgical resection. Pneumonectomy is associated with significant postoperative morbidity and mortality, whereas the use of sleeve resection and arterioplasty has reduced complications. However, lobectomy is considered the standard of care for localized lung cancer. Lung-sparing procedures such as a segmentectomy or wedge resection are considered alternatives for older patients. When wedge resection is compared with lobectomy, no significant difference in local recurrence and overall survival exists, but wedge resection had a reduction in postoperative complications, making it a reasonable alternative for older patients with high operative risk, comorbid diseases, or other cardiopulmonary problems. Video-assisted thoracic surgery was found to be beneficial in benign thoracic disorders and in several small trials in older adult patients with lung cancer. Larger randomized trials are needed to establish this type of surgery as standard care (Jaklitsch et al., 2003).

Patients with positive resection margins or incomplete resection should be considered for additional local treatment with further resection or radiation therapy. All patients undergoing resection should have an intraoperative mediastinal lymph node evaluation for accurate staging (Jaklitsch et al., 2003).

Radiation

Radiation therapy (RT) is the treatment of choice for patients unable to undergo surgery because of comorbid conditions such as poor pulmonary function or cardiac contraindications (Smythe & ACCP, 2003). Combined chemotherapy and RT have failed to demonstrate a significant survival benefit over RT alone for this population. Adjuvant chemotherapy and RT have been investigated postoperatively, but studies have failed to demonstrate a significant survival benefit (Gridelli, 2002b). At this time, neoadjuvant or adjuvant chemotherapy and adjuvant RT are not recommended outside the setting of a clinical trial for stage I or II NSCLC (Scott, Howington, & Movsas, 2003).

Non-Small Cell Lung Cancer Stage III

Almost half of patients with NSCLC have positive mediastinal lymph nodes. Patients with N2 have stage IIIA disease and are potential surgical candidates after preoperative chemoradiation. However, patients with N3 have stage IIIB disease and are not considered surgical candidates. Patients with N2 disease have a five-year survival of 30% compared with 5% for N3 disease. Therefore, distinguishing between N2 and

N3 disease plays a critical role in the management of patients with NSCLC (Gridelli, 2002b; Scott et al., 2003).

Patients older than 70 years of age with locally advanced NSCLC had comparable two- and five-year survival rates when compared with patients younger than 70 years of age in a study involving chemoradiotherapy (Schild et al., 2003). However, the older age group demonstrated more grade 4 or higher toxicities (81% of older patients versus 62% in younger patients, p = 0.007). Grade 4+ hematologic toxicities also were elevated in the older age group (56%, < 70 years of age versus 78%, > 70 years of age, p = 0.003), as was grade 4+ radiation pneumonitis (1%, < 70 years of age versus 6%, > 70 years of age, p = 0.02). However, the only prognostic factor identified was functional status; age was not a prognostic factor. Although this study did not evaluate the frequency of dosage reductions and other adjustments in therapy necessitated by toxicities, it indicates that age *per se* should not be a limiting factor in aggressive treatment of stage III NSCLC (Schild et al.).

Non-Small Cell Lung Cancer Stage IIIA

Surgery is the optimal treatment for patients with resectable stage IIIA disease. Neoadjuvant chemotherapy is being studied as a means of making "nonresectable" patients resectable by shrinking the tumor enough to make resection possible. The best approach for adjuvant therapy following surgery for these patients is under investigation. Preoperative cisplatin-based chemotherapy followed by postoperative radiotherapy was shown to result in superior survival when compared with surgery followed by radiotherapy in patients with stage IIIA disease (Goss, Paszat, Newman, Evans, & the Lung Cancer Disease Site Group, 1998). Local RT is used adjuvantly in patients with potentially curative resection for local control. Indications include positive surgical margins, positive regional lymph nodes (N1, N2), extracapsular lymph node invasion, and unresectable lesions. Patients with tumors confined to lung parenchyma or with negative nodes do not benefit from adjuvant RT. In fact, RT use has been controversial because of the lack of effect on long-term survival. Recent trials have shown a survival advantage with dose intensification with conventional fractionation or altered fractionation (Minna et al., 2001).

Non-Small Cell Lung Cancer Stage IIIB (without malignant pleural effusion)

Patients with large T4 tumors and multiple bulky nodal involvement (N2 or N3) are not eligible for resection. Treatment with chemotherapy and RT is recommended. However, the exact scheduling, whether sequential, concurrent, or rapidly alternating schedules, still is under investigation. RT can be administered as standard dose, hyperfractionated, accelerated, or continuous hyperfractionated RT or as a split course. A randomized trial showed improved survival of patients with continuous hyperfractionated, accelerated radiation therapy (CHART) over patients receiving standard therapy with 60 gray (Gy) in 30 fractions. Patients who have a performance status > 1, those unable to undergo induction chemotherapy and radiotherapy, or patients who prefer RT alone may be considered for CHART as part of a clinical trial. At this time, further randomized controlled trials are necessary to confirm the benefits of hyperfractionation radiotherapy, and insufficient data exist to recommend hyperfractionation over standard treatment. Cost of care and effect on quality of life of hyperfractionated RT have not been reviewed in most of the trials and need further exploration before recommendations can be made (Hayakawa et al., 2001; Kadono, Satoh, Homma, Ohtsuka, & Sekizawa, 2002; Yu et al., 2000). Triple therapy with induction chemotherapy followed by surgery and RT and/or chemotherapy has been studied with promising results, but the optimal combination of drugs for induction or adjuvant chemotherapy and/or subsequent radiotherapy dosages and schedules is far from clear (Detterbeck & Socinski, 2001).

Non-Small Cell Lung Cancer Stage IIIB (with malignant pleural effusion) and Stage IV

Survival rates of patients with stages IIIB and IV NSCLC are extremely poor. The median survival with best supportive care is approximately 16–17 weeks with a one-year survival rate of 10%–15%. Cisplatin-based therapy was shown to produce a 26% reduction in the rate of death and currently is considered to be the standard of care. The American Society of Clinical Oncology (ASCO, 1997) guidelines recommend a cisplatin-based regimen for the treatment of stage IV NSCLC in patients with good performance status (Eastern Cooperative Oncology Group [ECOG] 1 or 2). Approximately 20%–30% of patients, including many older adult patients, present with a poor performance status (≥ 2). Additionally, many older adult patients have comorbidities that would make it difficult to tolerate cisplatin (Hennessy et al., 2003). However, an ECOG study of stage IIIB or IV NSCLC in patients with good performance status compared outcomes of cisplatin chemotherapy in patients older than 70 with those in patients younger than 70. Although the older patients had more comorbidities and experienced more therapy-related toxicity than younger ones, no difference was seen in response rate or survival between the two groups (Langer et al., 2002). Additionally, a meta-analysis evaluating trials that compare chemotherapy versus best supportive care (BSC) found a statistical survival advantage for patients receiving chemotherapy even with a poor performance status (Gridelli, 2002a; Perrone, Gallo, & Gridelli, 2002). These findings support the notion that older adult patients with advanced NSCLC can benefit from aggressive treatment.

New chemotherapy regimens may be better tolerated in older adults. The ECOG recommended paclitaxel and carboplatin as a reference regimen for the treatment of older adult patients. In addition, ongoing studies of single-agent or combination chemotherapy or supportive care will better serve older adult patients with advanced NSCLC (Hennessy et al., 2003). The Elderly Lung Cancer Vinorelbine Italian Study trial (Gridelli, 2001) compared BSC with weekly vinorelbine plus BSC in patients with stage IV NSCLC who were older than 70. The median survival was significantly longer in the chemotherapy arm (28 versus 21 weeks), with a one-year survival of 32% in the vinorelbine arm versus 14% in the BSC alone arm. Additionally, the vinorelbine arm had a significantly improved quality of life as compared with BSC alone. The study concluded that it is appropriate to offer chemotherapy to older adult patients with a good performance status (ECOG 0–2). Single-agent therapy with vinorelbine has been demonstrated to be as effective as combination therapy and is a reasonable approach (Gridelli, Perrone, et al., 2003; Pfister et al., 2004).

Second-Line Therapy for Non-Small Cell Lung Cancer

Second-line therapy after failure of the first-line therapy may be an option for some older adult patients with a good performance status. A full discussion regarding the potential toxicities, limitations, and benefits should be provided. Other options include clinical trials involving new agents or regimens or BSC. Nurses should provide patients with information on all treatment options so they can make an educated decision (Hennessy et al., 2003; Sequist & Lynch, 2003).

Single-agent therapy with docetaxel is a reasonable second-line therapy. Docetaxel may result in improved quality of life and reduced disease-related symptoms when compared with BSC (Hennessy et al., 2003). Initial treatment with investigational regimens is appropriate for select patients with stage IV NSCLC as long as they are crossed over to an active treatment regimen when no response is evident after two cycles (Pfister et al., 2004). Concern exists regarding the clinical benefits versus economic cost of chemotherapy in this setting. However, data from a Canadian study found that systemic chemotherapy was more cost effective than BSC (Will, Berthelot, Nobrega, Flanagan, & Evans, 2001). Continued cost-benefit analysis is needed along with further research focusing on survival benefits and quality of life for all stages and types of lung cancer (Bunn & Lilenbaum, 2003; Manegold, 2001).

Recently, pemetrexed (Alimta®, Eli Lilly, Indianapolis, IN) was approved as single-agent second-line therapy for patients with locally advanced or metastatic NSCLC, with similar efficacy to docetaxel. It was previously approved for mesothelioma. This drug is an antifolate similar to methotrexate but with additional activity in folate-dependent pathways (Eli Lilly and Co., 2004).

Targeted Therapies

The only targeted therapies approved for NSCLC are gefitinib and erlotinib. Both gefitinib and erlotinib are tyrosine kinase inhibitors that work by inhibiting epidermal growth factor receptor (EGFR) signal transduction. Gefitinib was approved as monotherapy for the treatment of advanced NSCLC in patients who have progressed after platinum-based and docetaxel chemotherapy. This approval was based on the final results of the IDEAL 1 and 2 trials that showed evidence of tumor regression, improvement in symptoms, and overall benefit (Fukuoka et al., 2003; Kris et al., 2003). Response rates were similar to single-agent chemotherapy in the setting of second-line therapy. A comparison of the combination of gefitinib plus standard platinum-based chemotherapy against chemotherapy alone in chemo-naïve patients in the INTACT 1 and 2 trials did not show improved survival or other clinical end points for the gefitinib-containing regimen (Giaccone et al., 2004; Herbst et al., 2004). Preclinical data indicated that gefitinib was able to inhibit growth of cancer cells with a wide range of EGFR expression. Although subjects' tumors in the IDEAL 1 and 2 and INTACT 1 and 2 trials were not tested for EGFR overexpression, EGFR expression is widespread in NSCLC, and a lack of effect of gefitinib in the INTACT trials is surprising (Johnson & Arteaga, 2003). Interestingly, individual subjects had long-lasting responses to gefitinib, and the U.S. Food and Drug Administration (FDA) granted accelerated approval in May 2003. This type of approval requires the drug manufacturer to conduct additional studies to demonstrate efficacy (Cohen et al., 2004). Despite the promising initial study findings, data from recent clinical studies of gefitinib showed no significant survival benefit for the populations studied. Therefore, the FDA approved new labeling that limits the indication to patients who currently are benefiting or previously benefited from gefitinib and those enrolled in clinical trials approved by an institutional review board prior to June 2005. Ongoing clinical trials will determine the future role of gefitinib treatment (FDA Alert, 2005).

Erlotinib (Tarceva®, Genentech, Inc., South San Francisco, CA) was approved on November 18, 2004, for patients with NSCLC who have failed at least one previous chemotherapy regimen. A double-blind placebo-controlled trial showed that erlotinib given as monotherapy significantly increased survival, progression-free survival, and response duration when compared with placebo (Genentech, Inc., 2004).

Subsequently, biologic analysis of tumors from responders and nonresponders to gefitinib revealed that responders had an activating mutation in the cytoplasmic tail of EGFR such that antiapoptotic/survival pathways were activated. Evidently, the prosurvival activity of the mutated EGFR was responsible for tumor progression in these patients such that inhibition of the mutated EGFR produced a response (Lynch et al., 2004; Sordella, Bell, Haber, & Settleman, 2004). Interestingly, EGFR mutations in tumors sensitive to gefitinib or erlotinib were found in cases of NSCLC in "never smokers." Independent analysis of 15 tumors from "never smokers" and 81 tumors from former or current smokers revealed that tumors from the "never smokers" had a much higher rate of the same EGFR mutation. These data imply that "never smokers" develop genetically distinct NSCLC that is likely to be responsive to erlotinib or gefitinib (Pao et al., 2004).

Gefitinib is fairly well tolerated, with cutaneous side effects in the form of an acneform eruption on the face, anterior trunk, and back and diarrhea being the most common side effects. More rare side effects include desquamation as well as other skin reactions such as paronychia and ingrown nails. The mechanism by which gefitinib causes these side effects has not been elucidated. Gefitinib is well tolerated by older adult patients, even those heavily pretreated, with no grade 3 or 4 adverse events reported. Although experience with erlotinib is limited, its side-effect profile seems similar to gefitinib (Genentech, Inc., 2004).

Small Cell Lung Cancer

Case Study

T.H. is a 75-year-old white male with a 180 pack–year history of smoking and a 20-year history of hypertension. He had an MI five years ago, at which time he stopped smoking. Since his MI, he has had intermittently symptomatic CHF. He has chronic atrial fibrillation and takes sodium warfarin (Coumadin®, Bristol-Myers Squibb, Princeton, NJ). Additional current medications include an angiotensin converting enzyme inhibitor, a diuretic, and low-dose beta-blocker. A CT scan revealed a large right-sided mass with hilar and mediastinal lymphadenopathy. An enlarged right supraclavicular lymph node was biopsied and found to be infiltrated with SCLC. Two cardiothoracic surgeons saw the patient and informed him that chemotherapy and radiation were indicated for his extensive disease. A third surgeon who saw him offered to operate. When the chest wall was opened in preparation for a pneumonectomy, the surgeon decided that the cancer could not be resected and closed the patient's incision. Postoperatively, the patient could not be weaned from the ventilator and remained in the intensive care unit for two months without receiving chemotherapy or radiation.

At that point, he died from pneumonia and sepsis. This case demonstrates the need for patients with lung cancer to be treated on the basis of evidence, which shows that chemotherapy and radiation therapy are standard care for extensive SCLC.

Approximately 67% of patients with SCLC present with asymptomatic extensive disease. SCLC is very responsive to chemotherapy and RT, with partial response rates from 60%–70% and complete responses from 20%–30% (Simon et al., 2003). Unfortunately, the duration of response is not long, with progression-free survival lasting an average of 4 months for extensive disease and 12 months for limited SCLC. The median overall survival for patients with extensive disease is 9 months and 18 months for patients with limited SCLC (Paccagnella, Oniga, Favaretto, Biason, & Ghi, 2002; Simon et al., 2003).

Surgery generally is not indicated in SCLC unless for palliative reasons, and patients should be referred at diagnosis to radiation and medical oncologists for treatment. For the rare patient who presents with very early limited SCLC, a surgical resection may be considered, followed by chemotherapy. Consultation with experienced surgeons and medical oncologists is essential in making such a determination, as this case study illustrates (Simon et al., 2003).

Limited Small Cell Lung Cancer

SCLC is radiosensitive, and radiotherapy always is indicated in the treatment of limited SCLC. The addition of RT to chemotherapy was found to increase the three-year survival from 8.9% to 14.3%. Therefore, limited SCLC generally is treated with combined radiotherapy and chemotherapy. Older adult patients have similar outcomes compared with younger patients and should receive chemotherapy and RT if they have acceptable organ function and a good performance status. Platinum-based chemotherapy is considered the standard of care and should be offered to eligible older adult patients. Chemotherapy may include cisplatin and etoposide combined with radiotherapy once or twice daily. Carboplatin has been compared with cisplatin in combination with etoposide and found to be equally effective with fewer toxicities, with the exception of increased myelosuppression (Simon et al., 2003). Adding a third drug improved time to progression but added significant toxicity with no improvement in overall survival. If the older adult patient has a poor performance status, poor organ function, or serious comorbid conditions, chemotherapy still may be offered with dose adjustment for his or her condition (Simon et al.).

Several studies have examined the issue of the timing of thoracic RT and chemotherapy. Starting RT three to five weeks after chemotherapy has shown the most promising results. The longer the interval between the start of chemotherapy and the start of RT, the smaller the added benefit of chemoradiotherapy compared with chemotherapy alone. However, regimens involving alkylating agents and doxorubicin-based regimens showed no effect on the timing of RT and had long-term survival rates around 10%, which is comparable to chemotherapy alone (Simon et al., 2003). In addition, these regimens were associated with a significant toxicity. Moreover, concurrent RT with chemotherapy regimens containing platinum and etoposide were superior to sequential timing of therapies where RT was given after chemotherapy. Although the exact timing and dosing of RT and chemotherapy still are under investigation, little rationale exists for the combination of alkylating agents and radiotherapy (Simon et al.).

Recent randomized trials indicated that higher doses of thoracic RT (i.e., 30 Gy in 10 fractions or 45 Gy in 25 fractions) might provide better local control and progression-free survival. Other studies have evaluated fractionation involving two fractions per day at slightly smaller doses. Findings have been controversial, and hyperfractionated thoracic radiotherapy is not recommended at this time for SCLC outside of a clinical trial (Simon et al., 2003).

Extensive Small Cell Lung Cancer

Patients with extensive SCLC can be treated in the same manner as limited SCLC, with combination chemotherapy and radiotherapy or chemotherapy alone (Minna et al., 2001). If brain metastases are present, whole-brain irradiation is recommended unless immediate systemic therapy is needed. RT may be administered after chemotherapy in asymptomatic patients. Patients who relapse within three months of first-line therapy are considered refractory, whereas patients who relapse after three months are considered sensitive and can be retreated with the same regimen. All patients, including older adults, who have relapsed or are refractory to first-line chemotherapy should be offered additional treatment. At this time, the evidence does not support maintenance, dose dense/intense, or neoadjuvant chemotherapy for those with limited or extensive SCLC, but patients should be encouraged to participate in clinical trials and in trials specifically for older adults (Simon et al., 2003).

Lung Cancer Biology

Cancer is a genetic disease caused by multiple mutations in oncogenes whose protein products promote growth or tumor suppressor genes whose protein products repair damage to DNA, inhibit progression through the cell cycle, or regulate programmed cell death (apoptosis). If a gene is mutated, every protein molecule encoded by that gene will be defective, resulting in a nonfunctioning or dysfunctional protein. Oncogenes, which encode protein products that promote cell division and growth, usually are mutated in one of two ways. First, the mutation may be such that the protein product is constitutively active so that growth is not properly regulated. Alternatively, the gene may be present in many copies in the cancer cell (gene amplification), resulting in overexpression of the protein product and consequent amplification of the growth signal. Either type of mutation in an oncogene leads to an unremitting, unregulated growth signal for the cancer cells (Ross, 1998).

Tumor suppressor genes frequently are mutated so that the function of the protein product is lost. Loss of DNA repair capability in cancer cells means that mutations will accumulate at an increased rate. Loss of function in proteins that inhibit progression through the cell cycle will produce unregulated cell division. Loss of function in proteins that promote apoptosis means that cells that normally would enter the apoptotic pathway remain alive and contribute to tumor growth and progression. The net result of constitutive activation of the growth-regulatory protein products of oncogenes and loss of function of protein products of tumor suppressor genes is unremitting growth with constantly accumulating mutations and immortality because of a lack of apoptosis (Bunn, Soriano, Johnson, & Healsey, 2000; Fong, Sekido, & Minna, 1999).

Studies have failed to show substantial genetic predisposition to lung cancer, indicating that relatively very few lung cancers are inherited. The genetic mutations that produce sporadic (nonhereditary) cancer occur in body cells during one's lifetime (somatic mutations) and are caused by exposure to carcinogens, including viruses, and chemical, dietary, and physical factors (Bunn et al., 2000).

Normal bronchial epithelium is composed of ciliated and nonciliated squamous or pseudostratified columnar cells, mucus-secreting goblet cells, basal cells, and neuroendocrine cells. NSCLC cells are thought to arise from bronchial epithelial cells lining the bronchi or peripherally in the bronchioles. NSCLC can be a carcinoma, arising from squamous or columnar epithelial cells, or adenocarcinoma, arising from glandular cells. SCLC is thought to arise from neuroendocrine cells (Minna et al., 2001).

Emphysema and chronic bronchitis are associated with morphologic changes in pulmonary epithelium. Epithelial thickening, mucous gland hypertrophy, and rupture of alveolar cells are frequently found in smokers. These cellular changes can progress to premalignant and finally to malignant changes. Smokers frequently exhibit bronchial epithelial changes that progress from hyperplasia to dysplasia and then to carcinoma in situ before becoming invasive, at which time they are considered to be frankly malignant (Minna et al., 2001).

Once a malignant cell is produced, it gives rise to a tumor whose cells are all progeny of that single mutated cell, a process known as clonal expansion. As the tumor develops, the cancer cells continue to mutate, gaining a growth advantage over normal cells. Progressively more mutated cancer cells are produced that are even more malignant in their behavior, resulting in further proliferation and development of a blood supply (angiogenesis), metastasis, and drug resistance. This process, known as genetic carcinogenesis, is a continuum beginning with dysplasia and ending with an advanced malignancy (Minna et al., 2001). The more the bronchiogenic carcinoma cells differ in appearance and behavior from their original cell of origin (i.e., the more undifferentiated), the poorer the prognosis and the greater the likelihood that the cancer will develop resistance to therapy (ACS, 2004b).

Biologic Prognostic Factors

The stage of disease gives the greatest prognostic information for lung cancer. Other negative prognostic factors include degree of weight loss, male sex, elevated serum lactic dehydrogenase, and presence of liver or bone metastasis. In older adults, good performance status is a favorable prognostic indicator, but age alone does not have prognostic value (Pfister et al., 2004). In the future, molecular characteristics of an individual's tumor may predict what type of treatment that particular patient will respond to. As mentioned previously, the first such marker, a mutated EGFR, recently has been described as a requirement for response to gefitinib or erlotinib. A variety of additional molecular markers has been studied, but the findings remain controversial. Some of the markers under investigation include blood group A, precursors of blood antigens, the laminin receptor, c-*erbB1*/EGFR, c-*erbB2* or *HER2/neu, bcl-2,* and the *p53* tumor suppressor gene. These markers were evaluated in 515 cases with stage I NSCLC. However, none was an independent predictor of survival (Pastorino et al., 1997). Even if these markers are not found to be important predictors of survival, they have been found to be ideal targets for development of targeted therapies. EGFR/c-*erbB1* is targeted by the tyrosine kinase inhibitors gefitinib and erlotinib.

Many other molecules are under investigation as drug targets (Bunn et al., 2000; Kimura et al., 2001; Pastorino et al.).

New Therapies Under Investigation

The goal of targeted therapy is to affect the cancer cell by targeting the machinery involved in unremitting proliferation or resistance to apoptosis of that particular tumor so that it can be destroyed or controlled with minimal or no effect on normal cells. Imatinib mesylate (Gleevec®, Novartis, East Hanover, NJ) was the first such drug that targeted the specific mutation involved in chronic myeloid leukemia. This therapy now has been applied to multiple other malignancies (Bunn, 2002; Bunn et al., 2000).

A greater difficulty may exist in developing targeted therapies for solid tumors, including lung cancer, because solid tumors are genetically very heterogeneous among patients. Moreover, as a tumor grows, it gains additional mutations such that each individual's tumor may have a unique set of mutations. This makes it difficult to design a specific targeted therapy that would affect all lung cancers. In the future, researchers may have to identify and treat numerous cellular targets simultaneously (Bunn et al., 2000; Hinton & Sandler, 2002). This chapter's review of new therapies for lung cancer is not all-inclusive but meant to give examples of different approaches currently under investigation (see Table 10-4).

Table 10-4. Examples of New Therapies Under Investigation

Proposed Mechanism of Action	Therapies Under Investigation
Signal transduction inhibitors/cell cycle inhibitors	Farnesyl transferase inhibitors Flavopyridole UCN-101
Receptor targeted therapy	*erbB1* (*HER1*) Tyrosine kinase inhibitors Gefitinib (Iressa®, ZD 1839) Erlotinib (Tarceva®, OSI-774) Monoclonal antibody Cetuximab (C225, Erbitux®) *erbB2* (*HER2/neu*) Monoclonal antibody Trastuzumab (Herceptin®)
Gene therapy	Wild type *p53* Ad-*p53* Antisense
Anti-angiogenesis	Natural inhibitors Angiostatin, endostatin Growth factor receptor inhibitors Anti-vascular endothelial growth factor Bevacizumab (Avastin®) Tyrosine kinase inhibitors Matrix metalloproteinase inhibitors Nonspecific inhibitors Thalidomide, shark cartilage

Note. Based on information from Aberle & McLeskey, 2003; Bunn, 2002.

Signal Transduction Inhibitors/Cell Cycle Inhibitors

Signal transduction refers to the process of communicating growth signals from the extracellular environment to the nucleus inside the cell (see Figure 10-2). Growth factors, sometimes called ligands, are released from other cells and bind with growth factor receptors (GFRs) on the cell surface. Epidermal growth factor (EGF) and transforming growth factor alpha (TGF-α) are examples of specific ligands that bind to EGFR and activate it. The activated receptor is an intracellular tyrosine kinase that places a phosphate group on

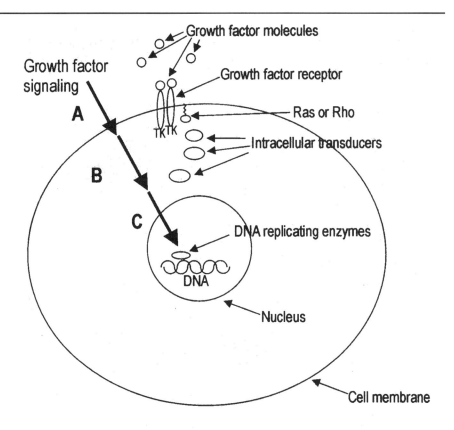

Growth factor signaling begins outside the cell (A), where molecules of growth factors are present. The signal is transmitted to the inside of the cell when growth factor molecules (e.g., epidermal growth factor) bind to growth factor receptors (e.g., epidermal growth factor receptor). Growth factor receptors are tyrosine kinase (TK) enzymes that are activated when growth factor is bound. The TK activity is a signal that activates adjacent small molecules called Ras or Rho. These molecules, in turn, activate cytosolic signaling molecules (transducers) that transmit the growth factor signal to the nucleus (B). In the nucleus, the receipt of the growth factor signal (C) causes a series of events, including duplication of the chromosomes by DNA replicating enzymes and culminating in mitosis, the splitting of the parent cell into two daughter cells.

Figure 10-2. Growth Factor Signaling Pathway

Note. From "Biology of Lung Cancer With Implications for New Therapies," by M.F. Aberle and S.W. McLeskey, 2003, *Oncology Nursing Forum, 30,* p. 275. Copyright 2003 by the Oncology Nursing Society. Adapted with permission.

nearby small molecules in the cytoplasm of the cell (phosphorylation). Two nearby small molecules that might be phosphorylated by the tyrosine kinase activity of EGFR are Ras and Rho. When either Ras or Rho has a phosphate group attached to it, it becomes active and can, in turn, activate other cytoplasmic molecules called transducers, which then can transmit a signal to the nucleus of the cell resulting in chromosomal duplication and cell division (proliferation) (Normanno, Maiello, & De Luca, 2002; Thomas, 2003).

Activating Ras mutations are found in 20%–40% of NSCLC but rarely are seen with SCLC and have been associated with poor prognosis. The mutant *ras* gene's protein product is constitutively activated (always turned on) and sends a growth signal to the nucleus independent of GFR phosphorylation. Both the normal Ras protein and the mutant one use an enzyme called farnesyl transferase to become attached to the inner aspect of the plasma membrane where they function to transmit the growth signal. If the normal or mutant Ras cannot be attached to the cell membrane by farnesylation, it cannot transmit the growth signal. Several farnesyl transferase inhibitors are under investigation that will inhibit farnesyl transferase enzymes. Use of these drugs would mean that even though mutant *ras* oncogenes continue to make Ras proteins, the protein cannot attach to the plasma membrane and therefore could not direct the cell to proliferate. This would interfere with the unremitting growth signal transmitted by the mutant Ras (Bunn et al., 2000; Cooper, 2001).

Cyclin-dependent kinases (CDKs) are an important set of enzymes that help to regulate cell growth and division. Their genes commonly are mutated in malignancies, producing a loss of cell cycle control (Bunn et al., 2000). Direct CDK modulators produce cell cycle arrest and apoptosis and also may produce differentiation and/or have antiangiogenic properties. Flavopyridole and UCN-01 (7-hydroxystaurosporine) are examples of CDK modulators currently in early-phase clinical trials (Senderowicz, 2003; Shapiro, Koestner, Matranga, & Rollins, 1999).

Receptor-Targeted Therapy

As mentioned in the discussion of gefitinib and erlotinib, new therapies are targeting GFRs. Growth factors and GFRs are types of oncogenes that are mutated or inappropriately overexpressed in cancer. The erbB family of GFRs (also known as HER family) has four known members: (a) *erbB1* (EGFR or *HER1*), (b) *erbB2* (*HER2/neu*), (c) *erbB3* (*HER3*), and (d) *erbB4* (*HER4*). As is true of the first member, EGFR, all of these GFRs are tyrosine kinases and are important mediators of cell growth, survival, and differentiation (Baselga & Hammond, 2002). These GFRs are membrane-spanning glycoproteins composed of an extracellular ligand-binding domain, a hydrophobic transmembrane region, and a cytoplasmic domain that contains both the tyrosine kinase domain and a regulatory carboxy-terminal region that is involved in binding of proteins such as Ras and Rho (see Figure 10-3) (Normanno et al., 2002).

Therapies have been developed to target the extracellular domain of GFRs with monoclonal antibodies, which bind to the GFR and somehow prevent it from becoming active. Trastuzumab is an example of such a drug that is approved for breast cancer and is being investigated for lung cancer. Small molecule therapies, such as gefitinib and erlotinib, have been designed to work in the intracellular domain by inhibiting the tyrosine kinase ability. Different therapies have been developed to target individual or multiple receptors in the ErbB family. Targeting multiple receptors might be advantageous in lung cancer because coexpression of *erbB1*, *erbB3*, or expression of three of more of the ErbB family of receptors has been shown to correlate with lung cancer recurrence.

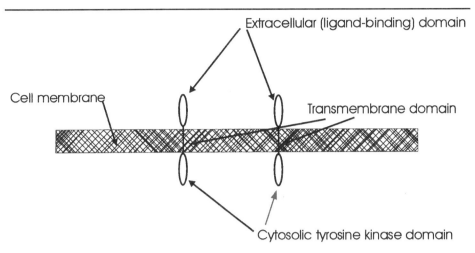

Growth factor receptors are large protein molecules that contain an extracellular domain that binds a specific growth factor, a transmembrane domain that anchors the molecule to the plasma membrane, and cytosolic domain that has tyrosine kinase activity and binding sites for interacting molecules such as Ras and Rho. The cytosolic domain's tyrosine kinase does not become active unless the appropriate growth factor is bound to the receptor. New antibody drugs such as cetuximab or trastuzumab bind to the extracellular domain of the particular receptor (EGFR or *erbB2* or *HER2/neu*) that they target. Tyrosine kinase inhibitors such as gefitinib and erlotinib bind to the tyrosine kinase domain (of EGFR) and inhibit its activity. Other drugs under development may inhibit a particular growth factor receptor's ability to interact with other molecules that convey the growth signal to the nucleus.

Figure 10-3. Structure of Growth Factor Receptors

Note. Figure courtesy of Sandra W. McLeskey, PhD, RN. Used with permission.

Further study will help to identify the clinical importance of coexpression of the ErbB family and highlight opportunities for potential therapies (Lai et al., 2001).

Epidermal Growth Factor Receptor

Although EGFR expression is found in normal epithelial cells in the basal layer of the bronchial and other epithelium, when epithelial dysplasia develops, tumor cells may develop overexpression of EGFR. Overexpression leads to upregulation of the growth signal communicated to the nucleus by signal transduction, which leads to increased proliferation (Baselga & Hammond, 2002). Overexpression of EGFR has correlated with poor prognosis in some types of cancer, whereas in other types of cancer, no association was found. This discrepancy may be related to differences in how EGFR overexpression was detected and the level of expression that was deemed excessive (Bunn, 2002).

Cetuximab (Erbitux®, Bristol-Myers Squibb) is a therapeutic antibody that has been developed to compete for binding of EGF to the extracellular domain of EGFR. Cetuximab was approved for use in the treatment of colorectal cancer in February 2004 (Bristol-Myers Squibb, 2004) and has shown activity in renal cell carcinoma. Studies now are being conducted in lung cancer (Bunn et al., 2000).

Numerous other antibodies and inhibitors targeting EGFR, in addition to gefitinib, erlotinib, and cetuximab, are in development and are showing promise as potential future therapies (Green, Murray, & Hortobagyi, 2000; Sekine & Saijo, 2001).

HER2/neu

Approximately 20%–50% of NSCLCs overexpress the receptor *erbB2* (*HER2/neu*), which is associated with unfavorable prognosis (Langer, Stephenson, Thor, Vangel, & Johnson, 2004). Trastuzumab is a monoclonal antibody against the extracellular domain of *HER2/neu*. Phase II trials of trastuzumab in lung cancer have revealed variable responses from no improvement to a partial response of 42% (Ferrone & Motl, 2003). Additional clinical trials currently are under way to identify efficacy of this monoclonal antibody and others targeting the *HER2/neu* GFR or other GFRs (Bunn et al., 2000).

Gene Therapy

Tumor suppressor genes normally suppress malignant transformation. A loss of tumor suppressor genes has been found in many epithelial cancers, including lung cancer. For instance, inactivation of *p53* was present in 80% of lung cancers, although these findings are controversial (Huncharek, Kupelnick, Geschwind, & Caubet, 2000). Inactivation of *p53* may be related to tobacco smoke, which causes specific *p53* mutations, leading to inactive protein products. If inactivation of *p53* is responsible for malignant behavior of lung cancer cells, supplying a nonmutated gene that would produce a functional protein product might revert the malignant behavior of the cancer cells toward normal (Aberle & McLeskey, 2003; Bunn et al., 2000).

Phase I and II gene therapy trials of *p53* gene replacement in NSCLC have demonstrated that *p53* gene transfer is associated with little toxicity, and evidence of antitumor activity exists. Phase III trials are necessary to evaluate whether this therapy will impact overall survival (Swisher & Roth, 2002). However, the biggest obstacle remains the efficient delivery of gene therapy to tumors that may lie deep within the body (Aberle & McLeskey, 2003; Bunn et al., 2000).

A second type of gene therapy is called antisense. This strategy targets genes such as GFR genes that are overexpressed in cancer. For a gene to be expressed as a protein, the genetic code that comprises that gene (made up of A [adenosine], G [guanosine], C [cytosine], and T [thymosine]) is copied out as a single strand, known as messenger RNA (mRNA). mRNA is a sense genetic sequence made up of A, C, G, and U (uracil, which replaces T in RNA), which can be translated according to the genetic code into a string of amino acids in proper sequence to form the particular protein encoded by the gene. Scientists can make a strand of RNA that is the complementary copy of the mRNA for a particular gene. Every place where an A exists in the mRNA, scientists place a U in the complementary copy so that As are replaced with Us, Us with As, Gs with Cs, and Cs with Gs. This complementary strand is called the antisense strand. Shorter antisense RNAs or DNAs to correspond to different portions of the mRNA also can be made in a laboratory. Drugs consisting of these antisense molecules are designed to bind to mRNAs of target genes so that the genetic code in the RNA cannot be translated into protein. This stops production of the overexpressed proteins (Rieger, 2003). In the case of GFRs that are overexpressed, antisense therapy would stop the overexpression and lessen the growth signal that the cancer cell was receiving. Antisense therapies currently are in preclinical and early trials for lung cancer (Rieger).

Angiogenesis Inhibitors

Tumors must have the ability to develop a blood supply, a process called angiogenesis, to grow and metastasize to distant sites. A variety of angiogenesis inhibitors are in clinical trials, including natural inhibitors such as endostatin and angiostatin, monoclonal antibodies against molecules important in angiogenesis, tyrosine kinase inhibitors that target GFRs on blood vessel cells, and nonspecific inhibitors such as thalidomide and shark cartilage (Bunn, 2002).

Vascular endothelial growth factor (VEGF) binds to one of two VEGF receptors (VEGFRs) on the endothelial cell membrane and stimulates blood vessel cell growth. Inhibitors of VEGF or VEGFRs are thought to inhibit angiogenesis in lung and other cancers, which increases their VEGF expression as they become progressively more aggressive. Many therapeutic antibodies and tyrosine kinase inhibitors that target VEGF or VEGFRs are being investigated. One of the antibodies for VEGF, bevacizumab, recently was approved for metastatic colorectal cancer in combination with irinotecan (Braun et al., 2004; Bunn et al., 2000).

Matrix Metalloproteinases

Matrix metalloproteinases (MMPs) are enzymes used by tumor cells to destroy the basement membrane confining them to their original site. These enzymes may function in both invasion of nearby tissues and in metastasis. Lung cancer cells can produce MMPs and induce their neighboring cells to do so as well. If a drug were to inhibit MMPs, it might prevent invasion and/or metastasis of cancer cells. MMP inhibitors currently are being studied in clinical trials (Aberle & McLeskey, 2003; Bunn et al., 2000).

Case Study

D.H. was a pleasant 74-year-old female who presented with stage IB NSCLC in December 1998. Following geriatric assessment that indicated good functional status and no severe comorbidities, she underwent a left upper lobectomy. She did well until February 1999, when a follow-up CT scan showed haziness in her left upper lobe. A CT guided biopsy showed poorly differentiated NSCLC. The patient agreed to participate in a randomized clinical trial involving an investigational agent (MMPI) versus placebo in combination with chemotherapy. She started treatment in March. She completed six cycles of paclitaxel and carboplatin in June and tolerated the chemotherapy well. In August 1999, the clinical trial was closed because of a lack of response in the treatment arm. D.H. was "unblinded" and found to be on the MMPI. She and her physician made the decision to request compassionate use of the drug and continue with treatment. D.H. did well until December 2000, when she was found to have recurrent disease. She was treated with four cycles of docetaxel but died in April 2001. This case study illustrates the individual treatment options that each patient should be afforded. D.H. participated in a clinical trial knowing that she personally may not benefit from the drug but may be able to help future patients with lung cancer by helping scientists to discover and develop new therapies.

Summary

Many new therapies for lung cancer that target biologic characteristics of tumor cells are under investigation (see Table 10-4). However, questions remain to be answered concerning the application of these therapies to lung and other cancers; including timing of their use as initial, adjuvant, or salvage therapies; optimal treatment regimens that might include conventional chemotherapy or RT as well as the biologic therapy; and the side effects and high cost of these therapies.

Follow-Up and Usual Disease Progression

Lung cancer is naturally aggressive and most often fatal within five years, as evidenced by the 15% overall five-year survival rate. Typically, patients will have local invasion of the surrounding structures followed by regional invasion. When it gains access to the bloodstream, lung cancer most often spreads to the liver, adrenal glands, bones, and brain (Minna et al., 2001). Patients who have been treated with a curative intent should be followed by the appropriate specialist for three to six months and then be reevaluated by the multidisciplinary tumor board for entry into an appropriate surveillance program (Colice, Rubins, & Unger, 2003). Specific recommendations concerning surveillance are an area of controversy. For NSCLC cases where surgery with curative intent has been accomplished, NCCN guidelines recommend physical examination and CXR every three to four months for two years, every six months for the next three years, and annually thereafter. Additionally, low-dose spiral (helical) CT scans are recommended annually (NCCN, 2005c). For SCLC, NCCN (2005d) guidelines recommend that following a complete response to therapy, oncology follow-up visits take place every two to three months during the first year, every three to four months during the second and third years, every four to six months during years four and five, and then annually. Oncology visits should consist of history and physical, chest imaging, and blood work as clinically indicated (NCCN, 2005b). Other authorities recommend CT scans or CXR every six months for two years, then yearly or sooner if clinically indicated. Patients should be educated on symptoms that are associated with recurrence requiring medical attention. PET scanning, tumor markers, fluorescence bronchoscopy, and sputum cytology currently are not recommended for surveillance (Colice et al.).

Case Study

M.H. was a 71-year-old female who was newly diagnosed with advanced NSCLC with significant bony metastasis. M.H. had received one cycle of chemotherapy when she suddenly died at home. Her family appropriately called 911. Emergency medical services arrived and began CPR. The patient could not be successfully resuscitated, but the family heard the patient's bones crack under the chest compression and witnessed the patient bleed from her mouth and nose. Afterward, the police questioned the family as to the patient's sudden death, and they were extremely distraught during the questioning. This type of scenario can be avoided if the patient and family are educated on the patient's prognosis, advance directives, and state laws. These strategies might allow the patient to die without futile last-minute medical interventions.

Summary

Because most lung cancer presents at an advanced stage, outcomes are not likely to be favorable. However, one-year survival rates have improved from 34% in 1975 to

41% in 1994. This improvement is attributed to improved surgical techniques. The five-year survival rates for all stages of lung cancer combined remain a disheartening 15%. This is most likely because 84% of lung cancers will present at an advanced stage (ACS, 2004b). Therefore, it is important that healthcare practitioners address likely outcomes with patients and their families at early time points in the diagnostic and treatment process.

Palliative Care

Most patients with lung cancer will succumb to their disease and, in the process, suffer symptoms that require aggressive management. Moreover, more than two-thirds of patients dying of lung cancer are older than age 65 and may have special needs, such as caregiver, polypharmacy, financial, and social issues. Older adult patients will benefit from care planning by a multidisciplinary team. Incorporation of palliative care throughout the illness will enhance quality of life. Moreover, ongoing discussion about appropriate goals for treatment should include the patient and family members (Kvale et al., 2003).

It is especially important to avoid or plan for procedures that might result in respiratory compromise, because emergent placement of the patient on a ventilator may result in difficult or impossible weaning. If a patient needs such a procedure to palliate symptoms, frank discussion with the patient and family prior to the procedure may result in the patient and family expressing the desire to avoid intubation or limit the time on the ventilator prior to a terminal wean. Prolonged mechanical ventilation should be discouraged because of poor outcomes in all patients with lung cancer regardless of their age (Ingle, 2000).

Many older patients do not have prescription coverage. Some pharmaceutical companies provide indigent programs, but these may take four to six weeks for processing. Even middle-class patients may have cash-flow problems because of fixed retirement incomes. Patients with cancer may need information on strategies to improve cash flow while still providing for adequate living arrangements and day-to-day expenses (Henschke et al., 2001; Ingle, 2000).

Patients and their loved ones must be informed about and participate in decisions about therapy, including the transition from a curative approach to control or palliation. Discussions about care planning should occur early and recur as conditions change. The patient and family must understand options for palliative care and the benefits of hospice care in order to choose a setting for end-of-life care should curative therapy not be possible. This understanding may assist the family in decisions about end-of-life care and may facilitate earlier referrals to hospice (Henschke et al., 2001; Ingle, 2000).

Unfortunately, many times the referral to hospice does not occur until days or even hours before a patient's death. However, hospice programs provide highly trained physicians, nurses, social workers, and chaplains who work as a team to prepare patients and their families for death. Nurses can advocate for more timely referrals to hospice. Some hospice programs will allow patients to enter their program while receiving treatment if the goal is palliation and a cure is not possible. Home care with hospice support allows the patient to stay at home with less cost. However, not all families are able to care for their loved ones at home, and other alternatives, such as inpatient hospice, should be explored (Henschke et al., 2001; Ingle, 2000).

As soon as a diagnosis of lung cancer is made, patients should be screened for advance directives. They should be educated on the differences among advanced directives or living wills, do not resuscitate (DNR) orders, and medical power of attorney. An outpatient DNR order is required by many states to prevent resuscitation efforts if emergency medical services are called (Griffin et al., 2003; Ingle, 2000).

Ethics committees can be an excellent resource in the inpatient setting if questions or concerns exist about the interpretation or validity of an advance directive or if a concern arises about a patient's care. Nurses can advocate for patients by opening a dialogue among patients, families, and physicians (Griffin et al., 2003).

Symptom Control

Patients with lung cancer and their families must be educated on how to manage their symptoms because most therapy occurs on an outpatient basis, and patients will experience effects of therapy and their disease at home (Ingle, 2000). Patients should receive an individualized symptom control plan and be active participants. The symptom management plan should be simple and noninvasive when possible (Griffin et al., 2003).

Pain

Older adult patients with lung cancer present difficult pain management challenges because of metastatic disease in ribs, the spine, and other bones. Treatment of these metastatic sites may be effective in alleviating pain or at least making it more manageable. The patient should receive an individualized pain control plan and be an active participant in the planning. The pain management plan should be simple, as noninvasive as possible, and reevaluated on a frequent basis (Griffin et al., 2003). See Chapter 19 for a comprehensive discussion of pain management in older adults with cancer.

Bone Metastasis

Many patients with lung cancer develop bone metastasis. External beam RT is indicated to control local pain. For most, a single, large fraction of RT will provide pain relief to the localized site. Systemic corticosteroids (prednisone 20–40 mg/d) with RT may augment pain relief. If the patient does not respond to the steroid and RT, adding a bisphosphonate or calcitonin may be beneficial. Radiopharmaceuticals also are available to treat pain and should be considered for patients with bone metastasis who do not respond to conventional approaches. Surgical fixation may be considered for weight-bearing bones to stabilize fractures or to minimize the potential for fracture if the patient has a life expectancy of more than one month (Kvale et al., 2003).

Brain Metastasis

Patients with symptomatic brain metastasis should be treated with dexamethasone, 16 mg daily for four weeks, with concomitant whole-brain irradiation followed by a rapid taper of steroids upon completion of the RT. For patients with intracranial metastases that are not surgically accessible, the presence of two to four lesions, or with intracranial recurrence after surgery, stereotactic radiosurgery accompanied by whole-brain RT also can be offered (Kvale et al., 2003).

Spinal Cord Metastasis

Spinal cord compression (SCC) is an oncologic emergency requiring immediate attention. In patients with lung cancer, 70% of SCC involves the thoracic vertebrae, 20% the lumbar vertebrae, and 10% the cervical vertebrae (Keller & Benton, 2001). Most patients will present with central or radicular neck or back pain followed by weakness, numbness, and paresthesias. Bowel and/or bladder dysfunction and paralysis are late findings. If patients are asymptomatic or have minimal neurologic impairment at presentation, 60%–70% will be able to maintain function. However, if the patient presents with paraplegia, the prognosis is poor, and less than 55% will be able to walk again even with therapy (Keller & Benton).

If the patient is found to have epidural SCC but has no symptoms, RT should be administered. Ambulatory patients should immediately receive high-dose steroids and RT to retain or restore function. Surgical stabilization is required if an instability of the spine, rapidly progressive neurologic symptoms, uncontrolled pain, or treatment failure is present. If the patient has not received RT, has spinal instability, has bony compression, or has neurologic symptoms, surgery should be performed first. Steroids always should be started with suspicion of an SCC and then stopped if ruled out (Coleman & Rubens, 2004; Kvale et al., 2003).

A randomized clinical trial reported at the 2003 ASCO annual meeting evaluated patients with SCC treated with surgery followed by RT compared with those treated with RT alone. Those treated with dual therapy retained the ability to walk significantly longer than those treated with RT alone (129 days versus 100 days) (Patchell et al., 2003).

Dyspnea and Cough

Many patients suffer from dyspnea and cough that could be controlled. Causes include pleural effusions, localized obstruction of a major airway, or exacerbation of comorbid conditions, such as chronic obstructive pulmonary disease or asthma. If a pleural effusion is present, thoracentesis can provide immediate relief of symptoms. Recurrent pleural effusion may be treated effectively in 75%–85% of cases with pleurodesis, which involves fusing the pleural layers with inflammation produced by injection of a chemical agent such as bleomycin or sterilized talc into the pleural space. An indwelling Tenckhoff catheter, which can be drained by the patient, family member, or home healthcare personnel, is another option for managing recurrent malignant pleural effusions. However, this involves placing the catheter into the pleural cavity with the patient in the operating room under anesthesia (Works & Maxwell, 2000).

Bronchoscopy can be used therapeutically to remove an intraluminal tumor that is causing central bronchiolar obstruction. Bronchial stent placement can relieve dyspnea as well as help to manage sites of hemoptysis. Laser cautery, electrocautery, argon plasma coagulation, cryotherapy, brachytherapy, and photodynamic therapies are other effective modalities for bronchial obstruction but have a slower onset for relief of symptoms (Kvale et al., 2003).

Patients in respiratory failure, whether from cancer or other reasons, experience acute discomfort and anxiety that sometimes cannot be relieved by therapeutic maneuvers to improve respiratory function. In these instances, morphine and other opioids have been found to be very effective in controlling dyspnea and are recommended as the treatment of choice for cough suppression. Benzodiazepine tranquilizers and/or oxygen therapy can relieve symptoms of anxiety as well as dyspnea. Nonpharmacologic therapies such as a fan, cooler room, or relaxation therapy also may be helpful (Kvale et al., 2003; NCCN, 2004).

Distress

Distress is defined as " . . . a multifactorial unpleasant emotional experience of a psychological (cognitive, behavioral, emotional), social, and/or spiritual nature that may interfere with the ability to cope effectively with cancer, its physical symptoms and its treatment" (NCCN, 2005a). Distress can encompass any feeling of vulnerability or sadness or may progress to more disabling disorders of depression, anxiety, or panic. Feelings of distress are almost universal in patients with cancer (NCCN, 2005a).

Every patient with lung cancer, including older adults, should be evaluated routinely for distress. The NCCN (2005a) guidelines include a distress assessment tool. Measures to relieve distress can be directed against the cancer, the therapy, or an underlying psychiatric disorder that may become evident as a result of the cancer or therapy. Assessment of distress should include differentiation among delirium, dementia, or a mood disorder. Mood disorders can include depression or anxiety (NCCN, 2005a).

Depression is extremely common in patients with lung cancer. In a study of 987 patients with lung cancer, 33% self-reported depression before treatment, and 50% reported persistent depression after treatment. Multivariate analysis showed that functional impairment was the most important risk factor for depression, with pretreatment physical symptom burden, fatigue, and performance status also as independent predictors of depression. Lung cancer type (NSCLC or SCLC) was not a predictor of depression (Hopwood & Stephens, 2000).

Special considerations should be taken when prescribing antidepressants, especially in older patients. The healthcare provider should check for drug interactions, anticholinergic side effects, and other potential problems before instituting therapy. Additionally, ongoing monitoring of side effects and response to therapy is essential. Referral to a mental health practitioner may be needed in some cases; however, such referrals may add to the patient's burden and might be reserved for patients who are most affected by depression (Henschke et al., 2002).

Clinical Practice Guidelines for Lung Cancer

Several organizations have developed clinical practice guidelines for lung cancer. NCCN provides evidence-based clinical practice guidelines for treatment of NSCLC and SCLC, as well as guidelines for supportive care, including cancer- and treatment-related anemia, emesis, cancer-related fatigue, cancer pain, distress management, fever and neutropenia, palliative care, and senior adult oncology. ACCP, ASCO, and other organizations provide clinical practice guidelines for lung cancer, which are available online.

The ACCP conducted a systematic review of the literature to identify published guidelines and evaluate their quality. Fifty-one relevant guidelines were identified for evaluation using the Appraisal of Guidelines for Research and Evaluation instrument. This instrument evaluates six domains, including stakeholder involvement; rigor of development; clarity and presentation; applicability; editorial independence; and scope and purpose. Only 53% of the guidelines evaluated were found to be evidence-based. Based on the domain scores, only 19 guidelines were recommended by reviewers. This study identifies the importance of evidence-based guidelines and encourages clinicians to evaluate clinical practice guidelines critically and use them as a tool for guiding care. Practitioners must understand that no single guideline addresses all issues and that each patient should be treated as an individual. Treatment decisions should be based on evidence and patient choice (Harpole et al., 2003).

Nursing Care Issues

Over the next 20–30 years, the population of older adults with lung cancer is expected to become much larger. Although age is not a prognostic factor in outcomes of treatment, older patients are treated less aggressively than younger ones (Gillani & Grunberg, 2004). These findings imply that age bias prevents oncology practitioners from providing effective treatment to older adults. Nurses must recognize any biases they may have about the treatment of older patients and continually educate themselves and their patients about evidence-based cancer care. Older adult patients with lung cancer present unique challenges that require the expertise of oncology nurses to advocate for the best treatment options, symptom management, and palliative care throughout the illness continuum. In particular, nurses play a key role in symptom management and therefore may be most responsible for patients' quality of life during the illness. Nurses must educate patients on resources and provide information on participation in clinical trials. Table 10-5 provides a list of resources for patients with lung cancer and their families.

Conclusion

Lung cancer has reached epidemic proportions in the United States and remains the leading cause of cancer-related death. The typical patient presenting with lung cancer is older, with 60% of newly diagnosed patients older than age 65 and 50% older than age 70. Most patients will have advanced disease at the time of diagnosis, and their chance of five-year survival is less than 15% (ACS, 2004b). Because most newly diagnosed patients present with advanced disease, treatment has had limited effects on overall survival. New understanding of the biology and pathogenesis of lung cancer must be gained through research. Unfortunately, less than 5% of all adult patients with cancer participate in clinical trials, making the process of discovering new therapies difficult. Clinicians should educate themselves and their patients on the option of participation in clinical trials. Nurse researchers are well qualified and positioned to study symptom management and quality-of-life issues. Energies need to be continually directed toward smoking cessation and development of effective screening strategies. The potential for new therapies in lung cancer is tremendous and exciting.

Table 10-5. Resources for Patients With Lung Cancer

Organization	Contact Information
ALCASE: Alliance for Lung Cancer Advocacy, Support, and Education National not-for-profit organization dedicated to patients with lung cancer or those at risk	Available online: www.alcase.org Phone: 800-298-2436
National Cancer Institute's Cancer Information Service Offers specific information on lung cancer through the Physician Data Query as well as available clinical trials	Available online: www.cancer.gov/cancertopics/types/lung Phone: 800-4-CANCER
CancerCARE Offers educational information on cancer	Available online: www.cancercare.org Phone: 800-813-HOPE
American Cancer Society Provides general information on lung cancer, clinical trials, and other cancer-related subjects	Available online: www.cancer.org Phone: 800-ACS-2345
It's Time to Focus on Lung Cancer Established in fall 2000 by a group of nonprofit organizations, this lung cancer awareness campaign is dedicated to improving care for those with lung cancer. Provides information and support; e-mail questions via the Web site, and questions will be answered within 48 hours.	Available online: www.lungcancer.org Phone: 877-646-LUNG
People Living with Cancer (American Society of Clinical Oncology) Information on types of cancer, clinical trials, coping, and side effects of treatment. "Find an oncologist" database, a drug database, and patient support organizations database. Online chats and message boards.	Available online: www.peoplelivingwithcancer.org

Note. Based on information from Henschke et al., 1999.

References

Aberle, M., & McLeskey, S. (2003). Biology of lung cancer with implications for new therapies. *Oncology Nursing Forum, 30,* 273–278.

Aelony, Y., Bonnet, R., Colt, H., & Potkin, R. (2002). *Position paper on thoracoscopy.* California Thoracic Society and American Lung Association. Retrieved April 25, 2004, from http://www.thoracic.org/ca.html

American Cancer Society. (2004a). *Cigarette smoking. Prevention and early detection.* Retrieved April 25, 2004, from http://www.cancer.org/docroot/PED/content/PED_10_2X_Cigarette_Smoking.asp?sitearea=PED

American Cancer Society. (2004b). *Lung cancer.* Retrieved April 25, 2004, from http://www.cancer.org/downloads/PRO/1

American Cancer Society. (2005). *Cancer facts and figures, 2005.* Retrieved May 5, 2005, from http://www.cancer.org/downloads/STT/CAFF2005f4PWSecured.pdf

American Society of Clinical Oncology. (1997). Clinical practice guidelines for the treatment of unresectable non-small-cell lung cancer. *Journal of Clinical Oncology, 15,* 2996–3018.

Bach, P.B., Niewoehner, D.E., & Black, W.C. (2003). Screening for lung cancer: The guidelines. *Chest, 123*(Suppl. 1), 83S–88S.

Baselga, J., & Hammond, L. (2002). HER-targeted tyrosine-kinase inhibitors. *Oncology, 63*(Suppl. 1), 6–16.

Beckles, M.A., Spiro, S.G., Colice, G.L., & Rudd, R.M. (2003). Initial evaluation of the patient with lung cancer: Symptoms, signs, laboratory tests, and paraneoplastic syndromes. *Chest, 123*(Suppl. 1), 97S–104S.

Borges, M., Sculier, J.P., Paesmans, M., Richez, M., Bureau, G., Dabouis, G., et al. (1996). Prognostic factors for response to chemotherapy containing platinum derivatives in patients with unresectable non-small cell lung cancer (NSCLC). *Lung Cancer, 16*(1), 21–33.

Braun, A.H., Achterrath, W., Wilke, H., Vanhoefer, U., Harstrick, A., & Preusser, P. (2004). New systemic frontline treatment for metastatic colorectal carcinoma. *Cancer, 100,* 1558–1577.

Bristol-Myers Squibb. (2004). Erbitux® [Prescribing information]. Retrieved November 22, 2004, from http://www.fda.gov/cder/foi/label/2004/125084lbl.pdf

Bunn, P. (2002). New targeted therapies for lung cancer: Expectations and reality. *Medscape General Medicine, 4*(3). Retrieved April 27, 2004, from http://www.medscape.com/viewarticle/439357

Bunn, P.A., Jr., & Lilenbaum, R. (2003). Chemotherapy for elderly patients with advanced non-small-cell lung cancer. *Journal of the National Cancer Institute, 95,* 341–342.

Bunn, P., Soriano, A., Johnson, G., & Healsey, L. (2000). New therapeutic strategies for the treatment of lung cancer. *Chest, 117*(4 Suppl. 1), 163S–168S.

Centers for Disease Control and Prevention. (2003). *Tobacco/smoking.* Retrieved March 8, 2004, from http://www.cdc.gov/nceh/dls/tobacco.htm

Centers for Medicare and Medicaid Services. (2004). *Medicare expands coverage of PET scans.* Retrieved April 25, 2004, from http://www.cms.hhs.gov/default.asp?fromhcfadotgov=true

Cohen, M.H., Williams, G.A., Sridhara, R., Chen, G., McGuinn, W.D., Jr., Morse, D., et al. (2004). United States Food and Drug Administration drug approval summary: Gefitinib (ZD1839; Iressa) tablets. *Clinical Cancer Research, 10,* 1212–1218.

Cohen, V., & Khuri, F.R. (2003). Progress in lung cancer chemoprevention. *Cancer Control, 10,* 315–324.

Coleman, R.E., & Rubens, R.D. (2004). Bone metastases. In M.D. Abeloff, J.O. Armitage, J.E. Niederhuber, M.B. Kastan, & W.G. McKenna (Eds.), *Clinical oncology* (3rd ed., pp. 1122–1123). Philadelphia: Elsevier.

Colice, G.L., Rubins, J., & Unger, M. (2003). Follow-up and surveillance of the lung cancer patient following curative-intent therapy. *Chest, 123*(Suppl. 1), 272S–283S.

Conti, B., Brega Massone, P.P., Lequaglie, C., Magnani, B., & Cataldo, I. (2002). Major surgery in lung cancer in elderly patients? Risk factors analysis and long-term results. *Minerva Chirurgica, 57,* 317–321.

Cooper, M.R. (2001). Systemic therapy. In R. Lenhard, R. Osteen, & T. Gansler (Eds.), *The American Cancer Society's clinical oncology* (pp. 210–220). Atlanta, GA: American Cancer Society.

Curran, M.P., & Plosker, G.L. (2002). Vinorelbine: A review of its use in elderly patients with advanced non-small cell lung cancer. *Drugs and Aging, 19,* 695–721.

Detterbeck, F.C., DeCamp, M.M., Jr., Kohman, L.J., & Silvestri, G.A. (2003). Lung cancer. Invasive staging: The guidelines. *Chest, 123*(Suppl. 1), 167S–175S.

Detterbeck, F.C., & Socinski, M.A. (2001). Induction therapy and surgery for I-IIIA, B non-small cell lung cancer. In F.C. Detterbeck, M.P. Rivera, M.A. Socinski, & J.G. Rosenman (Eds.), *Diagnosis and treatment of lung cancer: An evidence-based guide for the practicing clinician* (pp. 267–282). Philadelphia: Saunders.

Dragnev, K., Stover, D., & Dmitrovsky, E. (2003). Lung cancer. Prevention: The guidelines. *Chest, 123*(Suppl. 1), 60S–71S.

Edwards, B.K., Howe, H.L., Ries, L.A., Thun, M.J., Rosenberg, H.M., Yancik, R., et al. (2002). Annual report to the nation on the status of cancer, 1973–1999, featuring implications of age and aging on U.S. cancer burden. *Cancer, 94,* 2766–2792.

Eli Lilly and Co. (2004). Alimta® [Prescribing information]. Retrieved December 5, 2004, from http://www.fda.gov/cder/foi/label/2004/021677lbl.pdf

Environmental Protection Agency. (2003). *Indoor air—Radon. Assessment of risks from radon in homes.* Retrieved March 8, 2004, from http://www.epa.gov/radon/risk_assessment.html

FDA Alert for Healthcare Professionals. (2005). *Gefitinib.* Retrieved September 22, 2005, from http://www.fda.gov/cder/drug/infosheets/hcp/gefitinibHCP.pdf

Ferrone, M., & Motl, S.E. (2003). Trastuzumab for the treatment of non-small-cell lung cancer. *Annals of Pharmacotherapy, 37,* 1904–1908.

Fong, K., Sekido, Y., & Minna, J. (1999). Molecular pathogenesis of lung cancer. *Journal of Thoracic and Cardiovascular Surgery, 118,* 1136–1152.

Fretz, P., & Peterson, M. (2004). *Lung tumors: A multidisciplinary database: Clinical presentation and initial evaluation. Tissue diagnosis.* Retrieved April 25, 2004, from http://www.vh.org/adult/provider/radiology/LungTumors

Fukuoka, M., Yano, S., Giaccone, G., Tamura, T., Nakagawa, K., Douillard, J.Y., et al. (2003). Multi-institutional randomized phase II trial of gefitinib for previously treated patients with advanced non-small-cell lung cancer. *Journal of Clinical Oncology, 21,* 2237–2246.

Genentech, Inc. (2004). Tarceva® [Package insert]. Retrieved November 22, 2004, from http://www.fda.gov/cder/foi/label/2004/021743lbl.pdf

Giaccone, G., Herbst, R.S., Manegold, C., Scagliotti, G., Rosell, R., Miller, V., et al. (2004). Gefitinib in combination with gemcitabine and cisplatin in advanced non-small-cell lung cancer: A phase III trial—INTACT 1. *Journal of Clinical Oncology, 22,* 777–784.

Gillani, A.A., & Grunberg, S.M. (2004). Aerorespiratory tract cancer in older patients. *Seminars in Oncology, 31,* 220–233.

Ginsberg, R. (1998). Continuing controversies in staging NSCLC: An analysis of the revised 1997 staging system. *Oncology, 12*(1 Suppl. 2), 51–54.

Goodman, G.E., Thornquist, M.D., Balmes, J., Cullen, M.R., Meyskens, F.L., Omenn, G.S., et al. (2004). The Beta-Carotene and Retinol Efficacy Trial: Incidence of lung cancer and cardiovascular disease mortality during 6-year follow-up after stopping beta-carotene and retinol supplements. *Journal of the National Cancer Institute, 96,* 1743–1750.

Goss, G., Paszat, L., Newman, T., Evans, W.K., & the Lung Cancer Disease Site Group. (1998). Use of preoperative chemotherapy with or without postoperative radiotherapy in technically resectable stage IIIA non-small cell lung cancer. *Cancer Prevention and Control, 2,* 32–39.

Green, M., Murray, J., & Hortobagyi, G. (2000). Monoclonal antibody therapy for solid tumors. *Cancer Treatment Reviews, 26,* 269–286.

Greene, F.L., Page, D.L., Fleming, I.D., Fritz, A., Balch, C.M., Haller, D.G., et al. (Eds.). (2002). *AJCC cancer staging manual* (6th ed.). New York: Springer-Verlag.

Gridelli, C. (2001). The ELVIS trial: A phase III study of single-agent vinorelbine as first-line treatment in elderly patients with advanced non-small cell lung cancer. Elderly Lung Cancer Vinorelbine Italian Study. *Oncologist, 6*(Suppl. 1), 4–7.

Gridelli, C. (2002a). Chemotherapy of non-small cell lung cancer in the elderly. *Lung Cancer, 38*(Suppl. 3), S67–S70.

Gridelli, C. (2002b). Does chemotherapy have a role as palliative therapy for unfit or elderly patients with non-small-cell lung cancer? *Lung Cancer, 38*(Suppl. 2), S45–S50.

Gridelli, C., De Vivo, R., & Monfardini, S. (2002). Management of small-cell lung cancer in the elderly. *Critical Reviews in Oncology/Hematology, 41,* 79–88.

Gridelli, C., Maione, P., Castaldo, V., & Rossi, A. (2003). Gefitinib in elderly and unfit patients affected by advanced non-small-cell lung cancer. *British Journal of Cancer, 89,* 1827–1829.

Gridelli, C., Perrone, F., Gallo, C., Cigolari, S., Rossi, A., Piantedosi, F., et al. (2003). Chemotherapy for elderly patients with advanced non-small-cell lung cancer: The Multicenter Italian Lung Cancer in the Elderly Study (MILES) phase III randomized trial. *Journal of the National Cancer Institute, 95,* 362–372.

Griffin, J.P., Nelson, J.E., Koch, K.A., Niell, H.B., Ackerman, T.F., Thompson, M., et al. (2003). End-of-life care in patients with lung cancer. *Chest, 123*(Suppl. 1), 312S–331S.

Harpole, L., Kelley, M., Schreiber, G., Toloza, E., Kolimaga, J., & McCrory, C. (2003). Assessment and scope of the quality of the clinical practice guidelines in lung cancer. *Chest, 123*(Suppl. 1), 7S–20S.

Hayakawa, K., Mitsuhashi, N., Katano, S., Saito, Y., Nakayama, Y., Sakurai, H., et al. (2001). High-dose radiation therapy for elderly patients with inoperable or unresectable non-small cell lung cancer. *Lung Cancer, 32,* 81–88.

Hennessy, B.T., Hanrahan, E.O., & Breathnach, O.S. (2003). Chemotherapy options for the elderly patient with advanced non-small cell lung cancer. *Oncologist, 8,* 270–277.

Henschke, C.I., McCarthy, P., & Wernick, S. (2002). *Lung cancer: Myths, facts and choices—and hope.* New York: Norton.

Henschke, C.I., McCauley, D.I., Yankelevitz, D.F., Naidich, D.P., McGuinness, G., Miettinen, O.S., et al. (1999). Early Lung Cancer Action Project: Overall design and findings from baseline screening. *Lancet, 354,* 99–105.

Henschke, C.I., McCauley, D.I., Yankelevitz, D.F., Naidich, D.P., McGuinness, G., Miettinen, O.S., et al. (2001). Early Lung Cancer Action Project: A summary of the findings on baseline screening. *Oncologist, 6,* 147–152.

Herbst, R.S., Giaccone, G., Schiller, J.H., Natale, R.B., Miller, V., Manegold, C., et al. (2004). Gefitinib in combination with paclitaxel and carboplatin in advanced non-small-cell lung cancer: A phase III trial—INTACT 2. *Journal of Clinical Oncology, 22,* 785–794.

Hinton, S., & Sandler, A. (2002). Lung cancer in the elderly: Current and future chemotherapeutic options. *Drugs and Aging, 19,* 365–375.

Hopwood, P., & Stephens, R. (2000). Depression in patients with lung cancer: Prevalence and risk factors derived from quality-of-life data. *Journal of Clinical Oncology, 18,* 893–903.

Huncharek, M., Kupelnick, B., Geschwind, J.F., & Caubet, J.F. (2000). Prognostic significance of p53 mutations in non-small cell lung cancer: A meta-analysis of 829 cases from eight published studies. *Cancer Letters, 153,* 219–226.

Hurria, A., & Kris, M.G. (2003). Management of lung cancer in older adults. *CA: A Cancer Journal for Clinicians, 53,* 325–341.

Ishida, T., Yokoyama, H., Kaneko, S., Sugio, K., & Sugimachi, K. (1990). Long-term results of operation for non-small cell lung cancer in the elderly. *Annals of Thoracic Surgery, 50,* 919–922.

Jaklitsch, M.T., Mery, C.M., & Audisio, R.A. (2003). The use of surgery to treat lung cancer in elderly patients. *Lancet Oncology, 4,* 463–471.

Jemal, A., Chu, K.C., & Tarone, R.E. (2001). Recent trends in lung cancer mortality in the United States. *Journal of the National Cancer Institute, 93,* 277–283.

Johnson, D.H., & Arteaga, C.L. (2003). Gefitinib in recurrent non-small-cell lung cancer: An IDEAL trial? *Journal of Clinical Oncology, 21,* 2227–2229.

Johnson, K. (2003). Gefitinib (Iressa) trials in non-small cell lung cancer. *Lung Cancer, 41*(Suppl. 1), S23–S28.

Kadono, K., Satoh, H., Homma, T., Ohtsuka, M., & Sekizawa, K. (2002). Radiotherapy for elderly non-small cell lung cancer patients. *Oncology Reports, 9,* 1273–1276.

Keller, J.W., & Benton, J.B. (2001). Oncologic emergencies. In P. Rubin & J. Williams (Eds.), *Clinical oncology: A multidisciplinary approach for physicians and students* (8th ed., pp. 208–219). Philadelphia: Saunders.

Kennedy, T.C., Lam, S., & Hirsch, F.R. (2001). Review of recent advances in fluorescence bronchoscopy in early localization of central airway lung cancer. *Oncologist, 6,* 257–262.

Kimura, T., Kudoh, S., Hirata, K., Takifuji, N., Negoro, S., & Yoshikawa, J. (2001). Prognostic factors in elderly patients with unresectable non-small cell lung cancer. *Anticancer Research, 21,* 1379–1383.

Knop, C.S. (2005). Lung cancer. In C.H. Yarbro, M.H. Frogge, M. Goodman, & S.L. Groenwald (Eds.), *Cancer nursing: Principles and practice* (6th ed., pp. 1379–1413). Sudbury, MA: Jones and Bartlett.

Koizumi, K., Haraguchi, S., Hirata, T., Hirai, K., Mikami, I., Fukushima, M., et al. (2002). Video-assisted lobectomy in elderly lung cancer patients. *Japanese Journal of Thoracic and Cardiovascular Surgery, 50,* 15–22.

Kris, M.G., Natale, R.B., Herbst, R.S., Lynch, T.J., Jr., Prager, D., Belani, C.P., et al. (2003). Efficacy of gefitinib, an inhibitor of the epidermal growth factor receptor tyrosine kinase, in symptomatic patients with non-small cell lung cancer: A randomized trial. *JAMA, 290,* 2149–2158.

Kvale, P.A., Simoff, M., & Prakash, U.B. (2003). Lung cancer: Palliative care. *Chest, 123*(Suppl. 1), 284S–311S.

Lai, W., Chen, F., Wu, J., Chow, N., Su, W., Ma, M., et al. (2001). Immunohistochemical analysis of epidermal growth factor receptor family members in stage I non-small cell lung cancer. *Annals of Thoracic Surgery, 72,* 1868–1876.

Langer, C.J. (2002). Elderly patients with lung cancer: Biases and evidence. *Current Treatment Options in Oncology, 3,* 85–102.

Langer, C.J., Manola, J., Bernardo, P., Kugler, J.W., Bonomi, P., Cella, D., et al. (2002). Cisplatin-based therapy for elderly patients with advanced non-small-cell lung cancer: Implications of Eastern Cooperative Oncology Group 5592, a randomized trial. *Journal of the National Cancer Institute, 94,* 173–181.

Langer, C.J., Stephenson, P., Thor, A., Vangel, M., & Johnson, D.H. (2004). Trastuzumab in the treatment of advanced non-small-cell lung cancer: Is there a role? Focus on Eastern Cooperative Oncology Group study 2598. *Journal of Clinical Oncology, 22,* 1180–1187.

Lea, D.H., Calzone, K.A., Masny, A., & Bush, A.M. (2002). *Genetics and cancer care: A guide for oncology nurses.* Pittsburgh, PA: Oncology Nursing Society.

Lynch, T.J., Bell, D.W., Sordella, R., Gurubhagavatula, S., Okimoto, R.A., Brannigan, B.W., et al. (2004). Activating mutations in the epidermal growth factor receptor underlying responsiveness of non-small-cell lung cancer to gefitinib. *New England Journal of Medicine, 350,* 2129–2139.

Manegold, C. (2001). Treatment of elderly patients with non-small-cell lung cancer. *Oncology (Huntington), 15*(3 Suppl. 6), 46–51.

Marcus, P.M., Bergstralh, E.J., Fagerstrom, R.M., Williams, D.E., Fontana, R., Taylor, W.F., et al. (2000). Lung cancer mortality in the Mayo Lung Project: Impact of extended follow-up. *Journal of the National Cancer Institute, 92,* 1308–1316.

Matsui, K., Masuda, N., Yana, T., Takada, Y., Kobayashi, M., Nitta, T., et al. (2001). Carboplatin calculated with Chatelut's formula plus etoposide for elderly patients with small-cell lung cancer. *Internal Medicine, 40,* 603–606.

Minna, J., Dekido, Y., Fong, K., & Gazdar, A. (2001). Cancer of the lung. In V. DeVita, S. Hellman, & S. Rosenberg (Eds.), *Cancer: Principles and practice of oncology* (6th ed., pp. 123–127). Philadelphia: Lippincott Williams & Wilkins.

National Cancer Institute. (2004). *Cancer screening overview. Levels of evidence.* Retrieved March 8, 2004, from http://www.cancer.gov/templates/page_print.aspx?viewid=6155397B-A57F-45BC-8898-4E5C290E0411&version=healthprofessional

National Comprehensive Cancer Network. (2004). *Clinical practice guidelines in oncology: Palliative care.* Retrieved September 21, 2005, from http://www.nccn.org/professionals/physician_gls/PDF/palliative.pdf

National Comprehensive Cancer Network. (2005a). *Clinical practice guidelines in oncology: Distress management.* Retrieved September 21, 2005, from http://www.nccn.org/professionals/physician_gls/PDF/distress.pdf

National Comprehensive Cancer Network. (2005b). *Clinical practice guidelines in oncology: Senior adult oncology.* Retrieved September 21, 2005, from http://www.nccn.org/professionals/physician_gls/PDF/senior.pdf

National Comprehensive Cancer Network. (2005c). *Clinical practice guidelines in oncology: Non-small cell lung cancer.* Retrieved September 21, 2005, from http://www.nccn.org/professionals/physician_gls/PDF/nscl.pdf

National Comprehensive Cancer Network. (2005d). *Clinical practice guidelines in oncology: Small cell lung cancer.* Retrieved September 21, 2005, from http://www.nccn.org/professionals/physician_gls/PDF/sclc.pdf

Normanno, N., Maiello, M., & De Luca, A. (2002). Epidermal growth factor receptor tyrosine kinase inhibitors (EGFR-TKIs): Simple drugs with a complex mechanism of action? *Journal of Cellular Physiology, 194,* 13–19.

North-Eastern Italian Oncology Group. (1990). Clinical characteristics, diagnosis and treatment of elderly patients with lung cancer at non-surgical institutions: A multicenter study. *Tumori, 76,* 429–433.

O'Rourke, M.A., Feussner, J.R., Feigl, P., & Laszlo, J. (1987). Age trends of lung cancer stage at diagnosis. Implications for lung cancer screening in the elderly. *JAMA, 258,* 921–926.

Paccagnella, A., Oniga, F., Favaretto, A., Biason, R., & Ghi, M.G. (2002). Elderly patients with small cell lung cancer. *Tumori, 88*(1 Suppl. 1), S145–S147.

Pao, W., Miller, V., Zakowski, M., Doherty, J., Politi, K., Sarkaria, I., et al. (2004). EGF receptor gene mutations are common in lung cancers from "never smokers" and are associated with sensitivity of tumors to gefitinib and erlotinib. *Proceedings of the National Academy of Sciences USA, 101,* 13306–13311.

Pastorino, U., Andreola, S., Tagliabue, E., Pezzella, F., Incarbone, M., Sozzi, G., et al. (1997). Immunocytochemical markers in stage I lung cancer: Relevance to prognosis. *Journal of Clinical Oncology, 15,* 2858–2865.

Patchell, R., Tibbs, P., Regine, W., Payne, R., Saris, S., Kryskio, R., et al. (2003). A randomized trial of direct decompressive surgical resection in the treatment of spinal cord compression caused by metastasis [Abstract 2]. *Proceedings of the American Society of Clinical Oncology, 22,* 1.

Perrone, F., Gallo, C., & Gridelli, C. (2002). Re: Cisplatin-based therapy for elderly patients with advanced non-small-cell lung cancer: Implications of Eastern Cooperative Oncology Group 5592, a randomized trial. *Journal of the National Cancer Institute, 94,* 1029–1030.

Pfister, D., Johnson, D., Azzoli, C., Sause, W., Smith, T., Baker, S., et al. (2004). American Society of Clinical Oncology treatment of unresectable non-small-cell lung cancer guideline: Update 2003. *Journal of Clinical Oncology, 22,* 330–353.

Rieger, P. (2003). The impact of genetic information in the management of cancer. In A. Trainin, A. Masny, & J. Jenkins (Eds.), *Genetics in oncology practice: Cancer risk assessment* (pp. 167–169). Pittsburgh, PA: Oncology Nursing Society.

Ries, L.A.G., Eisner, M.P., Kosary, C.L., Hankey, B.F., Miller, B.A., Clegg, L., et al. (2004). *SEER cancer statistics review, 1975–2001.* Retrieved December 5, 2004, from http://seer.cancer.gov/csr/1975_2001/results_merged/sect_15_lung_bronchus.pdf

Rivera, M.P., Detterbeck, F., Mehta, A.C., & the American College of Chest Physicians. (2003). Diagnosis of lung cancer; the guidelines. *Chest, 123*(Suppl. 1), 129S–136S.

Ross, D.W. (1998). *Introduction to oncogenes and molecular cancer medicine.* New York: Springer.

Schild, S.E., Stella, P.J., Geyer, S.M., Bonner, J.A., McGinnis, W.L., Mailliard, J.A., et al. (2003). The outcome of combined-modality therapy for stage III non-small-cell lung cancer in the elderly. *Journal of Clinical Oncology, 21,* 3201–3206.

Scott, W.J., Howington, J., & Movsas, B. (2003). Treatment of stage II non-small cell lung cancer. *Chest, 123*(Suppl. 1), 188S–201S.

Sekine, I., & Saijo, N. (2001). Growth-stimulating pathways in lung cancer: Implications for targets of therapy. *Clinical Lung Cancer, 2,* 299–306.

Senderowicz, A. (2003). The cell cycle as a target for cancer therapy: Basic and clinical findings with the small molecule inhibitors Flavopyridole and UCN-01. *Oncologist, 7*(Suppl. 3), 12–19.

Sequist, L.V., & Lynch, T.J. (2003). Aggressive treatment for the fit elderly with non-small-cell lung cancer? Yes! *Journal of Clinical Oncology, 21,* 3186–3188.

Shapiro, G.I., Koestner, D.A., Matranga, C.B., & Rollins, B.J. (1999). Flavopyridole induces cell cycle arrest and p53-independent apoptosis in non-small cell lung cancer cell lines. *Clinical Cancer Research, 5,* 2925–2938.

Silvestri, G., Tanoue, L., Margolis, M., Barker, J., & Detterbeck, F. (2003). The noninvasive staging of non-small cell lung cancer: The guidelines. *Chest, 123*(Suppl. 1), 147S–156S.

Simon, G.R., Wagner, H., & the American College of Chest Physicians. (2003). Small cell lung cancer. *Chest, 123*(Suppl. 1), 259S–271S.

Smythe, W.R., & the American College of Chest Physicians. (2003). Treatment of stage 1 non-small cell lung carcinoma. *Chest, 123*(Suppl. 1), 181S–187S.

Sordella, R., Bell, D.W., Haber, D.A., & Settleman, J. (2004). Gefitinib-sensitizing EGFR mutations in lung cancer activate anti-apoptotic pathways. *Science, 305,* 1163–1167.

Swisher, S.G., & Roth J.A. (2002). Clinical update of Ad-p53 gene therapy for lung cancer. *Surgical Oncology Clinics of North America, 11,* 521–535.

Syrigos, K., & Dionellis, G. (2003). Management of elderly patients with lung cancer. *Pneumonologic, 16,* 337–340.

Thomas, M. (2003). Epidermal growth factor receptor tyrosine kinase inhibitors: Application in non-small cell lung cancer. *Cancer Nursing, 26*(Suppl. 6), 21S–25S.

Van Houtte, P., McDonald, S., Chang, A., & Salazar, O. (2001). Lung cancer. In P. Rubin & J.P. Williams (Eds.), *Clinical oncology: A multidisciplinary approach for physicians and students* (8th ed., pp. 823–844). Philadelphia: Saunders.

van Rens, M.T., de la Riviere, A.B., Elbers, H.R., & van Den Bosch, J.M. (2000). Prognostic assessment of 2,361 patients who underwent pulmonary resection for non-small cell lung cancer, stage I, II, and IIIA. *Chest, 117,* 374–379.

Will, B.P., Berthelot, J.M., Nobrega, K.M., Flanagan, W., & Evans, W.K. (2001). Canada's Population Health Model (POHEM): A tool for performing economic evaluations of cancer control interventions. *European Journal of Cancer, 37,* 1797–1804.

Works, C., & Maxwell, M. (2000). Malignant effusions and edemas. In C.H. Yarbro, M.H. Frogge, M. Goodman, & S.L. Groenwald (Eds.), *Cancer nursing: Principles and practice* (5th ed., pp. 813–815). Sudbury, MA: Jones and Bartlett.

Yamamoto, K., Padilla Alarcon, J., Calvo Medina, V., Garcia-Zarza, A., Pastor Guillen, J., Blasco Armengod, E., et al. (2003). Surgical results of stage I non-small cell lung cancer: Comparison between elderly and younger patients. *European Journal of Cardiothoracic Surgery, 23,* 21–25.

Yu, E., Lochrin, C., Dixon, P., Ung, Y.C., Gagliardi, A., Evans, W.K., et al. (2000). Altered fractionation of radical radiation therapy in the management of unresectable non-small-cell lung cancer. *Current Oncology, 7,* 98–109.

CHAPTER 11

The Older Adult With Prostate Cancer

Maureen E. O'Rourke, RN, PhD

Introduction

Prostate cancer is a significant health problem for older men in the United States and is the most frequently diagnosed noncutaneous male cancer in the United States, with an estimated 232,090 new cases expected to be diagnosed in 2005 (American Cancer Society ([ACS], 2005). Incidence rates are expected to rise dramatically, with an expected 380,000 new cases per year in 2025 as the baby boom population ages (Scardino, 2003). More than 75% of all prostate cancers are diagnosed in men 65 years of age or older, and 90% of deaths occur in this age group, making age a particularly significant risk factor (Stanford et al., 2004). Autopsy studies have demonstrated that at least 30% of men older than age 50 have some evidence of adenocarcinoma of the prostate, and by age 90, that percentage rises to 57% (Scott, Mutchnik, Laskowski, & Schmalhorst, 1969). This chapter will present incidence rates, risk factors, screening recommendations, clinical manifestations, treatment options, and research issues for the older adult with prostate cancer.

Incidence

Prostate cancer is the sixth most commonly occurring cancer worldwide. Within the United States, prostate cancer incidence increased steadily from 1988–1992, coinciding with the advent of widespread prostate cancer screening using the prostate-specific antigen (PSA) test. From 1992–1995, however, sharp declines in incidence were noted, followed by a gradual leveling off through 1999. An American male has a 10% lifetime risk of developing prostate cancer but only a 3% risk of dying of the disease (Steinberg, Bales, & Brendler, 1998). The highest incidence and mortality rates worldwide occur among African Americans.

Prostate cancer accounts for one-third of all male cancer deaths; 30,350 deaths are expected in the United States in 2005 (ACS, 2005). Since 1974, five-year survival rates have steadily improved for both Whites and African Americans; however, African Americans continue to have lower five-year survival rates for all stages of prostate cancer. The relative five-year survival within the United States is 98% for Whites and is 93% for African Americans (Brawley & Barnes, 2001).

Risk Factors

The cause of prostate cancer remains unknown. Age, race, ethnicity, and family history are the only well-established risk factors. The highest incidence rates worldwide are among African Americans. Hormonal factors have been suggested as an explanation for the differential incidence and mortality rates. Higher rates of bioavailable testosterone have been noted among African Americans, as well as a higher incidence of mutations in the prostate cancer susceptibility gene. Different ethnic groups experience different rates of incidence. Americans of Northern European origin have higher rates of incidence than Native Americans, Mexican Americans, or Chinese Americans. Prostate cancer is rare in developing countries. Although Japanese men have one of the lowest incidence rates, incidence rates become similar to those of Caucasian American males after only two generations of living within the United States (Brawley & Barnes, 2001).

Links between prostate cancer and lifestyle have been postulated, although no conclusive evidence exists at this point. In one prospective cohort study involving 51,529 men, increased fat intake, consumption of red meat, and increased animal fat intake were positively correlated with increases in prostate cancer risk (Giovannucci et al., 1993). More recent studies also suggest a correlation between increased prostate cancer risk and high intake of saturated fats (Kolonel, Nomura, & Cooney, 1999; Kushi & Giovannucci, 2002). Diets high in vitamins E and D, selenium, and lycopene have been suggested to be protective, yet evidence is not conclusive (Gann et al., 1999). Vitamin D has shown promise as a chemopreventive agent based on epidemiologic data. African American men who have more melanin deposition have higher rates of prostate cancer. Melanin inhibits vitamin D synthesis. Men living in higher latitudes with less sun exposure (a major source of vitamin D) have higher incidence rates of prostate cancer. Additionally, older men, who are also often vitamin D deficient, have higher incidence rates (Polek & Weigel, 2002). Phase II clinical trials suggest that vitamin D can slow the rate of PSA rise among men with prostate cancer who have had biochemical failure following treatment; however, the risk of hypercalcemia and renal calculi were limiting factors (Gross, Stamey, Hancock, & Feldman, 1998). One clinical trial demonstrated that men fed tomato-based pasta dishes for three weeks prior to radical prostatectomy had increased lycopene levels in both the prostate gland and in the blood and had reductions in both serum PSA levels and oxidative DNA damage (Chen et al., 2001).

Occupational exposure to chemicals and pesticides used in farming, as well as exposure to cadmium during welding and battery manufacturing, also have been linked with an increased risk for the development of prostate cancer (Brawley & Barnes, 2001), but conclusions are lacking, and no prescriptive recommendations can be made at this point.

A variety of genetic links have been suggested. A possible susceptibility locus noted on chromosome 1 is thought to be responsible for up to 33% of hereditary prostate cancers overall. At present, however, heredity is estimated to account for only 3% of prostate cancers overall (Cooney et al., 1997). Genetic mutations associated with the development of breast cancer, *BRCA1* and *BRCA2,* also have been implicated in prostate cancer (Ekman, 1999). Strong familial associations have been noted, although it is unclear if these represent purely genetic links or a combination of environmental and genetic factors. Men with a first-degree relative, such as their brother or father, affected by prostate cancer are two to three times more likely to develop the disease themselves. Men with a first-degree relative and a second-degree relative with the disease are six times more likely to develop prostate cancer themselves (Zlotta & Schulman, 1998).

The presence of high-grade prostatic intraepithelial neoplasia (PIN) is a marker for the development of adenocarcinoma. PIN only is detected on biopsy and does not significantly elevate serum PSA. It is not detectable on ultrasound. PIN is highly predictive for the development of adenocarcinoma of the prostate within 10 years (Bostwick, 2000).

Numerous other suspected linkages are reported in the literature, including early sexual experiences, venereal disease, and multiple sexual partners. These associations have been weak and inconclusive, with contradictory evidence at times. Additionally, research has not been able to substantiate the suspected link between vasectomy and prostate cancer incidence.

Pathophysiology

The prostate is a small muscular organ, measuring approximately 4 cm in diameter and located posterior to the symphysis pubis, inferior to the bladder, and in front of the rectum (Martini, Timmons, & McKinley, 2000). The gland encircles the urethra as it exits the bladder and is composed of three zones: transitional, central, and peripheral. The prostate gland functions as a secondary sex organ, secreting a component of seminal fluid.

Most malignancies develop within the peripheral zone, and malignant growth spreads locally to the seminal vesicles, bladder, and peritoneum. Hematogenous spread typically involves the lungs, liver, kidney, and bones. Lymphatic node invasion is common (Nelson et al., 2004). Adenocarcinomas comprise 95% of all prostate cancers, with the remaining 5% consisting of sarcomas and transitional cell carcinomas (Frank, Granham, & Neighbors, 1991).

Screening

On both the national and international levels, a high level of controversy surrounds prostate cancer screening, with the central issue being an understanding that screening may reveal clinically insignificant tumors that are subsequently unnecessarily treated. Treatment results in significant side effects and diminished quality of life (QOL).

Few randomized controlled trials (RCTs) have been conducted to answer the ultimate question: Does screening result in decreased prostate cancer mortality? One such study was the Quebec Screening Study, which randomly assigned men to screening or no screening and then compared mortality over time. Men were screened with PSA and digital rectal examination (DRE) and only had transrectal ultrasound if PSA levels were > 3.0 ng/ml. The trial demonstrated a reduction in prostate cancer mortality among the screened men of up to 70% compared with those who were not screened (Labrie et al., 1999). The trial has been widely criticized, however, because of its methodologic flaws. Although 46,193 men were eligible to participate, only 31,000 actually were invited to participate, and of these, only 7,100 were screened. Randomization was compromised and statistical power was inadequate. Additionally, a lag time of up to three years occurred between "randomization" and actual screening.

Perron, Moore, Bairati, Bernard, and Meyer (2002) examined whether the decline in prostate cancer incidence in Quebec could be attributed to PSA screening. The change in incidence rates between 1989 and 1993 was compared with the change in prostate cancer mortality between 1995 and 1999. Fifteen birth cohorts in 15 regions of Quebec were studied. The authors concluded that increased screening rates in Quebec did not correlate with the subsequent declining prostate cancer mortality rate.

Clearly, the verdict is still out. Until well-designed RCTs are conducted wherein the screened and nonscreened groups are similar in baseline characteristics, the question remains unanswered. Such trials currently are under way in Europe and the United States. Presently, major healthcare organizations have not formed a clear consensus regarding prostate screening recommendations. The U.S. Preventive Services Task Force (2002) found "good" evidence that PSA screening can detect early-stage prostate cancer but "mixed and inconclusive evidence" that early detection improves overall health outcomes. In light of this, it does not endorse routine PSA screening.

Despite disagreement among major healthcare groups, ACS guidelines regarding testing for early prostate cancer recommend that PSA tests and DREs should be offered beginning at age 50 to men having a life expectancy of 10 years or more (Smith, Cokkinides, & Eyre, 2003). ACS further suggests that prior to testing, men should fully discuss with their healthcare provider the risks and benefits in order to make an informed decision. Men at high risk, including men of African descent and men with a first-degree relative affected by prostate cancer, should begin testing at age 45. For men with a history of numerous first-degree relatives with prostate cancer, testing should be initiated at age 40 (Smith et al.). Routine screening generally is not recommended for males older than 75 years of age because early detection is unlikely to affect survival, and PSA values can increase with age because of increasing prostate volume and benign prostatic hypertrophy, resulting in false positives (Raghavan & Skinner, 2004).

The pros and cons of prostate cancer screening have been detailed in the lay literature as well. When considering screening in the older adult male, factors that should be reviewed include the patient's general health status and life expectancy. Each man must make his own decision after consulting with his primary healthcare provider to discuss controversies and benefits of screening. Factors cited in favor of prostate cancer screening include the fact that advanced prostate cancer is not curable. Men who are screened have a greater likelihood of being diagnosed at an earlier stage that is more conducive to cure. Factors that have been cited in the arguments against routine screening include the fact that many men die with the disease versus of the disease (Steinberg et al., 1998), and a lack of clear scientific evidence exists to conclude that screening decreases a man's risk of dying from prostate cancer.

Clinical Presentation

Men with early-stage prostate cancer often are symptom free because the majority of prostatic malignancies arise in the peripheral zone. Most prostate cancers are detected following routine screening using PSA testing. A total serum PSA concentration > 4.0 ng/ml is considered abnormal in most assays and generally is suspicious for malignancy (Mettlin et al., 1994). It should be noted, however, that some men with PSA levels < 4.0 ng/ml will have prostate cancer. Among 2,950 men (aged 62–91 years) in the control group of the Prostate Cancer Prevention Study who had PSA levels < 4.0 ng/ml and who lacked any suspicious finding on DREs during the seven-year course of the study, 15% were found to have prostate cancer on biopsy at the conclusion of the study. The prevalence of high-grade cancers with Gleason scores of 7 or higher was 25% among men with cancer at PSA levels of 3.1–4.0 ng/ml (Thompson et al., 2004). Age-specific PSA reference ranges have been suggested to decrease unnecessary biopsies; however, this still is controversial (National Comprehensive Cancer Network [NCCN], 2005a; Raghavan & Skinner, 2004).

Although symptoms may be present in early-stage disease, urinary frequency, hesitancy, and incomplete emptying of the bladder are seen more often with disease progression. Progression also may cause blood in the semen with decreased ejaculatory volume and, less commonly, impotence as the tumor encroaches upon the neurovascular bundles in periprostatic tissue. Bone pain, pathologic fractures, spinal cord compression, hematuria, and anemia are signs of advanced disease.

Staging

As in the case of any malignancy, diagnosis is only definitively established via biopsy. Men either present for evaluation because of bothersome symptoms or following an elevated PSA or suspicious DRE. A DRE that reveals asymmetry, nodules, or areas of induration raises the suspicion for malignancy. In the presence of symptoms or questionable screening test results, a biopsy generally is performed. Biopsies are performed transrectally under transrectal ultrasound to facilitate visualization of the gland. A spring-loaded biopsy gun is used to obtain multiple samples (generally six) from all regions of the prostate gland. Although sextant biopsy has long been standard, extended biopsy protocol sampling gradually is replacing the procedure, with emphasis on sampling the lateral aspects of the gland. Investigators have reported higher detection rates when using more than six samples (Presti, Chang, Bhargava, & Shinohara, 2000). In one study of 483 men with PSA levels of 4.0 ng/ml, lateral biopsies of the peripheral zone in addition to the routine sextant protocol for a total of 10 biopsies detected 96% of cancers, as opposed to the traditional sextant biopsy protocol, which detected only 80% of cancers (Presti et al.). The more extensive schema has not been associated with more pain but is associated with more frequent bloody stools (hematochezia) and hematospermia. The extended 10-core biopsy scheme has been demonstrated to be significantly superior to sextant biopsies in predicting the underlying pathologic Gleason score for prostate cancer. In particular, it significantly improves detection of an underlying high-grade component. This finding may be of critical clinical importance, and King, McNeal, Gil, and Presti (2004) suggested that the extended biopsy scheme should become the standard of care.

Patient education at the time of biopsy includes instructions regarding anticipatable side effects: hematuria, hematochezia, and hematospermia, which may occur for several days to several weeks postprocedure. Men should contact their urologist in the presence of an elevated temperature, excessive or prolonged bleeding, or increased urinary difficulties.

Other diagnostic tests may be employed. Magnetic resonance imaging (MRI) may be used to evaluate extracapsular penetration beyond the prostate gland itself and possible lymph node metastasis. Evaluation of the use of endorectal coil MRI is under way. In one study of men with clinical stage T1 or T2 lesions, with PSA levels of 10–20 ng/ml and Gleason scores ≤ 7, or those who underwent radical prostatectomy, the addition of endorectal coil MRI to preoperative staging would have correctly predicted extracapsular spread (D'Amico, Schnall, et al., 1998). This finding is significant because these men would not have been candidates for surgery. Endorectal MRI may become a useful tool in helping to make more evidence-based recommendations for surgery versus radiation therapy (RT).

Computed tomography (CT) scans also may be used to evaluate prostate size and lymph node status. The NCCN guidelines recommend radionucleotide bone scans for T1 or T2 disease only if PSA levels are > 20 ng/ml, Gleason score is ≥ 8, presence of signs or symptoms consistent with bony metastases, or any clinical T3 or T4 disease (NCCN, 2004). These scans are performed to assess possible bone metastasis but are interpreted with caution, as they may yield false-positive results signaling activity at sites of old trauma or arthritis. In males with low- or moderate-risk disease, bone and CT scans usually are not necessary (Raghavan & Skinner, 2004).

Prostate cancer is staged as a means of describing the extent of the disease and determining the appropriate type of therapy. The American Joint Committee on Cancer has updated the tumor-node-metastasis (TNM) staging system for prostate cancer (Greene et al., 2002) (see Figure 11-1).

Prostate cancer is graded according to the level of cellular differentiation noted among the malignant specimens taken from biopsies. The most common system employed for the grading of prostate cancer is the Gleason score. Two scores are assigned. The two most common malignant cellular patterns noted under microscopic examination are graded on a score of 1–5. Scores for each then are summed. Total scores range from 2–10, with higher scores indicating more aggressive disease and subsequently poorer prognosis (Gleason & Mellinger, 1974; Stoller & Carroll, 2003).

Treatment

Currently, men generally are presented with three main treatment options for early-stage prostate cancer: radical prostatectomy, RT (either external beam or brachytherapy), or the "watchful waiting" or expectant management approach (see Figure 11-2). Hormone therapy also may be considered in the frail or older adult male. Recently, the option of cryotherapy is becoming more available in some regions, although it remains investigational and without long-term outcome data. Neoadjuvant hormonal therapy may be offered prior to surgical or radiotherapy treatments.

Many factors are involved in decision making regarding treatment selection for early-stage cancer. The process of deciding on the most appropriate prostate cancer treatment is a truly collaborative process among the patient, his partner, and the

TNM definitions

Primary tumor (T)
- TX: Primary tumor cannot be assessed
- T0: No evidence of primary tumor
- T1: Clinically inapparent tumor not palpable nor visible by imaging
  - T1a: Tumor incidental histologic finding in 5% or less of tissue resected
  - T1b: Tumor incidental histologic finding in more than 5% of tissue resected
  - T1c: Tumor identified by needle biopsy (e.g., because of elevated prostate-specific antigen)
- T2: Tumor confined within prostate*
  - T2a: Tumor involves one-half of one lobe or less
  - T2b: Tumor involves more than one-half of one lobe but not both lobes
  - T2c: Tumor involves both lobes
- T3: Tumor extends through the prostate capsule**
  - T3a: Extracapsular extension (unilateral or bilateral)
  - T3b: Tumor invades seminal vesicle(s)
- T4: Tumor is fixed or invades adjacent structures other than seminal vesicles: bladder neck, external sphincter, rectum, levator muscles, and/or pelvic wall

Note: Tumor found in one or both lobes by needle biopsy, but not palpable or reliably visible by imaging, is classified as T1c.

**Note:* Invasion into the prostatic apex or into (but not beyond) the prostatic capsule is not classified as T3 but as T2.

Regional lymph nodes (N)
- NX: Regional lymph nodes were not assessed
- N0: No regional lymph node metastasis
- N1: Metastasis in regional lymph node(s)

Distant metastasis (M)*
- MX: Distant metastasis cannot be assessed (not evaluated by any modality)
- M0: No distant metastasis
- M1: Distant metastasis
  - M1a: Nonregional lymph node(s)
  - M1b: Bone(s)
  - M1c: Other site(s) with or without bone disease

Note: When more than one site of metastasis is present, the most advanced category (pM1c) is used.

Histopathologic grade (G)
- GX: Grade cannot be assessed
- G1: Well-differentiated (slight anaplasia) (Gleason 2–4)
- G2: Moderately differentiated (moderate anaplasia) (Gleason 5–6)
- G3-4: Poorly differentiated or undifferentiated (marked anaplasia) (Gleason 7–10)

American Joint Committee on Cancer stage groupings
Stage I
- T1a, N0, M0, G1

Stage II
- T1a, N0, M0, G2, Gleason 3–4
- T1b, N0, M0, any G
- T1c, N0, M0, any G
- T1, N0, M0, any G
- T2, N0, M0, any G

Stage III
- T3, N0, M0, any G

Stage IV
- T4, N0, M0, any G
- Any T, N1, M0, any G
- Any T, any N, M1, any G

Figure 11-1. Prostate Cancer Staging

Note. Data from "Prostate Cancer Treatment," by the National Cancer Institute, 2004. Retrieved July 8, 2004, from http://www.cancer.gov/cancertopics/pdq/treatment/prostate/HealthProfessional

healthcare team. No true consensus exists within the scientific community as to which, if any, treatment is optimal for early-stage prostate cancer. The ultimate decision is affected by medical considerations and the patient's general health status, life expectancy, comorbidities, and unique preferences. Numerous medical

---

- Radical prostatectomy
- Radiation therapy
- Watchful waiting
- Hormone therapy (consideration for older adult male)

Figure 11-2. Treatment Options for Early-Stage Prostate Cancer

---

decision-making guides have been developed both for physicians and for men and their partners. Key factors in these decision-enhancement models include patient age, projected survival, coexisting medical conditions, stage of disease, and Gleason score. Patient factors include his personal preferences and biases toward or against particular treatment modalities, personal and vicarious experiences with cancer and cancer treatments, concerns about potential side effects of therapy and their effects on QOL, costs of treatment, lost work time, and tolerance of uncertainty (O'Rourke, 2001).

Aside from the aforementioned factors, risk classifications have been proposed based upon clinical stage, Gleason score, and PSA to determine the likelihood of future metastases and assist in treatment decision making (NCCN, 2005b; Raghavan & Skinner, 2004). NCCN has developed guidelines for those with a low, moderate, or high risk for recurrence. *Low risk of recurrence* is defined as men with T1 to T2 prostate cancer, a Gleason score between 2 and 6, and a PSA value $\leq$ 10 ng/ml. Healthcare providers recommend treatment based on predicted estimates of life expectancy. For low-risk men whose life expectancy is < 10 years, the recommended treatment includes observation or RT in the form of brachytherapy or three-dimensional conformal external-beam radiotherapy (3DCRT). If the estimated life expectancy is 10–20 years, the treatment recommendations are unchanged, with the exception of the addition of radical prostatectomy with or without lymph node dissection as a third treatment option (NCCN, 2005b).

NCCN (2005b) defined *intermediate risk of recurrence* as T2b to T2c disease or any Gleason score of 7 or PSA value of 10–20 ng/ml. For these men, the recommended initial treatment strategy also is based on estimated life expectancy. For men having a life expectancy of < 10 years, treatment options include observation, 3DCRT with or without brachytherapy, or radical prostatectomy with or without pelvic lymphadenectomy. For those men having a life expectancy > 10 years, treatment recommendations are similar, although observation is no longer recommended (NCCN, 2005b).

NCCN (2005b) defined men at *high risk of recurrence* as those with T3a to T3b disease, a Gleason score of 8–10, or a PSA value > 20 ng/ml. Active intervention is recommended for men having life expectancies > 5 years. Three treatment options are proposed for this group: neoadjuvant androgen deprivation followed by 3DCRT with androgen deprivation; 3DCRT alone for patients with T3a to T3b cancer but Gleason scores < 7 and PSA values < 10 ng/ml; and radical prostatectomy for selected patients with low-volume disease and no fixation to the pelvis.

An analysis of data from 3,073 participants in the National Cancer Institute Prostate Cancer Outcomes Study from 1994–1995 indicated that radical prostatectomy was the most common treatment for early-stage prostate cancer and was the initial treatment for 47.6% of newly diagnosed patients. RT was the second most common treatment for early-stage prostate cancer, with 23.4% of men choosing this option. RT was the most common treatment for men age 70–80 years. Among men in this sample, 10.5%

chose hormonal therapy, and 18.5% elected watchful waiting (Harlan et al., 2001). Men age 75 or older were more likely to receive conservative treatment, with 57.9% of men age 50–75 receiving watchful waiting or hormonal therapy alone, and 82% of men age 80 or older receiving the same. Conservative treatment was associated with unmarried status, high PSA levels, history of myocardial infarction, baseline history of incontinence or impotence, and geographic location. Treatment was noted to vary considerably by geographic location, with men in the Atlanta and Connecticut regions being more likely to receive RT than men in the other regions studied (New Mexico, Los Angeles, Utah, and Seattle). Racial variations also were noted. Older African American men were significantly less likely to receive any treatment at all—surgical, RT, or hormonal. Although African American men as a group have a tendency toward more coexisting diseases, these treatment deficits were noted even after controlling for these conditions (Harlan et al.).

For all men, comprehensive, accurate information from credible sources is the critical factor in decision making. For the older adult, complications of local treatment should be considered when making treatment decisions (Raghavan & Skinner, 2004). A trusting relationship with healthcare providers and assistance in sorting through the wide array of patient education products now available on the market and on the Internet represent areas where nurses play a pivotal professional role.

Radical Prostatectomy

The gold standard for comparing the efficacy of treatment options is the prospective randomized controlled trial (RCT). To date, only one RCT has directly compared radical prostatectomy and watchful waiting in men with early-stage, clinically localized prostate cancer (Holmberg et al., 2002). In this prospective study, 695 men with clinical stage T1–2 prostate cancer were randomly assigned to radical prostatectomy or watchful waiting. After eight years of follow-up, 7.1% of the radical prostatectomy group had died of prostate cancer as opposed to 13.6% of men in the watchful waiting group. Local progression was significantly more likely among men in the watchful waiting group as well—60% versus 20%. Of note, however, is the fact that 75% of the participants in this study had palpable tumors on diagnosis, and participants were not obtained from a screening population, thereby making them different than the majority of newly diagnosed men. Despite the impressive disease-specific survival rates associated with radical prostatectomy, surgery had no significant influence on overall survival. The two treatment groups were similar in overall survival. Significantly fewer men undergoing radical prostatectomy experienced disease metastasis at eight years (13% versus 27%), and this effect alone may translate into better overall survival with longer follow-up.

Currently, no RCTs are directly comparing radical prostatectomy with radiotherapy. Comparison between the two modalities is hampered by the fact that patients undergoing RT are only clinically staged, as men can only be pathologically staged based on findings during surgery, making understaging a problem among men undergoing RT alone. In a retrospective series of patients with clinically localized disease, cure rates with external beam RT are comparable to those for radical prostatectomy, at least for the first five to eight years (Kanumaru et al., 1998; Kuban et al., 2003). However, as noted previously, such comparisons are difficult because patients undergoing RT are not typically pathologically staged, and no randomized, prospective trials have been performed directly comparing RT with radical prostatectomy.

Within the United States, the mainstay of treatment is the radical retropubic prostatectomy, which includes the complete removal of the prostate gland, with lymph node sampling. The anatomic nerve-sparing approach, introduced in 1982, involves isolation of the neurovascular bundles responsible for innervation of the corpus cavernosa of the penis, necessary for erection, thereby maintaining potency postoperatively (Walsh & Donker, 1982). The procedure is performed under general or spinal anesthesia, and an incision is made from the umbilicus to the pubis. Removal of one or both of the neurovascular bundles is sometimes necessary to facilitate removal of all visible cancer. Care is taken to protect the urethral sphincter. The vas deferens and seminal vesicles are removed, and the bladder neck then is reconnected to the urethra. Pelvic drains are placed for several days to prevent urinary leakage from the bladder neck and urethral attachment site. A Foley catheter is inserted and remains in place for 10–21 days (Marschke, 2001).

Recent surgical advances include the use of a laparoscopic approach to prostatectomy. This surgical option offers the advantage of being minimally invasive with significantly less intra-operative blood loss and early return to full activity levels. However, initial data suggest variable rates of erectile dysfunction, higher positive margins and rectal injury rates, and slower return to urinary continence (Abbou et al., 2000; Guillonneau et al., 2003; Rassweiler et al., 2003). Robotic laparoscopic prostatectomy currently is under investigation as well.

In general, radical prostatectomy is recommended for men younger than 70 years of age and is only offered to men older than 75 years of age who are considered to be in good health, because prostatectomy is believed to benefit only those patients with a 10-year life expectancy (Raghavan & Skinner, 2004). If the older adult male possesses good cardiac function, no alterations are made in the surgical technique.

Nursing Care

Although nursing care of the patient following prostatectomy is not guided by RCTs, one published study examined the effects of shortened length of stay following radical prostatectomy on adverse surgical outcomes, cost, and patient satisfaction (Klein et al., 1996). Postoperative procedural changes included the use of on-demand morphine sulfate plus bupivacaine via epidural catheter for 24 hours followed by ketorolac tromehaline (Toradol®, Roche Pharmaceuticals, Nutley, NJ) via the IV route or ibuprofen via the oral route, as needed. Foley catheters and incision staples were removed seven days following discharge. Length of stay was shortened to a mean of two nights versus seven; 30-day mortality and 30-day readmission rates remained constant. Patient satisfaction was high at 83%, and the cost savings were 43% per case.

Nursing priorities for postprostatectomy care include vigilant pain assessment and the prevention of postoperative complications such as thrombophlebitis and pulmonary emboli, which may be more common among older men. Early ambulation on the first postoperative day and the performance of dorsiflexion exercises are advised. The use of an incentive spirometer, compression hose, or sequential compression devices also may be indicated. Pillow splinting may facilitate comfort during coughing and deep breathing exercises. Fluid intake should be encouraged to maintain a minimum urine output of 30 cc/hr or more. Rectal manipulation, including rectal temperatures and suppositories, is to be avoided because of the close proximity of the prostate gland to the rectal wall and the risk of rectal injury.

Additional nursing priorities focus on patient and partner education. Management of the Foley catheter in the home setting, including procedures for switching from the daytime leg bag to bedside drainage overnight, monitoring and reporting temperature elevations of $\geq 101°F$, and avoiding lifting anything 10 pounds or greater, should be emphasized prior to discharge and in follow-up phone contacts. Patients also should be instructed regarding maintenance of adequate fluid intake.

Prior to discharge, patients generally are instructed on the performance of pelvic floor muscle strengthening exercises. A review of 10 clinical trials conducted among men who had either radical prostatectomy or transurethral resection of the prostate concluded that five of the studies demonstrated "some value" to the use of conservative management of urinary incontinence (UI) via Kegel exercises and biofeedback. Evidence was inconclusive regarding pelvic muscle strengthening exercises alone, transcutaneous electrical nerve stimulation, and rectal electrical stimulation (Hunter, Moore, Cody, & Glazener, 2004).

Radiation Therapy

External Beam

No published randomized trials directly compare radical prostatectomy with RT among men with early prostate cancer, although one large-scale RCT is in progress. The SPIRIT trial, which randomly assigned low-risk men with early-stage prostate cancer (T1c or T2a) to brachytherapy or surgery, recently has closed to patient accrual. Analysis is planned at six-month intervals for up to five years post-treatment and then annually until death. No data are yet available (American College of Surgeons Oncology Group, 2004). Unfortunately, this trial does not have an external beam RT arm.

Nonrandomized retrospective reviews have demonstrated comparable cure rates with external beam RT and radical prostatectomy, with five to eight years of follow-up (Kanumaru et al., 1998; Kuban et al., 2003; Kupelian et al., 1997). RT remains a viable potentially curative treatment option for men with early-stage prostate cancer.

RT also is useful in the management of advanced disease for palliation of painful bone metastasis and other symptoms such as urethral or rectal obstruction, lymphatic blockage, or spinal cord compression. RT may be recommended for men experiencing locally recurrent disease documented by a rising PSA with or without symptoms.

Nursing Care

Nursing considerations for men undergoing RT focus on symptom management. Acute side effects include diarrhea, proctitis, cystitis, fatigue, and local skin reactions. The management of adequate nutritional intake and hydration status are important nursing foci. Low-residue diets and antidiarrheal medications are indicated. Topical rectal steroid products and sitz baths may be prescribed to provide relief from proctitis. No RCTs are available to guide interventions in this area. One review summarized the results of six RCTs for the management of chronic proctitis. Although evidence was insufficient to draw definite conclusions, the use of rectal sucralfate and the addition of metronidazole to an anti-inflammatory regimen showed promise with outcomes of decreased rectal bleeding, erythema, and ulceration (Denton, Forbes, Andreyev, & Maher, 2002).

Although the exact mechanism of radiation-induced fatigue has not been explained, contributing factors may include anemia, cytokine activation, psychological distress, and medication effects. Management should focus on correcting potential etiologies and symptom relief. Evidence based on the results of two RCTs suggested that moderate aerobic exercise during RT may attenuate the effects of fatigue (Mock et al., 1997; Windsor, Nicol, & Potter, 2004). Windsor et al. tested the effects of a home-based 30-minute walking program (three days per week) among men undergoing RT for localized prostate cancer. Participants in the exercise program had significantly less fatigue and improved physical functioning at the conclusion of four weeks of treatment.

Brachytherapy

Brachytherapy is the delivery of RT through the implantation of radioactive seeds, and it may be used as a solo treatment or in combination with external beam RT and/or hormonal therapy. No prospective randomized trials are available that compare brachytherapy to either radical prostatectomy or external beam RT, although several retrospective series are available for review. Based on these retrospective reviews, some evidence shows that brachytherapy is equivalent to external beam RT and radical prostatectomy for men with low-risk disease but may be associated with inferior outcomes in men with high-grade disease and men with higher pretreatment PSA levels. One meta-analysis that reviewed 13 case series and three cohort studies concluded that brachytherapy was comparable to radical prostatectomy in men with a low risk of recurrence (clinical stage T1–T2, Gleason score ≤ 6, and serum PSA level < 10 ng/ml) (Crook, Lukka, Klotz, Bestic, & Johnston, 2001). Results were similar for men with low-risk disease in a retrospective cohort study of 1,872 men who underwent radical prostatectomy, RT, or brachytherapy. However, among men with a high risk of recurrent disease, defined in this study as stage T2c, serum PSA > 20 ng/ml, or a Gleason score ≥ 8, men undergoing brachytherapy did significantly worse than men treated with prostatectomy. The addition of hormonal therapy did not improve outcomes. This held true for men with intermediate risk of recurrent disease (defined in this study as stage T2b, a Gleason score of 7, or serum PSA > 10 ng/ml) as well (D'Amico, Whittington, et al., 1998).

A single study demonstrated that RT and brachytherapy are equally effective for low-risk patients having T1 or T2 disease with Gleason scores < 6 and PSA < 10 ng/ml, but for patients with Gleason scores of 8–10 or PSA 10–20 ng/ml, brachytherapy was less effective than RT. Neither RT nor brachytherapy were particularly effective for those patients presenting with PSA levels > 20 ng/ml (Beyer & Brachman, 2000).

Finally, although no prospective randomized trials are yet available for review, studies are under way that compare brachytherapy alone with brachytherapy and external beam RT as a means of dose intensification to periprostatic tissues (Critz et al., 2000).

For men with prostate cancer, brachytherapy generally is performed as a same-day surgical procedure under general or spinal anesthesia. Radioactive seeds are implanted into the gland through a perineal approach guided by transrectal ultrasound. The most common isotopes used include Iodine[125] or Palladium[103]. The procedure takes one to two hours, and the patient is discharged at the end of the day. Patients may be discharged with an indwelling Foley catheter, generally for a period of 24–48 hours.

Nursing Care

Nursing care includes teaching and management of symptoms similar to those associated with external beam RT: cystitis, proctitis, and fatigue. Additional considerations include assessment and teaching regarding potential infection and instruction regarding prophylactic antibiotic use. Perineal pain, ecchymoses, and scrotal edema may be treated with ice packs and analgesic administration.

The radioactive seed implants into the prostate gland are permanent. Radioactivity dissipates over time, but precautions are required to minimize exposure to others during the radioisotope degradation period. Initially, men are instructed to strain their urine for one to two weeks in case a migratory radioactive seed is passed. Although recommendations vary, patients usually are told to retrieve the seed with tweezers, place it in a sealed container, and return it to the radiation oncology department. Body fluids are not radioactive, and the presence of the implanted seeds will not set off metal detectors.

Precautions are advised for a period of three weeks for men with Palladium[103] seed implants, or two months for Iodine[125], which has a longer half-life. Radiation safety guidelines vary by institution and state standards. Patients are advised to refrain from close contact with young children and pregnant women. Abstinence from sexual intercourse is advised for a two-week period. Condoms should be worn for the first six ejaculations, and patients should be informed that they may observe a brownish or bloody tinge to their semen during this period.

Watchful Waiting or Expectant Management

Watchful waiting, also known as expectant management, observation, or surveillance, has been defined as initial surveillance followed by active treatment in the presence of bothersome symptoms (Adolfsson, 1995). The rationale for this option for early-stage prostate cancer is based on the observation that prostate cancer incidence rates far exceed prostate cancer death rates, and more men die with the disease than of the disease (Steinberg et al., 1998). Although no RCTs exist, the most appropriate candidate for this treatment approach is the asymptomatic older adult male with low-risk disease (Raghavan & Skinner, 2004). Proponents of this strategy have cited two retrospective studies (Goodman, Busttil, & Chisholm, 1988; Johansson, Holmberg, Johansson, Bergstrom, & Adami, 1997) as evidence that watchful waiting is a reasonable alternative to aggressive treatment for men with localized disease. Adolfsson reviewed various end points from 12 studies, including overall survival, progression-free survival, and disease-specific survival. He concluded that overall survival at 10 years among patients with prostate cancer choosing watchful waiting ranged from 35%–72%. Disease-specific survival rates among this series ranged from 74%–87% at 10 years.

Two early randomized clinical trials comparing watchful waiting with radical prostatectomy found no statistically significant differences in survival between the two groups at 15 and 23 years, respectively (Graversen, Nielsen, Gasser, Corle, & Madsen, 1990; Iversen, Madsen, & Corle, 1995). However, both studies had small samples and limited statistical power. More recently, Holmberg et al. (2002) reported the results of a large RCT comparing watchful waiting to radical prostatectomy (reviewed earlier in this chapter) among 689 men with early-stage prostate cancer. Their findings did not lend support to the watchful waiting option. At eight-year follow-up, the researchers found a 50% reduction in cancer-specific mortality (7% versus 14%) and distant metastasis (13% versus 27%) in the patients with radical prostatectomy as compared to the watchful waiting group. Palliative RT was necessary twice as often in the watchful waiting group, who had a higher incidence of bony metastasis resulting in spinal cord compression requiring laminectomy. Additionally, local progression and increased morbidity, including urinary obstruction, was greater in the watchful waiting group compared with the radical prostatectomy group (61% versus 19%).

Although the study by Holmberg et al. (2002) is the largest RCT to date comparing watchful waiting with radical prostatectomy, it does not settle the question definitively. In this study, 75% of the patients had palpable disease, and only 10% of the cases were diagnosed following an elevated PSA level. These men, therefore, are not representative of most patients with prostate cancer seen in the United States, wherein the vast majority of men (75%) have nonpalpable disease and are only biopsied because of elevated PSA levels (Walsh, 2002). Although the Scandinavian trial provides evidence suggesting that treatment of early-stage prostate cancer reduces mortality, until results of RCTs based on contemporary diagnostic patterns (PSA screening) are available, a definite conclusion cannot be made.

Nursing Care

Nursing considerations for men who select watchful waiting basically consist of continuous assessment of QOL, including both the physiologic and psychosocial dimensions. Care can be guided by knowledge of which aspects of QOL are most affected. Although proponents of the watchful waiting option highlight the potential for better QOL based on the absence of treatment-related side effects, this has not been substantiated by research. Although the majority of literature published in the past 10 years has focused on QOL comparisons among men who underwent active treatment with RT, radical prostatectomy, or brachytherapy, some data are available regarding QOL in men choosing watchful waiting.

In a companion to the largest randomized clinical trial to date comparing watchful waiting with radical prostatectomy, Steineck et al. (2002) examined QOL in both groups. Although overall QOL, anxiety, depression, well-being, and bowel function were similar, erectile dysfunction and urinary leakage were more common among men who had radical prostatectomy. The higher rates of erectile dysfunction reported may have been related to the lack of use of nerve-sparing surgical techniques. Additionally, many of the men undergoing surgery were older than 65 and, thus, more likely to become impotent and incontinent, and 28% of the men received antiandrogen therapy during the follow-up period, known to cause erectile dysfunction. Steineck et al. also found higher rates of erectile and urinary dysfunction than would be expected in a control population, suggesting that local tumor progression, which occurred in 60% of the patients in the watchful waiting group, also can be a detriment to QOL.

Two nursing investigations of QOL involving men choosing watchful waiting are worth noting. Galbraith, Ramirez, and Pedro (2001) examined health-related QOL and prostate-specific symptoms among 185 men with localized prostate cancer who were enrolled in four treatment groups: radical prostatectomy, watchful waiting, RT, or a combination RT protocol. Although no significant differences in overall health-related QOL were observed, post hoc analyses revealed more gastrointestinal symptoms among patients receiving RT and more sexual dysfunction among the men receiving surgery. Men in the watchful waiting group had poorer general health overall. Wallace (2003) reported that the QOL of 21 men surveyed who had elected watchful waiting was negatively affected by anxiety, uncertainty, and a perception of danger. Cumulatively, the research indicates that if the goal of watchful waiting is to maintain QOL, nursing interventions to attenuate the negative aspects of uncertainty should be a high research priority.

In the nursing literature, Bailey and Mishel (1997) and O'Rourke (1997, 1999) reported that men and their spouses used a variety of cognitive schemas to reframe uncertainty. One such strategy was reframing treatment as negative, with a focus on the potential adverse side effects. Other strategies included upward social comparisons, with men choosing watchful waiting focusing on how much better off they were than others, as well as attempts to minimize the cancer threat by focusing on the small size of the tumor, their low PSA levels, and/or low Gleason scores (O'Rourke, 1997). The use of prayer, reflection, spending more time with family, and working harder physically also have been reported with varying levels of efficacy (Hedestig, Sandman, & Widmark, 2003).

Mishel et al. (2002) reported the effects of an uncertainty management intervention delivered by telephone to 239 men who had been treated for localized prostate cancer with either RT or radical prostatectomy. The individualized interventions were directed at the management of their disease and treatment side effects, and no watchful waiting patients were included in the sample. The treatment groups showed significant improvement in two uncertainty management strategies, problem solving and cognitive reframing. The impact of incontinence and impotence was modified for some men in the treatment group, with improvement of control over urine flow and satisfaction with sexual functioning. Testing a modified intervention targeted to men who choose watchful waiting would be beneficial.

Given that no studies specifically test nursing interventions for men electing watchful waiting, clinicians can be guided by the previous findings. Encouraging the use of spiritual resources, active problem solving, positive social comparisons, and reframing may be beneficial. Patients and partners need reassurance that although no active treatment is being employed, the patient is being closely followed. Additionally, the decision to watch and wait is not irrevocable, and treatment can be initiated if their desire or condition changes.

Hormonal Therapy

Hormonal therapy is based on the rationale that androgens regulate prostate tissue growth. Four major types of hormonal manipulation are used in the treatment of prostate cancer, each aimed at disruption of androgen stimulation: bilateral removal of the testicles (orchiectomy), the use of luteinizing hormone-releasing hormones (LHRH), antiandrogens, and estrogen therapy. Another approach is total androgen blockade via orchiectomy plus an antiandrogen or the combination of an LHRH agonist with the use of an antiandrogen. The efficacy of androgen deprivation as adjuvant therapy in improving overall survival and reducing clinical recurrence has been demonstrated in two well-designed RCTs (Ganfors, Modig, Damber, & Tomic, 1998; Schmidt, Gibbons, Murphy, & Bartolucci, 1996).

Androgen deprivation therapy traditionally has been reserved for metastatic disease. Although limited research exists on hormonal therapy in the adult male older than 70 years of age with advanced prostate cancer, this is a reasonable option given the relatively low toxicity profile (Raghavan & Skinner, 2004). Toxicities that may impact QOL include hot flashes, impotence, and the development of osteoporosis in more sedentary older adults.

Androgen deprivation therapy is increasingly being employed in nonmetastatic disease at the point of biochemical recurrence as measured by rising PSA levels. Neoadjuvant hormonal therapy also is being used to shrink tumor mass prior to surgery. Two RCTs have demonstrated significant reduction in cancer-positive surgical margins in men treated with neoadjuvant hormonal therapy prior to prostatectomy versus control group (prostatectomy alone) (33.8% versus 7.8% and 45.5% versus 23.6%, respectively) (Aus et al., 1998; Labrie et al., 1997). However, at three-year post-prostatectomy follow-up, Aus et al. noted that the addition of neoadjuvant hormonal therapy did not result in any significant difference in progression-free survival.

Nursing Care

Nursing care of men receiving hormonal therapy is aimed at patient education, psychosocial support, recognition of side effects, and effective symptom management. Higano (2003) presented an excellent review of the side effects of androgen deprivation and recommendations for monitoring and minimizing toxicity.

Anemia is associated with androgen deprivation therapy and can be severe in up to 13% of patients and correctable with recombinant human erythropoietin (Strum, McDermed, Scholz, Johnson, & Tisman, 1997). Anemia is associated with functional loss among older patients, and NCCN guidelines (2005b) recommend maintaining a hemoglobin level of 12 g/dl.

Loss of bone density also has been documented and requires quantitative monitoring. Other metabolic changes include hyperlipidemia, which may require statin therapy (Higano, 2003).

The management of hot flashes in men treated with androgen deprivation has not been well researched. Venlafaxine (Effexor®, Wyeth, Philadelphia, PA) has demonstrated promise in one pilot study (Quella et al., 1999). Although megestrol acetate was found to decrease hot flashes by 85% in one trial (Loprinzi et al., 1994), further investigation demonstrated that it is associated with elevated PSA levels even at low doses (Sartor & Eastham, 1999). The efficacy of clonidine for androgen deprivation–induced hot flashes is not validated in the research literature. Black cohosh (*Actaea racemosa*) is a popular alternative remedy for menopausal symptoms, although definitive evidence on efficacy is not available, and one systematic review concluded that the product seemed safe (Huntley & Ernst, 2003). It is unclear if research findings from menopausal women can be transferred to this population. Currently, phase II clinical trials are under way testing the efficacy and safety of gabapentin for men receiving hormonal therapy to alleviate distressing hot flashes (National Cancer Institute, 2004).

Chemotherapy

Treatment of advanced prostate cancer remains problematic. The mainstay of treatment is hormonal manipulation through the use of orchiectomy, LHRH, antiandrogens, and estrogen therapy. Recently, ketoconazole has been added to the armament mainly for its adrenal testosterone suppression properties (O'Rourke, 2003). RT is indicated for palliative purposes, especially in the case of bone metastasis and for emergent treatment of spinal cord compression. Treatment for hormone-refractory prostate cancer also remains controversial without clear evidence-based treatment guidelines. Few chemotherapy regimens are available for the treatment of prostate cancer. Mitoxantrone has been the most researched agent to date, although these studies have not addressed age-related issues (Raghavan & Skinner, 2004). Therapies that lower the body's level of testosterone are the mainstay of treatment of prostate cancer that has spread to other organs. Unfortunately, many patients become resistant to hormonal therapies after two to three years of treatment, and no other therapies have been available to stop disease progression at that point. Results of two multicenter, phase III clinical trials involving 1,776 men with advanced prostate cancer recently have been reported (Petrylak et al., 2004; Tannock et al., 2004). In the first RCT, docetaxel plus estramustine was compared to mitoxantrone plus prednisone in men with progressive androgen-independent prostate cancer (Petrylak et al.). The median age for each arm was 70 years of age, and the majority of participants had bone metastases. In the docetaxel plus estramustine group, the overall survival was 17.5 months compared to 15.6 months in the mitoxantrone plus prednisone group. Statistically significant higher rates of neutropenic fever, nausea and vomiting, and cardiovascular events were reported in patients receiving docetaxel plus estramustine. In the second RCT, docetaxel plus prednisone was compared to mitoxantrone plus prednisone in men with advanced, hormone-refractory prostate cancer (Tannock et al.). Patients were randomized to receive docetaxel every three weeks or weekly or mitoxantrone every three weeks. The median age for each arm was 68 years, and the majority of participants had bone metastases. The median survival was 16.5 months for the mitoxantrone group, 18.9 months for the every three-week docetaxel group, and 17.4 months for the weekly docetaxel group. Adverse events were higher in the docetaxel group, with a higher incidence of cardiac events documented in the mitoxantrone group. These clinical trial results are the first to suggest that chemotherapy can improve survival in advanced prostate cancer.

Nursing Care Issues

Urinary Incontinence

Dysfunction in either the storage of urine or in the process of emptying urine can result in incontinence. UI is particularly significant because it is associated with embarrassment and the potential for social isolation, diminished QOL, and depression. UI also may be associated with skin breakdown. The actual incidence of UI following prostatectomy or radiation treatments is difficult to determine in the literature, and reports vary from 2%–87% (Palmer, 2000). This wide range is related to measurement methods and differences in definitions of incontinence. Differences in UI rates have been reported to be associated with age, with men younger than age 65 reporting less UI at both 3 and 12 months after radical prostatectomy compared with similarly treated men older than 65 years. The difference could not be explained by pretreatment status. No association was found between tumor volume, tumor stage, or type of surgery (nerve sparing or non-nerve sparing) (Catalona, Carvalhal, Mager, & Smith, 1999).

Medical interventions for prostatectomy-induced incontinence include the use of anticholinergic or alpha-sympathomimetic medications combined with pelvic floor strengthening exercises (Kegels). Although conflicting reports exist in the literature, a meta-analysis of 10 clinical trials concluded that evidence was lacking to support the use of these exercises as a solo treatment for postprostatectomy incontinence (Hunter et al., 2004). Persistent incontinence may require surgical intervention for the placement of an artificial sphincter. Other management strategies include the use of pads, scheduled bladder emptying, sitting to void to facilitate complete emptying, and the use of penile clamps. Patients may benefit from restricting potential bladder irritants in their diets, including alcohol, carbonated beverages, caffeine, citrus products, tomato-based products, and artificial sweeteners (Robinson, 2000), although no research is available to support these recommendations. The use of stool softeners and increased dietary fiber intake may lessen bowel pressure on the bladder.

Radiation-induced cystitis (acute) occurs within six months of RT and is associated with dysuria, urinary frequency, urgency, nocturia, bladder spasms, and hematuria. This is caused by an acute inflammatory reaction and generally is self-limiting. Treatment is symptomatic and includes the use of anticholinergic medications such as oxybutynin and urinary analgesics.

Erectile Dysfunction

For both men and their partners, erectile dysfunction is a distressing treatment-related side effect. Additionally, erectile dysfunction is influenced by concomitant medical conditions and pharmacologic agents such as the use of beta-blockers, which is common among older men. As in the case of treatment-related UI, interpretation of incidence rates following prostate cancer treatment is hampered by the lack of standard definitions and reliance on self-report. Lim et al. (1995) reported significantly higher rates of impotence following radical prostatectomy compared with RT, whereas Walsh, Marsche, Ricker, and Burnett (2000) reported potency rates of 38%, 54%, 73%, and 86% at 3, 6, 12, and 18 months post–radical prostatectomy, respectively. In their retrospective review of 269 men who underwent radical prostatectomy and 142 men undergoing brachytherapy, Davis, Kuban, Lynch, and Schellhammer (2001) reported that prostatectomy was associated with significantly worse sexual function than brachytherapy.

Patient assessment and education are primary nursing responsibilities. Both patients and their partners need assurance that this condition can be effectively dealt with and does not signal the end of their sexual relationship. Interventions are both medical and psychological. The use of sildenafil (Viagra®, Pfizer, New York, NY) in men following RT for the treatment of prostate cancer has been supported by a single RCT (Incrocci, Hop, & Slob, 2003). Although no RCTs have been published testing the efficacy of sildenafil following radical prostatectomy, one retrospective study was located. Of the 174 patients followed, 104 (59.8%) had undergone a bilateral nerve-sparing procedure, 28 (16.1%) had undergone a unilateral nerve-sparing procedure, and 42 (24.1%) had undergone a non–nerve-sparing procedure. Four factors were significantly associated statistically with a successful outcome: the presence of at least one neurovascular bundle, preoperative potency, age 65 or younger, and an interval from radical prostatectomy to drug use of more than six months (Raina et al., 2004).

Nonpharmacologic strategies for the management of erectile dysfunction include the use of vasoconstrictive devices such as penile vacuum pumps and counseling. Other interventions include the use of intraurethral prostaglandin suppositories or the use of intercavernosal penile injections to attain erections, although none of these are associated with high levels of patient satisfaction. Erectile dysfunction may be treated surgically with penile implants.

Bone Metastasis

Bone involvement is the most frequent site of prostate cancer metastasis. As a result, patients may experience pain, weakness, and loss of function, with an increased risk of bone fractures and bone complications secondary to the bone lesions. Patients should be evaluated for palliative RT and provided with analgesic pain management. Zoledronic acid is an option to decrease the risk of bone complications. Saad et al. (2002) conducted a study involving the use of zoledronic acid in 770 men with metastatic prostate cancer to the bone. Results indicated that the use of zoledronic acid significantly reduced the incidence of bone fractures and complications in comparison to placebo. Zoledronic acid has limited side effects and, therefore, should be considered for all patients with bone metastasis to prevent morbidity associated with bone metastasis.

Areas for Future Research

No shortage of research exists regarding issues with prevention, screening, and treatment of prostate cancer. Some key areas for future study include longitudinal RCTs examining dietary and lifestyle changes and the prevention of prostate cancer. The need for well-designed RCTs examining the efficacy of PSA screening cannot be overstated. Definitive RCTs examining the efficacy of radical prostatectomy versus external beam RT, brachytherapy, and watchful waiting for early-stage prostate cancer is critical. Definitive RCTs examining treatment options and outcomes for the older adult male highlighting stage of disease, comorbidities, and performance status also are critical. Nurses are in a pivotal position to develop the symptom management knowledge base with respect to the treatment of hormone-induced hot flashes and the management of treatment-induced incontinence and impotence. Optimal management of erectile dysfunction and urinary dysfunction has not been established. Interventions aimed at assisting patients and their partners to deal effectively with these treatment-related side effects are nursing priorities. Further investigation of decision making and the management of uncertainty are warranted. The question remains unanswered as to how to best support men who are newly diagnosed with prostate cancer. Are they best served in support groups, or are men better served in a different setting? Should men who elect watchful waiting participate in support groups with men who have undergone or are undergoing active treatment for their prostate cancer? Nurses can and must participate in the design and execution of research that will develop a substantive knowledge base so that the practice truly is evidence based.

Case Study

A.H. is a 73-year-old African American male diagnosed with clinical stage T2 prostate cancer by biopsy following the finding of an elevated PSA on routine annual screening. His Gleason score was 5. In relating his history, he shared that he had never really discussed the implications of PSA testing with his primary care provider but had been monitoring his PSA levels over the past five years. His initial PSA was 3, and subsequently rose to 4 and then to 7 over a period of five years. The diagnosis came as a shock despite the fact that his older brother had died of prostate cancer some years earlier. His initial DRE was remarkable for a "knot," but following the biopsy, the urologist had told him that his transrectal ultrasound had been unremarkable.

Both the patient and his wife met with the urologist for consultation and discussion of treatment options. At that time they stated that the urologist advised them to "do nothing" because of his advanced age. The patient had no comorbid conditions and was quite concerned about the high mortality rates among African Americans. He had no other medical conditions and was taking no medication. At this point, the patient was certain that he wanted immediate surgery and believed that this was the optimal curative treatment.

Dissatisfied with being told that the best option was for him to "watch and wait," the patient opted to pursue a second opinion at a major medical center in New York City. He was hopeful that the doctors there would be "more up to date," and he anticipated being scheduled for surgery. To his dismay, the consulting urologist did not recommend surgery and referred him to a radiation oncologist who presented brachytherapy as an option. After extensive discussion and consultation with his wife and son, he decided to pursue brachytherapy, yet he stated, "I would still vote for surgery, but no one will do it. They think I am too old." He shared that this was upsetting because he was healthy and felt that he had many good years ahead of him. He boasted about his activity level and the fact that some family members had lived to be 100 years old, and he planned to as well. He stated, "I am not going to sit and watch and wait to die." One of the contradictions that was evident is that this patient viewed himself in terms of his physiologic age, whereas his physicians viewed him in terms of his chronologic age. One of the most upsetting things for him was that his second opinion did not recommend what he had hoped. He felt that having brachytherapy was not the optimal treatment but rather the one he would settle for.

Ultimately, the patient was treated with brachytherapy in New York. The implants were done as an inpatient procedure, and he was discharged the following day. Three months post-treatment, the patient's PSA level was 0.8 ng/ml. He was unable to sustain an erection adequate for intercourse but was interested in investigating sildenafil. He continued to have irritative urinary symptoms, characterized by urinary frequency and nocturia requiring pads. Subjectively, he believed this was slowly improving.

At one-year follow-up, his PSA level was 0.6. He and his wife looked back at their experience and assessed the decision-making process to be the most difficult aspect. They felt far more uncertain having gone for a second opinion. They now believed that brachytherapy was by far "the superior option" and discussed the risks of surgical mortality and incontinence and impotence as factors that make surgery undesirable. This marked a change from their initial opinion that surgery was the best option for cure. Currently, the patient continues to experience some nocturia and frequency but less urgency than in the past. He is no longer reliant on pads. He has used sildenafil with success and is satisfied with the outcome of his treatment.

Conclusion

Prostate cancer is a significant public health problem among older men within the United States. With upcoming population shifts, this will become even more of a concern. Controversy continues regarding screening and treatment, although presently, best evidence suggests that the net benefit from PSA screening has not been established. Additionally, at present, moderate evidence suggests that radical prostatectomy offers some gain over both radiotherapy and the watchful waiting approach. Nurses are in a pivotal position to be leaders in the area of public education regarding these issues. The clear disparity in incidence and mortality rates among African Americans suggests an area for immediate nursing research. Care of patients undergoing treatment for prostate cancer must be family focused and requires expertise in symptom management and psychosocial support. The lack of evidence-based nursing interventions to guide the care of men diagnosed with prostate cancer is an area for immediate action.

References

Abbou, C.C., Salomon, L., Hoznek, A., Antiphon, P., Cicco, A., Saint, F., et al. (2000). Laparoscopic radical prostatectomy: Preliminary results. *Urology, 55,* 630–634.

Adolfsson, K. (1995). Deferred treatment for clinically localized prostate cancer. *European Journal of Surgical Oncology, 21,* 333–340.

American Cancer Society. (2005). *Cancer facts and figures, 2005.* Atlanta, GA: Author.

American College of Surgeons Oncology Group. (2004). *A randomized trial of radical prostatectomy versus brachytherapy for patients with T1c or T2a N0 M0 prostate cancer.* Retrieved August 22, 2004, from http://www.acosog.org/studies/synopses/Z0070_Synopsis.pdf

Aus, G., Abrahamsson, P.A., Ahlgren, G., Hugosson, J., Lundberg, S., Schain, M., et al. (1998). Hormonal therapy before radical prostatectomy: A 3-year followup. *Journal of Urology, 159,* 2013–2016.

Bailey, D.E., & Mishel, M.H. (1997). Uncertainty management strategies for men electing watchful waiting as a treatment option for prostate cancer [Abstract 156]. *Oncology Nursing Forum, 24,* 326.

Beyer, D.C., & Brachman, D.G. (2000). Failure free survival following brachytherapy alone for prostate cancer: Comparison with external beam radiotherapy. *Radiotherapy and Oncology: Journal of the European Society for Therapeutic Radiology and Oncology, 57,* 263–267.

Bostwick, D.G. (2000). Prostatic intraepithelial neoplasia. *Current Urology Report, 1*(1), 65–70.

Brawley, O.W., & Barnes, S. (2001). The epidemiology of prostate cancer in the United States. *Seminars in Oncology Nursing, 17,* 72–77.

Catalona, W.J., Carvalhal, G.F., Mager, D.E., & Smith, D.S. (1999). Potency, continence and complication rates in 1,870 consecutive radical retropubic prostatectomies. *Journal of Urology, 162,* 433–438.

Chen, L., Stacewicz-Sapuntzakis, M., Duncan, C., Sharifi, R., Ghosh, L., van Breemen, R., et al. (2001). Oxidative DNA damage in prostate cancer patients consuming tomato sauce-based entrees as a whole food intervention. *Journal of the National Cancer Institute, 93,* 1872–1879.

Cooney, K.A., McCarthy, J.D., Lange, E., Huang, L., Meisfeldt, S., Montie, J.E., et al. (1997). Prostate cancer susceptibility locus on chromosome 1q: A confirmatory study. *Journal of the National Cancer Institute, 89,* 955–959.

Critz, F.A., Williams, W.H., Levinson, A.K., Benton, J.B., Holladay, C.T., & Schnell, F.J. (2000). Simultaneous irradiation for prostate cancer: Intermediate results with modern techniques. *Urology, 164,* 738–741.

Crook, J., Lukka, H., Klotz, L., Bestic, N., & Johnston, M. (2001). Systematic overview of the evidence for brachytherapy in clinically localized prostate cancer. *Canadian Medical Association Journal, 164,* 975–981.

D'Amico, A.V., Schnall, M., Whittington, R., Malkowicz, S.B., Schultz, D., Tomaszewski, J.E., et al. (1998). Endorectal coil magnetic resonance imaging identifies locally advanced prostate cancer in select patients with clinically localized disease. *Urology, 51,* 449–454.

D'Amico, A.V., Whittington, R., Malkowicz, S.B., Schultz, D., Blank, K., Broderick, G.A., et al. (1998). Biochemical outcome after radical prostatectomy, external beam radiation therapy, or interstitial radiation therapy for clinically localized prostate cancer. *JAMA, 280,* 969–974.

Davis, J.W., Kuban, D.A., Lynch, D.F., & Schellhammer, P.F. (2001). Quality of life after treatment for localized prostate cancer: Differences based on treatment modality. *Journal of Urology, 166,* 947–952.

Denton, A., Forbes, A., Andreyev, J., & Maher, E.J. (2002). Non-surgical interventions for late radiation proctitis in patients who have received radiotherapy to the pelvis. *Cochrane Database Systematic Reviews, 1,* CD003455.

Ekman, P. (1999). Genetic and environmental factors in prostate cancer genesis: Identifying high-risk cohorts. *European Urology, 35,* 362–369.

Frank, I., Granham, S., & Neighbors, W. (1991). Urologic and male genital cancers. In A. Holleb, D. Fink, & G. Murphy (Eds.), *American Cancer Society textbook of clinical oncology* (pp. 271–289). Atlanta, GA: American Cancer Society.

Galbraith, M.E., Ramirez, J.M., & Pedro, L.W. (2001). Quality of life, health outcomes, and identity for patients with prostate cancer in five different treatment groups. *Oncology Nursing Forum, 28,* 55–60.

Ganfors, T., Modig, H., Damber, J.E., & Tomic, R. (1998). Combined orchiectomy and external radiotherapy versus radiotherapy alone for non-metastatic prostate cancer with or without pelvic node involvement: A prospective randomized study. *Journal of Urology, 159,* 2030–2034.

Gann, P.H., Ma, J., Giovannuccci, E., Willett, W., Sacks, F.M., Hennekens, C.H., et al. (1999). Lower prostate risk in men with elevated plasma lycopene levels: Results of a prospective analysis. *Cancer Research, 59,* 1225–1230.

Giovannucci, E., Rimm, E.B., Colditz, G.A., Stampfer, M.J., Ascherrio, A., Chute, C.C., et al. (1993). A prospective study of dietary fat and risk of prostate cancer. *Journal of the National Cancer Institute, 85,* 1571–1579.

Gleason, D., & Mellinger, G. (1974). Prediction of prognosis for prostatic adenocarcinoma by combined histological grading and clinical staging. *Journal of Urology, 11,* 58–64.

Goodman, C.M., Busttil, A., & Chisholm, G.D. (1998). Age, size, and grade of tumor predict prognosis in incidentally diagnosed carcinoma of the prostate. *British Journal of Urology, 62,* 576–580.

Graversen, P.H., Nielsen, K.T., Gasser, T.C., Corle, D.K., & Madsen, P.O. (1990). Radical prostatectomy versus expectant treatment in stages I and II prostate cancer. A fifteen-year follow-up. *Urology, 36,* 493–498.

Greene, F.L., Page, D.L., Flemming, I.D., Fritz, A.G., Balch, C.M., Haller, D.G., et al. (2002). *AJCC cancer staging manual* (6th ed.). New York: Springer-Verlag.

Gross, C., Stamey, T., Hancock, S., & Feldman, D. (1998). Treatment of early recurrent prostate cancer with 1,25 dihydroxyvitamin D3 (calcitriol). *Journal of Urology, 159,* 2035–2039.

Guillonneau, B., el-Fettouh, H., Baumert, H., Cathelineau, X., Doublet, J.D., Fromont, G., et al. (2003). Laparoscopic radical prostatectomy: Oncological evaluation after 1,000 cases at Montsouris Institute. *Journal of Urology, 169,* 1261–1266.

Harlan, L.C., Potosky, A., Gilliland, F.D., Hoffman, R., Albertsen, P.C., Hamilton, A.S., et al. (2001). Factors associated with initial therapy for clinically localized prostate cancer: Prostate cancer outcomes study. *Journal of the National Cancer Institute, 93,* 1864–1871.

Hedestig, O., Sandman, P.O., & Widmark, A. (2003). Living with untreated localized prostate cancer: A qualitative analysis of patient narratives. *Cancer Nursing, 26,* 55–60.

Higano, C.S. (2003). Side effects of androgen deprivation therapy: Monitoring and minimizing toxicity. *Urology, 61*(2 Suppl. 1), 32–38.

Holmberg, L., Bill-Axelsoon, A., Helgessen, F., Sato, J.O., Folmerz, P., Haggman, M., et al. (2002). A randomized trial comparing radical prostatectomy with watchful waiting in early prostate cancer. *New England Journal of Medicine, 347,* 781–796.

Hunter, K.F., Moore, K.N., Cody, D.J., & Glazener, C.M. (2004). Conservative management of post prostatectomy incontinence. *Cochrane Database Systematic Reviews, 2,* CD001843.

Huntley, A., & Ernst, E. (2003). A systematic review of the safety of black cohosh. *Menopause, 10,* 58–64.

Incrocci, L., Hop, W.C., & Slob, A.K. (2003). Efficacy of sildenafil in an open-label study as a continuation of a double-blind study in the treatment of erectile dysfunction after radiotherapy for prostate cancer. *Urology, 62,* 116–120.

Iversen, P., Madsen, P.O., & Corle, D.K. (1995). Radical prostatectomy versus expectant treatment for early carcinoma of the prostate. Twenty-three year follow-up of a prospective randomized study. *Scandinavian Journal of Urology and Nephrology, 172*(Suppl.), 65–72.

Johansson, J.E., Holmberg, L., Johansson, S., Bergstrom, R., & Adami, H.O. (1997). Fifteen-year survival in prostate cancer: Results and identification of high-risk patient population. *JAMA, 277,* 467–471.

Kanumaru, H., Arai, Y., Moroi, S., Yoshida, H., Yoshimura, K., & Okada, K. (1998). Long term results of definitive treatment in elderly patients with localized prostate cancer. *International Journal of Urology, 5,* 546–549.

King, C.R., McNeal, J.E., Gil, I.H., & Presti, J.C., Jr. (2004). Extended prostate biopsy scheme improves reliability of Gleason grading: Implications for radiotherapy patients. *International Journal of Radiation Oncology, Biology, Physics, 59,* 386–391.

Klein, E.A., Grass, J.A., Calabrese, D.A., Kay, R.A., Sargeant, W., & O'Hara, J.F. (1996). Maintaining quality of care and patient satisfaction with radical prostatectomy in the era of cost containment. *Urology, 48,* 269–276.

Kolonel, L., Nomura, A., & Cooney, R. (1999). Dietary fat and prostate cancer: Current status. *Journal of the National Cancer Institute, 91,* 414–428.

Kuban, D.A., Thames, H.D., Levy, L.B., Horowitz, E.M., Kupelian, P.A., Martinez, A.A., et al. (2003). Long-term multi-institutional analysis of stage T1-T2 prostate cancer treated with radiotherapy in the PSA era. *International Journal of Radiation Oncology, Biology, Physics, 57,* 915–928.

Kupelian, P., Katcher, J., Levin, H., Zippe, C., Suh, J., Macklis, R., et al. (1997). External beam radiotherapy versus radical prostatectomy for clinical stage T1-2 prostate cancer: Therapeutic implications of stratification by pretreatment PSA levels and biopsy Gleason scores. *Cancer Journal From Scientific American, 3,* 78–87.

Kushi, L., & Giovannucci, E. (2002). Dietary fat and cancer. *American Journal of Medicine, 113*(Suppl.), 63S–70S.

Labrie, F., Candas, B., Dupont, A., Cusan, L., Gomez, J.L., Suburu, R.R., et al. (1999). Screening decreases prostate cancer death: First analysis of the 1988 Quebec prospective randomized controlled trial. *Prostate, 38*(2), 83–91.

Labrie, F., Cusan, L., Gomez, J.L., Diamond, P., Suburu, R., Lemay, M., et al. (1997). Neoadjuvant hormonal therapy: The Canadian experience. *Urology, 49*(Suppl. 3A), 56–64.

Lim, A.J., Brandon, A.H., Fiedler, J., Brickman, A.L., Boyer, C.I., Raub, W.A., et al. (1995). Quality of life: Radical prostatectomy versus radiation therapy for prostate cancer. *Journal of Urology, 154,* 1420–1425.

Loprinzi, C.L., Michalak, J.C., Quella, S.K., O'Fallon, J.R., Hatfield, A.K., Nelimark, R.A., et al. (1994). Megestrol acetate for the prevention of hot flashes. *New England Journal of Medicine, 332,* 347–352.

Marschke, P.S. (2001). The role of surgery in the treatment of prostate cancer. *Seminars in Oncology Nursing, 17,* 85–89.

Martini, F.H., Timmons, M.J., & McKinley, M.P. (Eds.). (2000). *Human anatomy* (3rd ed.). Upper Saddle River, NJ: Prentice Hall.

Mettlin, C., Littrup, P.J., Kane, R.A., Murphy, G.P., Lee, F., Chesley, A., et al. (1994). Relative sensitivity and specificity of serum prostate specific antigen (PSA) level compared with age-referenced PSA, PSA density, and PSA change. Data from the American Cancer Society National Prostate Cancer Detection Project. *Cancer, 74,* 1615–1620.

Mishel, M.H., Belyea, M., Germino, B.B., Stewart, J.L., Bailey, D.E., Robertson, C., et al. (2002). Helping patients with localized prostate carcinoma manage uncertainty and treatment side effects. *Cancer, 94,* 1854–1866.

Mock, V., Dow, K.H., Meares, C.J., Grimm, P.M., Dienemann, J.A., Haisfield-Wolfe, M.E., et al. (1997). Effects of exercise on fatigue, physical functioning, and emotional distress during radiation therapy for breast cancer. *Oncology Nursing Forum, 24,* 991–1000.

National Cancer Institute. (2004). *Gabapentin in treating hot flashes in patients with prostate cancer.* Retrieved September 5, 2004, from http://www.nci.nih.gov/search/ViewClinicalTrials. aspx?cdrid=69107&version=patient&protocolsearchid=1125631

National Comprehensive Cancer Network. (2005a). *Clinical practice guidelines in oncology: Prostate cancer early detection.* Retrieved September 21, 2005, from http://www.nccn.org/professionals/ physician_gls/PDF/prostate_detection.pdf

National Comprehensive Cancer Network. (2005b). *Clinical practice guidelines in oncology: Prostate cancer.* Retrieved September 21, 2005, from http://www.nccn.org/professionals/physician_gls/ PDF/prostate.pdf

Nelson, W.G., Carter, H.B., DeWeese, T.L., Bajaj, G., Thompson, T.L., & Eisenberger, M.A. (2004). Prostate cancer. In M.D. Abeloff, J.O. Armitage, J.E. Niederhuber, M.B. Kastan, & W.G. McKenna (Eds.), *Clinical oncology* (3rd ed., pp. 2085–2148). Philadelphia: Churchill Livingstone.

O'Rourke, M.E. (1997). *Prostate cancer treatment selection: The family decision process.* Doctoral dissertation, University of North Carolina, Chapel Hill.

O'Rourke, M.E. (1999). Narrowing the options: The process of deciding on prostate cancer treatment. *Cancer Investigation, 17,* 349–359.

O'Rourke, M.E. (2001). Decision making and prostate cancer treatment selection: A review of the issues. *Seminars in Oncology Nursing, 17,* 108–117.

O'Rourke, M.E. (2003). Ketoconazole in treatment of prostate cancer. *Clinical Journal of Oncology Nursing, 7,* 235–236.

Palmer, M.H. (2000). Postprostatectomy incontinence: The magnitude of the problem. *Journal of Wound, Ostomy, and Continence Nursing, 27,* 129–137.

Perron, L., Moore, L., Bairati, I., Bernard, P.M., & Meyer, F. (2002). PSA screening and prostate cancer mortality. *Canadian Medical Association Journal, 166,* 586–591.

Petrylak, D.P., Tangen, C.M., Hussain, M.H.A., Lara, P.N., Jones, J.A., & Taplin, M. (2004). Docetaxel and estramustine compared with mitoxantrone and prednisone for advanced refractory prostate cancer. *New England Journal of Medicine, 351,* 1513–1520.

Polek, T.C., & Weigel, N.L. (2002). Vitamin D and prostate cancer. *Journal of Andrology, 23,* 9–17.

Presti, J.C., Jr., Chang, J.J., Bhargava, V., & Shinohara, K. (2000). The optimal systematic prostate biopsy scheme should include 8 rather than 6 biopsies: Results of a prospective clinical trial. *Journal of Urology, 163,* 163–166.

Quella, S.K., Loprinzi, C.L., Sloan, J., Novotny, P., Perez, E.A., Burch, P.A., et al. (1999). Pilot evaluation of venlafaxine for the treatment of hot flashes in men undergoing androgen ablation therapy for prostate cancer. *Journal of Urology, 162,* 98–102.

Raghavan, D., & Skinner, E. (2004). Genitourinary cancer in the elderly. *Seminars in Oncology, 31,* 249–263.

Raina, R., Lakin, M.M., Agarwal, A., Mascha, E., Montague, D.K., Klein, E., et al. (2004). Efficacy and factors associated with successful outcome of sildenafil citrate use for erectile dysfunction after radical prostatectomy. *Urology, 63,* 960–966.

Rassweiler, J., Seemann, O., Schulze, M., Teber, D., Hatzinger, M., & Fede, T. (2003). Laparoscopic versus open radical prostatectomy: A comparative study at a single institution. *Journal of Urology, 169,* 1689–1693.

Robinson, J.P. (2000). Managing urinary incontinence following radical prostatectomy. *Journal of Wound, Ostomy, and Continence Nursing, 27,* 138–145.

Saad, F., Gleason, D.M., Murray, R., Tchekmedyian, S., Venner, P., Lacombe, L., et al. (2002). A randomized placebo-controlled trial of zoledronic acid in patients with hormone refractory metastatic prostate carcinoma. *Journal of the National Cancer Institute, 9,* 1458–1468.

Sartor, O., & Eastham, J.A. (1999). Progressive prostate cancer associated with use of megestrol acetate administered for control of hot flashes. *Southern Medical Journal, 92,* 415–416.

Scardino, P. (2003). The prevention of prostate cancer—The dilemma continues. *New England Journal of Medicine, 349,* 297–299.

Schmidt, J.D., Gibbons, R.P., Murphy, G.P., & Bartolucci, A. (1996). Evaluation of adjuvant estramustine phosphate, cyclophosphamide, and observation only for node positive patients following radical prostatectomy and definitive radiation. *Prostate, 28,* 51–57.

Scott, R., Mutchnik, D.L., Laskowski, T.Z., & Schmalhorst, W.R. (1969). Carcinoma of the prostate in elderly men: Incidence, growth characteristics and clinical significance. *Journal of Urology, 101,* 602–607.

Smith, R.A., Cokkinides, V., & Eyre, H.J. (2003). American Cancer Society guidelines for the early detection of cancer, 2003. *CA: A Cancer Journal for Clinicians, 53,* 27–43.

Stanford, J.L., Stephenson, R.A., Coyle, L.M., Cerhan, J., Correa, R., Eley, J.W., et al. (2004). *Prostate cancer trends, 1973–1995.* SEER Program, National Cancer Institute. Retrieved August 1, 2004, from http://seer.cancer.gov/publications/prostate/

Steinberg, G.D., Bales, G.T., & Brendler, C.B. (1998). An analysis of watchful waiting for clinically localized prostate cancer. *Journal of Urology, 159,* 1431–1436.

Steineck, G., Helgesen, F., Adolfsson, J., Dickman, P.W., Johansson, J.E., Norlen, B.J., et al. (2002). Quality of life after radical prostatectomy or watchful waiting. *New England Journal of Medicine, 347,* 790–796.

Stoller, M.L., & Carroll, R.R. (2003). Urology. In I.M. Tierney, S.J. McPhee, & M.A. Papdakis (Eds.), *Current medical diagnosis and treatment* (42nd ed., pp. 903–945). New York: Appleton and Lange.

Strum, S.B., McDermed, J.E., Scholz, M.C., Johnson, H., & Tisman, G. (1997). Anaemia associated with androgen deprivation in patients with prostate cancer receiving combined hormone blockade. *British Journal of Urology, 79,* 933–941.

Tannock, I.F., de Wit, R., Berry, W.R., Horti, J., Pluzanska, A., Chi, K.N., et al. (2004). Docetaxel plus prednisone or mitoxantrone plus prednisone for advanced prostate cancer. *New England Journal of Medicine, 351,* 1502–1512.

Thompson, I.M., Pauler, D.K., Goodman, P.J., Tangem, C.M., Lucia, M.S., Parnes, H.L., et al. (2004). Prevalence of prostate cancer among men with a prostate-specific antigen level ≤ 4 ng per milliliter. *New England Journal of Medicine, 350,* 2239–2246.

U.S. Preventive Services Task Force. (2002). Screening for prostate cancer: Recommendation and rationale. *Annals of Internal Medicine, 137,* 915–916.

Wallace, M. (2003). Uncertainty and quality of life of older men who undergo watchful waiting for prostate cancer. *Oncology Nursing Forum, 30,* 303–309.

Walsh, P.C. (2002). Surgery and the reduction of mortality from prostate cancer [Editorial]. *New England Journal of Medicine, 347,* 839–840.

Walsh, P.C., & Donker, P.J. (1982). Impotence following radial prostatectomy: Insight into etiology and prevention. *Journal of Urology, 152,* 492–497.

Walsh, P.C., Marsche, P., Ricker, D., & Burnett, A.L. (2000). Patient-reported urinary continence and sexual function after anatomic radical prostatectomy. *Urology, 55,* 58–61.

Windsor, P.M., Nicol, K.F., & Potter, J. (2004). A randomized, controlled trial of aerobic exercise for treatment-related fatigue in men receiving radical external beam radiotherapy for localized prostate carcinoma. *Cancer, 101,* 550–557.

Zlotta, A.R., & Schulman, C.C. (1998). Etiology and diagnosis of prostate cancer: What's new? A review. *European Urology, 33,* 351–358.

CHAPTER 12

The Older Adult With Non-Hodgkin Lymphoma

Cheryl D. Kosits, RN, MSN, OCN®, CCRC

Introduction

Non-Hodgkin lymphoma (NHL) is a malignancy of the B and T lymphocytes and is the sixth most common newly diagnosed cancer in the United States. An estimated 56,390 new cases of NHL, including 29,070 in men and 27,320 in women, will be diagnosed in 2005, and 19,200 people with NHL will die (Jemal et al., 2005). NHL is one of the few malignancies that has increased in incidence between 1975 and 2000. The relative five-year survival rate between 1974 and 2000 also has significantly increased from 47% to 59% (Groves, Linet, Travis, & Devesa, 2000; Jemal et al.). Between the ages of 60–79 years, the probability of developing NHL is 1 in 76 for men and 1 in 100 for women. In comparison, between the ages of 40–59 years, the probability of developing NHL for men is 1 in 217 and for women is 1 in 328 (Jemal et al.). Between 1996 and 2000, 54% of NHL cases were diagnosed in patients older than 65 years, with 30% being in those older than 75 years of age. The median age of people with NHL has risen in the last two decades from those in their late 50s to their early 60s (Groves et al.). The median age at diagnosis for NHL is 64 years for men and 69 years for women. Survival rate of NHL is lower in people older than 65 years (Ries, Reichman, Lewis, Hankey, & Edwards, 2003). The reasons for the increased incidence of NHL are largely unknown (Bilodeau & Fessele, 1998; Dalla-Favera & Gaidano, 2001; Groves et al.). People age 65 and older represented 11.4% of the total population in 1980, and this number is anticipated to rise to 20% by 2030 (Yancik, 1997). In addition, age shifts within the 65 and older population have resulted in a greater number of people older than 75 years of age; by 2030, this age group is estimated to account for just fewer than 50% of the total group older than age 65. This chapter will present the etiology, pathophysiology, clinical manifestations, diagnosis, and treatment of NHL, highlighting the special needs and care of the older adult.

Risk Factors

As the size of America's older population increases, so increases the risk of lymphoma; however, this only can account for a small increase in the NHL incidence (Armitage, Mauch, Harris, & Bierman, 2001; Dalla-Favera & Gaidano, 2001). Groves et al. (2000) looked at the patterns and trends of NHL subtypes in a large population–based study and found differing demographic patterns and incidence trends.

- Therapeutic immunosuppression for transplant-associated NHL accounted for only a very small fraction.
- NHL-related autoimmune diseases are unlikely to contribute to the rising trends in NHL because the incidence has not increased over time.
- The rarity of congenital immunodeficiency disorders also does not add to the increasing incidence of NHL.
- Patients with AIDS secondary to HIV infection are at a 59- to104-fold risk of NHL; however, AIDS accounts for a very small fraction of NHL.
- The relationship between hepatitis C virus and NHL is mixed and not well established.
- In the United States, the rarity of human T-lymphotropic virus type I, the declining prevalence of *Helicobacter pylori,* and the prevalence of the Epstein-Barr virus suggest that these agents are unlikely to explain the increases in NHL.
- Blood transfusions, which may transmit infectious agents and other immune-modulating antigenic exposures, have not been associated with NHL.
- The small number of people with NHL that has been exposed to pesticides, crops, and livestock only accounts for a small fraction of the NHL increase in the general population.
- Relatively few studies have addressed lifestyle risk factors (e.g., diet, smoking) for NHL and have not firmly established the increasing trends.
- Genetic lesions characterizing certain NHL subtypes and familial occurrence do not account for the rising incidence.

Despite previous reports of disorders of the immune system, infectious agents, blood transfusions, agricultural and pesticide exposures, lifestyle factors, and genetic factors being linked to the increased incidence of NHL, Groves et al. (2000) found the numbers to be small, accounting for only a fraction of the cases of this malignancy and, therefore, did not account for or explain the rising incidence of NHL. More research is needed to determine other possible causes.

Pathophysiology

The knowledge about NHL has increased over the past 10 years. This is due, in part, to an evolving accurate classification of NHL that has enabled a better understanding of the clinical aspects of lymphoma (Armitage et al., 2001; Dalla-Favera & Gaidano, 2001; Kosits & Callaghan, 2000; Treseler, n.d.). NHL may be classified on the basis of morphology, natural history, and immunophenotypic and molecular characteristics. Currently, three classification systems are used: the World Health Organization system, the Revised European-American Lymphoma system, and the International Working Formulation (IWF) system (Dalla-Favera & Gaidano; National Comprehensive Cancer Network [NCCN], 2005). The IWF system is the most common lymphoma classification used in the United States for clinical purposes. It organizes NHL types into three major categories that include low grade, intermediate grade, and high grade. Table 12-1 presents a summary of the classification systems and categories. Armitage and Weisenburger (1998) presented the work of the International Lymphoma Classification Project and found 90% of the cases of NHL in the United States are from subtypes, as detailed in Table 12-2. B-cell lineage subtypes comprise 80%–90% of NHL, and the remaining 10%–20% are from the T-cell lineage (Treseler; Walker & Dang, 2004).

Table 12-1. Summary of Classification Systems for Selected Entities and Variant Forms of Non-Hodgkin Lymphoma

Working Formulation	REAL/WHO B-Cell Neoplasms	REAL/WHO T-Cell Neoplasms
Low grade		
A. Small lymphocytic	*Indolent* B-cell chronic lymphocytic leukemia	T-cell chronic lymphocytic leukemia
B. Follicular, predominantly small cleaved cell	Mantle zone; marginal zone; follicular center, follicular grade 1	–
C. Follicular, mixed small cleaved and large cell	Follicular center; follicular, grade II; marginal zone/mucosa-associated lymphoid tissue (MALT)	–
Intermediate grade		
D. Follicular, large cell	*Aggressive* Follicular center; follicular, grade III	–
E. Diffuse, small cleaved cell	Mantle cell; follicle center, diffused small cell; marginal zone/MALT	Peripheral T cell, unspecified; mycosis fungoides/Sezary syndrome; adult T-cell lymphoma/leukemia (HTLV-1 associated)
F. Diffuse, mixed small and large cell	Marginal zone/MALT; mantle cell	Peripheral T cell, unspecified; angiocentric; angioimmunoblastic
G. Diffuse, large cell	*Aggressive* Diffuse large B cell	Peripheral T cell, unspecified
High grade		
H. Large cell immunoblastic	Diffuse large B cell	Peripheral T cell, unspecified; intestinal T cell
I. Lymphoblastic	B-precursor lymphoblastic	Precursor T-lymphoblastic
J. Small noncleaved cell Burkitt, non-Burkitt	Burkitt; high-grade B cell, Burkitt-like	

REAL—Revised European-American Lymphoma (system); WHO—World Health Organization

Note. Based on information from Armitage et al., 2001; Bilodeau & Fessele, 1998; Frizzera, 1995; Kosits & Callaghan, 2000; Treseler, n.d.

Table 12-2. Incidence by Type of Cases of Non-Hodgkin Lymphoma in the United States

Type	Incidence
Diffuse large B cell	31%
Follicular lymphoma	22%
Small lymphocytic lymphoma	6%
Mantle cell lymphoma	6%
Peripheral T-cell lymphoma	6%
Marginal zone B-cell lymphoma, MALT (mucosa-associated lymphoid tissue) type	5%
Remaining subtypes	< 2%

Note. Based on information from Armitage & Weisenburger, 1998.

In addition to the classification of NHL as a predictor of clinical outcome, the International Non-Hodgkin's Lymphoma Prognostic Factors Project (1993) developed a model for predicting outcome in patients with aggressive NHL on the basis of the person's clinical characteristics. The International Prognostic Index (IPI) is used to stratify people older than 60 years of age with aggressive NHL into better or worse prognostic groups (see Table 12-3). The IPI also is used to individualize treatment and aids in the design and interpretation of clinical trials (Armitage et al., 2001; International Non-Hodgkin's Lymphoma Prognostic Factors Project; Shipp, 1994).

Clinical Presentation

People with NHL generally present with localized or generalized lymphadenopathy, which they may report as having waxed and waned over a period of several months. Lymphomatous nodes tend to be firm or hard and rubbery, sometimes matted to one another or fixed on examination. Early involvement of the oropharyngeal lymphoid tissue or infiltration of the bone marrow is common. With gastrointestinal involvement, an abdominal mass may be detected or the person may describe vague symptoms of back pain or abdominal discomfort. Other nonspecific generalized symptoms, which can include fatigue, often are reported at routine physicals. Approximately 20%–30% of people with NHL also present with systemic "B" symptoms, which include night sweats, fever, chills, fatigue, itching, and/or weight loss, and approximately one-third will have splenomegaly or hepatomegaly. Often, people with NHL report shortness of breath or cough and/or difficulty swallowing (Armitage et al., 2001; Bilodeau & Fessele, 1998).

Staging

Many of the assessments for the diagnosis and therapy of the various NHL types are similar. A careful patient and family history and physical examination, which includes performance status, duration of symptoms, pace of progression, presence of specific

Table 12-3. International Prognostic Index Risk Factors

Factor	Adverse Risk	Score
Age of patient	Greater than 60 years	
Lactic dehydrogenase (LDH) blood levels	Greater than 1 x normal	
Performance status	2–4	
Stage of lymphoma	III or IV	
The number of extranodal sites	Greater than 1	

Total Score	Risk Group	Overall Survival
0–1	Low	73%
2	Low intermediate	51%
3	High intermediate	43%
4–5	High	26%

Note. Based on information from the International Non-Hodgkin's Lymphoma Prognostic Factors Project, 1993; Shipp, 1994.

B symptoms, history of comorbidities, examination of lymph node bearing areas, and evaluation of areas to rule out hepatomegaly, splenomegaly, pleural effusion, cutaneous lesions, testicular mass, and thyroid mass, are required to determine the extent of the disease, determine further studies, and plan treatment. Laboratory studies should include complete blood count and comprehensive chemistry studies, including lactic dehydrogenase (LDH), to aid in determining the prognosis and identify abnormalities in other organ systems that might complicate treatment (Armitage et al., 2001; Dalla-Favera & Gaidano, 2001; NCCN, 2005).

For all cases, the most important first step is to make an accurate pathologic diagnosis. An incisional or excisional lymph node biopsy is recommended to establish the diagnosis of NHL (NCCN, 2005). The addition of immunophenotyping by immunohistochemistry, immunofluorescence, and flow cytometry, cytogenetics, and molecular analysis can be helpful and often is necessary for correct subclassification. Approximately 80%–90% of lymphomas are B-cell lymphomas; the remainder are T cell and other subtypes (Armitage et al., 2001; Leonard, 2004).

Once the pathologic diagnosis and cell type has been completed, a healthcare professional should adequately determine the extent of cancer. Unilateral or bilateral bone marrow biopsies and/or aspirate may be required to establish disseminated disease. Positive bone marrow findings vary among different subtypes of NHL. In patients with the blastic variant, aggressive, testicular, and/or HIV positive, lumbar puncture is performed to evaluate the spinal fluid for involvement. In the highly aggressive lymphomas, HIV serology should be part of the diagnostic workup. The use of computed tomography of the chest, abdomen, and pelvis has been applied to the initial staging of NHL, and they represent today's standard diagnostic examinations, replacing lymphangiography for the evaluation of retroperitoneal lymphadenopathy (Armitage et al., 2001; Bilodeau & Fessele, 1998; NCCN, 2005). Magnetic resonance imaging may be useful in identifying bone, bone marrow, and central nervous system involvement, but further studies are needed to confirm its routine use. Gallium scans and positron emission tomographic scan may be helpful in identifying occult sites of disease and have a role in diffuse large B-cell lymphomas, but they remain to be verified in larger prospective studies for other lymphomas (Armitage et al., 2001; Friedberg & Chengazi, 2003; Kostakoglu, Leonard, Coleman, & Goldsmith, 2004; NCCN). The Ann Arbor staging system initially was developed in 1971 to describe the extent of Hodgkin disease in patients (Bilodeau & Fessele). The Ann Arbor system for NHL (see Table 12-4) and the IPI provide a basis for treatment planning (Armitage et al., 2001). The Ann Arbor system has limited utility in determining prognosis (Westin & Longo, 2004), and controversy exists regarding the role of the IPI in predicting survival for the older adult (Cuttner, Wallenstein, & Troy, 2002; Maartense et al., 2002).

Table 12-4. Ann Arbor Staging

Stage	Description
I	Involvement of single lymph node region
I_E	Localized involvement of a single extralymphatic organ or site in the absence of any lymph node involvement
II	Involvement of two or more lymph node regions on the same side of the diaphragm
II_E	Localized involvement of a single extralymphatic organ or site in association with regional lymph node involvement with or without involvement of other lymph node regions on the same side of the diaphragm involvement
III	Involvement of lymph node regions on both sides of the diaphragm
III_E	Also may be accompanied by extralymphatic extension in association with adjacent lymph node involvement
III_S	Or by involvement of the spleen
IV	Diffuse or disseminated involvement of one or more extralymphatic organs, with or without associated lymph node involvement; or isolated extralymphatic organ involvement in the absence of adjacent regional lymph node involvement, but in conjunction with disease in distant site(s). Any involvement of the liver or bone marrow or nodular involvement of the lung(s). By designating the specific site, the location of stage IV disease is identified further.

Note. Based on information from the National Cancer Institute, 2004.

Factors That Influence Treatment in the Older Person With Non-Hodgkin Lymphoma

Chronologic Versus Physiologic Age

Clinical decisions for older people often are complicated by comorbid conditions, diminished organ function, altered drug metabolism, irregular drug clearance rates, symptom confusion, and performance and functional status, which correlate poorly with chronologic age (Balducci & Extermann, 1997; Bertini, Boccomini, & Calvi, 2001; Kagan, 2004; Reuben, 1997; Yancik et al., 2001). Chronologic versus physiologic age is an important issue in clinical decision making and has been difficult to quantify in clinical research. Chronologic age influences study design, sample selection, and findings (Kagan).

Some of the clinical factors that have been used to predict curability of NHL are the prognostic effect of clinical variables such as age, stage, performance status, serum LDH, and specific sites of involvement. Sonneveld et al. (1995) found that unfavorable prognostic factors at diagnosis of advanced NHL include high serum LDH level, bulky mass, and low performance status, but not age.

Kouroukis, Browman, Esmail, and Meyer (2002), in their systematic review of 12 randomized treatment trials, found that older patients were defined as those older than 60 years of age. They concluded that "age is a continuous prognostic variable because patients older than 70 years of age have inferior outcomes compared with patients 60 to 70 years of age" (p. 149). They further suggested that treatment in the older adult should be based on the "balance of treatment benefits versus toxicity" (p. 150). Clinical research studies, however, often do not address the benefits versus toxicity or the care needs of the older person living with NHL. Balducci and Yates (2000) noted, in their work on the management of older patients with cancer, that much of the work on age as a contraindication to chemotherapy cannot be generalized because these studies did not generally include people older than 80 years, adults older than 80 were highly selected, and many of the treatment regimens had lower dose intensity than in current use. However, they also noted that many lymphoma studies have been specifically directed to an older patient population and have used treatment regimens of moderate and consistent dose intensity.

In an early review of two randomized trials of 307 patients by Dixon et al. (1986), the effect of age on therapeutic outcome was addressed in advanced diffuse lymphoma. Survival rates declined significantly with age; however, no association was found between age and frequency of toxicity, and the inferiority of outcomes for older adults may have resulted, in part, from less-intensive chemotherapy. They also recommended that further treatment trials enroll all eligible patients irrespective of age and focus on severity of treatment-related toxicities and causes of all deaths. Other studies (Armitage et al., 2001; Coiffier et al., 2002; Dale, 2003; Kouroukis et al., 2002; Meyer et al., 1995; Sonneveld et al., 1995; Zinzani et al., 1997, 1999) that examined treatment in the older adult with NHL supported these findings. Gomez et al. (1998) evaluated the influence of pretreatment variables on treatment-related death in a retrospective study of 267 older adults with aggressive NHL and concluded that for older people treated with doxorubicin-based chemotherapy, their risk for treatment-related death was associated with poor performance status rather than with increased chronologic age.

In a number of studies reviewed by Shipp (1994), healthcare professionals had a tendency to treat older adults with lower doses of chemotherapy to reduce treatment-related toxicity, and yet older patients benefited from full-dose therapy. Findings suggested that although people older than 60 years of age treated for aggressive NHL had complete response rates that were similar or only slightly lower than those of patients younger than 60 years, older adults were much less likely to maintain their complete remissions. Shipp further suggested that people older than 60 years may have had less durable complete responses because they received less-intensive treatment, and with full support to reduce the toxicity of chemotherapy with hematopoietic growth factors, prophylactic antibiotics, and platelet support, treating older patients with full-dose regimens would be easier. Balducci (2003), Dale (2003), and Kennedy (1997) supported Shipp's findings in that older adults with NHL have been treated less aggressively, inadequately, or not at all. Voelker et al. (2004) also looked at age bias in a study of factors associated with the first course of chemotherapy in older people with diffuse large cell NHL. They found that only 68% of patients older than age 65 received chemotherapy, and those older than 85 years were significantly less likely to receive chemotherapy. Further research is needed to explore the different histologic findings, different risk groups, and factors associated with maintaining complete responses to facilitate treatment planning for the older adult with NHL.

Comorbidity

An assessment of comorbidity is an important part of a comprehensive assessment of an older adult. The number of comorbidities significantly rises with increasing age (Yancik, 1997). A patient with lymphoma between the ages of 70 and 80 may be expected to have three to four comorbidities (Yancik et al., 2001). Kouroukis et al. (2002) further concluded that age alone should not be used to determine therapy for patients who have no significant comorbidities. Also, even though comorbidities had no effect on initial performance status, comorbidities were associated with significantly worse overall survival.

Socioeconomic Factors

Assessment of other factors that may increase the risk of complications is important. Assessment of socioeconomic conditions that may prevent compliance with NHL treatment or enhance the risk of complications facilitates proactive interventions. The recognition of frailty and assessment of emotional and cognitive conditions also may contribute to an older person's well-being and survival and warrants further investigation (Balducci & Yates, 2000). Nurses are encouraged to become familiar with and use screening tools and assessment tools beyond performance status and comorbidities in decision analysis for older people with NHL (Balducci & Yates; Dale, 2003; Duhamel & Dupuis, 2004; Hood, 2003; Hurria & Kris, 2003; Kagan, 2004; Kennedy, 1997; Repetto, 2003; Yancik et al., 2001). Recommended elements to assess in the older adult with NHL can be found in Table 12-5.

Toxicity

Older adults may be more susceptible to a number of NHL treatment-related toxicities, including hematologic toxicity, mucositis, neurotoxicity, tumor lysis syndrome, and cardiomyopathy, compromising their recovery from chemotherapy (Balducci & Extermann, 1997; Balducci & Yates, 2000; Bertini et al., 2001; Dorr & Von Hoff, 1994; Hood, 2003; Repetto, 2003). Table 12-6 lists selected therapeutic agents available for NHL treatment and special considerations in the older population. Evidence-based strategies for managing these toxicities are of significant importance in this population.

Table 12-5. Assessment Elements for Older Adults With Non-Hodgkin Lymphoma

Assessment	Elements
Functional status	Independent performance of activities of daily living Instrumental activities of daily living, including transportation, money management, medication management, meal preparation, and fulfillment of societal roles Performance status Hearing and visual impairment
Comorbidities	Number and severity of comorbid conditions
Nutritional status	Weight loss of greater than 5%, body mass index less than 22 kg/m^2, and low serum albumin
Socioeconomic status	Social support, including caregivers Neglect and abuse Access to transportation Home safety Financial issues
Psychological	Screen for dementia/depression Adjustment to diagnosis Vision, gait, balance, and hearing assessment
Polypharmacy	Number of medications and potential drug-drug interactions

Note. Based on data from Balducci, 2003; Balducci & Yates, 2000; Hurria & Kris, 2003; Repetto, 2003; Reuben, 1997.

Cardiac Toxicity

Cardiac toxicity in the older adult can be a severe dose-limiting toxicity of NHL therapy. Older people are uniquely at risk for developing cardiac dysfunction during treatment and after therapy. Anthracyclines are used to treat NHL and are the agents most widely associated with irreversible cardiomyopathy (Bertini et al., 2001; Chanan-Khan, Srinivasan, & Czuczman, 2004; Loerzel & Dow, 2003). Anthracycline-induced cardiac toxicity varies from 2%–23%. The increased risk factors for anthracycline-induced cardiac toxicity in the older adult with NHL are age (i.e., older than 65 years), preexisting heart disease or hypertension, previous anthracycline therapy, concomitant cyclophosphamide administration, and previous history or concurrent administration of radiation therapy (RT) to the chest and mediastinum (Loerzel & Dow). Rituximab, a monoclonal antibody approved for the treatment of NHL, also is associated with rare cardiovascular events, including reversible or transient infusion-related hypotension and arrhythmia, as well as acute myocardial infarction, ventricular fibrillation, and cardiogenic shock (Chanan-Khan et al.).

RT for the treatment of NHL can affect the cells of the myocardium when the heart is in or near the treatment field. When mediastinal radiation is combined with anthracyclines and cyclophosphamide, cardiac toxicity may occur at lower radiation doses. Many advances in RT now limit the amount of exposure to the heart. Three-dimensional conformal tangential irradiation and intensity-modulated RT have been shown to spare normal tissue from RT-induced cardiac dysfunction (Chanan-Khan et al., 2004; Loerzel & Dow, 2003).

Table 12-6. Selected Therapeutic Agents Available for Non-Hodgkin Lymphoma and Special Considerations for the Older Adult

Agent	Special Considerations
Anthracyclines	At risk for acute and chronic congestive heart failure. Monitor closely in people with a cardiac ejection fraction < 50%. Significant myelosuppression, mucositis, nausea, and emesis potential Increased risk for extravasation
Cyclophosphamide	Elimination decreased in patients with impaired renal function Increased risk for hemorrhagic cystitis May block metabolism of barbiturates, increasing sedative effects At risk for congestive heart failure
Vincristine	Monitor carefully for neurotoxicity. At risk for autonomic cardioneuropathy At risk for bowel dysfunction Increased risk for extravasation
Prednisone	May mask infections Monitor for hypertension, depression, fragile skin, loss of muscle mass, osteoporosis, visual acuity, and thromboembolism.
Rituximab	Monitor for hypotension, hypertension, arrhythmia, and bronchospasm.
Ibritumomab tiuxetan	At risk for increased thrombocytopenia with delayed recovery
Tositumomab	At risk for increased myelosuppression with delayed recovery
Alemtuzumab	Monitor for hypotension, hypertension, and arrhythmia.
Denileukin diftitox	Monitor for vascular leak syndrome. At risk for increased skin reactions
Bleomycin	Pulmonary toxicity increases for those older than age 70.
Mitoxantrone	At risk for congestive heart failure At risk for increased mucositis Increased risk for extravasation
Etoposide	At risk for increased hypotension Monitor dose in patients with renal dysfunction.
Methotrexate	At risk for increased mucositis and renal tubular necrosis
Cisplatin	At risk for increased renal and cardiac toxicity
Fludarabine	Use caution in patients with preexisting neurologic disorders. At increased risk for cumulative myelosuppression, treatment-related myelodysplasia, and acute leukemia. Elimination is decreased in patients with impaired renal function. Monitor for hypotension, edema, and pericardial effusion.
Procarbazine	Interactions with certain drugs and food At risk for hypotension and pneumonitis

Note. Based on data from Balducci & Extermann, 1997; Beveridge, 2003; Camp-Sorrell, 1999; Chanan-Khan et al., 2004; Dorr & Von Hoff, 1994; Holmes & Muss, 2003; Hood, 2003; Repetto, 2003; Vose, 2004; Walker & Dang, 2004.

Nursing Implications

Cardioprotective measures begin with assessment of the older adult prior to start of therapy, taking into consideration the current cardiac status, any history of cardiac dysfunction, prior cardiotoxic treatment regimens, and current cardiac medications (Chanan-Khan et al., 2004). Evaluation of the cardiac wall motion and the left ventricular ejection fraction (LVEF) are standard tools to assess cardiac function. An early decline in LVEF values of more than 4% after lower cumulative doses of doxorubicin (200 mg/m^2) were administered was predictive of doxorubicin toxicity in patients with lymphoma (Loerzel & Dow, 2003).

Patient assessment during treatment focuses on identifying symptoms of cardiac changes associated with chemotherapy, monoclonal antibodies, and RT. Patients need to be evaluated for angina, dysrhythmias, dyspnea at rest and with activity, hypotension, hypertension, diaphoresis, venous jugular distention, peripheral edema, electrocardiogram changes, and third and fourth heart sounds. Therapy may need to be stopped until symptoms resolve or discontinued until symptoms are further assessed. Patient assessment after treatment ends includes continued monitoring for cardiotoxicity, educating patients about long-term risk of cardiac toxicity, and instructing them to inform their oncology team of any changes (Chanan-Khan et al., 2004; Loerzel & Dow, 2003).

Treatment

The options for treatment of NHL have changed dramatically in the past 10 years. Treatment options traditionally have been based on the clinical presentation and classification of the lymphoma into one of the three IWF types: low (indolent), intermediate, and high grades (aggressive). NCCN provides practice guidelines for the treatment of NHL on the Internet. Clinical trials have demonstrated that older people can tolerate treatment for NHL as well as younger people, with careful attention to supportive care (Dixon et al., 1986; Zinzani et al., 1997, 1999). Older adults treated for NHL over time may receive single-agent or combination chemotherapy, local RT, biologic therapy, or a combination of these in addition to participation in clinical trials, however limited they may be. A number of single-agent therapies are available, along with new therapies and new combinations of old therapies in refractory or relapsed disease. Monoclonal antibody therapy has changed the mode of treatment for older adults with NHL. Researchers are studying several new chemotherapeutic agents in phase I and II trials. Table 12-6 lists a number of therapeutic agents available for the treatment of NHL (Kosits & Callaghan, 2000).

Low-Grade Non-Hodgkin Lymphoma

Many effective treatment options exist for older people with low-grade NHL. Many patients receive a series of systemic treatments that often begin with low-dose and relatively well-tolerated oral agents (Hainsworth et al., 2002). Some patients require little or no treatment initially (watchful waiting) (Westin & Longo, 2004). In a randomized controlled trial of 309 patients, Ardeshna et al. (2003) found that in some patients with indolent disease, treatment may not be necessary until signs of progression appear, especially in those older than 70 years of age. Chronic indolent disease usually is felt to be incurable, with patients experiencing shorter periods of remission over time (Bilodeau & Fessele, 1998; Hainsworth et al.). Conventional chemotherapy and dose-intense regimens have brought high response rates and prolonged duration of response but have failed to demonstrate prolonged survival (Dalla-Favera & Gaidano, 2001; Meyer et al., 1995). Response to treatment can change over time; what worked initially may be ineffective the next time. In recent clinical trials, Hainsworth et al. and Piro et al. (1999) found that extended use of rituximab in older adults, who typically have a poor prognosis, resulted in a good response rate and tolerance of therapy. In another study that included 58 people up to 81 years of age, Davis et al. (2000) found that people with low-grade and intermediate-grade follicular NHL can be treated safely and effectively with multiple courses of rituximab. In a review of oral abstracts during the 2003 meeting of the American Society of Clinical Oncology, Coleman (2003) reported that the concurrent use of a chemotherapy regimen of fludarabine, mitoxantrone, and dexamethasone with rituximab is safe and effective for people with indolent lymphomas; however, neither the age range nor the results stratified by age were reported.

Follicular Lymphoma

A standard first-line treatment for follicular lymphoma does not exist. In follicular as well as the other indolent types of lymphoma, the initial approach depends on the clinical situation. Patients may be observed without treatment (also known as watch and wait), or they may be treated with rituximab alone. Fludarabine has been used for second-line therapy or later relapses (Sweetenhan, 1999). A number of studies suggest that, at least in the short term, the addition of rituximab to chemotherapy in the treatment of indolent lymphomas can extend the time to progression and the duration of response in comparison to chemotherapy alone (Hainsworth et al., 2002). Whether this result translates to a survival benefit is not yet known.

High-Grade Lymphoma

Diffuse large B-cell lymphoma, the most common of the aggressive lymphomas, occurs in approximately 36% of older adults with NHL (Bertini et al., 2001). It is curable in approximately 50% of patients younger than 65 years of age but has significantly lower cure rates in older people. Chemotherapy is the primary therapeutic modality for aggressive lymphomas (Bertini et al.; Dalla-Favera & Gaidano, 2001; Riley & Byar, 2004; Walker & Dang, 2004). The standard first-line therapy that has been critical to improving survival and cure rates is generally the myelosuppressive regimen with cyclophosphamide, doxorubicin, vincristine, and prednisone (CHOP) plus rituximab (Coiffier et al., 2002; Crawford, 2004). Bertini et al. reported on a number of studies that showed encouraging results for intensive chemotherapy followed by autologous stem cell transplantation in a highly selected group of people older than 60 years with aggressive NHL histology, a good performance status, no comorbidity, good multi-geriatric scale assessment, and a poor IPI rating. The collection of a sufficient number of stem cells for transplantation was not an obstacle for older adults considering treatment in these studies.

Progressive Disease

Treatment with salvage chemotherapy for older adults who have relapsed from complete remission or failed to achieve an initial remission is based on the goal of treatment. Armitage et al. (2001) looked at three randomized studies and found that patients who progressed on the previous chemotherapy regimen had a poorer outlook than those who had stable or partially responding disease. They also noted that in the older adult with extensive disease and poor performance status, the likelihood of cure was less. They further suggested that in the older adult considering the goal of cure, less-intensive palliative treatments should be considered.

Stem Cell Transplantation

Nonmyeloablative allogeneic stem cell transplantation (NST) is an emerging treatment for NHL. NST is based on a graft-versus-lymphoma effect. Khouri and Champlin (2001) in a review of NST for NHL studies found that NST would not be recommended for first-line treatment for diffuse large B-cell lymphoma, newly diagnosed patients, disease that has transformed or is refractory, or mantle cell and follicular lymphoma. However, NST should be considered irrespective of the person's age if his or her disease is sensitive to chemotherapy. Randomized studies need to be conducted to determine whether NST is more effective than conventional allogeneic stem cell transplantation, and long-term follow-up data are needed.

Rituximab

Rituximab, a chimeric murine-human monoclonal antibody to the CD20 antigen, was the first monoclonal antibody approved for treatment of patients with relapsed or refractory low-grade or follicular CD20-positive B-cell NHL (Maloney et al., 1994). The average duration of response to rituximab is in the range of approximately one year (Cheson, 2000). However, some patients and some subsets can have responses extending to several years. A number of different maintenance therapy schedules also have been studied with this approach aiming to prolong treatment in order to sustain remission and extend the response (Hainsworth et al., 2002; Leonard, 2004). Most of the side effects are well tolerated and limited to the first infusion and include fevers, chills, nausea (mild), asthenia, and headache. Severe side effects that may be associated with rituximab include hypersensitivity reactions, cardiac events, rare tumor lysis syndrome, and desquamating mucocutaneous reactions (Cheson; Hainsworth et al.; Kosits & Callaghan, 2000; Leonard; Maloney et al.).

Tositumomab and Radioimmunoconjugates

Two radioimmunoconjugates have been approved for treatment of patients with B-cell NHL. Both Iodine[131] (^{131}I) tositumomab (Bexxar®, Corixa, Seattle, WA) and Yttrium-90 (^{90}Y) ibritumomab tiuxetan (Zevalin®, Biogen Idec, Cambridge, MA) have been approved as therapy for follicular NHL that has relapsed or failed to respond to chemotherapy and are being investigated for the earlier treatment of low-grade NHL (Biogen Idec, 2005; Byar & Fernando, 2004; Corixa, 2003; Riley & Byar, 2004; Vose, 2004; Witzig et al., 2003). Both therapies have been found to produce overall response rates of approximately 80% in patients with NHL. However, in people older than 60 years of age, the response rate is approximately 60% (Vose, 2004). In older adults who may have been heavily pretreated, both agents have been reported to be relatively well tolerated, with delayed myelosuppression being common with both agents (Hendrix, 2004; Riley & Byar; Vose, 2004; Witzig et al.). Patients, however, may be at increased risk for treatment-related myelodysplasia and acute leukemia (Armitage et al., 2003; Witzig et al.). Post-treatment education for the family and the older adult receiving Zevalin includes instructions to clean any spilled urine, properly dispose of any materials contaminated with body fluids, and wash hands thoroughly after toilet use (Byar, 2004; Hendrix). Post-treatment education for the family and the older adult receiving Bexxar includes the prevention of radiation exposure by avoiding sleeping in a common bed for more than six hours and avoiding close contact with infants or pregnant women by minimizing the time of exposure and maximizing the distance from the patient (Riley & Byar; Vose, 2004).

Denileukin Diftitox

Denileukin diftitox is a genetically engineered fusion protein that targets the interleukin-2 receptor on cell surfaces while sparing nonexpressing cells. It is approved for the treatment of cutaneous T-cell lymphoma and is active in the treatment of B-cell lymphoma (Walker & Dang, 2004). In a pivotal study of 71 patients with cutaneous T-cell lymphoma (Olsen et al., 2001), the adverse events were not reported by age; however, the two potential side effects of skin reactions (20%–30%) and vascular leak syndrome (17%–25%) may be of special concern to older adults, depending on other comorbidities.

Investigational Therapies

New directions for the management of NHL currently in clinical trials are targeted and vaccine therapies. Oblimersen sodium blocks the action of *bcl-2*, a protein produced by the body that works to prevent cell death, and bortezomib, a proteasome inhibitor that delays tumor growth, may have less nonspecific toxicities compared with chemotherapy. Targeting resistance pathways may reduce or reverse chemoresistance (Coleman, 2003). Stimulation of the immune system to treat lymphoma is demonstrated in several new therapies, including vaccine therapy. Types of vaccines currently under study are tumor-specific idiotype hybridoma, idiotype recombinant, lymphoma CD40-L, CLL/CD40-L-adenovirus, and idiotype heat shock protein. Vaccine therapy for the treatment of low-grade NHL is promising because it is slow growing, which permits sufficient time to manufacture the patient-specific vaccine and offer new treatment options for older adults with NHL (Vose, 2001).

Nursing Care Issues

Nursing and clinical empirical evidence is lacking for much of the nursing management of the older adult with NHL. Nursing management often is based on generalizations, tradition, care setting practices, theoretical considerations, or expediency. As the incidence of NHL increases, the scope of evidence-based nursing practice also must increase (Larson & Nirenberg, 2004). For the purpose of this review, the following nursing management categories with selected issues will be discussed: assessment, symptoms, and patient and family education.

Assessment

As previously discussed, the assessment of comorbidity, socioeconomic conditions, the recognition of frailty, emotional and cognitive conditions, the burden of care, availability of resources, and performance and functional status are important parts of a comprehensive assessment of the older adult. Table 12-5 lists suggested assessments to be performed at every visit in the older population for specific therapeutic agents during treatment. Other nursing assessments include self-care learning readiness and recognition of signs and symptoms of tumor lysis syndrome, peripheral neuropathy (PN), delayed toxicities, superior vena cava syndrome, spinal cord compression, progressive radiation myelopathy, and second malignancies as part of ongoing care for early detection and prevention of severe outcomes for the older adult with NHL (Dodd, 1999; Yarbro, 2000).

Symptoms

The nursing management of NHL-related and treatment-related symptoms should focus on prevention and comfort and relief measures. However, clinical research studies often do not address the benefits versus toxicity or the care needs of the older person living with NHL. Significant treatment-related symptoms and toxicities are cardiac toxicity, neutropenia, anemia, infusion-related reactions (as previously discussed), B symptoms, tumor lysis syndrome, and PN.

Night sweats, fever, chills, fatigue, itching, and weight loss are common presenting systemic symptoms that merit appropriate management to promote comfort and increase quality of life while the treatment plan is being developed. A balance of bed coverings for night sweats, treatment with antipyretics for fever, adequate clothing and a warm environment free of drafts to prevent chills, warm blankets to stop shivering, rest and activity periods for fatigue, and nutritional support to decrease weight loss often will offer relief until the treatment of NHL becomes effective (Cunningham, 2004; Nail, 2004; Yarbro & Seiz, 2004).

Tumor lysis syndrome is a potentially fatal but preventable complication occurring in patients with high tumor burdens who may be expected to have a rapid response to treatment. The recognition of at-risk populations is the most important nursing intervention, which includes assessing for tumors with high growth fractions (elevated white blood count) or bulky disease (> 8–10 cm), splenomegaly, and elevated LDH. Assessment for signs of hyperkalemia, hyperphosphatemia, hypocalcemia, and hyperuricemia and the initiation of medical management with increased hydration and prophylactic allopurinol is important in the early management and prevention of renal failure. Late management measures include the continued monitoring of electrolytes and renal function for a period of three to seven days after initiation of cytotoxic therapy, medical treatment, and comfort measures for symptoms of hyperkalemia, hyperphosphatemia, hypocalcemia, hyperuricemia, and dialysis for those unresponsive to maintenance measures (Richerson, 2004).

PN is a common complication occurring in patients with NHL treated with vinca alkaloids and podophyllotoxins. The older adult is at increased risk because of other possible comorbidities, such as preexisting PN, diabetes, alcoholism, or malnutrition. Prevention generally is not possible; however, progression to severe or permanent PN can be prevented by cessation of the chemotherapy. Early identification of PN with a complete nursing assessment includes sensory perception, presence of numbness and tingling, presence of painful sensations, and alterations in sensations that affect activities of daily living. Treatment is symptomatic and directed toward support and relief of pain, injury, and disability. Home safety, physical therapy, assistive devices, medications for pain relief, and self-care measures to prevent constipation are a few key therapeutic approaches to be included in nursing management of the older adult with PN (Wilkes, 2004).

Patient and Family Education

Nurses play a significant role in assessing not only the older adult's and family members' ability to acquire knowledge but also their ability to manage the patient's self-care. Unless the older adult and family members are prepared to assess and manage the toxicities of treatment, the resulting morbidity may require a change in the treatment goals, which may reduce the chance for cure or prolong survival and a diminishing quality of life. Ongoing assessment of readiness to learn, knowledge of the situation, and belief and ability for self-care are required before effective management can be instituted (Dodd, 1999).

Dodd (1999), in a review of studies, discussed the important topics for patient and family education as those focused on prevention and early-stage and late-stage self-care. For the older adult undergoing treatment for NHL, educational goals that can prevent or diminish the occurrence of disease symptoms include understanding the risks of developing side effects, monitoring for potential side effects, and initiating timely self-care activities. Early-stage, immediate essential information would include knowledge and skills for potentially life-threatening events, such as fever and infection.

Patient and family education should include the procedures for monitoring fevers and contacting the healthcare provider in a timely manner. Early self-care includes teaching patients and families about care before it is needed. Later self-care includes the sustained performance of activities by the patient and families and measuring the depth of their abilities.

Fatigue, PN, disease progression and recurrence, the watch and wait method for indolent disease, and clinical trials are just a few key areas in which nurses may offer patient and family education that can lead to patient and family empowerment and control. When the depth of patients' and families' abilities are limited, the role of the nurse is critical in augmenting their skills through clinical experience and knowledge of current literature.

Current Research Issues

It has frequently been reported in the literature that age has emerged as an important risk factor for aggressive NHL (Bertini et al., 2001; Dixon et al., 1986; Sonneveld et al., 1995; Zinzani et al., 1997, 1999). In a systematic review of 12 randomized trials that compared chemotherapeutic regimens for the treatment of older people with newly diagnosed, advanced-stage, aggressive NHL, the analysis demonstrated that survival and disease control were improved when an anthracycline-containing regimen such as CHOP or cyclophosphamide, teniposide, prednisone, and pirarubicin was compared with a regimen that omitted the anthracycline, used a substituted anthracycline, or was designed to be less toxic (Kouroukis et al., 2002). They also found that CHOP was associated with greater toxicity than some of the other regimens. Caggiano, Morrison, Fridman, and Delgado (2004) recently reviewed factors associated with reduced chemotherapy dose intensity in patients with NHL or breast cancer. Increased age, comorbidity, low body surface area, and no preemptive growth factor in cycle one were associated with increased risk for delivery of reduced chemotherapy dose intensity in cycles one through three.

In an early study of 38 people older than 65, Meyer et al. (1995) found that dose-intense CHOP did not increase overall survival when compared to standard CHOP in older people with aggressive NHL. Coleman (2003) supported the findings that a shortened interval was found to be inferior to the standard interval for people older than 60 years when an age-based subanalysis was conducted.

The use of growth factors, such as granulocyte–colony-stimulating factor (G-CSF), has been shown in a number of studies as a means of reducing the degree of neutropenia, the incidence of infections, and length of hospital stay for febrile neutropenia in older people being treated for NHL (Balducci & Yates, 2000; Chrischilles et al., 2002; Kouroukis et al., 2002; Morrison et al., 2001; Voelker et al., 2004). Although the American Society of Clinical Oncology (Ozer et al., 2000) recommendations for the use of hematopoietic colony-stimulating factors (CSFs) do not specifically address older patients with NHL, the NCCN (2005) guidelines recommend prophylactic G-CSF for all patients age 65 or older treated with CHOP or CHOP-like chemotherapy. The use of epoetin, however, is recommended as a treatment option for patients with chemotherapy-associated anemia and a hemoglobin concentration that has declined to a level less than 10 g/dl. The Infectious Disease Society of America (Hughes et al., 2002) has identified neutropenic patients older than 60 years to be at greater risk for fever, which also was supported in the studies by Balducci and Yates and Chrischilles et al. Dubois, Pinto, Bernal, Badamgarav, and Lyman (2004), in their review of 24 studies looking at special populations for the use of CSFs, found that older adults, people undergoing myelosuppressive chemotherapy, and those with low performance status were at increased risk for febrile neutropenia and may benefit from first-cycle CSF administration. NCCN also recommended that older adults with NHL should receive CSF support during the first cycle of CHOP (Crawford, 2004). The impact of dose-intense chemotherapy on survival and the use of CSFs in the older adult are yet to be fully studied.

Clinical Trials

Knowledge about the optimal treatment and survival experience for people older than 65 with NHL is limited by their underrepresentation in clinical trials (Anderson & Gillespie, 2004; Hurria & Kris, 2003; Unger et al., 2004; Yancik, 1997). Chronic comorbidities affect older people in greater numbers and often are exclusion criteria for participation in clinical trials (Holmes & Muss, 2003; Repetto, 2003). The lack of participation of older people with NHL in clinical trials, physician bias as to which older adults are offered participation, and the fact that many trials do not evaluate younger versus older people suggest that the optimal strategies being designed for patients with NHL are not generalizable to the older adult population (Hurria & Kris; Yancik). The quality of life of older people associated with different treatment regimens and chemotherapy dose delays also has received limited attention in clinical research (Bertini et al., 2001).

Burden of Care

Involvement of family caregivers is essential for optimal treatment of older people receiving treatment for cancer, especially in ensuring treatment compliance, continuity of care, and social support (Glajchen, 2004; Haley, 2003). Studies on the burden of care looked at the effect of cancer on the productivity of family members of patients with cancer. Shih and Zhao (2004) found that cancer affects the productivity of American families through work loss of patients with cancer and their family caregivers. Families with cancer with employed family caregivers had a significantly higher number of work-loss days than noncancer families. As noted by Duhamel and Dupuis (2004), family members usually are comfortable with providing physical care but may have difficulty with addressing emotional needs and concerns. One of the most important roles for caregivers is assisting with pain management (Glajchen). Comorbidities of the patient with cancer, especially in the older adult with NHL, also may increase the burden of care, particularly because the caregiver also may be elderly with a number of comorbidities (Haley). Evidence-based interventions for nurses to employ with family caregivers to facilitate communication and to meet caregivers' needs are essential to support practice. Failure to incorporate the effect of cancer on family caregivers in research may underestimate the economic, physical, psychological, social, and spiritual burdens of cancer (Glajchen; Haley; Hodgson & Given, 2004; Shih & Zhao).

Older Adult Clinical Outcomes

Clinical decision making for older people with cancer often is complicated by limited information from clinical trials. Concerns about toxicities and comorbidities and the inability to select people who might tolerate more intensive therapy often are based on age (Holmes & Muss, 2003; Kagan, 2004; Repetto, 2003). Gillespie et al. (2004) and Ribeiro et al. (2004) found in their studies of chronologic age in people with NHL that age alone is a poor predictor of dose reductions, dose delays, toxicities, or ability to complete therapy, and the Screening Geriatric Assessment tool may serve to promote use of standard-of-care and improve outcomes in older adults. Current recommendations by NCCN include the use of screening tools and a geriatric assessment tool in developing care plans for all patients with cancer aged 70 and older (Balducci & Yates, 2000). No current assessment tool has emerged as the preferred choice. However, performance status alone is not an adequate assessment of functional status (Holmes & Muss; Hurria & Kris, 2003; Kagan; Repetto). For example, performance status scales reflect fewer and less varied domains of functioning, such as self-care and ability to ambulate. Hodgson and Given (2004) found that psychological well-being was a significant factor in functional recovery in older people after surgery. Thome, Dykes, Gunnars, and Hallberg (2003) conducted a descriptive study of 41 people (5 with NHL) older than 75 years of age with a cancer diagnosed within the past five years. They concluded that healthcare providers' support of the person's choice was very important. To ensure evidence-based practice, further studies of interventions aimed at psychological symptoms in the older person with NHL need to be completed.

Older adults treated for NHL with alkylating chemotherapy and RT are at increased risk for treatment-related dysplasia and leukemia because of their longer and more frequent exposure to leukemogenic agents (Armitage et al., 2003).

Areas for Future Research

As the aging population increases, NHL will affect a significant number of older people. Further research is needed to explore treatment decisions, disease prognosis, and nursing implication strategies in older adults with NHL in selected areas, as listed in Figure 12-1. The results from randomized trials suggest that in the absence of

- Biologic difference
- Gene expression profiles
- Treatment preferences
- Geriatric assessment
- Ageist attitudes among nurses
- Impact of comorbid illnesses
- Maximize treatment efficacy
- Cancer-related functional loss
- Care delivery in a fragmented healthcare environment
- Appropriate supportive measures to minimize toxicity
- Targeted therapies
- Burden of care
- Functional recovery after treatment
- Impact of chemotherapy delays on quality of life
- Management of persistent symptoms

Figure 12-1. Selected Areas of Research for Older Adults With Non-Hodgkin Lymphoma

significant comorbid illness or strong patient preferences, age should not be used as a variable to modify therapy and that older patients with NHL should be offered the same standard therapy as younger people. Adherence to evidence-based guidelines can standardize clinical care and potentially improve outcomes in older adults with NHL. Compliance with standards can promote optimal therapy and completion of the treatment plan, avoiding dose reductions and decision making based primarily on chronologic age. Major issues remain to be addressed with the development of new therapies in older people with NHL. Randomized controlled trials evaluating treatment options targeting older adults with comorbidities are needed (Westin & Longo, 2004). The number of older adults with NHL participating in clinical trials needs to increase so that newer and more effective therapies can be identified more rapidly and be made available for the treatment of this population. Older people with NHL should be asked what they prefer and be included in treatment planning, supportive care needs, family caregiver needs, clinical trials, and nursing research.

Case Study

R.S. is a 72-year-old Caucasian male who is a retired U.S. Navy nuclear physicist. He has been a widower for two years but remains active with golf, friends, and neighbors. R.S. has a son who lives outside of the area and a daughter who lives nearby; both are very much a part of his life and involved in his care. He has a past history of atrial fibrillation, hypertension, gastric resection for benign tumor, and transurethral resection of the prostate. His baseline medications include daily multivitamins, hydrochlorothiazide, and aspirin. He is a nonsmoker, consumes a minimal amount of alcohol, and has no known allergies.

He presented to the emergency department with the second episode of constipation within the past three months. His latest episode was associated with symptomatic, recurrent, increasing abdominal pain. On examination, his abdomen was mildly distended, and a CT of the abdomen and pelvis revealed mesenteric, retroperitoneal, and retrocrural lymphadenopathy, with the largest nodal mass measuring approximately

4.4 cm x 5.9 cm. His prostate gland was enlarged; he had bilateral renal cysts and two right renal stones. He had no B symptomatology, such as unexplained fevers, night sweats, or weight loss, but recently had experienced fatigue. A fine needle aspirate of a perirenal mass was sent to pathology for cytology and flow cytometry, which revealed 10% medium to large abnormal lymphoid cells with irregular nuclei, a monoclonal kappa, and CD10 positive B-cell follicular small cleave low-grade NHL. Laboratory results were notable for an elevated white blood cell count of 11,700/µl, with an absolute lymphocyte count of 3,100, hemoglobin 15.9 g/dl, hematocrit 45.7%, and platelet count of 290,000/µl. His chemistries, including a liver panel, were normal. He then was referred to the oncology department. His medical and social history were reviewed, and a complete physical exam revealed normal findings, including no lymphadenopathy. A CT of the chest as well as a bone marrow biopsy were discussed with the patient to complete his staging for treatment planning. He was supported in his decision to go for a second opinion as soon as possible so that he could get started on therapy without delay.

Two months later, he returned to the oncology department with a 10-pound weight loss, intermittent constipation, and increased pelvic pain. He had taken the time for consultation with another oncologist who confirmed his diagnosis and supported aggressive therapy. He elected to proceed with the completion of his staging and treatment planning. The interpretation on the repeat flow cytometry analysis of the bone marrow aspirate was consistent with chronic lymphocytic leukemia/small lymphocytic lymphoma; however, the bone marrow biopsy and aspirate revealed no evidence of malignant lymphoma and did not support the presence of an abnormal lymphoid population. Echocardiogram showed a normal LVEF of 69% and a normal sinus rhythm. CT scans of the abdomen and pelvis were repeated and demonstrated no significant interval change and no extranodal lesions. However, the CT of the thorax demonstrated mild mediastinal adenopathy. Laboratory tests also were repeated, with notable findings of a slightly elevated LDH of 273 U/L and a white count of 12,800/µl. The completion of his evaluations included an assessment of current medications, comorbidities, and functional, nutritional, socioeconomic, and psychological status. He was diagnosed with a stage III, low-grade NHL with an IPI score of 2 and was determined to be an excellent candidate for aggressive management. He and his family were presented with the findings and were offered the opportunity to participate in a clinical trial evaluating the efficacy and safety of rituximab in combination therapy with six cycles of rituximab and CHOP followed by rituximab maintenance every six months for two years. R.S. and his daughter asked questions about his cancer, treatment details, related symptoms, and side effects and were very much included in the treatment planning and decision making. R.S., fully aware that his risk of recurrence would be high even after initial therapy, agreed to consider aggressive therapy. After initial discussion, further information, and education with the research nurse, informed consent was obtained, and treatment was begun four months after his initial presentation and diagnosis.

R.S. completed six cycles of full-dose rituximab and CHOP with supportive care, including standard antiemetics and CSFs. His daughter accompanied him to all appointments, and he received emotional support and possible resources as needed from the staff. R.S. received support from his friends and neighbors with frequent fellowship and meals. After cycle 2, R.S. reported feeling great, able to play golf again with excellent energy. His abdominal pain and constipation were resolved, and LDH levels were within normal limits. After cycle 3, he reported a drop in energy, poor appetite, and a weight loss of five pounds. His serum albumin and total protein were low. A dietary consult was ordered, and the need for added nutritional support was discussed. R.S., being a very independent person, elected to make arrangements for meal service in his home during "chemo" week. After cycle 4, the CT scans were repeated and showed a significant decrease in adenopathy. During the last two cycles, R.S. developed a grade 1 neuropathy in his fingertips and grade 1 hyperglycemia, which was closely followed. Nursing management included collaboration with the clinical research nurse, close monitoring of his blood counts and chemistries, assessment of the burden of care and support for his family, thorough detailed review of toxicities, and clinical assessment at each visit. Other strategies included assessment of availability of resources, assessment of changing emotional concerns, and support for his decisions and choices. At the end of cycle 6, his CT scans showed no adenopathy, he was regaining his energy, his neuropathy continued, and his hyperglycemia had resolved. R.S. required no dose reduction or dose delays during his therapy. His first rituximab maintenance dose was given per protocol, four weeks after the completion of cycle 6.

Six months following initial therapy, one small lymph node was identified in the mesentery. After two cycles of maintenance rituximab, he had residual resolving neuropathy, mild granulocytopenia, and low normal serum albumin and total protein. With each maintenance dose of rituximab, he experienced mild fatigue but continued with his regular activities. R.S. regularly played golf, traveled, and continued to enjoy friends and family. The treatment plan was to continue with rituximab maintenance per protocol for two more cycles, with CT scans every six months and follow-up as clinically indicated.

R.S. is an ideal example of an older person with a diagnosis of NHL with treatment based on disease status, IPI, and a complete and comprehensive assessment, with consideration of the goals of the patient and family. R.S. was offered the opportunity to participate in a clinical trial, and he and his family were included in the treatment planning, with caregiver support included in the care plan. R.S. and his family will continue to require assistance and information from the healthcare team and revision of the care plan as needed to ensure their well-being, care, and treatment goals.

Conclusion

With the projected growth of the aging population, the incidence of NHL in the older adult is expected to rise. Thorough assessment of the older adult, highlighting physiologic age versus chronologic age, is critical in determining treatment options. Studies suggest that older adults can tolerate treatment for NHL as well as younger individuals. Nurses have a key role in assessment, education, and supportive care for patients and caregivers. Further research is needed exploring assessment, treatment, symptom management, and supportive care for the older adult with NHL.

References

Anderson, K.A., & Gillespie, T.W. (2004, May). *Ageist attitudes among nurses: Implications for long-term nursing care for elder clients with cancer.* Abstract presented at the 29th Annual Congress of the Oncology Nursing Society, Anaheim, CA.

Ardeshna, K.M., Smith, P., Norton, A., Hancock, P.J., Hoskin, P.J., MacLennan, K.A., et al. (2003). Long-term effect of a watch and wait policy versus immediate systemic treatment for asymptomatic advanced-stage non-Hodgkin lymphoma: A randomized trial. *Lancet, 362,* 516–522.

Armitage, J.O., Carbone, P.P., Connors, J.M., Levine, A., Bennett, J.M., & Kroll, S. (2003). Treatment-related myelodysplasia and acute leukemia in non-Hodgkin's lymphoma patients. *Journal of Clinical Oncology, 21,* 897–906.

Armitage, J.O., Mauch, P.M., Harris, N.L., & Bierman, P. (2001). Non-Hodgkin's lymphomas. In V. DeVita, S. Hellman, & S. Rosenberg (Eds.), *Cancer: Principles and practice of oncology* (6th ed., pp. 2256–2316). Philadelphia: Lippincott Williams & Wilkins.

Armitage, J.O., & Weisenburger, D.D. (1998). New approach to classifying non-Hodgkin's lymphomas: Clinical features of the major histologic subtypes. Non-Hodgkin's Lymphoma Classification Project. *Journal of Clinical Oncology, 16,* 2780–2795.

Balducci, L. (2003). New paradigms for treating elderly patients with cancer: The comprehensive geriatric assessment and guidelines for supportive care. *Journal of Supportive Oncology, 1*(4 Suppl. 2), 30–37.

Balducci, L., & Extermann, M. (1997). Cancer chemotherapy in the older patient. *Cancer, 80,* 1317–1322.

Balducci, L., & Yates, J. (2000). General guidelines for the management of older patients with cancer. *Oncology, 14,* 221–227.

Bertini, M., Boccomini, C., & Calvi, R. (2001). The influence of advanced age on the treatment and prognosis of diffuse large-cell lymphoma. *Clinical Lymphoma, 1,* 278–283.

Beveridge, R.A. (2003). *Guide to selected cancer chemotherapy regimens and associated adverse events* (4th ed.). Thousand Oaks, CA: Amgen.

Bilodeau, B.A., & Fessele, K. (1998). Non-Hodgkin's lymphoma. *Seminars in Oncology Nursing, 14,* 273–283.

Biogen Idec. (2005). Zevalin (ibritumomab tiuxetan) [Package insert]. Cambridge, MA: Author.

Byar, K. (2004). Educating patients about radioimmunotherapy with yttrium 90 ibritumomab tiuxetan (Zevalin). *Seminars in Oncology Nursing, 20,* 20–25.

Byar, K., & Fernando, D. (2004, May). *Second-line therapy with Zevalin® produces higher response rates and more durable responses in patients with B-cell NHL: Implications for nursing practice.* Abstract presented at the 29th Annual Congress of the Oncology Nursing Society, Anaheim, CA.

Caggiano, V., Morrison, V.A., Fridman, M., & Delgado, D.J. (2004, June). *A model to predict delivery of reduced chemotherapy dose intensity in the first three cycles of treatment among patients with non-Hodgkin's lymphoma and breast cancer.* Abstract presented at the 40th Annual Meeting of the American Society of Clinical Oncology, New Orleans, LA.

Camp-Sorrell, D. (1999). Surviving the cancer, surviving the treatment: Acute cardiac and pulmonary toxicity. *Oncology Nursing Forum, 26,* 983–990.

Chanan-Khan, A., Srinivasan, S., & Czuczman, M.S. (2004). Prevention and management of cardiotoxicity from antineoplastic therapy. *Journal of Supportive Oncology, 2,* 251–256.

Cheson, B.D. (2000). Rituximab in the next millennium. *Biological Therapy of Lymphoma, 2,* 10–13.

Chrischilles, E., Delgado, D.J., Stolshek, B.S., Lawless, G., Moshe, F., & Carter, W.B. (2002). Impact of age and colony-stimulating factor use on hospital length of stay for febrile neutropenia in CHOP-treated non-Hodgkin's lymphoma. *Cancer Control, 9,* 203–211.

Coiffier, B., Lepage, E., Briere, J., Herbrecht, R., Tilly, H., Bouabdallah, R., et al. (2002). CHOP chemotherapy plus rituximab compared with CHOP alone in elderly patients with diffuse large B-cell lymphoma. *New England Journal of Medicine, 346,* 235–242.

Coleman, M. (2003). Lymphoma/myeloma. In D.H. Johnson (Ed.), *2003 annual meeting summaries* (pp. 144–150). Alexandria, VA: American Society of Clinical Oncology.

Corixa. (2003). Bexxar (tositumomab and iodine I[131] tositumomab) [Package insert]. Seattle, WA: Author.

Crawford, J. (2004). Improving the management of chemotherapy-induced neutropenia. *Journal of Supportive Oncology, 2*(Suppl. 2), 11–17.

Cunningham, R.S. (2004). Anorexia-cachexia syndrome. In C.H. Yarbro, M.H. Frogge, & M. Goodman (Eds.), *Cancer symptom management* (3rd ed., pp. 137–168). Sudbury, MA: Jones and Bartlett.

Cuttner, J., Wallenstein, S., & Troy, K. (2002). Non-Hodgkin's lymphoma in patients 70 years of age or older: Factors associated with survival. *Leukemia Research, 26,* 447–450.

Dale, D. (2003). Poor prognosis in elderly patients with cancer: The role of bias and undertreatment. *Journal of Supportive Oncology, 1*(4 Suppl. 2), 11–17.

Dalla-Favera, R., & Gaidano, G. (2001). Lymphomas. In V. DeVita, S. Hellman, & S. Rosenberg (Eds.), *Cancer: Principles and practice of oncology* (6th ed., pp. 2215–2338). Philadelphia: Lippincott Williams & Wilkins.

Davis, T., Grillo-Lopez, A.J., White, C.A., McLaughlin, P., Czuczman, M.S., Link, B., et al. (2000). Rituximab anti-CD20 monoclonal antibody therapy in non-Hodgkin's lymphoma: Safety and efficacy of re-treatment. *Journal of Clinical Oncology, 18,* 3135–3143.

Dixon, D.O., Neilan, B., Jones, S.E., Lipschitz, D.A., Miller, T.P., Grozea, P.N., et al. (1986). Effect of age on therapeutic outcome in advanced diffuse histiocytic lymphoma: The Southwest Oncology Group Experience. *Journal of Clinical Oncology, 4,* 295–305.

Dodd, M.J. (1999). Self-care and patient/family teaching. In C.H. Yarbro, M.H. Frogge, & M. Goodman (Eds.), *Cancer symptom management* (2nd ed., pp. 20–29). Sudbury, MA: Jones and Bartlett.

Dorr, R.T., & Von Hoff, D.D. (1994). *Cancer chemotherapy handbook* (2nd ed.). Norwalk, CT: Appleton & Lange.

Dubois, R.W., Pinto, L., Bernal, M., Badamgarav, E., & Lyman, G.H. (2004, June). *Review of special populations for the use of colony-stimulating factors.* Abstract presented at the 40th Annual Meeting of the American Society of Clinical Oncology, New Orleans, LA.

Duhamel, F., & Dupuis, F. (2004). Guaranteed returns: Investing in conversations with families of patients with cancer. *Clinical Journal of Oncology Nursing, 8,* 68–71.

Friedberg, J.W., & Chengazi, V. (2003). PET scans in the staging of lymphoma: Current status. *Oncologist, 8,* 438–447.

Frizzera, G. (1995). Non-Hodgkin lymphomas: Pathologic features and clinical correlations. In R. Hoffman, E. Benz, Jr., S. Shattil, B. Furie, H. Cohen, & L. Silberstein (Eds.), *Hematology: Basic principles and practice* (2nd ed., pp. 1247–1278). New York: Churchill Livingstone.

Gillespie, T.W., Patterson, H., Harris, W.B., Shumate, M., Nadella, P., Jacobs, J., et al. (2004, June). *Improving clinical outcomes in elderly oncology patients.* Poster session presented at the 40th Annual Meeting of the American Society of Clinical Oncology, New Orleans, LA.

Glajchen, M. (2004). The emerging role and needs of family caregivers in cancer care. *Journal of Supportive Oncology, 2,* 145–155.

Gomez, H., Hidalgo, M., Casanova, L., Colomer, R., Pen, D.L., Otero, J., et al. (1998). Risk factors for treatment-related death in elderly patients with aggressive non-Hodgkin's lymphoma: Results of a multivariate analysis. *Journal of Clinical Oncology, 16,* 2065–2069.

Groves, F.D., Linet, M.S., Travis, L.B., & Devesa, S.S. (2000). Cancer surveillance series: Non-Hodgkin's lymphoma incidence by histologic subtype in the United States from 1978 through 1995. *Journal of the National Cancer Institute, 92,* 1240–1251.

Hainsworth, J.D., Litchy, S., Burris, H.A., Scullin, D.C., Carso, S.W., Yardley, C.A., et al. (2002). Rituximab as first-line and maintenance therapy for patients with indolent non-Hodgkin's lymphoma. *Journal of Clinical Oncology, 20,* 4261–4267.

Haley, W.E. (2003). Family caregivers of elderly patients with cancer: Understanding and minimizing the burden of care. *Journal of Supportive Oncology, 1*(4 Suppl. 2), 25–29.

Hendrix, C. (2004). Radiation safety guidelines for radioimmunotherapy with yttrium 90 ibritumomab tiuxetan. *Clinical Journal of Oncology Nursing, 8,* 31–34.

Hodgson, N.A., & Given, C.W. (2004). Determinants of functional recovery in older adults surgically treated for cancer. *Cancer Nursing, 27,* 10–16.

Holmes, C.E., & Muss, H.B. (2003). Diagnosis and treatment of breast cancer in the elderly. *CA: A Cancer Journal for Clinicians, 53,* 227–244.

Hood, L.E. (2003). Chemotherapy in the elderly: Supportive measures for chemotherapy-induced myelotoxicity. *Clinical Journal of Oncology Nursing, 7,* 185–190.

Hughes, W.T., Armstrong, D., Bodey, G.P., Bow, E.J., Brown, A.E., Calandra, T., et al. (2002). 2002 guidelines for the use of antimicrobial agents in neutropenic patients with cancer. *Clinical Infectious Diseases, 34,* 730–751.

Hurria, A., & Kris, M.G. (2003). Management of lung cancer in older adults. *CA: A Cancer Journal for Clinicians, 53,* 325–341.

International Non-Hodgkin's Lymphoma Prognostic Factors Project. (1993). A predictive model for aggressive non-Hodgkin's lymphoma. *New England Journal of Medicine, 329,* 987–994.

Jemal, A., Murray, T., Ward, E., Samuels, A., Tiwari, R.C., Ghafoor, A., et al. (2005). Cancer statistics, 2005. *CA: A Cancer Journal for Clinicians, 55,* 10–30.

Kagan, S.H. (2004). Gero-oncology nursing research. *Oncology Nursing Forum, 31,* 293–297.

Kennedy, B.J. (1997). Aging and cancer. *Cancer, 80,* 1270–1272.

Khouri, I.F., & Champlin, R.E. (2001, Spring). Non-myeloablative allogeneic stem cell transplantation for lymphoid malignancies. *Lymphoma Update,* pp. 15–21.

Kosits, C., & Callaghan, M. (2000). Rituximab: A new monoclonal antibody therapy for non-Hodgkin's lymphoma. *Oncology Nursing Forum, 27,* 51–59.

Kostakoglu, L., Leonard, J.P., Coleman, M., & Goldsmith, S.J. (2004). The role of FDG-PET imaging in the management of lymphoma. *Clinical Advances in Hematology and Oncology, 2,* 115–121.

Kouroukis, C.T., Browman, G.P., Esmail, R., & Meyer, R.M. (2002). Chemotherapy for older patients with newly diagnosed, advanced-stage, aggressive-histology non-Hodgkin lymphoma: A systematic review. *Annals of Internal Medicine, 136,* 144–152.

Larson, E., & Nirenberg, A. (2004). Evidence-based nursing practice to prevent infection in hospitalized neutropenic patients with cancer. *Oncology Nursing Forum, 31,* 717–723.

Leonard, J.P. (2004). Antibodies in the treatment of lymphoma. *Clinical Advances in Hematology and Oncology, 2,* 210–211.

Loerzel, V.W., & Dow, K.H. (2003). Cardiac toxicity related to cancer treatment. *Clinical Journal of Oncology Nursing, 7,* 557–562.

Maartense, E., Le Cessie, S., Kluin-Nelemans, H.C., Kluin, P.M., Snijder, S., Wijermans, P.W., et al. (2002). Age-related differences among patients with follicular lymphoma and the importance of prognostic scoring systems: Analysis from a population-based non-Hodgkin's lymphoma registry. *Annals of Oncology, 13,* 1275–1284.

Maloney, D.G., Liles, T.M., Gzerwinski, D.K., Waldichuk, C., Rosenberg, J., Grillo-Lopez, A., et al. (1994). Phase I clinical trial using escalating single-dose infusion of chimeric anti-CD20 monoclonal antibody (IDEC-CS88) in patients with recurrent B-cell lymphoma. *Blood, 84,* 2457–2466.

Meyer, R.M., Browman, G.P., Samosh, M.L., Benger, A.M., Bryant-Lukosius, D., Wilson, W.E., et al. (1995). Randomized phase II comparison of standard CHOP with weekly CHOP in elderly patients with non-Hodgkin's lymphoma. *Journal of Clinical Oncology, 13,* 2386–2393.

Morrison, V.A., Picozzi, V., Scott, S., Pohlman, B., Dickman, E., Lee, M., et al. (2001). The impact of age on delivered dose intensity and hospitalizations for febrile neutropenia in patients with intermediate-grade non-Hodgkin's lymphoma receiving initial CHOP chemotherapy: A risk factor analysis. *Clinical Lymphoma, 2,* 47–56.

Nail, L.M. (2004). Fatigue. In C.H. Yarbro, M.H. Frogge, & M. Goodman (Eds.), *Cancer symptom management* (3rd ed., pp. 47–61). Sudbury, MA: Jones and Bartlett.

National Cancer Institute. (2004). *Adult non-Hodgkin's lymphoma treatment.* Retrieved July 23, 2004, from http://www.cancer.gov/cancertopics/pdq/treatment/adult-non-hodgkins/HealthProfessional

National Comprehensive Cancer Network. (2005). *Clinical practice guidelines in oncology.* Retrieved September 21, 2005, from http://www.nccn.org/physician_gls/f_guidelines.html

Olsen, E., Duvic, M., Frankel, A., Kim, Y., Martin, A., Vonderheid, E., et al. (2001). Pivotal phase III trial of two dose levels of denileukin diftitox for the treatment of cutaneous T-cell lymphoma. *Journal of Clinical Oncology, 19,* 376–388.

Ozer, H., Armitage, J.O., Bennett, C., Crawford, J., Demetri, G.D., Pizzo, P.A., et al. (2000). 2000 update of recommendations for the use of hematopoietic colony-stimulating factors: Evidence-based, clinical practice guidelines. *Journal of Clinical Oncology, 18,* 3558–3585.

Piro, L.D., White, C.D., Grillo-Lopez, A.J., Janakiraman, N., Saven, A., Beck, T.M., et al. (1999). Extended rituximab (anti-CD20 monoclonal antibody) therapy for relapsed or refractory low-grade or follicular non-Hodgkin's lymphoma. *Annals of Oncology, 10,* 655–661.

Repetto, L. (2003). Greater risks of chemotherapy toxicity in elderly patients with cancer. *Journal of Supportive Oncology, 1*(4 Suppl. 2), 18–24.

Reuben, D.B. (1997). Geriatric assessment in oncology. *Cancer, 80,* 1311–1316.

Ribeiro, M.J., Patterson, H., Shumate, M., Harris, W.B., Nadella, J., & Gillespie, T.W. (2004, June). *Compliance with guidelines for elderly patients undergoing cancer therapy.* Abstract presented at the 40th Annual Meeting of the American Society of Clinical Oncology, New Orleans, LA.

Richerson, M.T. (2004). Electrolyte imbalances. In C.H. Yarbro, M.H. Frogge, & M. Goodman (Eds.), *Cancer symptom management* (3rd ed., pp. 440–461). Sudbury, MA: Jones and Bartlett.

Ries, L.A., Reichman, M.E., Lewis, D.R., Hankey, B.F., & Edwards, B.K. (2003). Cancer survival and incidence from the Surveillance, Epidemiology, and End Results (SEER) program. *Oncologist, 8,* 541–552.

Riley, M.B., & Byar, K. (2004). The rationale for and background of radioimmunotherapy: An emerging therapy for B-cell non-Hodgkin's lymphoma. *Seminars in Oncology Nursing, 20*(Suppl. 1), 1–7.

Shih, Y.C., & Zhao, L. (2004, June). *Impact of cancer on the productivity of American families.* Poster session presented at the 40th Annual Meeting of the American Society of Clinical Oncology, New Orleans, LA.

Shipp, M.A. (1994). Prognostic factors in aggressive non-Hodgkin's lymphoma: Who has "high-risk" disease? *Blood, 83,* 1165–1173.

Sonneveld, P., de Ridder, M., van der Lelie, H., Nieuwenhuis, K., Schouten, H., Mulder, A., et al. (1995). Comparison of doxorubicin and mitoxantrone in the treatment of elderly patients with advanced diffuse non-Hodgkin's lymphoma using CHOP versus CNOP chemotherapy. *Journal of Clinical Oncology, 13,* 2530–2539.

Sweetenhan, J. (1999). Economic analysis of the use of rituximab in comparison with CHOP and fludarabine in patients with indolent B-cell non-Hodgkin's lymphoma. *Biological Therapy of Lymphoma, 2,* 9–12.

Thome, B., Dykes, A., Gunnars, B., & Hallberg, I.R. (2003). The experiences of older people living with cancer. *Cancer Nursing, 26,* 85–96.

Treseler, P.A. (n.d.). *Who's W.H.O. in lymphomas: A practical clinical approach to the new lymphoma classifications.* Retrieved February 17, 2004, from http://www.addr.com/~pathmax/who.html

Unger, J.M., Crowley, J.J., Coltman, C.A., Hutchins, L.F., Martino, S., MacDonald, J.S., et al. (2004, June). *Accrual patterns of the Southwest Oncology Group (SWOG) by sex, race/ethnicity, and age: Updated and expanded analyses.* Poster discussion presented at the 40th Annual Meeting of the American Society of Clinical Oncology, New Orleans, LA.

Voelker, M.D., Chrischilles, E.A., Wright, K.B., Link, B.K., Park, T.R., & Celagado, D.J. (2004, June). *Factors associated with first course chemotherapy among older patients with newly diagnosed non-Hodgkin's lymphoma.* Abstract presented at the 40th Annual Meeting of the American Society of Clinical Oncology, New Orleans, LA.

Vose, J.M. (2001, Spring). Vaccination trials for non-Hodgkin's lymphoma. *Lymphoma Update,* pp. 22–26.

Vose, J.M. (2004). Bexxar®: Novel radioimmunotherapy for the treatment of low-grade and transformed low-grade non-Hodgkin's lymphoma. *Oncologist, 9,* 160–172.

Walker, P., & Dang, N.H. (2004). Denileukin diftitox as novel targeted therapy in non-Hodgkin's lymphoma. *Clinical Journal of Oncology Nursing, 8,* 169–174.

Westin, E.H., & Longo, D.L. (2004). Lymphoma and myeloma in older patients. *Seminars in Oncology, 31,* 198–205.

Wilkes, G.M. (2004). Symptoms of neurological disturbances. In C.H. Yarbro, M.H. Frogge, & M. Goodman (Eds.), *Cancer symptom management* (3rd ed., pp. 331–398). Sudbury, MA: Jones and Bartlett.

Witzig, T.E., White, C.A., Gordon, L.I., Wiseman, G.A., Emmanouilides, C., Murray, J.L., et al. (2003). Safety of yttrium-90 ibritumomab tiuxetan radioimmunotherapy for relapsed low-grade, follicular, or transformed non-Hodgkin's lymphoma. *Journal of Clinical Oncology, 21,* 1263–1270.

Yancik, R. (1997). Cancer burden in the aged: An epidemiologic and demographic overview. *Cancer, 80,* 1273–1283.

Yancik, R., Wesley, M.N., Ries, L.A., Havlik, R.J., Edwards, B.K., & Yates, J.W. (2001). Effect of age and comorbidity in postmenopausal breast cancer patients aged 55 years and older. *JAMA, 285,* 885–892.

Yarbro, C.H. (2000). Malignant lymphomas. In C.H. Yarbro, M.H. Frogge, M. Goodman, & S.L. Groenwald (Eds.), *Cancer nursing: Principles and practice* (5th ed., pp. 1329–1353). Sudbury, MA: Jones and Bartlett.

Yarbro, C.H., & Seiz, A.M. (2004). Pruritus. In C.H. Yarbro, M.H. Frogge, & M. Goodman (Eds.), *Cancer symptom management* (3rd ed., pp. 97–111). Sudbury, MA: Jones and Bartlett.

Zinzani, P.L., Pavone, E., Storti, S., Moretti, L., Fattori, P.P., Guardigni, L., et al. (1997). Randomized trial with or without granulocyte colony-stimulating factor as adjunct to induction VNCOP-B treatment of elderly high-grade non-Hodgkin's lymphoma. *Blood, 89,* 3974–3979.

Zinzani, P.L., Storti, S., Zaccaria, A., Moretti, L., Magagnoli, M., Pavone, E., et al. (1999). Elderly aggressive-histology non-Hodgkin's lymphoma: First-line VNCOP-B regimen experience on 350 patients. *Blood, 94,* 33–38.

CHAPTER 13

The Older Adult With Hematologic Malignancies and Disorders

Sandra A. Mitchell, CRNP, MScN, AOCN®

Introduction

The acute and chronic leukemias and myelodysplastic syndromes (MDSs) are a group of clonal neoplastic hematologic disorders characterized by disordered proliferation and maturation in lymphocyte or myeloid cell hematopoietic cell lines, resulting in the accumulation of immature hematopoietic cells in the bone marrow and peripheral blood and inhibition of normal hematopoiesis. Figure 13-1 presents a conceptual organization of the leukemias and MDS based on the cell lineage. *Acute leukemias* are marked by abnormal proliferation of highly immature blood cells, whereas *chronic leukemias* have an excessive accumulation of more mature-appearing but still ineffective blood cells. Chronic myeloid leukemia (CML) may transform over time to an acute blastic phase and, thereafter, more closely resembles an acute leukemia in its biology and clinical course. The accumulation of immature neoplastic cells results in crowding of other marrow elements and infiltration of proliferating lymphocytes into various organs of the body in patterns characteristic of particular subtypes of leukemia. The primary sites of disease are the bone marrow and blood and extramedullary, or sanctuary sites of disease, which may include the central nervous system (CNS), lymph nodes, skin, and testes. The signs and symptoms that result from the increased production of malignant cells, along with the reduction in the number of the mature red cells, platelets, and neutrophils, include bone marrow failure and the consequences of anemia, hemorrhage, and infection.

Effective treatment of leukemia or MDS requires a multifaceted approach, including aggressive management of cytopenias and other clinical manifestations of disease, prevention and treatment of the side effects of therapy, and meticulous supportive care. In the older adult, careful attention to the provision of a high standard of general medical care for any coexisting diseases and the application of a systematic approach to supportive care (Lichtman, 2003) will help to ensure the length and quality of survival of the older adult with a hematologic malignancy. This chapter presents

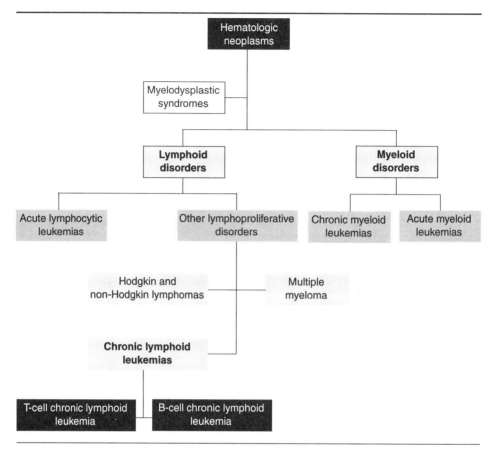

Figure 13-1. Conceptual Organization of the Hematologic Malignancies

Note. Based on information from Bennett et al., 2004; Scheinberg et al., 2001; Souhami & Tobias, 1998.

an overview of epidemiology, classification, evaluation, treatment, and supportive management of the older adult with an acute or chronic leukemia or MDS.

Classifications

Acute leukemia is broadly classified into acute myeloid leukemia (AML) and acute lymphoid leukemia (ALL) based on the cell lineage. AML is a clonal abnormality of the myeloid committed stem cell. ALL is a clonal abnormality of the lymphoid committed stem cell. Subtypes of AML, such as acute promyelocytic leukemia, and ALL can be further defined based on biologic features of the leukemic cells. Chronic leukemias frequently encountered in the older adult include CML and chronic lymphoid leukemia, of which B-cell chronic lymphocytic leukemia is the most common variant. MDS can be defined as a clonal neoplastic disease of the bone marrow characterized by clinical manifestations of bone marrow failure together with a tendency to transform into an acute leukemic phase. The disorders that comprise MDS are characterized by peripheral cytopenias, hypercellular bone marrow, and dysplastic changes (such as ringed sideroblasts, megaloblastic erythroid precursors, hypogranulation/hyposegmentation of the granulocytes, and micromegakaryocytes) in all cell lines. The abnormal clone of MDS is thought to arise in the pluripotent stem cell and may involve both myeloid and lymphoid cell lines.

The Challenge of Treating Acute or Chronic Leukemias or Myelodysplastic Syndromes in the Older Adult

The treatment of a leukemia or MDS in the older adult presents formidable challenges to achieving long-term disease-free survival while at the same time preserving an optimal functional status and an acceptable quality of life. Older patients may have reduced bone marrow regenerative capacity and may be less able to tolerate long periods of pancytopenia and malnutrition. Renal insufficiency or cardiopulmonary disease may make it more difficult for the older adult patient to tolerate the cardiac effects of anthracyclines or mitoxantrone or the cumulative nephrotoxicity associated with treatment effects, such as tumor lysis syndrome or the use of multiple concurrent antimicrobial agents. However, improvements in supportive care, including the introduction of less toxic antimicrobial agents, potent antiemetics with an improved side-effect profile, and a greater range of options for cytokine support to limit neutropenia and anemia (Stone, 2002), have greatly enhanced treatment tolerance in the older adult, and most older adult patients can tolerate intensive induction chemotherapy (Schiffer, 2002). However, leukemia and MDS in the older adult have an unfavorable disease biology, including the presence of chromosomal abnormalities presumed to cause chemoresistance (Appelbaum, 2005; Hiddemann et al., 1999; Lichtman & Rowe, 2004), and this remains the critical impediment.

Despite these challenges, the older individual with a good functional status, favorable cytogenetics, and no comorbid illnesses who makes the decision to proceed with therapy may be offered intensive therapy with curative intent because this offers the highest chance for achievement of remission and progression-free survival (Hiddemann et al., 1999; Lancet & Karp, 2003; Latagliata, Petti, & Mandelli, 1999; Lichtman & Rowe, 2004). For others, participation in a clinical trial of one of the new molecularly targeted therapies may represent the best treatment direction (Schiffer, 2002). For some patients, cytoreductive therapy with hydroxyurea or low-dose Ara-C (cytosine arabinoside) may represent a reasonable option (Sekeres & Stone, 2002). All older adult patients with leukemia or MDS benefit from aggressive supportive management and vigorous efforts to promote and maintain an optimal functional status.

Acute Leukemias

AML is the most common acute leukemia in the older adult, with a median age of onset of 64 years of age and an increasing incidence with advanced age. Acute leukemia in the older adult often emerges secondary to myelodysplasia or the treatment of a previous malignancy and is associated with a high incidence of unfavorable cytogenetic abnormalities (Buchner, 1998; Rowe, 2000). ALL has a bimodal distribution, with an initial peak incidence at age three to five years. The incidence remains low until approximately age 50, when the incidence increases steadily with age and reaches nearly 1.5 cases per 100,000 people in those older than 65 years (Redaelli, Laskin, Stephens, Botteman, & Pashos, 2005).

Risk Factors

For most patients with acute leukemia, the cause of the disease is unknown. In a minority of patients, the cause of the leukemia may be a prior history of radiation therapy or chemotherapy. Such secondary leukemias, more than 90% of which are myeloid leukemias, are extremely difficult to treat. Chemotherapeutic agents associated with a risk of secondary leukemia include nitrogen mustard, procarbazine, cyclophosphamide, lomustine, etoposide, and chlorambucil (Larson & Le Beau, 2005). Therefore, patients at greatest risk for the development of a therapy-induced leukemia include patients with non-Hodgkin lymphoma, Hodgkin lymphoma, acute or chronic leukemias, including childhood leukemia, and breast, ovarian, or testicular cancers, because the chemotherapeutic agents associated with secondary leukemias are ones that are commonly used in the treatment of these tumors. A secondary leukemia generally occurs between two and nine years after therapy (Scheinberg, Maslak, & Weiss, 2001).

Occupational and environmental exposure to chemicals or ionizing radiation is hypothesized to be a contributing factor to the development of acute leukemia. A clear relationship exists between the exposure to ionizing radiation at high levels, such as those that occurred at Chernobyl and Hiroshima, and leukemia, and this has led to the exploration of a possible leukemogenic role for other potential carcinogens in the environment, including low-dose radiation, chemicals, cigarette smoke, and electromagnetic radiation. Although electromagnetic fields have received considerable attention as a possible carcinogen, the actual risk of leukemia from exposure to commercial and residential power fields remains controversial, with a large number of conflicting reports. Cigarette smoking has been linked to AML, and, in fact, as many as 20% of AML cases may be attributable to smoking (Korte, Hertz-Picciotto, Schulz, Ball, & Duell, 2000). Occupational exposure to benzene has been established as a cause of AML. Two viruses, human T-cell leukemia viruses I and II, are known to cause T-cell leukemia, a very rare form of lymphocytic leukemia, in humans. However, only a small percentage of people who are infected with these viruses develop cancer. Although virus-related leukemia is rare in humans, incidences in other animal species, such as cats, chickens, and mice, are quite common. Perhaps in humans, the viral infection provides a setting in which a second oncogenic event, such as oncogene activity, can result in clonal neoplastic proliferation (Scheinberg et al., 2001).

Prognostic Factors

Acute leukemias in the older adult have biologic characteristics that make successful treatment more challenging (Hiddemann et al., 1999; Lancet & Karp, 2003; Latagliata et al., 1999; Rowe, 2000; Sekeres & Stone, 2002). When compared with acute leukemias occurring at a younger age, older adults often have had an antecedent hematologic disorder and may present with involvement of more than one hematopoietic cell lineage, suggesting that in the older adult, acute leukemia arises from a clonal abnormality of the most primitive pluripotent hematopoietic stem cell (Hiddemann et al.). Older adults with AML also have a lower incidence of favorable chromosomal abnormalities and a higher incidence of unfavorable abnormalities when compared with younger adults and children with AML (Appelbaum, 2005). Older adults with AML also have increased frequency of drug-resistant phenotypes, such as overexpression of multidrug resistance glycoprotein (MDR1). MDR1 gene expression mediates the P-glycoprotein chemotherapy efflux pump, resulting in cellular resistance to daunorubicin, and is associated with lower rates of complete remission and more chemotherapy-resistant disease (Rowe). MDR1 was expressed in the leukemia cells of more than 70% of patients with AML who were older than 55 years of age but only was expressed by 30% of patients younger than 55 years of age (Appelbaum, 2005; Sekeres & Stone).

Researchers can identify a subset of older adults with AML with relatively favorable prognostic features (Leith et al., 1997; Wahlin, Markevarn, Golovleva, & Nilsson, 2001), and with aggressive supportive care, studies suggest that these individuals may derive benefit from standard remission induction therapy (Estey, 2000a; Hiddemann et al., 1999; Leith et al.). In fact, a randomized trial by the European Organization for Research and Treatment of Cancer found that patients older than age 65 with good performance status and relatively preserved organ function not only lived approximately two months longer if given standard treatment rather than supportive care alone, but, perhaps more importantly, they also required fewer hospitalizations (Lowenberg et al., 1989). Estey (2000a) proposed a risk-adapted treatment strategy for AML in the older adult based on the presence of adverse clinical and cytogenetic prognostic features. The adverse prognostic features of AML and ALL are presented in Table 13-1.

Table 13-1. Adverse Prognostic Features of Acute Myeloid Leukemia and Acute Lymphoid Leukemia in Adults

Feature	Acute Myeloid Leukemia	Acute Lymphoid Leukemia
Age	Age older than 60 years	Age older than 60 years
White blood cell (WBC) count	Antecedent myelodysplasia WBC > 100,000/mm^3	WBC > 30,000/mm^3
Lactic dehydrogenase level (LDH)	Elevated LDH	–
Morphology	M0, M6, M7	Mature B-cell phenotype (FAB-L-3; World Health Organization Burkitt type leukemia)
Markers	CD34+, mdr-1+, Flt-3+	–
Cytogenetics	Adverse cytogenetics: deletions/trisomy of chromosome 5 or 7 (7q, 5q) T (6;9) T (11q23) T (11q23, 3q21, 3q26) or other complex cytogenetic abnormalities	Adverse cytogenetics: T (9;22) or *bcr-abl* gene rearrangement T (4;11) T (8;14)
Clinical features	Poor performance status	Poor performance status Lack of mediastinal lymphadenopathy

Note. Based on information from Grimwade, 2001; Kebriaei et al., 2003; Lichtman & Rowe, 2004; Lichtman & Kolitz, 2000; Scheinberg et al., 2001; Wahlin et al., 2001; Winton & Langston, 2004.

Acute Leukemias

Although the signs and symptoms are relatively nonspecific, the diagnosis of an acute leukemia usually is made based on the history, physical examination, and an examination of the peripheral smear and bone marrow aspirate smear. Additional laboratory examinations such as the complete blood count, coagulation profile, and basic metabolic panel and additional diagnostic imaging such as computed tomography scans are important in the management of the disease but usually are not necessary for the initial diagnosis. Figure 13-2 summarizes the findings typically seen at the time of presentation with an acute leukemia.

- Fatigue for more than one to three months
- Bone marrow failure
- Hemorrhage
- Infection/fever
- Easy bruising
- Hepatic/splenic enlargement
- Lymphadenopathy
- White blood cell count up or down
- Chest mass (T-cell acute lymphoblastic leukemia [ALL])
- Organ infiltration (ALL)
- Gingival infiltration (acute myeloid leukemia, M-5)
- Minimal to moderate weight loss
- Bone pain
- Fibrinogen is down
- Prothrombin time and partial thromboplastin time up
- Blasts on peripheral smear

Figure 13-2. Presenting Signs and Symptoms of Acute Leukemia

Clinical Presentation

Patients with acute leukemia often report a one- to three-month history of fatigue or malaise, easy bruisability or frank bleeding, dyspnea, minimal to modest weight loss, fever, bone pain, or abdominal pain. Excessive bleeding after a minor dental procedure or severe epistaxis may be a presenting feature. Physical examination typically shows pallor consistent with anemia and hemorrhage from the gums, nose, gut, and skin as manifested by petechiae or fundal hemorrhage. Less commonly, hepatic or splenic enlargement and lymphadenopathy are present. Instances of fever or infection, usually of respiratory origin, are frequent, and sepsis may occur. Neurologic signs and symptoms occur more commonly with ALL and may include cranial neuropathies, nausea and vomiting, visual disturbances, and headache. Bone pain is infrequent in adults with AML, although some individuals describe sternal discomfort or tenderness, occasionally with aching in the long bones. This may be especially severe in the lower extremities because of expansion of the medullary cavity by the proliferation of leukemic cells. Discomfort also may occur secondary to lymphadenopathy or hepatosplenomegaly.

The laboratory examination usually reveals anemia and severe thrombocytopenia, with a platelet count less than 50,000/μl. The white blood cell (WBC) count may be normal, reduced, or elevated. Examination of the peripheral blood smear shows blasts in almost all cases. Peripheral blood myeloblasts in excess of $100,000/mm^3$ represent a medical emergency requiring prompt leukapheresis to prevent leukostasis. Prothrombin time and partial thromboplastin time may be elevated, and in acute promyelocytic leukemia, this coagulopathy often is associated with reduced fibrinogen and other evidence of disseminated intravascular coagulation (DIC). This is another medical emergency that must be treated urgently. Subclinical DIC may be present in many forms of acute leukemia. Blood chemistries typically are normal at the time of presentation with an acute leukemia. However, in patients with high cell turnover, such as those with L-3 ALL, there may be evidence of tumor lysis syndrome, with elevated phosphate, potassium, and uric acid levels accompanied by low levels of calcium, elevated lactic dehydrogenase, and renal insufficiency. The clinical presentation of AML usually cannot be distinguished from ALL without examination of the blasts for morphology and immunophenotype. Some signs and symptoms, however, are more frequent with certain disease subgroups than with others. For example, bone pain is more common in ALL, as are signs and symptoms of CNS involvement. Lymph node involvement and hepatosplenomegaly are more common in ALL and in monocytic subtypes of AML. Gingival leukemic infiltrates are seen most frequently in the French-American-British (FAB) group M-5 AML, and mediastinal masses are found in more than 50% of patients with T-cell ALL (Chang et al., 2004; Onishi et al., 2004).

Diagnostic Evaluation

The diagnosis and classification of acute leukemias integrate clinical information with morphologic assessment of blood and bone marrow smears, supplemented by cytochemistry, immunophenotyping, metaphase cytogenetics, and molecular genetic analysis (Swirsky & Richards, 2001). These strands of information are complementary, and together they provide the diagnosis, determine the dimensions for monitoring response to treatment, and indicate the most sensitive method to evaluate for the presence of minimal residual disease.

The peripheral blood smear and the bone marrow aspirate and biopsy are the foundational components of the evaluation of a patient with an acute leukemia. Examination of the peripheral blood and bone marrow provides an evaluation of the morphology or microscopic appearance of the leukemia cells, provides tissue for immunohistochemistry to identify the lineage of the cell, provides material for flow cytometry to determine the percentage of highly immature cells and the cell surface markers, and provides tissue for cytogenetics to determine if a structural chromosomal abnormality such as deletion, inversion, duplication, or translocation exists (Swirsky & Richards, 2001). The diagnosis of acute leukemia usually is made based on the morphology or microscopic appearance of the cells, with an excess of immature cells, also called blasts, and the appearance of dysplasia in more mature cells.

Immunohistochemistries are used to assist in the classification of the lineage of the cell. For example, myeloperoxidase and Sudan Black are the immunohistochemical stains used to confirm the myeloid origin of the blast cells (Swirsky & Richards, 2001). Other immunohistochemical stains include PAS (periodic acid-Schiff) and toluidine blue. Flow cytometry or immunophenotyping is based on knowledge of the normal distribution and strength of expression of membrane antigens on all hematopoietic cells. Certain antigens appear and disappear in an orderly sequence as myeloid and lymphoid cells mature and differentiate. For example, flow cytometry on a patient with a poorly differentiated AML may be distinguished by a high proportion of cells expressing CD34, CD13, CD33, CD117, HLA-DR, and TdT. This information may be useful in monitoring for minimal residual disease after treatment and also may be useful in prognostication. For example, AML characterized by a CD7+, TdT+ overexpression phenotype is associated with a poorer prognosis (Swirsky & Richards).

Cytogenetics and other molecular diagnostic techniques, such as fluorescence in situ hybridization (FISH), reverse transcriptase-polymerase chain reaction, and polymerase chain reaction (PCR), also are essential techniques in the evaluation of an acute leukemia. They can offer important information about both prognosis and clinical decision making regarding whether to proceed to allogeneic transplantation, and they facilitate the earliest detection of relapse and evaluate for the presence of minimal residual disease (Baer, 1998; Grimwade, 2001; Swirsky & Richards, 2001). Although many patients attain a complete remission morphologically based on what is seen under the microscope, flow cytometry and molecular diagnostics are sensitive methods for detecting residual leukemic blasts that still may be present at the end of treatment. The presence of aberrant antigen expression phenotypes by flow cytometry or the continued presence of a cytogenetic or molecular abnormality by Southern blot, FISH, or PCR may help to distinguish those patients who would benefit from further treatment and assist in monitoring patients for early relapse.

Because the treatment of ALL and AML may differ significantly, the most important first step in the diagnostic process is to clarify whether the lymphoid or myeloid lineages or both lineages are involved. FAB offers a widely used classification system of eight different types of AML and three types of ALL based on morphology and cytochemistry. The World Health Organization (WHO) also has developed a new classification system for both ALL and AML. Both the WHO and FAB classification systems are based on the morphology and immunohistochemistry features; however, the WHO classification system also incorporates cytogenetic and molecular features (Heaney & Golde, 2000; Iovino & Camacho, 2003). Studies have shown that cytogenetic analysis can identify biologically distinct subsets of acute leukemia, and cytogenetic profiles are increasingly thought to have a role in tailoring the design of remission induction and postremission therapies, particularly in older adult patients with AML (Grimwade, 2001). For ALL, the FAB classification relies on morphology, dividing blasts into L1, L2, and L3 by their appearance. In the WHO classification system, ALL blasts are specified as derived from either B-cell or T-cell lineages, as determined by cell surface and other markers. Table 13-2 compares the FAB and WHO classification systems for ALL and AML.

Chronic Leukemias

The chronic leukemias are a group of disorders characterized by the neoplastic proliferation of relatively mature myelocytes or lymphocytes, with involvement of both the peripheral blood and the bone marrow. Numerous subvarieties of chronic leukemia exist, including CML, B-cell chronic lymphoid leukemia (B-CLL), and the chronic myeloproliferative disorders, such as essential thrombocythemia, idiopathic myelofibrosis, and polycythemia vera (Breed, 2003).

Table 13-2. Comparison of French-American-British and World Health Organization Classification Systems for Myeloid and Lymphoid Leukemias

System	Classifications
FAB Classification for Acute Myeloid Leukemias (AMLs)	M0: minimally differentiated M1: myeloblastic leukemia without maturation M2: myeloblastic leukemia with maturation M3: hypergranular promyelocytic leukemia M4: myelomonocytic leukemia M4Eo: variant, increase in marrow eosinophils M5: monocytic leukemia M6: erythroleukemia (DiGuglielmo disease) M7: megakaryoblastic leukemia
WHO Classification for Acute Myeloid Leukemias	AML with recurrent cytogenetic translocations • AML with T(8;21)(q22;q22) AML1/CBFα/ETO • Acute promyelocytic leukemia: AML with T(15;17)(q22;q12) and variants PML/RARα • AML with abnormal bone marrow eosinophils inv(16)(p13;q22) vagy T(16;16)(p13;q22) CBFbeta/MYH1 • AML with 11q23 MLL abnormalities AML with multilineage dysplasia • With prior myelodysplastic syndrome (MDS) • Without prior MDS AML with MDS, therapy-related • Alkylating agent–related • Epipodophyllotoxin-related • Other types AML not otherwise categorized • AML minimally differentiated • AML without maturation • AML with maturation • Acute myelomonocytic leukemia • Acute monocytic leukemia
FAB Classification for Acute Lympho-cytic Leukemia (ALL)	FAB L-1 (small cells with almost no cytoplasm, round to cleaved nuclei, and perinuclear chromatin) FAB L-2 (larger cells with 20% cytoplasm; nucleoli more prominent) FAB L-3 (Burkitt-type ALL) (large cells with cytoplasmic vacuolization)
WHO Classification for Lymphoid Leukemias	Precursor T-cell acute lymphoblastic leukemia Precursor B-cell acute lymphoblastic leukemia Burkitt-cell leukemia

Chronic Myeloid Leukemia

CML is a disorder characterized by proliferation and accumulation of myeloid elements at all stages of differentiation. CML has three clinical phases. The first phase, or chronic phase, is characterized by a proliferation of myeloid cells showing a full range of maturation. Eventually a decrease in myeloid differentiation occurs, and the disease enters an accelerated phase, followed by a blast crisis phase, which is characterized by more than 30% blasts in the peripheral blood and bone marrow and carries a very poor prognosis. In this late stage, usual survival without aggressive treatment is only a few months. Survival in the accelerated phase also is limited, usually between one and two years.

CML is associated with a specific cytogenetic abnormality characterized by a translocation between chromosomes 9 and 22, also called the Philadelphia chromosome. This genetic alteration results in the formation of an oncogene called *bcr-abl*. *Bcr-abl* is constitutively active as a tyrosine kinase, activating multiple signal transduction pathways shared by many cellular growth factors and resulting in cell cycle dysregulation, enhanced cellular proliferation, and reduced apoptosis (programmed cell death), thus leading to excess production of myeloid cellular elements.

The onset of CML usually is insidious, with most patients presenting in chronic phase. Patients may be asymptomatic, and the disease may be detected on a routine CBC, demonstrating neutrophilic leukocytosis and basophilia. Thrombocytosis also may be present. Other patients will present with fevers, sweats, bone pain, weight loss, fatigue, or signs of extramedullary hematopoietic involvement (splenomegaly and left upper quadrant discomfort) or with leukemia infiltration of the skin, bleeding, thrombosis, or arthralgias.

Chronic Lymphocytic Leukemia

B-CLL occurs predominantly in older adults, with a median age of onset between 60 and 70 years of age. B-CLL is characterized by the proliferation and accumulation of small immunoincompetent B lymphocytes. The clinical course is highly variable, with some patients dying soon after diagnosis and others living with their disease for more than 15 years without major complications (Reilly, 1998). The median survival is approximately five years, and unfavorable prognostic factors include a diffuse pattern of CLL infiltration of the bone marrow, an initial peripheral lymphocyte count > 50,000 x 10^9/liter, serum beta-2 microglobulin > 3.5 mg/liter, and specific chromosomal and molecular abnormalities such as deletion of chromosome 11 or the presence of *p53* mutations (Lichtman & Kolitz, 2000). Approximately 50% of patients present with an incidental finding of an elevated lymphocyte count of greater than 10,000 x 10^9/liter. Other initial disease manifestations may include lassitude, weight loss, dyspnea, and night sweats. Hypogammaglobulinemia also may be seen, and infections, including bronchopneumonia, sinusitis, urinary tract infections, staphylococcal abscesses, and skin infections, are other common presenting signs (Pangalis et al., 2002). Splenomegaly and lymphadenopathy involving the cervical, inguinal, and axillary regions often are present. The staging criteria for B-CLL are presented in Table 13-3.

Myelodysplastic Syndromes

MDS is a group of hematologic malignancies that manifest as cytopenias and occur almost exclusively in the older adult population (median age 60–75 years) (Reilly, 1998). It is now generally accepted that they represent early stages of AML. The bone marrow may be normocellular or even hypercellular. Cytogenetic abnormalities, usually involving the loss of chromosomal material, are reported in approximately 40%–70% of patients with MDS.

In 1982, the FAB Cooperative Group proposed diagnostic criteria for this heterogeneous group of disorders. The classification system is depicted in Table 13-4 and depends on the percentage of ringed sideroblasts and blasts in the bone marrow and the absolute peripheral monocyte count. In 2001, WHO published new classification schemes for neoplasms of the hematopoietic and lymphoid tissues. The WHO classification scheme for MDS is depicted in Table 13-5.

Table 13-3. Binet and Rai Staging Criteria for Chronic Lymphocytic Leukemia

Binet Staging Criteria for CLL

Stage	Characteristics*+	Median Survival
A	Characterized by no anemia or thrombocytopenia and fewer than three areas of lymphoid involvement	> 10 years
B	Characterized by no anemia or thrombocytopenia with three or more areas of lymphoid involvement	7 years
C	Characterized by anemia and/or thrombocytopenia regardless of the number of areas of lymphoid enlargement	2 years

*Each of the following counts as one area: lymph node > 1 cm in the neck, axillae, groins, spleen, and liver.
+ Secondary causes of anemia (iron deficiency, folate, or B_{12} deficiency), as well as autoimmune cytopenias must be identified and treated prior to staging.

Note. Based on information from Scheinberg et al., 2001.

Rai System for Clinical Staging of CLL

Stage	Extent of Disease
0	Lymphocytosis in blood and bone marrow
I	Lymphocytosis plus lymphadenopathy (local or generalized, small nodes or bulky)
II	Lymphocytosis plus enlarged spleen and/or liver (nodes may or may not be enlarged)
III	Lymphocytosis plus anemia (hemoglobin less than 11 g/dl). Enlarged nodes, spleen, or liver may or may not be present.
IV	Lymphocytosis plus thrombocytopenia (platelet count less than 100 x 10^9/L). Anemia and enlarged nodes, spleen, and liver may or may not be present.

Note. Based on information from Keating, 2002.

The clinical signs and symptoms of MDS are related to progressive bone marrow failure. Half of the patients identified will be asymptomatic in terms of symptoms of MDS at the time of presentation. Others will present with symptoms related to anemia, bacterial infection (secondary to neutropenia or to neutrophil dysfunction), or bleeding. Patients with chronic myelomonocytic leukemia and peripheral monocytosis may have splenomegaly, skin infiltrations, or serous effusions. Prognosis is variable, and those with the poorest prognosis include those with more than 10% blasts in the bone marrow and trilinear cytopenias (List, 2004; List, Vardiman, Issa, & DeWitte, 2004).

Risk factors for developing MDS include being older than age 50, environmental exposures to benzene and possibly other industrial solvents, and prior therapy for cancer, including radiation therapy or chemotherapy with an alkylating agent (e.g., chlorambucil, cyclophosphamide, melphalan) or an epipodophyllotoxin (e.g., etoposide, teniposide) (Rund & Ben-Yehuda, 2004). For alkylating agents, the risk of developing a secondary MDS or AML begins at the end of therapy and peaks at 4 years, with a plateau at 10 years. For epipodophyllotoxins, the latency period to development of MDS/AML is almost always less than five years, with a shorter latency of transition from MDS to AML.

Table 13-4. French-American-British Classification and Prognosis of Myelodysplastic Syndromes

Type	Peripheral Blood	Bone Marrow	Median Survival
Refractory anemia (RA)	< 1% blasts	Dyshematopoiesis in one, two, or three lineages, < 5% blasts	53 months
RA with ringed sidero-blasts (RAS)	< 1% blasts	As RA with ringed sidero-blasts representing at least 15% of erythroblasts	76 months
RA with excess of blasts (RAEB)	< 5% blasts	As with RA, with 5%–20% blasts	10.5 months
RAEB in transformation (RAEBt)	< 5% blasts	As with RA, with 20%–30% blasts	5 months
Chronic myelomonocytic leukemia (CMML)	> 1 x 10^9/L mono-cytes	As any of the above, with monocyte precursors	22 months

Note. Based on information from Saba, 1996, 2001.

Table 13-5. World Health Organization Classification of Myelodysplastic Syndromes and Myelodysplastic/Myeloproliferative Diseases

Disease	Blood Findings	Bone Marrow Findings
Refractory anemia (RA)	Anemia No or rare blasts < 1 x 10^9/L monocytes	Erythroid dysplasia only < 10% granulocytes or megakaryocytes dysplastic < 5% blasts < 15% ringed sideroblasts
Refractory anemia with ringed sidero-blasts (RARS)	Anemia No blasts	Erythroid dysplasia only < 10% granulocytes or megakaryocytes dysplastic ≥ 15% ringed sideroblasts < 5% blasts
Refractory cyto-penias with multi-lineage dysplasia (RCMD)	Cytopenias (bicytopenia or pancytopenia) No or rare blasts No Auer rods < 1 x 10^9/L monocytes	Dysplasia in ≥ 10% of cells in two or more myeloid cell lines < 5% blasts in marrow No Auer rods < 15% ringed sideroblasts
Refractory cytopenias with multilineage dysplasia and ringed sideroblasts (RCMD-RS)	Cytopenias (bicytopenia or pancytopenia) No or rare blasts No Auer rods < 1 x 10^9/L monocytes	Dysplasia in ≥10% of cells in two or more myeloid cell lines < 5% blasts in marrow No Auer rods ≥ 15% ringed sideroblasts
Refractory anemia with excess blasts-1 (RAEB-1)	Cytopenias < 5% blasts No Auer rods < 1 x 10^9/L monocytes	Unilineage or multilineage dysplasia 5%–9% blasts No Auer rods

(Continued on next page)

Table 13-5. World Health Organization Classification of Myelodysplastic Syndromes and Myelodysplastic/Myeloproliferative Diseases *(Continued)*

Disease	Blood Findings	Bone Marrow Findings
Refractory anemia with excess blasts-2 (RAEB-2)	Cytopenias 5%–19% blasts Auer rods +/– < 1 x 10⁹/L monocytes	Unilineage or multilineage dysplasia 10%–19% blasts Auer rods +/–
Myelodysplastic syndrome, unclassified (MDS-U)	Cytopenias No or rare blasts No Auer rods	Unilineage granulocyte or megakaryocyte dysplasia < 5% blasts No Auer rods
MDS associated with isolated deletion (5q)	Anemia < 5% blasts Platelets normal or increased	Normal to increased megakaryocytes with hypolobulated nuclei < 5% blasts No Auer rods Isolated deletion (5q)
Chronic myelomonocytic leukemia (CMML)	Persistent peripheral blood monocytosis greater than 1 x 10⁹/L No Philadelphia chromosome or *bcr-abl* fusion gene Fewer than 20% blasts (myeloblasts, monoblasts, and promonocytes) in the blood	No Philadelphia chromosome or *bcr-abl* fusion gene Fewer than 20% blasts (myeloblasts, monoblasts, and promonocytes) in the bone marrow Dysplasia in one or more myeloid lineages. If myelodysplasia is absent or minimal, the diagnosis of chronic myelomonocytic leukemia still may be made if the other requirements are present and an acquired, clonal cytogenetic abnormality is present in the marrow cells, or the monocytosis has been persistent for at least three months and all other causes of monocytosis have been excluded. Diagnose CMML-1 when blasts are fewer than 5% in blood and fewer than 10% in bone marrow. Diagnose CMML-2 when blasts are 5%–19% in blood or 10%–19% in marrow, or if the Auer rods are present and blasts are fewer than 20% in blood or marrow. Diagnose CMML-1 or CMML-2 with eosinophilia when the criteria listed previously are present and when the eosinophil count in the peripheral blood is greater than 1.5 x 10⁹/L.

Note. Based on information from Bain, 2004; List et al., 2004; Vardiman et al., 2002.

Initial Evaluation of the Patient With Leukemia or Myelodysplastic Syndrome

The initial evaluation of the adult with leukemia or MDS helps to develop the plan for ongoing treatment. Some of the common physical findings in the patient with an acute leukemia are presented in Table 13-6. The history and review of systems should include attention to a history of prior hematologic disorder (e.g., myeloproliferative disorder, myelodysplastic syndrome) or a history of malignancy treated with

Table 13-6. Common Manifestations of Acute Leukemia

Site	Symptoms
Head, ears, eyes, nose, throat	Mucosal bleeding, mucositis, oral cavity infection, sinus tenderness, epistaxis, gingival hypertrophy, periorbital ecchymoses, conjunctival/scleral hemorrhages, fundal hemorrhages, papilledema secondary to increased intracranial pressure and leukostasis
Lymphatics	Lymphadenopathy more common in acute lymphoblastic leukemia (ALL)
Pulmonary	Tachypnea, adventitious sounds, hypoxemia, dyspnea on exertion
Cardiovascular	Murmur, tachycardia
Abdomen	Hepatosplenomegaly more common in ALL
Skin	Petechiae, ecchymoses, frank bleeding, leukemic infiltrates in skin, erythema, tenderness or edema suggest infection
Rectal	Circumanal ulceration, tenderness or erythema suggest infection, abscess or fissure
Musculoskeletal	Myalgias and muscle tenderness may indicate infection. Erythema and diminished or painful range of motion may indicate bleeding into joint. Arthralgias and periarticular joint swelling are common with ALL meningeal leukemic infiltrates.
Central nervous system	Cranial nerve abnormality or paresthesias secondary to leukemic infiltrates more common in ALL. Cerebral bleeding may occur in acute promyelocytic leukemia with disseminated intravascular coagulation.
Constitutional	Fever, fatigue, weight loss, malaise
Hematologic	Signs of bone marrow failure, coagulopathy, hypogammaglobulinemia, disseminated intravascular coagulation

Note. Based on information from Henderson & McArthur, 2002.

chemotherapy or radiation therapy. Occupational exposure to chemicals or ionizing radiation should be noted, as should the presence of symptoms such as headache, visual changes, or neurologic abnormalities that might suggest CNS involvement. Multiple comorbidities, such as cardiovascular disease, diabetes mellitus, renal insufficiency, or pulmonary disorders, may increase the risk of adverse outcomes. Such patients may have more difficulty tolerating intensive chemotherapy and its attendant complications and will require expert general medical management and may benefit from involvement of specialists in cardiology, endocrinology, pulmonology, and internal medicine. Attention also should be paid to prior infections or bleeding episodes and the number of prior transfusions, because these may presage difficulties with recurrent infection or with platelet alloimmunization (National Comprehensive Cancer Network [NCCN], 2005b).

Physical examination should include a thorough neurologic examination to exclude cranial neuropathies or paresthesias that might suggest CNS leukemic involvement, funduscopic examination to assess for retinal hemorrhage, and evaluation for extramedullary evidence of leukemic involvement, including lymphadenopathy and hepatosplenomegaly, or testicular masses. Screening for dental and nutritional problems also should be performed. Comprehensive geriatric assessment is a useful tool for gauging tolerance to treatment, systematically evaluating functional status, and identifying comorbidities and reversible factors that may interfere with cancer treatment, including depression, malnutrition, and suboptimal caregiver support (Balducci, 2003; Chen, Kenefick, Tang, & McCorkle, 2004; Extermann, 2003). The components that should be considered in the initial evaluation of the older adult patient with leukemia or MDS are outlined in Figure 13-3.

- Physical examination and family history
- Dental evaluation
- Viral serologies, including herpes simplex virus, cytomegalovirus, hepatitis, and HIV
- Cardiac status evaluation with multiple-gated acquisition scan or echocardiogram (if starting anthracycline chemotherapy or cardiac disease at baseline)
- Evaluation of pulmonary, renal, and hepatic function
- Leukapheresis if white blood cell count > 100,000 or symptomatic
- Screening for coagulopathy with prothrombin time and partial thromboplastin time, international normalized ratio, and fibrinogen
- Establish central venous access, if aggressive chemotherapy treatment or frequent transfusion support is anticipated
- Human leukocyte antigen (HLA)-typing to ensure availability of HLA-matched platelet transfusion support if platelet refractoriness develops and if it is being considered for possible allogeneic hematopoietic stem cell transplantation
- Comprehensive geriatric assessment, including functional status, comorbidity, socioeconomic issues, nutritional status, polypharmacy, and geriatric syndromes such as falls, incontinence, or delirium
- Nutritional assessment and ongoing follow-up
- Physical and occupational therapy assessment, treatment, and follow-up to optimize functional status and limit functional decline

Figure 13-3. Initial Evaluation of the Older Adult With Leukemia or Myelodysplastic Syndromes

Treatment of Acute Leukemia

Acute leukemia treatment generally is divided into remission induction therapy and postremission consolidation and maintenance therapy (Lechner, Geissler, Jager, Greinix, & Kalhs, 1999). The goal of remission induction is to achieve rapid clearing of leukemia cells from the peripheral blood with subsequent marrow aplasia. However, a substantial burden of leukemia cells can persist undetected (i.e., minimal residual disease), leading to relapse within a few weeks or months if no further postremission therapy is given. Postremission therapy is designed to eradicate these residual leukemic cells following remission induction chemotherapy.

Postremission therapy may be classified into consolidation, intensification, and maintenance. In consolidation, one or two courses of additional therapy are given using the same agents and same dose intensity as that used for initial induction. With intensification, different drugs, a different schedule, and higher dose intensity are used when compared with initial induction. Early intensification is given immediately following remission induction, whereas late intensification is given several months after remission induction. Maintenance treatment is given following consolidation or intensification and refers to intermittent treatment for a prolonged period of time using lower doses of either the same agents as those used in induction or other agents.

Acute Myeloid Leukemia

The most commonly used remission induction regimens for AML consist of combination chemotherapy with cytarabine and an anthracycline (Lowenberg, 2001; NCCN, 2005a; Tallman, Gilliland, & Rowe, in press). Another common induction strategy is high-dose cytarabine using cytarabine 1–3 g/m^2 every 12 hours for 6 days, plus anthracycline on days 1, 2, and 3. With good supportive care, older adults are able to withstand induction chemotherapy (Goldstone et al., 2001; Vey et al., 2004), and a small subset of older adult patients with AML who have favorable cytogenetics, a good functional status, and limited comorbidity will derive benefit from intensive chemotherapy (Buchner et al., 2001; Estey, 2000a; Ferrara, 2004; Gupta et al., 2005; Latagliata et al., 1999; Rowe, 2000; Sekeres & Stone, 2002; Vey et al.; Yoshida et al., 2001).

Following induction, postremission therapy is required to prevent disease relapse; however, many older adults in complete remission following induction are not good candidates for further postremission therapy, because of either prior medical problems or complications from the induction treatment (Seiter, 2002). The choice of consolidation therapy should be based on age and cytogenetic features, as well as functional status, performance status, and comorbidities (Sekeres & Stone, 2002; Winton & Langston, 2004). Considerable uncertainty and controversy remain about which approach to postremission therapy is preferable (Giles, Estey, & O'Brien, 2003; Lichtman & Rowe, 2004; Pinto, Zagonel, & Ferrara, 2001; Tallman, 2005; Wedding et al., 2004). Participation in a clinical trial of a new agent represents a potential postremission treatment option for selected patients (Schiffer, 2002; Stone, 2002; Tallman, 2005; Winton & Langston). In some situations (patients who have a suitable donor, are younger than 60–70 years, and have intermediate risk or high-risk cytogenetic features), autologous or allogeneic hematopoietic stem cell transplantation, including the possibility of a nonmyeloablative allogeneic stem cell transplant, may be included in the plan for consolidation therapy (Bertz, Potthoff, & Finke, 2003). A sample treatment regimen for a patient with AML is depicted in Table 13-7.

Patients who fail to achieve remission with one cycle of high-dose cytarabine or two cycles of standard-dose cytarabine are considered to have primary induction failure or refractory disease. If they are eligible to participate in a trial of hematopoietic stem cell transplantation and have a related or unrelated donor identified, they should be considered immediately for a related or a matched unrelated allogeneic stem cell transplant because a long-term disease-free survival rate of 25%–30% still can be achieved using stem cell transplant as a salvage therapy. For older adults with primary induction failure, treatment with an investigational or molecularly targeted agent (see Table 13-8), gemtuzumab ozogamicin (the toxin conjugated anti-CD33 monoclonal antibody) (Mylotarg®, Wyeth, Philadelphia, PA), low-dose

Table 13-7. Sample Treatment Regimen for Acute Myeloid Leukemia

	Induction			
	Drug	**Dosage**	**Administration**	**Duration**
	Cytarabine	100–200 mg/m^2	Continuous IV infusion	Days 1–7
+	Daunorubicin	45 mg/m^2	IV	Days 1–3
OR	Idarubicin	12 mg/m^2	IV	Days 1–3
OR	Mitoxantrone	12 mg/m^2	IV	Days 1–3
	Postremission			
	Drug	**Dosage**	**Administration**	**Length**
	Cytarabine	3 g/m^2 q 12 hours	IV over 3 hours	Days 1, 3, 5 (total 6 doses)
OR	Cytarabine	10 mg/m^2	Continuous IV infusion	Days 1–5
OR	Participation in a clinical trial of a new therapeutic agent			

Note. Based on information from National Comprehensive Cancer Network, 2005a; Tallman, 2001.

chemotherapy with drugs such as hydroxyurea or low-dose cytarabine, or supportive care all represent viable treatment options (Nabhan et al., 2005; Rathnasabapathy & Lancet, 2003; Rowe, 2000; Tallman, 2005; Tallman et al., in press). For patients who relapse following initial induction therapy, options for further treatment include treatment with an investigational protocol or with one of the novel molecularly targeted therapies that are under development, including agents that modulate multidrug resistance, angiogenesis inhibitors, and signal transduction inhibitors (see Table 13-8). Patients with a first complete remission lasting longer than 12 months may benefit from intensive salvage chemotherapy (Sekeres & Stone, 2002).

High-dose chemotherapy followed by autologous or allogeneic stem cell transplantation may represent a treatment option for selected older adults, although its role is undefined mainly because of exclusion of these patients from such trials (Rathnasabapathy & Lancet, 2003). Nonmyeloablative stem cell transplant regimens, which are believed to induce less treatment-related toxicity and can capitalize on the graft-versus-leukemia effect (Giralt et al., 1997), are being studied in an effort to expand the role of hematopoietic stem cell transplantation in the treatment of leukemia in the older adult (Bertz et al., 2003; Buchner et al., 2001; Maris et al., 2003).

Acute Promyelocytic Leukemia

For patients with acute promyelocytic leukemia (APL) (FAB M-3 AML; WHO acute promyelocytic leukemia), remission induction is achieved using all-trans-retinoic acid (ATRA) and an anthracycline (NCCN, 2005a; Randolph, 2000; Sanz et al., 2004; Tallman et al., in press). Some APL induction regimens also include cytarabine. This usually is

Table 13-8. New Therapeutics in the Treatment of Adult Acute Leukemia and Myelodysplastic Syndromes*

Molecular Target/Proposed Mechanism of Action**	Agent
Cells expressing CD33	Monoclonal antibody therapy with gemtuzumab ozogamicin (Mylotarg®)
Inhibit multidrug resistance P-glycoprotein (MDR-1/PGP)	Cyclosporine, PSC 833
Hypomethylating agent (induces reactivation of tumor suppressor genes silenced by leukemia)	5-azacitadine 5-aza-2'-deoxycytidine
Promote terminal differentiation	All-trans-retinoic acid (ATRA), topotecan (CPT-11), Bryostatin-1, TLK 199
Promote apoptosis (cell death)	*bcl-2* antisense oligonucleotide
Inhibit angiogenesis	Thalidomide, CC 5013, arsenic trioxide, bevacizumab
Inhibit Flt-3 tyrosine kinase	SU 5416, PKC 412, SU 11248, MLN518
Proteasome inhibitor	PSC 341 (Bortezomib®)
Histone deacetylase enzyme inhibitor	LAQ824, depsipeptide
Inhibition of tyrosine kinase (inhibits proliferation of cells containing *bcr-abl*)	BMS-354825
Farnesyltransferase inhibitors (block signaling pathways preventing cellular changes associated with malignant cell growth)	R115777 (Zarnestra®)
Cell cycle signal regulators (cyclin dependent kinase inhibitors)	Flavopiridol
New cytotoxic agents	Troxacitabine, clofarabine

*Information about active clinical trials can be obtained through www.cancer.gov/clinicaltrials
**Most of these drugs have multiple modes of action, and the headings used in this table are arbitrary and do not assume knowledge of the exact mechanisms of action, which for some of the agents described remains largely unknown.

Note. Based on information from Berman, 2000; Cortes & Kantarjian, 2000; Estey, 2000b; Faderl et al., 2005; Giles, 2002; Hoelzer & Gokbuget, 2000; Karp, 1998; Lancet & Karp, 2003; Levis, 2005; Lichtman & Rowe, 2004; List, 2002, 2004; Lowenberg, 2001; Nabhan et al., 2005; Radich & Sievers, 2000; Rathnasabapathy & Lancet, 2003; Ravandi et al., 2004; Sekeres & Stone, 2002; Stone, 1999; Tallman, 2005; Tallman et al., in press; Thomas et al., 2003; Wendtner et al., 2004.

followed by consolidation with two to three courses of cytarabine and an anthracycline. Maintenance therapy with ATRA plus a chemotherapy agent (such as mercaptopurine or methotrexate) is subsequently required. Patients receiving ATRA must be monitored closely for the development of a unique complication of ATRA called retinoic acid syndrome. This syndrome is characterized by pulmonary infiltrates, pleural effusion, weight gain, and fever. It is effectively managed by discontinuing ATRA therapy and administering dexamethasone (De Botton et al., 1998; Larson & Tallman, 2003).

For patients who fail to achieve a remission or who relapse early, arsenic trioxide can induce remission in approximately 80% of patients with relapsed and refractory APL. Patients who relapse 6–12 months or more following initial remission induction therapy may be reinduced with ATRA, plus an anthracycline and cytarabine. Following this, individuals younger than 60 years of age should be considered for consolidation with either allogeneic or autologous transplantation (NCCN, 2005a).

Acute Lymphocytic Leukemia

As illustrated in Table 13-9, the treatment of ALL generally is divided into four phases, with the total duration of therapy usually lasting two to three years.

No standard ALL regimen exists, and several are found in the literature (Hoelzer & Gokbuget, 2005; Hoelzer & Seipelt, 2000; NCCN, 2005a). A sample treatment regimen for ALL in the adult is depicted in Table 13-10. For patients who are younger, have high-risk disease features (e.g., Philadelphia chromosome positive ALL), and have a matched related or unrelated donor, allogeneic stem cell transplantation may be included in the recommendations for postremission therapy. Imatinib mesylate, given either for induction and consolidation or as consolidation following conventional induction, is a new therapeutic option for the substantial proportion of adult patients who have Philadelphia chromosome–positive ALL (Hoelzer & Gokbuget, 2005). Other options for treatment of ALL in the older adult include rituximab and alemtuzumab (Hoelzer & Gokbuget, 2005; Lynn, Williams, Sickler, & Burgess, 2003).

The prognostic significance and management of relapse of ALL are influenced by the duration of the first remission, the intensity of the initial regimen used, and

---

Table 13-9. Phases of Acute Lymphoid Leukemia Treatment

Phase	Treatment
Remission induction	Four- to five-drug regimen: • Anthracycline • Cyclophosphamide • L-asparaginase • Vincristine • Prednisone
Central nervous system prophylaxis	Intrathecal chemotherapy with methotrexate and/or cytarabine +/– craniospinal irradiation
Consolidation and intensification	Four- to five-drug regimen: • Cyclophosphamide • 6-mercaptopurine • L-asparaginase • Vincristine • Cytarabine (high dose) • Anthracycline
Maintenance	Three- to four-drug regimen given on monthly cycle for two years: • Vincristine (IV) • Prednisone (po) • Methotrexate (po) • 6-mercaptopurine (po)

Note. Based on information from Scheinberg et al., 2001.

Table 13-10. Sample Treatment Regimen for Adult Acute Lymphoblastic Leukemia

Treatment	Dosage	Administration	Duration
Induction			
Vincristine	2 mg	IV	Days 1, 8, 15, 22
Prednisone	60 mg/m²/day	IV	Days 1–21 (Days 1–7 if > 60 years old)
Daunorubicin	45 mg/m²	IV	Days 1, 2, 3
Cyclophosphamide	1,200 mg/m²	IV	Day 1
L-asparaginase	6,000 units/m²	SQ/IV/IM	Days 5, 8, 11, 15, 18, 22
Intensification (Two courses, each 28 days)			
IT methotrexate	15 mg	IT	Day 1
Cyclophosphamide	1,000 mg/m²	IV	Day 1
6-mercaptopurine	60 mg/m²	po	Days 1–14
Cytarabine	75 mg/m²/day	SQ	Days 1–4, 8–11
Vincristine	2 mg	IV	Days 15, 22
L-asparaginase	6,000 units/m²	SQ/IV/IM	Days 5, 18, 22, 25
Central Nervous System Prophylaxis			
Cranial irradiation	2,400 cGy	12 fractions	Three weeks
Intrathecal methotrexate	15 mg	IT	Days 1, 8, 15, 22, 29
6-mercaptopurine	60 mg	po	Days 1–70
Late Intensification			
Similar to intensification			
Maintenance (Four-week cycles; cycle generally continued to provide a total of 104 weeks of therapy)			
Vincristine	2 mg	IV	Day 1 of each month
Prednisone	60 mg/m²	po	Days 1–5 of each month
Methotrexate	20 mg/m²	po	Days 1, 8, 15, 22
6-mercaptopurine	60 mg/m²	po	Days 1–28

IM—intramuscular; IT—intrathecal; IV—intravenous; po—oral; SQ—subcutaneous

Note. Based on information from Scheinberg et al., 2001.

the site of relapse (i.e., systemic relapse or isolated extramedullary relapse in the CNS or testes). All patients who relapse require reinitiation of CNS-directed therapy in addition to systemic therapy. In addition, patients with isolated testicular relapse require testicular irradiation.

Patient Monitoring During Therapy

During therapy, patients are monitored with a CBC and relevant chemistries, which may include liver function tests; measures to detect tumor lysis such as uric acid, potassium, calcium, magnesium, and phosphorus levels; and kidney function tests, including blood urea nitrogen and creatinine. A bone marrow aspirate and biopsy should be performed 14–21 days after the start of treatment to determine whether the marrow has become profoundly hypocellular and the percentage of blasts has been reduced to less than 5%. Patients who still have more than 5% blasts in the bone marrow require reinduction or progression to a high-dose therapy maneuver with stem cell transplantation. Patients should be off granulocyte–colony-stimulating factors (G-CSFs) for at least seven days before obtaining the bone marrow aspirate and biopsy to document remission (NCCN, 2005a). The criteria for defining a complete and partial response to therapy for acute leukemia are depicted in Figure 13-4.

Complete Response
Absolute neutrophil count > 1,500/µl and platelets > 100,000/µl, no leukemic blasts in peripheral blood, and < 5% blasts in bone marrow, with > 15% normal erythropoiesis and > 25% granulopoiesis and a bone marrow cellularity of > 20%; no evidence of organ involvement

Partial Response
6%–25% blasts in bone marrow, with > 10% normal erythropoiesis and > 25% normal granulopoiesis

---

Figure 13-4. Response Criteria in Acute Leukemia

Note. Based on information from Scheinberg et al., 2001.

Once the patient has achieved a remission, ongoing monitoring with cytogenetics (if there is a cytogenetic abnormality) or other methods to detect minimal residual disease, such as molecular diagnostics using PCR or FISH techniques, should be used. The patient's response to treatment and tolerance of treated side effects is monitored through routine history and physical examination.

Supportive Nursing Care of the Patient Undergoing Treatment for Acute Leukemia

Supportive care measures for the patient with an acute leukemia begin at the time of diagnosis and are outlined in Figure 13-5. Significant controversies exist about the initiation of prophylactic antimicrobial therapy (NCCN, 2004; Yoshida & Ohno, 2004). Institutional protocols vary; however, at many institutions, prophylaxis of *Pneumocystis carinii* pneumonia (PCP) with cotrimoxazole; herpes simplex virus prophylaxis with valacyclovir, famciclovir, or acyclovir; and fungal prophylaxis with fluconazole, voriconazole, or amphotericin B generally are commenced (Gojo, Sarkodee-Adoo, Hakimian, Merz, & Karp, 2003). Steroid eye drops must be given with high-dose cytosine arabinoside treatment to prevent the development of conjunctivitis. Patients

---

- Hydration and allopurinol to prevent uric acid deposition in the kidney
- Prophylactic antimicrobials
- Steroid eye drops during treatment and for 24 hours following completion of high-dose cytosine arabinoside
- Cytokine support with erythropoietin, granulocyte–colony-stimulating factor, and granulocyte macrophage–colony-stimulating factor
- Blood products irradiated and leukoreduced

Figure 13-5. Supportive Care Measures for Patients With Acute Leukemia

---

Note. Based on information from Gojo et al., 2003; Murphy-Ende & Chernecky, 2002; NCCN, 2005a; Viele, 2003.

receiving high-dose cytosine arabinoside therapy, particularly those with impaired renal function or those older than 60 years of age, are at risk for cerebellar toxicity. Neurologic assessment, including evaluation for nystagmus, dysmetria, slurred speech, and impairment in the classic tests of cerebellar function, including Romberg, tandem gait, finger-to-nose and heel-to-shin tests, should be performed before each dose of cytosine arabinoside (Lundquist & Holmes, 1993; NCCN, 2005a). Patients with a new abnormality must have a cytosine arabinoside dose reduction and should not receive high-dose cytosine arabinoside as part of any subsequent therapy (Smith, Damon, Rugo, Ries, & Linker, 1997).

Support with G-CSF or granulocyte macrophage–colony-stimulating factor (GM-CSF) may permit optimal dose intensity by shortening the duration of severe neutropenia and allowing adherence to scheduled treatments, particularly in the older adult with acute leukemia (Buchner, 1998; Hood, 2003; NCCN, 2005a). Hematopoietic growth factors also may reduce mortality and infections in older adult patients with AML and promote a higher rate of remission and prolonged survival (Buchner; Hiddemann et al., 1999; Rowe, 2000).

Knowledge of the expected disease and treatment-related side effects in the older adult patient with leukemia or MDS allows the nurse to anticipate problems in this high-risk population. Neutropenia, thrombocytopenia, anemia, oral complications, electrolyte imbalances, and oncologic emergencies such as DIC, leukostasis, retinoic-acid syndrome, and tumor lysis syndrome require astute nursing assessment and timely management (Avvisati & Tallman, 2003; Eilers, 2004; Gojo et al., 2003; Mackey & Klemm, 2000; Murphy-Ende & Chernecky, 2002; Viele, 2003). Patients with leukemia or MDS also are at risk for the development of infection or bleeding. A thorough head-to-toe physical examination at regular intervals permits the earliest detection of evidence of infection or bleeding.

Patient and family education regarding diagnosis, treatment, and self-care strategies to prevent and manage disease and treatment side effects both in the hospital and at home is a crucial component of nursing care of the older adult with leukemia or MDS. Patients require information about the basic physiology of the bone marrow and explanations concerning the function of red blood cells, white blood cells, and platelets. Several Web sites offer an array of information regarding the pathophysiology, treatment, and supportive management of leukemia or MDS and may be very helpful in allowing patients and their families to efficiently gather up-to-date information (see Figure 13-6).

As the treatment plan is developed, an opportunity should be provided to both patients and family members to clarify with the team the goals of therapy, the expected side effects of treatment, and the potential benefits, risks, and alternatives of treatment

---

American Cancer Society: www.cancer.org
Cancer Consultants: http://patient.cancerconsultants.com
National Cancer Institute: www.cancer.gov/cancer_information/cancer_type/leukemia
Leukemia and Lymphoma Society: www.leukemia-lymphoma.org
Leukemia and Lymphoma Society of Canada: www.leukemia.ca
Leukemia Research Fund: www.lrf.org.uk/en/1/information.html
Medline Plus: www.nlm.nih.gov/medlineplus
National Comprehensive Cancer Network: www.nccn.org/patients/default.asp

---

Figure 13-6. Helpful Web Sites for Patient and Family Information

in terms of short- and long-term outcomes (Sekeres et al., 2004). Arrangements for family caregiving also should be addressed, because induction and consolidation chemotherapy treatments often require frequent hospital and clinic visits and adherence to a complex regimen of supportive care medications. The decision-making process for the older adult with leukemia or MDS is challenging and must balance issues of mortality, anticipated benefits of tolerance for aggressive therapy, and quality of life. A climate of trust, mutual respect, shared humanity, dialogue, and an understanding of the meaning of hope, autonomy, and control for the older adult are key components of healthcare team support in decision making (Shannon-Dorcy & Wolfe, 2003). Treatment planning discussions also should include an opportunity for patients and those important to them in their healthcare decision making to exchange information with the clinical team regarding the patient's wishes related to advanced cardiac life support. Such discussions also should include opportunities for the treatment team to clarify that "do not resuscitate" or "do not intubate" decisions are entirely consistent with full support of the patient during periods of pancytopenia and other complications that may occur following remission induction therapy.

New Strategies/Novel Targets for the Treatment of Acute Leukemia in the Older Adult

With increased understanding of the molecular events occurring during the development of acute leukemia, a number of new agents for the treatment of acute leukemia and MDS have emerged, some with novel molecular targets. Several of these new strategies are summarized in Table 13-8 and include (a) agents that target the immediate consequences of mutational events leading to acute leukemia, such as mutated FLT3 or multidrug resistance; (b) agents that target the adaptive nonmutational changes a leukemic cell must make to survive given the initial mutational event (e.g., increased *bcl-2* expression); and (c) agents that target cell surface antigens that distinguish leukemia cells from the normal hematopoietic stem cell (e.g., CD33+) (Appelbaum, 2003; Levis, 2005; List, 2004; Tallman et al., in press). The precise role of these novel agents, whether alone or in combination with conventional approaches to remission, induction, and maintenance therapy, requires further research (Larson, 2003; Stone, 2003). Clinical trials are ongoing to demonstrate their effectiveness and to define their role in the optimum treatment of the older adult with acute leukemia (Giles, 2002; Tallman et al.).

Treatment of Chronic Leukemia

Myeloid Leukemia

Interferon-alpha in combination with chemotherapy or, if eligible, allogeneic hematopoietic stem cell transplantation were the mainstays of therapy for CML for many years. More recently, a new targeted therapy, imatinib mesylate, has changed the management of CML in chronic or accelerated phase, particularly for those patients for whom allogeneic stem cell transplantation is not an option (Mughal & Goldman, 2004). Imatinib mesylate is a protein tyrosine kinase inhibitor that targets the abnormal tyrosine kinase protein, *bcr-abl,* which is created by the Philadelphia chromosome abnormality in CML. The *bcr-abl* oncoprotein activates multiple signal transduction pathways shared by many cell growth factors and promotes a number of cellular changes that contribute to the survival and proliferation of the CML cell, including reduced apoptosis (cell death), cell cycle dysregulation, and enhanced cellular proliferation (Gale, 2003). Imatinib inhibits cellular growth and proliferation and induces apoptosis in *bcr-abl*–positive CML cells.

The recommended dose of imatinib mesylate is 400 mg by mouth daily with food for patients in chronic phase and 600 mg by mouth daily for patients in accelerated phase or blast crisis. Doses of up to 800 mg/day in a divided dose have been administered to patients who do not enter a cytogenetic remission when treated at lower doses and to those who acquire resistance to imatinib (Cortes et al., 2003). Toxicities include myelosuppression, nausea, edema/fluid retention (including periorbital edema), fatigue, arthralgias, myalgias, diarrhea, hepatotoxicity, and skin rashes (Guilhot, 2004; Stone, 2004). Edema may be more common in older adults receiving imatinib mesylate. Key nursing responsibilities with the patient receiving imatinib include implementing interventions to maximize symptom relief; assess, prevent, and manage side effects; and provide education about medication precautions as effective self-management (Ault, Kaled, & Rios, 2003; Deininger, O'Brien, Ford, & Druker, 2003; Griffin, Amand, & Demetri, 2005; Hensley & Ford, 2003; Rule, O'Brien, & Crossman, 2002; Stull, 2003).

Because imatinib mesylate is metabolized in the liver via the cytochrome P450 system, drug-drug interactions can be significant (Breed, 2003). Concurrent administration with phenytoin can result in lower plasma levels of imatinib mesylate, whereas concurrent administration with cyclosporine, tacrolimus, fluconazole, itraconazole, azithromycin, erythromycin, and the antiretrovirals can result in higher plasma imatinib levels (Griffin et al., 2005). When administered concurrently with warfarin, close monitoring of the international normalized ratio is recommended. Coadministration with grapefruit juice is contraindicated because it is a potent inhibitor of CYP3A4 and may elevate plasma levels of imatinib mesylate. Although imatinib and its metabolites are not significantly excreted by the kidneys, plasma clearance of imatinib is decreased with worsening renal dysfunction (Guilhot, 2004). Therefore, careful monitoring is required when administering imatinib to patients with impaired renal function.

The response to treatment with imatinib is monitored with peripheral blood counts, cytogenetic analysis, and molecular diagnostics using quantitative PCR for *bcr-abl* messenger RNA (Goldman, 2004; O'Brien, 2004). More than 95% of patients in chronic phase CML achieve a complete hematologic response, and approximately 55% of these achieve a cytogenetic response (disappearance of the Philadelphia chromosome), although, in most cases, the *bcr-abl* transcript still is detectable by molecular diagnostic techniques such as FISH and PCR. A further challenge is the fact that some patients develop resistance to imatinib after an initial response (Druker, 2004). Several large-scale, prospective, randomized phase III trials of imatinib mesylate are ongoing, and although the results have not matured sufficiently to determine whether the imatinib-treated cohort experiences improved overall survival, progression-free survival was better in the imatinib-treated cohort when compared with a cohort treated with interferon-alpha and a cohort treated with cytarabine (O'Brien et al., 2003). Furthermore, no comparison has been made yet between treatment with imatinib mesylate and nonmyeloablative allogeneic hematopoietic stem cell transplantation. However, particularly for the older adult with CML who may not be a candidate for allogeneic hematopoietic stem cell transplantation, imatinib mesylate offers a treatment option for long-term disease control that generally is well tolerated (Stone, 2004). In patients who have achieved a good response, continued study is needed to answer the further questions regarding the duration of imatinib mesylate therapy (Cortes, O'Brien, & Kantarjian, 2004; Goldman).

B-Cell Chronic Lymphoid Leukemia

Patients with Binet stage A or Rai stages 0, I, or II usually are observed without treatment. New approaches to identifying patients with higher risk of disease progression and early mortality, such as zeta-associated protein-70 (ZAP-70) overexpression, may help in defining a subset of patients who would benefit from earlier treatment (Shanafelt & Call, 2004). Indications for the initiation of treatment include disease-related symptoms, the development of anemia, thrombocytopenia, autoimmune hemolysis or autoimmune thrombocytopenia, progressive splenomegaly, progressive bulky lymphadenopathy, or frequent bacterial infections (Pangalis et al., 2002; Spiers, 1998).

Chemotherapy agents used in the treatment of B-CLL include alkylating agents (CCNU/BCNU, busulfan, chlorambucil, cyclophosphamide), either as single agents or in combination with prednisone, doxorubicin, melphalan, or cytarabine. The inclusion of vincristine in a multiagent regimen for CLL should be avoided in the older adult because it has not shown effectiveness as a single agent and may cause unacceptable problems with peripheral neuropathy and constipation (Spiers, 1998). The purine analogs (pentostatin, fludarabine, and cladribine), alone or in combination with cyclophosphamide and rituximab, substantially improve survival and quality of life in patients with relapsed and refractory B-CLL (Hillmen, 2004; Nabhan, Gartenhaus, & Tallman, 2004). Local irradiation of a symptomatic lymph node mass or an enlarged spleen may provide acceptable palliation. Splenectomy also may be considered. Other therapies that may be used to treat CLL include monoclonal antibodies such as alemtuzumab (Campath-1H), rituximab, and other novel monoclonals in development, such as anti-CD23 monoclonal antibody (Liu & O'Brien, 2004; Lundin & Osterborg, 2004; Lynn et al., 2003) and new small molecules such as flavopyridole that inhibit the activity of cyclin-dependent kinases (Decker, Hipp, Hahntow, Schneller, & Peschel, 2004; Pangalis et al., 2002; Zhai, Senderowicz, Sausville, & Figg, 2002) or histone deacetylase enzyme-inhibiting agents such as depsipeptide (Wendtner, Eichorst, & Hallek, 2004), thus regulating cell proliferation and apoptosis (Weiss, 2001).

Patients with CLL are at risk for a number of disease-related complications, including infections, autoimmune disease, and transformation to large B-cell non-Hodgkin lymphoma (Shanafelt & Call, 2004). Infections in patients with CLL should be investigated and treated aggressively because patients with CLL have an increased incidence of bacterial, fungal, and viral infections because of both hypogammaglobulinemia and the neutropenia and deficiencies in T-lymphocyte function associated with the agents used to treat CLL (Stull, 2003). Fungal and PCP prophylaxis and monitoring for cytomegalovirus reactivation should be considered for patients receiving treatment with purine analogs or alemtuzumab because these produce profound deficits in T-lymphocyte function. Immunoglobulin replacement therapy is indicated for patients with hypogammaglobulinemia and a history of repeated infections (Pangalis et al., 2002). Autoimmune hemolytic anemia and idiopathic thrombocytopenia purpura (ITP) occur in 4%–11% and 2%–4%, respectively, in patients with CLL (Diehl & Ketchum, 1998). A bone marrow biopsy is helpful in evaluating anemia and distinguishing hemolytic anemia from progressive CLL. Treatment of autoimmune hemolytic anemia and ITP may include corticosteroids, gammaglobulin, rituximab, and splenectomy. Chemotherapy treatment of CLL also may help to treat these autoimmune complications.

Myelodysplastic Syndromes

Although allogeneic hematopoietic stem cell transplantation is the treatment of choice in younger patients with MDS, intensive chemotherapy treatment of MDS generally is ineffective and contraindicated in the older individual (Reilly, 1998). Supportive care, with transfusion of red cells and platelets combined with broad-spectrum antibiotics, remains the cornerstone of therapy for the older adult with MDS. Routine platelet transfusion support to treat chronic persistent thrombocytopenia leads to early platelet refractoriness and future problems in the management of bleeding. Platelet transfusions generally are indicated for episodes of acute hemorrhage or as prophylaxis prior to surgery or following chemotherapy (NCCN, 2005b). Infections in patients with MDS should be treated aggressively, and because dental and perirectal infections are particularly common, careful attention should be paid to preventive dental care and to proper bowel function and the avoidance of rectal fissures or hemorrhoidal inflammation (Erban, 1995). Vaccination of patients against pneumonoccocal pneumonia and influenza also is recommended (Erban).

In patients who show evidence of progressive MDS, low-dose chemotherapy, such as daily subcutaneous cytosine arabinoside ($20 \, mg/m^2$), for two to three weeks at a time or a combination of four days a week of oral 6-thioguanine ($25–50 \, mg/m^2$) and subcutaneous cytosine arabinoside ($70 \, mg/m^2$) once a week may help to control the disease (Saba, 2001). Oral etoposide, 6-mercaptopurine, and 6-thioguanine all can be effective agents in controlling peripheral leukocytosis (Saba, 2001). The combination of G-CSF and erythropoietin also may be effective, producing a well-tolerated and durable disease control in approximately one-third of patients with MDS subtypes, refractory anemia, refractory anemia with ringed sideroblasts, and refractory anemia with excess blasts (Pisani & Rainaldi, 2001). Efforts are under way to explore the effectiveness of therapies such as thalidomide, amifostine, or immunosuppressive therapy with antithymocyte globulin or cyclosporine A (List, 2002). Hypomethylating agents that induce hematopoietic progenitor cell differentiation, such as decitabine and 5-azacytidine, also are being studied in MDS, and preliminary results of phase I and II trials indicate that this class of agents may prolong survival, delay transformation to AML, and improve quality of life when compared with supportive care alone (Leone, Teofili, Voso, & Lubbert, 2002). Farnesyl transferase inhibitors such as tipifarnib (R115777) (Karp & Lancet, 2004), angiogenesis-inhibiting agents such as bevacizumab (SU5416), and thalidomide analogs such as CC-5013 are in clinical trials and show initial promise in patients with MDS (Langston, Walling, & Winton, 2004; List, 2002).

Post-Treatment Surveillance

Following the conclusion of therapy, all patients with an acute or chronic leukemia or MDS require close continued follow-up. The follow-up plan should consider the underlying disease, the nature of the prior therapy, the patient's response to therapy, and the expected timing and pattern of disease relapse, including measures for the evaluation of minimal residual disease. History and physical examination at regular intervals, together with laboratory evaluations to include CBC with differential, serum chemistries, and interval evaluation with bone marrow aspirate and biopsy to include cytogenetics and molecular diagnostics, offer an opportunity for the earliest detection of disease relapse. Patients and their families should be counseled on signs of relapse, and oncology providers must remain available for interim visits in the event of patient concerns. Follow-up from oncology providers at regular intervals also allows for the identification of late treatment complications, including atypical infections, oral complications, thyroid dysfunction, osteoporosis, and second malignancies (Baker et al., 2004).

Case Study

John O is a 66-year-old Caucasian male who presents to the family physician with a one-month history of low-grade fever, fatigue, mild weight loss, nausea, easy bruising, pallor, and shortness of breath. CBC reveals pancytopenia, with a WBC of 2.2 x 10^9/L, hemoglobin 8.7 g/dl, hematocrit 23.4%, platelets 33,000/mm^3, and 32% peripheral blasts on differential. An antecedent CBC done three months earlier as part of routine care showed a WBC of 6.8 x 10^9/L, hemoglobin of 15 g/dl, platelet count of 309,000/mm^3, and a normal differential. Physical examination is within expected limits, except for pallor, gingival bleeding, diffuse ecchymoses, and oral thrush.

Bone marrow aspirate and biopsy are performed, which demonstrate AML with 82% blasts and morphology suggestive of monocytic origin. Phenotyping of leukemic blasts demonstrates positivity for CD13, CD14, CD33, and CD34. Molecular diagnostics, including FISH and Southern Blot, reveal an 11q23 rearrangement. The FAB diagnostic classification is M-4, myelomonocytic leukemia; the WHO classification is AML with recurrent cytogenetic translocations. The diagnosis of AML M-4 is confirmed, and after considering his options for treatment, John has elected induction chemotherapy with idarubicin and cytosine arabinoside. Prior to chemotherapy, he undergoes a baseline multiple-gated acquisition scan to establish his ejection fraction (58%), and a double-lumen tunneled central venous catheter is placed. Human leukocyte antigen (HLA)-typing is performed in preparation for possible nonmyeloablative allogeneic hematopoietic stem cell transplantation; however, ultimately, John's two sisters were matched with him at only 4/6 HLA loci. Hydration is commenced with normal saline solution. Infection prophylaxis against PCP is initiated with trimethoprim-sulfamethoxazole three times a week. Induction chemotherapy with cytosine arabinoside 200 mg/m^2 by continuous IV infusion for seven consecutive days plus idarubicin 12 mg/m^2 IV for three consecutive days is administered.

The patient tolerates treatment with induction therapy fairly well, although his six-week hospital course is complicated by cytosine arabinoside cerebellar dysfunction (slurred speech and nystagmus requiring dose reduction of cytosine arabinoside), febrile neutropenia, severe epistaxis requiring nasal packing, grade III mucositis requiring narcotics and initiation of total parenteral nutrition, a 20-pound weight loss, as well as functional decline and diminished activity tolerance. He makes a slow recovery from these complications and, ultimately, is able to be discharged home by day +41 following remission induction. Bone marrow aspirate and biopsy at the time of count recovery at day +29 following induction therapy demonstrates tri-lineage hematopoiesis and no morphologic evidence of residual leukemia. FISH techniques continue to demonstrate the 11q23 rearrangement.

After considering the options for consolidation therapy, John elects consolidation treatment with Mylotarg. He tolerates treatment with Mylotarg well, although each course of therapy is complicated by deep cytopenias requiring transfusion support with platelets and packed cells and transient transaminitis and mild hyperbilirubinemia that resolve without intervention. John is able to be maintained as an outpatient, and although weakened by continued therapy, he is able to remain at home. Home physical therapy is helpful in improving his physical function, exercise tolerance, and independence in activities of daily living.

Bone marrow biopsies obtained on a monthly basis show continued remission morphologically, although molecular studies still show evidence of the 11q23 cytogenetic abnormality. After completing three cycles of Mylotarg consolidation therapy, John elects to participate in a phase II clinical trial of the farnesyl transferase–inhibiting agent R115777 for maintenance therapy. He tolerates this investigational treatment well and continues on therapy for nearly eight months. He undergoes evaluation with CBC and serum chemistries every two weeks, and a bone marrow biopsy is performed every other month. Although his blood counts are low, he experiences no intercurrent infections and no need for transfusion support.

Eleven months after initial diagnosis, John presents with cough, fever, and rigors. CBC demonstrates neutropenia, with an absolute neutrophil count of $800/mm^3$, and a chest CT demonstrates bilateral infiltrates. Broad-spectrum antimicrobial coverage is initiated. Bone marrow aspirate and biopsy confirm the presence of more than 25% blasts, and fungal cultures obtained during bronchoscopy reveal *Aspergillus fumigatus*. Immediate treatment with a liposomal amphotericin formulation is commenced. Options for further treatment offered to John include retreatment with Mylotarg or participation in another clinical trial. However, after discussions with his wife and daughter, John elects supportive treatment only, although he continues with daily liposomal amphotericin administered at home and requires intermittent transfusion support with platelets for symptomatic bleeding. John is discharged home, and hospice support is provided via a prehospice bridge program (a program provided by a hospice in collaboration with a home health agency that provides pain and symptom management as well as emotional support during a period when a patient with a life-limiting condition still may be pursuing active treatment). John dies peacefully in the company of his family approximately 10 days after discharge from the hospital.

Conclusion

The optimal treatment approach for leukemia or MDS in the older adult patient and the impact of the unique biology of these diseases in the older adult require further research (Schiffer, 2002). Although advances in supportive care have helped to make even intensive chemotherapy regimens more tolerable in older patients, drug resistance remains the critical impediment. A higher frequency of unfavorable biologic and prognostic factors, rather than age per se, is the major contributor to the inferior prognosis for the older adult with leukemia (Pinto et al., 2001). Advances in the treatment of this group of diseases will emerge from the development of new agents with better antileukemic effect and from improved understanding of the most rational approach to selecting, combining, and sequencing those new therapies to create a tailored treatment plan that is individualized to the disease biology, functional status, physiologic reserve, and preferences of the individual patient.

Nurses have an essential role in the care of the older adult with leukemia or MDS, particularly in relation to providing comprehensive education about diagnosis and treatment and support through the decision-making process. An important complement to the delivery of chemotherapy or investigational drug therapies for leukemia and MDS are supportive nursing care measures to prevent, promptly detect, and treat complications such as infection, anemia, and bleeding, symptoms such as fatigue, mucositis, nausea, nutritional compromise, fatigue, and depression and to promote optimal functional status. Ongoing emotional support of patients and family members throughout the process of diagnosis, treatment, and recovery or end-of-life care can promote a sense of control, autonomy, and, ultimately, hope in the face of fear and uncertainty.

References

Appelbaum, F.R. (2003). New targets for therapy in acute myeloid leukemia. *Leukemia, 17,* 492–495.

Appelbaum, F.R. (2005, Spring). Impact of age on the biology of acute leukemia. *American Society of Clinical Oncology Educational Book,* pp. 528–532.

Ault, S., Kaled, S., & Rios, M.B. (2003). Management of molecular-targeted therapy for chronic myelogenous leukemia. *Journal of the American Academy of Nurse Practitioners, 15,* 292–296.

Avvisati, G., & Tallman, M.S. (2003). All-trans retinoic acid in acute promyelocytic leukemia. *Best Practice in Research and Clinical Hematology, 16,* 419–432.

Baer, M. (1998). Assessment of minimal residual disease in patients with acute leukemia. *Current Opinion in Oncology, 10,* 17–22.

Bain, B. (2004). The WHO classification of the myelodysplastic syndromes. *Experimental Oncology, 26*(3), 166–169.

Baker, K.S., Gurney, J.G., Ness, K.K., Bhatia, R., Forman, S.J., Francisco, L., et al. (2004). Late effects in survivors of chronic myeloid leukemia treated with hematopoietic cell transplantation: Results from the Bone Marrow Transplant Survivor Study. *Blood, 104,* 1898–1906.

Balducci, L. (2003). New paradigms for treating elderly patients with cancer. *Journal of Supportive Oncology, 1*(Suppl. 2), 30–37.

Bennett, J.M., Komrokji, R., & Kouides, P. (2004). The myelodysplastic syndromes. In M. Abeloff, J. Armitage, J. Niederhuber, M. Kastan, & W. McKenna (Eds.), *Clinical oncology* (3rd ed., pp. 2849–2873). New York: Churchill Livingstone.

Berman, E. (2000). Recent advances in the treatment of acute leukemia. *Current Opinion in Hematology, 7,* 205–211.

Bertz, H., Potthoff, K., & Finke, J. (2003). Allogeneic stem cell transplantation from related and unrelated donors in older patients with myeloid leukemia. *Journal of Clinical Oncology, 21,* 1480–1484.

Breed, C. (2003). Diagnosis, treatment and nursing care of patients with chronic leukemia. *Seminars in Oncology Nursing, 19,* 109–117.

Buchner, T. (1998). Treatment of acute myeloid leukemia in older patients. In L. Balducci, G.H. Lyman, & W.B. Ershler (Eds.), *Comprehensive geriatric oncology* (pp. 545–549). Amsterdam, Netherlands: Harwood.

Buchner, T., Hiddemann, W., Schoch, C., Haferlach, T., Sauerland, M., & Heinecke, A. (2001). Acute myeloid leukemia (AML): Treatment in the older patient. *Best Practice and Research in Clinical Hematology, 14,* 139–151.

Chang, H., Brandwein, J., Yi, Q.L., Chun, K., Patterson, B., & Brien, B. (2004). Extramedullary infiltrates of AML are associated with CD56 expression, 11q23 abnormalities and inferior clinical outcome. *Leukemia Research, 28,* 1007–1011.

Chen, C.C., Kenefick, A.L., Tang, S.T., & McCorkle, R. (2004). Utilization of comprehensive geriatric assessment in cancer patients. *Critical Reviews in Oncology and Hematology, 49,* 53–67.

Cortes, J., Giles, F., O'Brien, S., Thomas, D., Albitar, M., Rios, M.B., et al. (2003). Results of high dose imatinib mesylate in patients with Philadelphia chromosome–positive chronic myeloid leukemia after failure of interferon alpha. *Blood, 102,* 83–86.

Cortes, J., & Kantarjian, H.M. (2000). Promising approaches in acute leukemia. *Investigational New Drugs, 18*(1), 57–82.

Cortes, J., O'Brien, S., & Kantarjian, H. (2004). Discontinuation of imatinib therapy after achieving a molecular response. *Blood, 104,* 2204–2205.

De Botton, S., Dombret, H., Sanz, M., Miguel, J.S., Caillot, D., Zittoun, R., et al. (1998). Incidence, clinical features, and outcome of all *trans*-retinoic acid syndrome in 413 cases of newly diagnosed acute promyelocytic leukemia. The European APL Group. *Blood, 92,* 2712–2718.

Decker, T., Hipp, S., Hahntow, I., Schneller, F., & Peschel, D. (2004). Expression of cyclin E in resting and activated B-chronic lymphocytic leukemia cells: Cyclin E/cdk2 as a potential therapeutic target. *British Journal of Hematology, 125,* 141–148.

Deininger, M.W., O'Brien, S.G., Ford, J.M., & Druker, B.J. (2003). Practical management of patients with chronic myeloid leukemia receiving imatinib. *Journal of Clinical Oncology, 21,* 1637–1647.

Diehl, L.F., & Ketchum, L.H. (1998). Autoimmune disease and chronic lymphocytic leukemia: Autoimmune hemolytic anemia, pure red cell aplasia, and autoimmune thrombocytopenia. *Seminars in Oncology, 25,* 80–87.

Druker, B.J. (2004). Imatinib as a paradigm of targeted therapies. *Advances in Cancer Research, 91,* 1–30.

Eilers, J. (2004). Nursing interventions and supportive care for the prevention and treatment of oral mucositis associated with cancer treatment. *Oncology Nursing Forum, 31,* 13–23.

Erban, J.K. (1995). Hematologic problems of the elderly. In W. Reichel, J. Gallo, J. Busby-Whitehead, J. Delfs, & J. Murphy (Eds.), *Care of the elderly: Clinical aspects of aging* (pp. 397–407). Baltimore: Williams & Wilkins.

Estey, E. (2000a). How I treat older patients with AML. *Blood, 96,* 1670–1673.

Estey, E. (2000b). New agents and new targets for the treatment of AML. *Hematology 2000,* pp. 70–74.

Extermann, M. (2003). Studies of comprehensive geriatric assessment in patients with cancer. *Cancer Control, 10,* 463–468.

Faderl, S., Gandhi, V., O'Brien, S., Bonate, P., Cortes, J., Estey, E., et al. (2005). Results of a phase 1–2 study of clofarabine in combination with cytarabine (ara-C) in relapsed and refractory acute leukemias. *Blood, 105,* 940–947.

Ferrara, F. (2004). Unanswered questions in acute myeloid leukemia. *Lancet Oncology, 5,* 443–450.

Gale, D. (2003). Molecular targets in cancer therapy. *Seminars in Oncology Nursing, 19,* 193–205.

Giles, F. (2002). Novel agents for the therapy of acute leukemia. *Current Opinion in Oncology, 14,* 3–9.

Giles, F., Estey, E., & O'Brien, S. (2003). Gemtuzumab ozogamicin in the treatment of acute myeloid leukemia. *Cancer, 98,* 2095–2104.

Giralt, S., Estey, E., Albitar, M., van Besien, K., Rondon, G., Anderlini, P., et al. (1997). Engraftment of allogeneic hematopoietic progenitor cells with purine analog-containing chemotherapy: Harnessing graft-versus-leukemia without myeloablative therapy. *Blood, 89,* 4531–4536.

Gojo, I., Sarkodee-Adoo, C., Hakimian, R., Merz, W., & Karp, J. (2003). Treatment strategies for hematological malignancies: Impact on host defenses and infection risk. In J. Wingard & R. Bowden (Eds.), *Management of infection in oncology patients* (pp. 17–36). New York: Martin Dunitz Group.

Goldman, J. (2004). Monitoring minimal residual disease in BCR-ABL-positive chronic myeloid leukemia in the imatinib era. *Current Opinion in Hematology, 12,* 33–39.

Goldstone, A., Burnett, A., Wheatley, K., Smith, A., Mutchinson, R.M., & Clark, R. (2001). Attempts to improve treatment outcomes in acute myeloid leukemia (AML) in older patients: The results of the United Kingdom Medical Research Council AML 11 trial. *Blood, 98,* 1302–1311.

Griffin, J.M., Amand, M., & Demetri, G. (2005). Nursing implications of imatinib as molecularly targeted therapy for gastrointestinal stromal tumors. *Clinical Journal of Oncology Nursing, 9,* 161–169.

Grimwade, D. (2001). The clinical significance of cytogenetic abnormalities in acute myeloid leukemia. *Best Practice and Research in Clinical Hematology, 14,* 497–529.

Guilhot, F. (2004). Indications for imatinib mesylate therapy and clinical management. *Oncologist, 9,* 271–281.

Gupta, V., Chun, K., Yi, Q.L., Minden, M., Schuh, A., Wells, R., et al. (2005). Disease biology rather than age is the most important determinant of survival of patients > or = 60 years with acute myeloid leukemia treated with uniform intensive therapy. *Cancer, 103,* 2082–2090.

Heaney, M., & Golde, D. (2000). Critical evaluation of the World Health Organization classification of myelodysplasia and acute myeloid leukemia. *Current Science, 2,* 140–143.

Henderson, E.S., & McArthur, J. (2002). Diagnosis, classification and assessment of response to treatment. In E.S. Henderson, T.A. Lister, & M.F. Greaves (Eds.), *Leukemia* (7th ed., pp. 227–248). Philadelphia: Elsevier Science.

Hensley, M.L., & Ford, J.M. (2003). Imatinib treatment: Specific issues related to safety, fertility and pregnancy. *Seminars in Hematology, 40*(Suppl. 2), 21–25.

Hiddemann, W., Kern, W., Schoch, C., Fonatsch, C., Heinecke, A., Wormann, B., et al. (1999). Management of acute myeloid leukemia in elderly patients. *Journal of Clinical Oncology, 17,* 3569–3576.

Hillmen, P. (2004). Advancing therapy for chronic lymphocytic leukemia—The role of rituximab. *Seminars in Oncology, 31*(Suppl. 2), 22–26.

Hoelzer, D., & Gokbuget, N. (2000). New approaches to acute lymphoblastic leukemia in adults: Where do we go? *Seminars in Oncology, 27,* 540–559.

Hoelzer, D., & Gokbuget, N. (2005, Spring). Treatment of elderly patients with acute lymphoblastic leukemia. *American Society of Clinical Oncology Educational Book,* pp. 533–539.

Hoelzer, D., & Seipelt, M. (2000). Leukemias. In F. Cavalli, H. Hansen, & S.B. Kaye (Eds.), *Textbook of medical oncology* (2nd ed., pp. 383–413). London: Martin Dunitz.

Hood, L. (2003). Chemotherapy in the elderly: Supportive measures for chemotherapy-induced myelotoxicity. *Clinical Journal of Oncology Nursing, 7,* 185–190.

Iovino, C., & Camacho, L. (2003). Acute myeloid leukemia: A classification and treatment update. *Clinical Journal of Oncology Nursing, 7,* 535–540.

Karp, J. (1998). Molecular pathogenesis and targets for therapy in myelodysplastic syndrome (MDS) and MDS-related leukemia. *Current Opinion in Oncology, 10,* 3–9.

Karp, J.E., & Lancet, J.E. (2004). Farnesyltransferase inhibitors (FTI) in myeloid malignancies. *Annals of Hematology, 83*(Suppl. 1), S87–S88.

Keating, M.J. (2002). Chronic lymphocytic leukemia. In E.S. Henderson, T.A. Lister, & M.F. Greaves (Eds.), *Leukemia* (7th ed., pp. 656–692). Philadelphia: Elsevier.

Kebriaei, P., Anastasi, J., & Larson, R. (2003). Acute lymphoblastic leukemia: Diagnosis and classification. *Best Practice and Research in Clinical Hematology, 15,* 597–621.

Korte, J.E., Hertz-Picciotto, I., Schulz, M.R., Ball, L.M., & Duell, E.J. (2000). The contribution of benzene to smoking-induced leukemia. *Environmental Health Perspectives, 108,* 333–339.

Lancet, J.E., & Karp, J.E. (2003). Toward more effective treatment of the elderly patient with acute myelogenous leukemia. *Clinical Geriatrics, 11*(6), 30–40.

Langston, A.A., Walling, R., & Winton, E.F. (2004). Update on myelodysplastic syndromes: New approaches to classification and therapy. *Seminars in Oncology, 31*(Suppl. 4), 72–79.

Larson, R.A. (2003). Is modulation of multidrug resistance a viable strategy for acute myeloid leukemia? *Leukemia, 17,* 488–491.

Larson, R.A., & Le Beau, M.M. (2005, May). Therapy-related myeloid leukaemia: A model for leukemogenesis in humans. *Chemico-Biological Interactions,* pp. 153–154, 187–195.

Larson, R.S., & Tallman, M.S. (2003). Retinoic acid syndrome: Manifestations, pathogenesis, and treatment. *Best Practice and Research in Clinical Hematology, 16,* 453–461.

Latagliata, R., Petti, M., & Mandelli, F. (1999). Acute myeloid leukemia in the elderly: Per aspera ad Astra? *Leukemia Research, 23,* 603–613.

Lechner, K., Geissler, K., Jager, U., Greinix, J., & Kalhs, P. (1999). Treatment of acute leukemia. *Annals of Oncology, 10*(Suppl. 6), 45–51.

Leith, C.P., Kopecky, K.J., Godwin, J., McConnell, T., Slovak, M.L., Chen, I.M., et al. (1997). Acute myeloid leukemia in the elderly: Assessment of multidrug resistance (MDR1) and cytogenetics distinguishes biologic subgroups with remarkably distinct responses to standard chemotherapy. A Southwest Oncology Group study. *Blood, 89,* 3323–3329.

Leone, G., Teofili, L., Voso, M.T., & Lubbert, M. (2002). DNA methylation and demethylating drugs in myelodysplastic syndromes and secondary leukemias. *Haematologica, 87,* 1324–1341.

Levis, M. (2005). Recent advances in the development of small-molecule inhibitors for the treatment of acute myeloid leukemia. *Current Opinion in Hematology, 12,* 55–61.

Lichtman, M.A., & Rowe, J.M. (2004). The relationship of patient age to the pathobiology of the clonal myeloid diseases. *Seminars in Oncology, 31,* 185–197.

Lichtman, S. (2003). Guidelines for the treatment of elderly cancer patients. *Cancer Control, 10,* 445–453.

Lichtman, S.M., & Kolitz, J.E. (2000). Leukemias, lymphomas, and myelomas. In C.P. Hunter, K.A. Johnson, & H.B. Muss (Eds.), *Cancer in the elderly* (pp. 361–418). New York: Marcel Dekker.

List, A. (2002). New approaches to the treatment of myelodysplasia. *Oncologist, 7,* 39–49.

List, A. (2004). Novel therapeutics for an orphan disease. *Hematology 2004,* pp. 297–317.

List, A., Vardiman, J., Issa, J.P., & DeWitte, T. (2004). Myelodysplastic syndromes. *Hematology 2004,* pp. 297–301.

Liu, N.S., & O'Brien, S. (2004). Monoclonal antibodies in the treatment of chronic lymphocytic leukemia. *Medical Oncology, 21,* 297–304.

Lowenberg, B. (2001). Managing therapy in older adult patients with acute myeloid leukemia. *Seminars in Hematology, 38*(3 Suppl. 6), 10–16.

Lowenberg, B., Zittoun, R., Kerkhofs, H., Jehn, U., Abels, J., Debusscher, L., et al. (1989). On the value of remission-induction chemotherapy in elderly patients of 65+ years with acute myeloid leukemia: A randomized phase III study of the European Organization for Research and Treatment of Cancer Leukemia Group. *Journal of Clinical Oncology, 7,* 1268–1274.

Lundin, J., & Osterborg, A. (2004). Advances in the use of monoclonal antibodies in the therapy of chronic lymphocytic leukemia. *Seminars in Hematology, 41,* 234–245.

Lundquist, D.M., & Holmes, W. (1993). Documentation of neurotoxicity resulting from high-dose cytosine arabinoside. *Oncology Nursing Forum, 20,* 1409–1413.

Lynn, A., Williams, M., Sickler, J., & Burgess, S. (2003). Treatment of chronic lymphocytic leukemia with alemtuzumab: A review for nurses. *Oncology Nursing Forum, 30,* 689–696.

Mackey, H.T., & Klemm, P. (2000, April). Leukemia. *American Journal of Nursing,* pp. 27–31, 52–54.

Maris, M., Niedwieser, D., Sandmaier, B., Storer, B., Stuart, M., Maloney, D., et al. (2003). HLA-matched unrelated donor hematopoietic cell transplantation after nonmyeloablative conditioning for patients with hematologic malignancies. *Blood, 102,* 2021–2030.

Mughal, T., & Goldman, J. (2004). Chronic myeloid leukemia: Current status and controversies. *Oncology, 18,* 837–854.

Murphy-Ende, K., & Chernecky, C. (2002). Assessing adults with leukemia. *Nurse Practitioner, 27,* 49–60.

Nabhan, C., Gartenhaus, R.B., & Tallman, M.S. (2004). Purine nucleoside analogues and combination therapies in B-cell chronic lymphocytic leukemia: Dawn of a new era. *Leukemia Research, 28,* 429–442.

Nabhan, C., Rundhaugen, L., Rile, M., Rademaker, A., Boehlke, L., Jatoi, M., et al. (2005). Phase II pilot trial of gemtuzumab ozogamicin (GO) as first line therapy in acute myeloid leukemia in patients age 65 or older. *Leukemia Research, 29,* 53–57.

National Comprehensive Cancer Network. (2004). *NCCN practice guidelines for fever and neutropenia.* Jenkintown, PA: Author.

National Comprehensive Cancer Network. (2005a). *NCCN practice guidelines for acute myeloid leukemia (AML).* Jenkintown, PA: Author.

National Comprehensive Cancer Network. (2005b). *NCCN practice guidelines for myelodysplastic syndromes (MDS).* Jenkintown, PA: Author.

O'Brien, S.G. (2004). Optimizing therapy in chronic myeloid leukemia. *Hematology 2004,* pp. 146–149.

O'Brien, S.G., Guilhot, F., Larson, R., Gathmann, I., Baccarani, M., Cervantes, F., et al. (2003). Imatinib compared with interferon and low-dose cytarabine for newly diagnosed chronic phase chronic myeloid leukemia. *New England Journal of Medicine, 348,* 994–1004.

Onishi, Y., Matsuno, Y., Tateishi, U., Maeshima, A.M., Kusumoto, M., Terauchi, T., et al. (2004). Two entities of precursor T-cell lymphoblastic leukemia/lymphoma based on radiologic and immunophenotypic findings. *International Journal of Hematology, 80,* 43–51.

Pangalis, G.A., Vassilakopoulos, T.P., Dimopoulou, M.N., Siakantaris, M.P., Kontopidou, F.N., & Angelopoulou, M.K. (2002). B-chronic lymphocytic leukemia: Practical aspects. *Hematological Oncology, 20,* 103–146.

Pinto, A., Zagonel, V., & Ferrara, F. (2001). Acute myeloid leukemia in the elderly: Biology and therapeutic strategies. *Critical Reviews in Oncology/Hematology, 39,* 275–287.

Pisani, F.D., & Rainaldi, A. (2001). Management of high-risk myelodysplastic syndromes. *Critical Reviews in Oncology and Hematology, 40,* 215–228.

Radich, J., & Sievers, E. (2000). New developments in the treatment of acute myeloid leukemia. *Oncology, 14,* 125–131.

Randolph, T.R. (2000). Acute promyelocytic leukemia (AML–M-3): Pathophysiology, clinical diagnosis, and differentiation therapy. *Clinical Laboratory Science, 13*(2), 98–105.

Rathnasabapathy, R., & Lancet, J. (2003). Management of acute myelogenous leukemia in the elderly. *Cancer Control, 10,* 469–477.

Ravandi, F., Kantarjian, H., Giles, F., & Cortes, J. (2004). New agents in acute myeloid leukemia and other myeloid disorders. *Cancer, 100,* 441–454.

Redaelli, A., Laskin, B.L., Stephens, J.M., Botteman, M.F., & Pashos, C.L. (2005). A systematic literature review of the clinical and epidemiologic burden of acute lymphoblastic leukemia. *European Journal of Cancer Care, 14,* 53–62.

Reilly, J.T. (1998). Haematological problems in elderly patients: An update. *Reviews in Clinical Gerontology, 8,* 141–154.

Rowe, J.M. (2000). Treatment of acute myelogenous leukemia in older adults. *Leukemia, 14,* 480–487.

Rule, S.A., O'Brien, S.G., & Crossman, L.C. (2002). Managing cutaneous reactions to imatinib therapy. *Blood, 100,* 3434–3435.

Rund, D., & Ben-Yehuda, D. (2004). Therapy-related leukemia and myelodysplasia: Evolving concepts of pathogenesis and treatment. *Hematology, 9*(3), 179–187.

Saba, H.I. (1996). Myelodysplastic syndromes in the elderly: The role of growth factors in management. *Leukemia Research, 20,* 203–219.

Saba, H.I. (2001). Myelodysplastic syndromes in the elderly. *Cancer Control, 8,* 79–102.

Sanz, M.A., Martin, G., Gonzalez, M., Leon, A., Rayon, C., Rivas, C., et al. (2004). Risk adapted treatment of acute promyelocytic leukemia with all-trans-retinoic acid and anthracycline monochemotherapy: A multicenter study by the PETHEMA group. *Blood, 103,* 1237–1243.

Scheinberg, D.A., Maslak, P., & Weiss, M. (2001). Acute leukemias. In V. DeVita, S. Hellman, & S. Rosenberg (Eds.), *Cancer: Principles and practice of oncology* (6th ed., pp. 2404–2432). Philadelphia: Lippincott.

Schiffer, C. (2002). Post-remission therapy in older adults with acute myeloid leukemia: An opportunity for new drug development. *Leukemia, 16,* 745–747.

Seiter, K. (2002). Treatment of acute myelogenous leukemia in the elderly patient. *Clinical Geriatrics, 10*(8), 41–46.

Sekeres, M., & Stone, R. (2002). The challenge of acute myeloid leukemia in older patients. *Current Opinion in Oncology, 14,* 24–30.

Sekeres, M.A., Stone, R.M., Zahrieh, D., Neuberg, D., Morrison, V., De Angelo, D.J., et al. (2004). Decision-making and quality of life in older adults with acute myeloid leukemia or advanced myelodysplastic syndrome. *Leukemia, 18,* 809–816.

Shanafelt, T., & Call, T. (2004). Current approach to diagnosis and management of chronic lymphocytic leukemia. *Mayo Clinic Proceedings, 79,* 388–398.

Shannon-Dorcy, K., & Wolfe, V. (2003). Decision-making in the diagnosis and treatment of leukemia. *Seminars in Oncology Nursing, 19,* 142–149.

Smith, G.A., Damon, L.E., Rugo, H.S., Ries, C.A., & Linker, C.A. (1997). High dose cytarabine dose modification reduces the incidence of neurotoxicity in patients with renal insufficiency. *Journal of Clinical Oncology, 15,* 833–839.

Souhami, R., & Tobias, J. (1998). Leukemia. In R. Souhami & J. Tobias (Eds.), *Cancer and its management* (pp. 483–500). London: Blackwell Science.

Spiers, A. (1998). Chronic lymphoid leukemias. In L. Balducci, G.H. Lyman, & W.B. Ershler (Eds.), *Comprehensive geriatric oncology* (pp. 551–564). Amsterdam, Netherlands: Harwood.

Stone, R. (1999). Leukemia in the elderly. *Hematology 1999,* pp. 510–516.

Stone, R. (2002). The difficult problem of acute myeloid leukemia in the older adult. *CA: A Cancer Journal for Clinicians, 52,* 363–371.

Stone, R. (2003). Induction and postremission therapy: New agents. *Leukemia, 17,* 496–498.

Stone, R. (2004). Optimizing treatment of chronic myelogenous leukemia. *Oncologist, 9,* 259–270.

Stull, D. (2003). Targeted therapies for the treatment of leukemia. *Seminars in Oncology Nursing, 19,* 90–97.

Swirsky, D., & Richards, S. (2001). Laboratory diagnosis of acute myeloid leukemia. *Best Practice and Research in Clinical Hematology, 14,* 1–17.

Tallman, M.S. (2001). Therapy of acute myeloid leukemia. *Cancer Control, 8,* 62–78.

Tallman, M. (2005, Spring). Treatment of the older patient with acute myeloid leukemia. *American Society of Clinical Oncology Educational Book,* pp. 540–546.

Tallman, M.S., Gilliland, D.G., & Rowe, J.M. (in press). Drug therapy in acute myeloid leukemia. *Blood.*

Thomas, D., Cortes, J., & Kantarjian, H. (2003). New agents in the treatment of acute lymphocytic leukemia. *Best Practice and Research in Clinical Hematology, 15,* 771–790.

Vardiman, J.W., Harris, N.L., & Brunning, R.D. (2002). The World Health Organization (WHO) classification of the myeloid neoplasms. *Blood, 100,* 2292–2302.

Vey, N., Coso, D., Bardou, V., Stoppa, A., Braud, A., Bouabdallah, R., et al. (2004). The benefit of induction chemotherapy in patients older than 75 years. *Cancer, 101,* 325–331.

Viele, C. (2003). Diagnosis, treatment and nursing care of acute leukemia. *Seminars in Oncology Nursing, 19,* 98–108.

Wahlin, A., Markevarn, B., Golovleva, I., & Nilsson, M. (2001). Prognostic significance of risk group stratification in elderly patients with acute myeloid leukemia. *British Journal of Haematology, 115,* 25–33.

Wedding, U., Bokemeyer, C., Meran, J.G., Working Group Geriatric Oncology of the German Society for Hematology and Oncology, Austrian Society for Haematology and Oncology, & German Society for Geriatrics. (2004). Elderly patients with acute myeloid leukemia: Characteristics in biology, patients and treatment. *Onkologie, 27*(1), 72–82.

Weiss, M.A. (2001). Novel treatment strategies in chronic lymphocytic leukemia. *Current Oncology Reports, 3,* 217–222.

Wendtner, C.M., Eichorst, B.F., & Hallek, M.H. (2004). Advances in chemotherapy for chronic lymphocytic leukemia. *Seminars in Hematology, 41,* 224–233.

Winton, E., & Langston, A. (2004). Update in acute leukemia 2003: A risk adapted approach to acute myeloblastic leukemia in adults. *Seminars in Oncology, 31*(Suppl. 4), 80–86.

Yoshida, M., & Ohno, R. (2004). Antimicrobial prophylaxis in febrile neutropenia. *Clinical Infectious Disease, 39*(Suppl. 1), 65–67.

Yoshida, S., Kuriyam, K., Miyazaki, Y., Taguchi, J., Fukushima, T., Honda, M., et al. (2001). De novo acute myeloid leukemia in the elderly: A consistent fraction of long-term survivors by standard-dose chemotherapy. *Leukemia Research, 25,* 33–38.

Zhai, S., Senderowicz, A., Sausville, E., & Figg, W. (2002). Flavopyridole, a novel cyclin-dependent kinase inhibitor, in clinical development. *Annals of Pharmacotherapy, 36,* 905–911.

CHAPTER 14

The Older Adult Receiving Radiation Therapy

Marilyn L. Haas, PhD, RN, CNS, ANP-C

Introduction

With a growing older adult population, it is not surprising that neoplasia is a disease of older adults. In the United States alone, 60% of all cancers occur in the older adult population (Maes, 2004). The median age for cancer has remained 70–74 years old (Ershler & Longo, 1997; Satariano & Muss, 2001). According to the Centers for Disease Control and Prevention's growth rates, individuals older than 85 will represent 20% of the population by the year 2020 (Jemal et al., 2004; Olmi, Cefaro, Balzi, Becciolini, & Geinitz, 1997). With life expectancy reaching 73 years of age for men and 80 years of age for women, cancer probably will not change in the hierarchy of diseases.

However, age alone should not be the deciding factor for cancer treatment in the older adult. Other factors such as Karnofsky Performance Scale (KPS), other comorbidities, and life expectancy should weigh heavier into the treatment decision process. Treatments that are safe and have favorable therapeutic indexes without impinging on the physiologic or psychological reserves of the older adult are important.

Radiation therapy is a local cancer treatment that can be effective for curative (either definitive or neoadjuvant treatment), prophylactic, control, or palliative purposes (Haas & Kuehn, 2001b). Typically, radiation therapy has limited systemic toxicities and, therefore, can be an excellent alternative to other modalities for the older adult. Although widely used, limited clinical trials are designed strictly for the older adult regarding its effectiveness, tolerance, and management. Therefore, it becomes imperative to explore the issue of radiotherapy in the older adult population. This chapter will discuss principles of radiotherapy, physical consequences of aging and radiotherapy, and special considerations, supportive care, and nursing interventions for the older adult receiving radiation. The chapter will conclude with a case study presentation of an older adult with lung cancer receiving radiotherapy.

Treatment Definition

Radiation therapy is the use of high-energy particles or waves, such as x-rays, gamma rays, electrons, and protons, to destroy or damage cancer cells. Other common names are radiotherapy, x-ray therapy, or irradiation. Several radiation modalities exist. Teletherapy, commonly referred to as external beam radiation, delivers radioactive energy at a distance from the treatment or target area. External beam is given daily, generally over two to seven weeks, depending on the purpose of treatment and total dose. Brachytherapy, also referred to as internal or implant radiation therapy, is a type of modality in which the radioactive source is placed on or within the tumor (interstitial, intracavitary, or systemic). Brachytherapy can be temporary or permanent, using low- or high-energy doses. Choosing which type of radiation depends on tumor type, size, and location.

Principles of Radiation Therapy

With the increasing incidence of cancer in the older adult, radiation therapy is a major treatment modality for this population. Approximately 60% of all individuals with cancer will be treated with radiation therapy at some point during the course of illness (Casey, Zachariah, & Balducci, 2003; Iwamoto, 2001). Radiation therapy delivers high doses of radiation to cancerous cells by either killing or damaging the cells so they cannot multiply or spread. The major effect is on the DNA, where some cells lose their proliferative ability and cause immediate cell death whereas others are indirectly affected by not being able to survive mitosis (Hall & Cox, 1994).

The radiosensitivity of cancer cells depends on four factors, commonly referred to as the four Rs in radiobiology: repopulation, reoxygenation, reassortment (redistribution), and repair of sublethal damage (Perez, Brady, Halperin, & Schmidt-Ullrich, 2004). During radiation therapy, growth rates can increase once cell killing with irradiation begins. This is known as repopulation. However, tumor cell proliferation decreases in the older adult, suggesting that radiosensitivity also might decrease with age (Balzi et al., 1992; Balzi, Becciolini, Mauri, Larosa, & Bechi, 1993; Balzi, Becciolini, Zanieri, et al., 1993; Balzi, Mauri, et al., 1993; Balzi et al., 1991; Becciolini et al., 1993). In addition, these same researchers suggested that older individuals may develop cancerous tumors with a more indolent, slower clinical course.

Oxygenation of the cells is required for maximal tumoricidal effect. Although no clinical studies directly correlate tumor reoxygenation and the older adult, decreased oxygenation because of circulatory changes in the older adult might affect tumor sensitivity. More studies are required to test this hypothesis.

Radiation therapy works best during certain phases in the cell cycles. Reassortment, or redistribution, has higher radiosensitivity for cells in the mitosis phase of the cell cycle than the cells in the late cell cycle, S phase. No clinical studies for the older adult directly investigate this dose-time ratio used in radiation delivery.

Repairing damaged portions of the cells caused by radiation occurs between each treatment. Normal cells repair quicker if smaller doses per fraction are given. Overall, tissue tolerances to therapeutic irradiation have been established so that treatment planning can minimize the possible complications or permanent damage. Normal tissue tolerance to irradiation is applicable to any age group. The radiosensitivity of cancer tumors and normal tissue is found in Table 14-1 (Emami et al., 1991).

Table 14-1. Radiosensitivity of Cancerous Tumors, Normal Tissues, and Cells

Organ	TD 5/5* (cGy)	TD 50/5** (cGy)	Selected Clinical End Points
Bladder	6,500	8,000	Symptomatic bladder contracture and volume loss
Bone			
• Femoral head	5,200	6,500	Necrosis
• Temporomandibular joint: mandible	6,000	7,200	Marked limited joint function
• Ribs	5,000	6,500	Pathologic fractures
Brain	4,500	6,000	Necrosis, infarction
Brain stem	5,000	6,500	Necrosis, infarction
Colon	4,500	5,500	Obstruction, perforation, fistula
Ear, middle/external	3,000	4,000	Acute serous otitis
Esophagus	5,500	6,800	Chronic stricture, perforation
Eye			
• Lens	1,000	1,800	Cataract requiring intervention
• Retina	4,500	6,500	Blindness
Heart	4,000	5,000	Pericarditis
Kidney	2,300	2,800	Clinical nephritis
Larynx	7,000	8,000	Cartilage necrosis
Liver	3,000	4,000	Liver failure
Lung	1,750	2,450	Pneumonitis
Optic nerve/chiasm	5,000	6,500	Blindness
Parotid	3,200	4,600	Xerostomia
Rectum	6,000	8,000	Severe proctitis, necrosis, fistula, stenosis
Skin	5,500	7,000	Telangiectasia, necrosis, ulceration
Small intestine	4,000	5,500	Obstruction, perforation, fistula
Spinal cord	4,700	7,000	Myelitis necrosis
Stomach	(20 cm)	(10 cm)	Ulceration, perforation
	5,000	6,500	

*TD 5/5 refers to the dose of radiation that could cause no more than a 5% severe complication rate within five years after treatment.

**TD 50/5 refers to the dose of radiation that could cause no more than a 50% severe complication rate within five years after treatment.

cGy—centiGray (100 centiGray = 1 Gray)

Note. From "Tolerance of Normal Tissue to Therapeutic Radiation," by B. Emami, J. Lyman, A. Brown, L. Coia, M. Goitein, J. Munzenrider, et al., 1991, *International Journal of Radiation Oncology, Biology, Physics, 21,* pp. 109–122. Copyright 1991 by Elsevier. Adapted with permission.

Radiotherapy and the Older Adult

Selecting the most appropriate radiotherapy modality for the older adult patient with cancer should be individualized. Although the overall purpose (cure versus palliative) is the utmost important consideration, two other factors weigh equally as important in the decision process: KPS and life expectancy (Olmi et al., 1997). KPS is an evaluation of cardiac function, pulmonary function, and exercise tolerance and is rated by multiples of ten, ranging from 10%–100%, with 10% representing the lowest level of functioning, where condition is moribund and disease is fatally progressing rapidly, and 100% representing normal level of functioning, no complaints, and no evidence of disease. Today, clinical trials offer older adults options based on their functional ability rather than strictly age.

Second, life expectancy ranks high in the consideration of radiotherapy modality. Comorbidities in reference to life expectancy are important factors in delivering radiotherapy in the older adult. Compromising quality of life and exacerbating other illnesses becomes very problematic and is not tolerated by older adults. Therefore, age of the person should be de-emphasized and should never be a contraindication to radiotherapy (Baumann, 1998; Fentiman et al., 1990; Zachariah et al., 1997).

Radiation therapy has its own distinct advantages and disadvantages. Radiotherapy's aim is loco-regional control, thereby limiting its effects to the treatment area and not producing systemic effects. For this reason alone, a strong therapeutic option for the older adult is radiation therapy. Older adults are relieved when informed this treatment does not automatically cause nausea and vomiting or loss of hair. Although mortality is rare, radiotherapy has definite acute toxicities, but these generally are manageable (see Table 14-2). With newer technology, such as 3-dimensional conformal radiation therapy (3DCRT) and intensity-modulated radiation therapy (IMRT), organ sparing usually can be maintained and better function preserved. In addition, improvement in medications can control acute symptomatology, improve radiosensitization, and offer radioprotection. Radiotherapy is definitely an alternative when surgery or chemotherapy is contraindicated.

Radiation therapy has the potential for acute and long-term side effects. The main disadvantage to radiotherapy is the long duration of treatment, especially when the intent is curative. Older adults can fatigue easily with daily treatments administered over a six- to seven-week time period. Second, the physiologic reserve diminishes with age, which affects the recovery of the older adult. Depending on the area being treated, site-related disturbances (toxicities) may be more pronounced in the older adult, which can impact quality of life and necessitate treatment interruptions and/or additional medical or surgical interventions or hospitalizations. Concerns for the older adult are present when therapy involves the whole brain (e.g., fear of neurologic sequelae, including dementia) or the pelvis (e.g., fear of marrow aplasia, radiation enteritis). Further research is needed to evaluate these hypotheses and side effects for the older adult receiving radiation therapy.

Physical Consequences of Aging and Radiotherapy

Physical aging affects the functioning of the human body. It reduces the viability at all levels (cells, molecules, tissues, organs, and organ systems) and increases the

Table 14-2. Physical Consequences of Aging in Patients Receiving Radiotherapy

Organ Site	Effects of Aging	Acute Toxicities of Radiation
Skin	Thinning of epidermis Unchanged stratum corneum, except moisture and cohesiveness Decreased melanocytes Decreased Langerhans cells Decreased fibroblasts Hypovascular endothelium Decreased mast cells	Mild to brisk erythema Dry desquamation Moist desquamation
Bone	Loss of bone density	Thrombocytopenia Neutropenia
Brain	Decrease in brain weight Loss of gray and white matter Changes in nerve cells	Cerebral edema Seizures Alopecia
Oral cavity	Less production of ptyalin and amylase in saliva glands Dry mouth (medication-induced) Decrease in olfactory senses Decrease in mastication muscles	Mucositis/stomatitis Acute xerostomia Taste changes Pharyngitis
Lung	Reduction in glandular epithelial cells Enlargement of alveoli and alveoli ducts Reduction in respiratory muscle functioning Ossification of costal cartilage	Increasing cough, dyspnea Pain (tumor) Esophagitis Hoarseness Skin reactions (see above)
Heart	Decreased heart rate Vascular stiffness Increased platelet adhesiveness Decreased aerobic capacity	Delayed acute pericarditis Delayed pericardial effusion Diffuse myocardial fibrosis Late coronary artery disease Conduction defects
Breast	Less glandular tissue, more connective and fat tissue	Breast pain, swelling, tenderness Radiodermatitis
Bladder	Loss of muscle tone, leading to incomplete bladder emptying Decreased bladder capacity	Frequency Urgency Dysuria Hesitancy Hematuria
Vagina/ovaries	Atrophy of organs	Hot flashes Vaginal dryness Dyspareunia
Prostate	Hyperplasia	Diarrhea Tenesmus Proctalgia Rectal bleeding Erectile dysfunction
Colon/rectum	Slow peristalsis Decreased muscle strength in abdomen	Abdominal cramping Diarrhea

Note. Based on information from Haas, 2004b.

vulnerability to diseases and comorbid conditions (Archley & Barusch, 2004). Age-associated factors can exacerbate radiation therapy side effects and cause physical changes and radiation consequences (see Table 14-2).

Skin

Certain aging changes should be recognized before assessing the effects of radiotherapy. Decreasing epidermal thickness in the older adult reduces the moisture content and cohesiveness of the stratum corneum (manifesting as dry, rough skin), decreases melanocyte numbers (loss of photoprotection), and reduces Langerhans cells (equates to loss of immune surveillance and increasing sensitivity to contact allergens). Aging affects the deeper layer, the dermis, by decreasing the number of fibroblasts (collagen protecting the tensile strength of the skin), reducing the amount of blood vessels within the reticular dermis (compromising blood flow), and decreasing the amount of mast cells, which explains urticaria (Tallis, Fillit, & Brocklehurst, 1998).

The basal layer of the epidermis is particularly sensitive to radiotherapy because it proliferates rapidly. Ionizing radiation essentially damages the mitotic ability of stem cells within the basal layer, thus preventing the process of repopulation and weakening the integrity of the skin. Repeated radiation impairs the cell division within the basal layer, so the degree to which a skin reaction develops is dependent on the survival of actively proliferating basal cells in the epidermis. Basal cell loss begins once the radiation dose reaches 20–25 Gray (Gy), and the maximum depletion of basal cells occurs when the patient has received a dose of 50 Gy (Perez et al., 2004).

In clinical practice, skin reactions tend to become visible around the second to third week of radiation therapy, reaching a peak at the end or within one week of completion of treatment. Therefore, assessment of the older adult at the beginning of radiation therapy is extremely important. Various skin reactions can manifest radiation changes to the skin (see Table 14-2). Assessing for early skin reactions would be appropriate in the older adult.

Bone

Bone loss starts between 35 and 40 years of age in both sexes and accelerates for women after menopause. As bone loss continues, osteoporosis becomes an issue. Several factors can contribute to bone loss: smoking, lack of physical activity, low dietary calcium intake, impaired metabolism of vitamin D, and steroid and estrogen replacement therapy.

When treating the skeletal system with radiation, the older adult frequently has metastatic disease to the bone. Bone marrow suppression is of concern when radiation is given to large volumes of active bone marrow (pelvis, spine, sternum, ribs, long bones, and skull). Generally, radiotherapy is very effective for treating painful bony metastases. Research has shown that single fractions can provide the necessary bone pain relief (Sze, Shelley, Held, Wilt, & Mason, 2003). Weekly blood counts may be indicated, especially if the older adult is receiving combined chemotherapy (Iwamoto, 2001). Transfusion of blood products during radiation is rare.

Brain

Advances in neuroimaging techniques (e.g., computed tomography, magnetic resonance imaging [MRI], position emission tomography [PET]) have resulted in more information about the changes in the brain as aging occurs and provides insight into problems of memory, intellect, or locomotion. Baseline assessment of mental deterioration (e.g., failing memory; emotional irritability; confusion, anxiety, depression, delusions, hallucinations, dementia) should be obtained at the onset of radiation therapy.

Once the brain is treated for a primary brain tumor, development of cerebral edema can quickly change the mental and physical status of the older adult, and distinctions need to be made rapidly. Symptoms of cerebral edema that can mimic mental deterioration are headache, nausea, vomiting, visual changes, changes in motor ability, slurred speech, confusion, and seizure activity.

Head and Neck/Oral Cavity

In normal physiology of aging, salivation in healthy older adults typically is unchanged, although 40% subjectively complain about dry mouth (Tallis et al., 1998). The salivary glands secrete less ptyalin and amylase, making the saliva more alkaline. The bony structure of the mouth shrinks, and tooth decay becomes problematic. The gustatory and olfactory sensations decrease, and the muscles used in mastication decrease, causing less chewing ability. Overall, the esophagus is unchanged.

Significant toxicities occur when giving radiation to the oral cavity, even if palliative doses are given (inoperable tumors typically require at least 45–50 Gy over five to six weeks) (Haas & Kuehn, 2001a). The older adult is extremely vulnerable to physiologic and psychological distress. Nutritional problems resulting from irradiation cause stomatitis, xerostomia, or alterations in taste buds. This affects the older adult's ability to complete therapy without treatment breaks. Inadequate nutrition can further exacerbate fatigue and depression for the older adult undergoing radiation treatments (Strohl, 1992).

Lung

Structural and functional changes in the respiratory system are associated with the aging body. A reduction in the number of glandular epithelial cells occurs, thus impairing the protective mechanism and defense capability. Alveoli and the alveoli ducts enlarge, decreasing lung volume and capacity. Respiratory muscles function less, impairing the strength and endurance. Ossification of costal cartilages changes the diameter of the thorax and impairs mobility.

Careful planning and limiting the dose to normal tissue is extremely important, especially when the older adult already may have a decreased capacity and comorbidities, such as asthma or chronic obstructive pulmonary disease. Pulmonary tests can be important predictors of a person's ability to withstand irradiation (Haas, 2004a). Treatments causing further dyspnea are very frightening for the older adult. Providing emotional support with consistent reinforcement that radiation opens blocked or narrow airways is very challenging for the radiation team. Recognition of acute airway distress and other respiratory toxicities caused by radiation requires immediate attention, especially for the older adult (see Table 14-2).

Heart

Age-related changes in cardiovascular functioning are interdependent on numerous factors: sedentary lifestyle, smoking, and development of comorbid diseases (e.g., coronary artery disease, congestive heart failure, hypertension). Changes in the heart's pumping ability and increasing atherosclerosis in the heart vessels cause a decrease in heart rate, a decrease in vascular elasticity (slowing blood flow), an increase in platelet adhesions (causing embolus formation), and an overall decrease in aerobic capacity.

Meticulous treatment planning is performed to limit the cardiac dose in the radiation treatment fields. With newer technologies (IMRT and 3DCRT), radiation oncologists are able to avoid treating heart muscle; however, healthcare professionals should monitor assessments in regard to cardiac status. Maintaining the highest level of cardiac functioning is of utmost importance for the older adult to be able to tolerate radiation therapy. Obviously, the more cardiac tissue or muscle involved in the treatment field, the higher the risk for pericardial disease and later effects of myocardial fibrosis, coronary artery disease, valvular disease, and conduction defects (Fajardo, Berthrong, & Anderson, 2001).

Breast

The changes in breast tissue are more evident after menopause because of hormonal changes. Less glandular tissue, reduced breast elasticity, and more connective tissue and fat cause the breast to sag in older age. Advancing age is certainly a risk factor for developing breast cancer. Most of the increase in the past two decades has occurred in women 47–74 years of age (Greenlee, Murray, Bolden, & Wingo, 2000). Fortunately, with advanced technology of mammograms and additionally with MRIs, healthcare professionals are detecting breast cancer at an earlier stage (Gibbs, Liney, Lowry, Kneeshaw, & Turnbull, 2004; Luciani et al., 2004).

Radiation therapy to the breast has played a significant role after breast conservation therapy (BCT) in early-stage breast cancer for women of any age. After BCT, whole breast radiation is administered for approximately seven weeks with external beam irradiation (National Comprehensive Cancer Network [NCCN], 2004a). Radiation to the breast causes mild skin darkening and shrinkening and thickening (firmness) of the tissue, although none of these changes is cosmetically noticeable (Perez et al., 2004).

In 2003, the U.S. Food and Drug Administration approved an exciting radiation therapy called the MammoSite® Radiation System. This is an accelerated partial breast irradiation system that treats only the breast tumor bed with radiation (Vicini et al., 2003). MammoSite offers a different radiation source by using a high-dose–rate remote afterloader, instilling a radioactive source for a brief period, twice a day, for approximately five days. The American Society of Breast Surgeons (2003) has identified patient selection criteria, which includes women older than 50 years of age, identified tumor type (invasive ductal carcinoma or ductal carcinoma in situ [DCIS]), total tumor size (invasive and DCIS) ≤ 2 cm, negative surgical margins of at least 2 mm in all directions, and negative axillary lymph node dissection or sentinel lymph node biopsy.

Bladder

During the aging process, the bladder tends to lose muscle tone and sometimes loses enough tone to result in incomplete emptying of the bladder. This places the older adult at higher risk for urinary retention and cystitis (Sale, 1995).

If the bladder is in the treatment field during pelvic irradiation, urinary tract symptoms are intensified and begin after 10 fractions or 20 Gy (Perez et al., 2004). Symptoms include dysuria, frequency, urgency, nocturia, hesitancy, and decreased urinary capacity. Baseline functioning for the older adult is essential before beginning radiation treatments to recognize differences between radiation-induced cystitis, aging effects, and bacterial infections.

Vagina and Ovaries

Aging changes in female genital tract organs accelerate after menopause (Moore-Higgs, 2000). The major change is atrophy, resulting in smaller and smoother structures, a flattened epithelial surface, and fibrous stomas, reducing the vascularity and fat content.

If the vaginal vault is in the treatment field during pelvic irradiation, vaginal stenosis may develop, if not already present because of aging. Ovarian failure occurs with small amounts of radiation, but this concern is not typical for older women, as they are already menopausal.

Prostate

The incidence of prostate cancer increases with age. A prostate change that occurs in the older male is predominantly enlargement. In older males, prostate cancer may manifest as a slow-growing local tumor or at the other extreme may act as an aggressive spreading disease that leads to painful and distressing death.

Depending on the staging of the disease, radiation can be offered in different modalities—external beam and brachytherapy (NCCN, 2004b). Clinical studies have shown more normal tissue sparing and equivalent if not higher control rates with 3DCRT and IMRT than with standard external beam radiation (Jani, Roeske, & Rash, 2003; Luxton, Hancock, & Boyer, 2004). Brachytherapy introduces radioactive seeds into the prostate gland, offering a predictable dose of radiation. Older males may find brachytherapy more appealing, as this can be performed as an outpatient procedure and not have the protracted time involved with external beam pelvic radiation. Ultimately, older men with prostate cancer should discuss treatment options (e.g., watchful waiting, hormonal external beam radiation, prostate seed implantation, combination of therapies) with the urologist, medical oncologist, and radiation oncologist.

Colon and Rectum

Nutritional absorption and digestion are decreased with advanced aging. Coupled with slow peristalsis and decreased muscular strength, constipation becomes a problem for older adults. Some older adults have problems with their anal sphincter because of hemorrhoids and anal ulcer, thus further aggravating constipation.

However, when the abdomen and pelvis receive radiation, the opposite occurs. Radiation irritates the mucosal lining and causes diarrhea. Although this is dose-limiting, it can become problematic where treatment breaks are required or, in a few cases, discontinued. Radiation-induced diarrhea for older adults can potentially cause nutritional problems of dehydration and electrolyte imbalances. Medications are available to control the gastrointestinal symptoms.

Supportive Care

The radiation therapy team members (radiation oncologists, nurse practitioners, radiation oncology nurses, radiation technologists, physicists, and dosimetrists) each have unique roles that impact the clinical outcome for the older adult receiving radiation therapy. Tumor staging along with a multidimensional evaluation of the older adult's functional status, cognitive and emotional functioning, comorbidities, life expectancy, socioeconomic resources, and family support should be done at the onset of diagnosis.

The radiation oncologist will decide the most appropriate treatment goal and regimen (combined modality or definitive radiation). Facts about the type of cancer and the role of radiotherapy are discussed with the older adult and family members. At the beginning of treatment planning, special attention is given to the patient's comorbidities. Conditions such as dementia, Parkinson disease, or other neurologic diseases may require additional or different immobilization aids. Kyphoscoliosis, arthritis, and other musculoskeletal problems may require special positions to make the older adult feel comfortable and safe.

The radiation oncology nurse practitioner (NP) can be involved with consults (history and physical examination) and close management of treatment-related symptoms while the patient is undergoing active treatment. The NP also can evaluate responses to and/or assess for treatment-related late effects or cancer recurrences in follow-ups.

Radiation oncology nurses should assist older patients and caregivers in anticipating the acute toxicities that may develop during therapy. Although evidence-based nursing interventions are scarce in radiation therapy, general principles can be shared about the nursing role. Recognizing that minimal acute side effects are associated with a palliative course of therapy (< 2,000–3,000 centigray [cGy] or 10 fractions or less), the nursing role then becomes one of an educator and facilitator. Curative treatments involve a longer course of therapy, generally lasting six to eight weeks, causing more intense site-specific reactions. For the older adult, this translates into more frequent nursing assessments and closer monitoring of interventions. For further discussion of specific nursing interventions for any acute and long-term side effects of radiation therapy, see Watkins Bruner, Haas, and Gosselin-Acomb (2005).

The radiation technologists deliver the radiation treatments and interact with the older adult every day. With possible sensory losses that accompany aging (vision and hearing), additional time may be needed to provide clear and direct instructions, to ensure glasses are returned to the patient if head molds are required, and to assist the older adult in transferring to the treatment table. With functional reserves possibly diminished, extra time may be allotted if using multiple treatment fields, thus protracting the treatment time. If older adults are hospitalized, special attention is needed while transferring the patient to the treatment table to protect the already thin skin from shearing, especially if the skin is in the treatment field. Extra blankets may be needed in the cold treatment room.

The radiation physicists and dosimetrists ensure optimum use of radiation to produce a stated diagnostic or therapeutic outcome. These individuals work closely with radiation oncologists to establish the measurement and characterization of radiation and the specification of dose delivered. Additional responsibilities include development and direction of quality assurance programs and assistance for practitioners to optimize the balance between the beneficial and deleterious effects of radiation (American College of Medical Physics, 2002). Most older adult patients will have very limited contact with these team members.

Each team member has a specific role in the delivery of radiation treatments. The physiologic changes of the older adult should be taken into consideration when developing an individualized plan of care; however, cure should never be compromised or confused with palliation. Radiation therapy is a stress on the body that is not always visualized. Careful attention is given to early changes in physical difficulties and behavior changes. Older adults should be encouraged to remain active during therapy, and suggestions can be offered to assist in maintaining their normal level of functioning. Explanations and education regarding radiation therapy and side effects should be offered in both written and verbal format in a relaxed environment. In addition, nurses play a key role in close monitoring for side effects and symptom management. Certainly, the older person who knows what to expect is better able to tolerate the radiotherapy and to maintain an optimal quality of life during therapy (Strohl, 1992).

Case Study

J.H.K., a 71-year-old white female, presented to the urgent care center complaining of cough, pain, dyspnea, wheezing, and recent hemoptysis. These symptoms began two weeks ago with no reported chest pain. She is among the 90% of individuals with lung cancer presenting with similar symptoms (Tan, Flaherty, Kazerooni, & Iannettoni, 2003). Additionally, she complained of facial swelling, possibly some swelling on the left side of her neck, and distended neck veins. At times, she has felt dizzy, experienced some blurred vision, and has had trouble swallowing. She reported no weight loss, despite the dysphagia. Her reported KPS was 90%, indicating that she was able to carry out normal activity with only minor signs of disease. Her past medical history includes adult-onset diabetes and atrial fibrillation, both well controlled with medications. She is married and lives with her husband. She denies drinking alcohol, but is a 20-pack/year smoker. She is a retired school teacher but remains very active volunteering.

A chest x-ray revealed a right hilar fullness, and she was sent to the local hospital's emergency room. J.H.K. had a computed tomography scan of the chest, which confirmed a 3.2 x 2.1 cm right hilar mass with a subcarinal lymph node measuring 3.3 x 2.0 cm. She had bilateral pleural effusions and right lower lobe consolidation. She was treated with steroids, antibiotics, and bronchodilators, and outpatient follow-up was arranged with a pulmonologist. A healthcare professional performed a bronchoscopy, noting normal mobile vocal cords, but a marked abnormality of the mucosa distal to the orifice of the superior segment of the right lower lobe was identified. Brushings and washings were obtained. Pathology returned revealing keratinizing squamous cell carcinoma. J.H.K.'s staging studies included a bone scan and MRI of the brain, which were both without evidence of disease. A PET scan was performed to rule out distant disease and aid in radiation therapy treatment planning. Fortunately, this also was found to be negative.

On exam, J.H.K. has left facial swelling with distended left neck veins. Lung assessment reveals rhonchi in the right lower lobe region with decreased breath sounds in the bases bilaterally, right greater than left. Pulse oximetry reveals a room air saturation of 92%. The rest of the physical examination was within normal limits.

J.H.K. was diagnosed with stage III non-small cell lung carcinoma (NSCLC) of the right lower lobe with superior vena cava syndrome. The role of radiation therapy in NSCLC is standard for individuals diagnosed with stage III disease. Introducing combined chemotherapy and radiation has improved outcomes in stage III. Current approaches include induction chemotherapy for several cycles followed by radiotherapy or concurrent chemoradiation. Cisplatin, vinblastine, carboplatin, and paclitaxel all have been used in clinical trials. Radiotherapy generally is given in a dose of 50–60 Gy over five to six weeks (Haas, 2004a). Because J.H.K. has a high KPS level and generally is in good health, the radiation oncologist offered definitive radiation therapy with concurrent chemotherapy.

The healthcare personnel caring for the older adult receiving radiation therapy must be able to recognize age-associated problems that affect the care during and after treatment. Although she has smoked for a long time, J.H.K. has not experienced any lung problems that impede her breathing capacity. Therefore, she was monitored for acute toxicities of esophagitis, skin reactions, and others identified in Table 14-2. Healthcare professionals will monitor late morbidity changes after radiation is complete (radiation fibrosis of the lung, esophageal stricture, skin changes, cardiac sequelae, spinal cord myelopathy, or brachial plexopathy [Haas, 2004a]).

J.H.K. received a total dose of 6,660 cGy in 37 fractions to the right lower lobe mass and ipsilateral mediastinum over a total elapsed treatment time of 60 days. Fields were planned with the aid of 3-dimensional computed tomography planning. J.H.K. received concurrent carboplatin/Taxol® (Bristol-Myers Squibb, Princeton, NJ) chemotherapy along with radiation therapy. Contralateral mediastinal nodes received a dose of 4,860 cGy. She tolerated radiation therapy well with minor complaints of odynophagia requiring liquid hydrocodone. She developed mild radiodermatitis, and aloe-based product was used that will continue to be applied until the skin reaction resolves. She had occasional nausea from the chemotherapy, requiring intermittent antiemetic therapy. Overall, she only lost two pounds, had some mild fatigue, and her reported KPS at completion was 80% (normal activity level with some effort and some signs of disease).

Conclusion

Radiation therapy may be given safely and effectively to older adults when the treatment is individualized and precautions are taken to minimize the complications of treatment. The risk of serious complications from radiation therapy is small. However, radiation therapy requires a multidisciplinary approach to offer the older adult all the different modalities and resources to ensure a quality outcome. Age alone never should be a deterrent in deciding if radiation therapy is appropriate for the older adult. As the population is growing older, more research is needed to assess the aggressive therapies for the older adult, including radiation and different treatment modalities. Emphasis on nursing interventions that help the older adult to tolerate the side effects and toxicities should be explored.

References

American College of Medical Physics. (2002, February). *Scope of practice of medical physics.* Reston, VA: Author.

American Society of Breast Surgeons. (2003, April). *Consensus statement for accelerated partial breast irradiation*. Columbia, MD: Author.

Archley, R., & Barusch, A. (2004). *Social forces and aging: An introduction to social gerontology* (10th ed.). Belmont, CA: Wadsworth, Thomson Learning.

Balzi, M., Becciolini, A., Mauri, P., Boanini, P., Zanieri, E., Ninu, M.B., et al. (1992). The prognostic role of thymidine labeling index in larynx carcinoma. *Cell Proliferation, 25,* 512.

Balzi, M., Becciolini, A., Mauri, P., Larosa, V., & Bechi, P. (1993). Proliferative activity in normal colon mucosa and tumor tissue: Clinical implications. *In Vivo, 7,* 635–638.

Balzi, M., Becciolini, A., Zanieri, E., Mauri, P., Maugeri, A., Melone, F., et al. (1993). TLI in superficial cancer of the bladder: Prognostic evaluation. *Cell Proliferation, 26,* 464.

Balzi, M., Mauri, P., Boanini, P., Giache, V., Ninu, M.B., Zarone, N., et al. (1993). Multivariate analysis of prognostic value of 3H-thymidine labeling index (TLI) in laryngeal carcinoma. *International Journal of Biology Markers, 8,* 42–44.

Balzi, M., Ninu, M., Becciolini, A., Scubia, E., Boanini, P., Gallina, E., et al. (1991). Labeling index in squamous cell carcinoma of the larynx. *Head and Neck, 13,* 344–348.

Baumann, M. (1998). Is curative radiation therapy in elderly patients limited by increased normal tissue toxicity? *Radiotherapy and Oncology, 46,* 225–227.

Becciolini, A., Balzi, M., Boanini, P., Maugeri, A., Pacini, P., Bianchi, S., et al. (1993). Cell kinetics in breast cancer. *In Vivo, 7,* 627–630.

Casey, L., Zachariah, B., & Balducci, L. (2003). Radiation therapy of older persons. In J. Overcash & L. Balducci (Eds.), *The older cancer patient* (pp. 131–143). New York: Springer.

Emami, B., Lyman, J., Brown, A., Coia, L., Goitein, M., Munzenrider, J., et al. (1991). Tolerance of normal tissue to therapeutic radiation. *International Journal of Radiation Oncology, Biology, Physics, 21,* 109–122.

Ershler, W., & Longo, D. (1997). The biology of aging. *Cancer, 80,* 1284–1293.

Fajardo, L., Berthrong, M., & Anderson, R. (2001). *Radiation pathology*. Oxford, England: Oxford University Press.

Fentiman, I., Tirelli, U., Monfardini, S., Schneider, M., Festen, J., Cognetti, F., et al. (1990). Cancer in the elderly: Why so badly treated? *Lancet, 335,* 1020–1022.

Gibbs, P., Liney, G., Lowry, M., Kneeshaw, P., & Turnbull, L. (2004). Differentiation of benign and malignant sub–1 cm breast lesions using dynamic contrast enhanced MRI. *Breast, 13*(2), 115–121.

Greenlee, R., Murray, T., Bolden, S., & Wingo, P. (2000). Cancer statistics, 2000. *CA: A Cancer Journal for Clinicians, 50,* 7–33.

Haas, M. (2004a). *Pocket guide to lung cancer*. Sudbury, MA: Jones and Bartlett.

Hass, M. (2004b). Utilizing geriatric skills in radiation oncology. *Geriatric Nursing, 25,* 355–360.

Haas, M., & Kuehn, E. (2001a). Head and neck cancers. In D. Watkins Bruner & M. Haas (Eds.), *Clinical outcomes in radiation therapy: Multidisciplinary approach* (pp. 195–213). Sudbury, MA: Jones and Bartlett.

Haas, M., & Kuehn, E. (2001b). Teletherapy: External radiation therapy. In D. Watkins Bruner & M. Haas (Eds.), *Clinical outcomes in radiation therapy: Multidisciplinary approach* (pp. 55–66). Sudbury, MA: Jones and Bartlett.

Hall, E., & Cox, J. (1994). Physical and biologic basis of radiation therapy. In J.D. Cox (Ed.), *Moss's radiation oncology: Rationale, technique, results* (7th ed., pp. 3–65). St. Louis, MO: Mosby.

Iwamoto, R. (2001). Radiation therapy. In S. Otto (Ed.), *Oncology nursing* (pp. 606–636). Philadelphia: Mosby.

Jani, A., Roeske, J., & Rash, C. (2003). Intensity-modulated radiation therapy for prostate cancer. *Clinical Prostate Cancer, 2,* 98–105.

Jemal, A., Tiwari, R.C., Murray, T., Ghafoor, A., Samuels, A., Ward, E., et al. (2004). Cancer statistics, 2004. *CA: A Cancer Journal for Clinicians, 54,* 8–29.

Luciani, A., Dao, T., Lapeyre, M., Schwarzinger, M., Debaecque, C., Lautieri, L., et al. (2004). Simultaneous bilateral breast and high-resolution axillary MRI of patients with breast cancer: Preliminary results. *American Journal of Roentgenology, 182,* 1059–1067.

Luxton, G., Hancock, S., & Boyer, A. (2004). Dosimetry and radiobiologic model comparison of IMRT and 3D conformal radiotherapy in treatment of carcinoma of the prostate. *International Journal of Radiation Oncology, Biology, Physics, 59,* 267–284.

Maes, S. (2004). Geriatric oncology nursing comes of age. *ONS News, 19*(2), 1, 4.

Moore-Higgs, G. (2000). *Women and cancer: A gynecological oncology nursing perspective*. Sudbury, MA: Jones and Bartlett.

National Comprehensive Cancer Network. (2004a). *Breast cancer clinical practice guidelines in oncology.* Retrieved September 5, 2004, from http://www.nccn.org/professional/physician_gls/PDF/breast .pdf

National Comprehensive Cancer Network. (2004b). *Prostate cancer clinical practice guidelines in oncology.* Retrieved September 5, 2004, from http://www.nccn.org/professional/physician_gls/ PDF/prostate.pdf

Olmi, P., Cefaro, A., Balzi, M., Becciolini, A., & Geinitz, H. (1997). Radiotherapy in the aged. *Clinics in Geriatric Medicine, 13*(1), 143–168.

Perez, C., Brady, L., Halperin, E., & Schmidt-Ullrich, P. (2004). *Principles and practice of radiation oncology* (4th ed.). Philadelphia: Lippincott.

Sale, P. (1995). Genitourinary infection in older women. *Journal of Obstetric, Gynecologic, and Neonatal Nursing, 24,* 769–775.

Satariano, W., & Muss, H. (2001). *Effects of comorbidity on cancer. Exploring the role of cancer centers for integrating aging and cancer research.* Washington, DC: National Institutes of Health.

Strohl, R.A. (1992). The elderly patient receiving radiation therapy: Treatment sequelae and nursing care. *Geriatric Nursing, 13,* 153–156.

Sze, W.M., Shelley, M.D., Held, I., Wilt, T.J., & Mason, M.D. (2003). Palliation of metastatic bone pain: Single fraction versus multifraction radiotherapy—A systematic review of randomized trials. *Clinical Oncology, 15,* 345–352.

Tallis, R., Fillit, H., & Brocklehurst, J. (1998). *Geriatric medicine and gerontology* (5th ed.). New York: Churchill Livingstone.

Tan, B.B., Flaherty, K.R., Kazerooni, E.A., & Iannettoni, M.D. (2003). The solitary pulmonary nodule. *Chest, 123*(Suppl. 1), 89S–96S.

Vicini, F., Kestin, L., Chen, P., Benitez, P., Goldstein, N., & Martinez, A. (2003). Limited-field radiation therapy in the management of early-stage breast cancer. *Journal of the National Cancer Institute, 95,* 120–121.

Watkins Bruner, D., Haas, M.L., & Gosselin-Acomb, T.K. (Eds.). (2005). *Manual for radiation oncology nursing practice and education* (3rd ed.). Pittsburgh, PA: Oncology Nursing Society.

Zachariah, B., Balducci, L., Venkattarmanabalaji, G.V., Casey, L., Greenberg, H.M., & DelRegato, J.A. (1997). Radiotherapy for cancer patients aged 80 and older: A study of effectiveness and side effects. *International Journal of Radiation Oncology, Biology, Physics, 39,* 1125–1129.

CHAPTER 15

The Older Adult With Myelosuppression and Anemia

Janet H. Van Cleave, MSN, ACNP-CS, AOCN®

Introduction

Compared with younger people, the population older than 65 has nearly 10 times the risk of developing cancer and a 16-fold greater risk of dying from cancer. With the shift toward an increased number of individuals 65 years of age or older in developed nations, the care of the older adult with cancer is an international public health concern (Yancik & Ries, 2004). A study of patients 65 years and older who died within one year of a diagnosis of lung, breast, colorectal, or other gastrointestinal cancer showed a trend toward increased use of aggressive treatment, including chemotherapy (Earle et al., 2004). To prevent and ameliorate treatment toxicities, the healthcare professional should understand chemotherapy-related hematologic toxicities in the older adult, especially myelotoxicity. Myelotoxicity is the most common toxicity of chemotherapy and is observed with increased frequency in older adults. It is a significant predictor of the development of febrile neutropenia and may contribute to a reluctance of administering chemotherapy to older adults (Pietropaolo, Gianni, Siliscavalli, Marigliano, & Repetto, 2003). This chapter addresses chemotherapy-related hematologic toxicities (CRHT) in the older adult patient with cancer. Physiologic effects of aging are described with assessment parameters and interventions to minimize complications related to CRHT in the older adult patient. Febrile neutropenia is discussed, and the chapter will conclude with a case study of a 72-year-old patient with non-Hodgkin lymphoma (NHL) undergoing chemotherapy.

Physiologic Effects of Aging

Aging is highly individualized, with frailty at the midpoint between independence and predeath (Lichtman, 2004). In the beginning of the aging process, physical activity has minimal limitations, and functional reserve is slightly reduced. Many individuals become somewhat vulnerable, leading to a critical reduction in functional reserve and functional limitations. At this point, reversibility of some conditions is possible. With advanced frailty, severe limitations are present with no significant recovery of functional reserve (Lichtman). Chronologic age often is used as a frame of reference but may poorly reflect the physiologic age of the individual (Balducci, 2000). Two chronologic ages, 70 and 85, are viewed as benchmarks for age-related changes. At age 70, age-related changes begin to increase. The age of 85 is considered a marker for risk of frailty because of hearing and vision deterioration, as well as greater functional dependence in the majority of people beyond this age. Also, some degree of dementia is present in more than 50% of individuals older than 85 (Balducci, 2000). In the aging process, functional declines occur in kidney and immune function, but the clinical consequences may be minimal or nonexistent in the absence of disease. Aging affects the bone marrow reserve, with fewer stem cells and less proliferative potential of progenitor cells (Harrison, 1979; Harrison, Astle, & Stone, 1989). Erythropoietin responses are blunted with advancing age, and low levels of anemia are common in otherwise healthy older adults.

Multiple theories exist on aging, yet no single theory is able to account for the complex aging process (Denduluri & Ershler, 2004) (see Table 15-1). These theories include models that approach aging as either exogenous or endogenous damage to DNA, causing mutations, decreased DNA repair, decreased neuronal and associated hormonal functions, as well as decreased immune function (Denduluri & Ershler).

Currently, experimental models supported with circumstantial evidence point toward carcinogenesis as a multistage process involving serial alterations of cellular genes. These alterations produce oncogenes and impaired tumor suppressor genes, which modify cell proliferation, as well as genes inhibiting apoptosis (programmed cell death) (Denduluri & Ershler, 2004). Viewing carcinogenesis as a multistage

---

Table 15-1. Theories of Aging

Intrinsic-stochastic	Somatic mutation
	Intrinsic mutagenesis
	Impaired DNA repair
	Error catastrophe
Extrinsic-stochastic	Ionizing radiation
	Free radical damage
Genetically determined	Neuroendocrine
	Immune

Note. From "Aging Biology and Cancer," by N. Denduluri and W.B. Ershler, 2004, *Seminars in Oncology, 31,* p. 139. Copyright 2004 by Saunders. Reprinted with permission.

process provides at least three hypotheses for the increasing incidence of cancer in the older adult. The first explanation is that the older person's tissues will have sustained the serial random events over time involved in carcinogenesis. The second theory is that the process of aging involves genetic events similar to those occurring early in carcinogenesis. The third theory is that the aging process provides time for the cancer to evolve in either path. Therefore, in older patients, an increased number of cells would be susceptible to the effects of late-stage carcinogenesis (Denduluri & Ershler).

The aging process affects older adults' response to pharmaceuticals; however, little information is available on older adults' drug tolerance. Although adults age 65 and older are the primary users of pharmaceuticals, pharmaceutical data typically come from studies on patients younger than 55 years of age (Lichtman, 2004). Therefore, the older adults' responses to cancer medications are theorized according to known age-related changes in pharmacodynamics and pharmacokinetics. The most significant age-related changes occur in the absorption, distribution, metabolism, and excretion systems (see Table 15-2).

Table 15-2. Physiologic Changes and Consequences of Chemotherapy Associated With Aging in Older Adult Patients With Cancer

Physiologic Change	Consequence of Chemotherapy
Slower repair of DNA damage	Prolonged toxicity
Reduced stem cell mass and hematopoiesis	Slow recovery of blood and mucosal cells
Reduced functional reserve of organ systems	Risk of organ failure with additional tissue loss
Reduced gastrointestinal absorptive surfaces, gastric motility, and gastric secretion	Reduced drug absorption
Reduced fat-free mass	Altered drug distribution
Greater anemia	Reduced drug metabolism
Decreased nephron mass	Reduced drug excretion

Note. From "Greater Risks of Chemotherapy Toxicity in Elderly Patients With Cancer," by L. Repetto, 2003, *Journal of Supportive Oncology, 1*(4 Suppl. 2), p. 19. Copyright 2003 by Elsevier. Reprinted with permission.

Absorption

The changes in the digestive system of the older adult may reduce the amount of drug absorbed in a unit of time. These changes include decreased gastrointestinal motility, decreased splanchnic blood flow, mucosal atrophy, and decreased secretion of digestive enzymes (Lichtman, 2004). With the emphasis on the IV route of chemotherapy, these physiologic changes have not been important in the past. However, oral chemotherapy is becoming more prominent in the clinical setting. Few data are available on age-related effects in oral chemotherapy (Carbone, 2000).

Distribution

The volume of distribution of drugs is a major factor in the drug toxicity in older patients with cancer. It is a function of body composition and the concentration of the serum albumin and red blood cells. A progressive loss of body protein and accumulation of body fat occurs until age 85, when generalized tissue atrophy occurs, as well as a possible progressive reduction in serum albumin and anemia. These changes can result in a reduced volume of distribution for water-soluble drugs, increased serum concentration, and increased toxicity, especially in anemic patients receiving anthracyclines, taxanes, and epipodophyllotoxins (Lichtman, 2004).

Excretion

Glomerular function decreases with age. A gradual loss in renal mass and glomerular sclerosis lead to loss of capacity to perform ultra filtration of plasma. Because of the loss of muscle mass from the aging process, the decreased glomerular filtration is not reflected in an increased serum creatinine (Lichtman, Skirvin, & Vemulapalli, 2003). The Cockcroft-Gault (Cockcroft & Gault, 1976) equation often is used to estimate creatinine clearance; however, these equations are less accurate in the older adult and in patients with severe renal failure or decreased muscle mass (Lichtman, 2004). Gelman and Taylor (1984) demonstrated that renally adjusted doses of cyclophosphamide and methotrexate in women 65 years of age or older with metastatic breast cancer had similar therapeutic responses with less myelotoxicity compared to younger patients who received full doses. Therefore, chemotherapy agents primarily excreted by the kidney should be used with caution, and dose adjustment may be needed, particularly in frail older adults (see Figure 15-1).

Metabolism

Age-related changes of decreased liver mass and blood flow appear to alter drug metabolism in older patients with cancer. Drug metabolism in the liver occurs in

Renal	Hepatic	Mixed
• Bleomycin	• Doxorubicin	• Epipodophyllotoxins
• Carboplatin	• Daunorubicin	• Mitomycin C
• Carmustine	• Epirubicin	
• Cisplatin	• Vinca alkaloids	
• 2-CDA	• Taxanes	
• Cytarabine		
• Dacarbazine		
• Fludarabine		
• Hydroxyurea		
• Ifosfamide		
• Melphalan		
• Methotrexate		

Figure 15-1. Chemotherapy Agents Associated With Renal or Hepatic Excretion

Note. From "Cancer Chemotherapy in the Older Patient: What the Medical Oncologist Needs to Know," by L. Balducci and M. Extermann, 1997, *Cancer, 80,* p. 1319. Copyright 1997 by Wiley. Adapted with permission.

phase I and II reactions. Phase I metabolism occurs primarily via the cytochrome P450 system consisting of oxidoreductive reactions that lead to activation and deactivation of drugs. Phase II reactions are primarily conjugation reactions that produce hydrosoluble compounds ready for renal and biliary excretion (Balducci & Corcoran, 2000). Phase I reactions are altered in the older patient with cancer, whereas it appears that phase II reactions are unaffected by age (Balducci & Corcoran; Lichtman, 2004). Currently, hepatic changes in the pharmacokinetics of drugs do not seem to have a significant effect on the tolerance of chemotherapy in the older adult. Future work with newer techniques may bring better clarity to the effect of altered phase I reactions in the older adult (Balducci & Corcoran; National Comprehensive Cancer Network [NCCN], 2004, 2005a).

Treatment Benefit

Although the older adult usually can tolerate surgery and radiation therapy, the decision to treat older adult patients with chemotherapy is more complex. Data associated with the older adult are limited (Hutchins, Unger, Crowley, Coltman, & Albain, 1999; Lewis et al., 2003; Teret, Albrand, & Droz, 2004). An analysis of data from a retrospective analysis of 28,766 people enrolled in 55 clinical trials from 1995–2002 investigating new medications or novel uses of approved drugs for leukemia, lymphoma, and cancers of the breast, lung, colon, ovary, pancreas, and central nervous system demonstrated that only 36% of patients enrolled were ages 65 and older. This unfavorably compares with the fact that 60% of the U.S. cancer population is 65 and older. Barriers to enrollment in these clinical trials included stringent eligibility criteria because of health limitations and concerns about ability to tolerate chemotherapy, causing debilitating side effects, healthcare costs, as well as lack of social and homecare support (Talarico, Chen, & Pazdur, 2004).

From the data, it appears that older adults benefit from standard treatment. This is demonstrated in the clinical trials in patients with NHL (Balducci, 2003b). In these clinical trials, the response rate to moderately aggressive chemotherapy was comparable to the response rate seen in younger patients. The ability of the older adult to tolerate chemotherapy is controversial. Some studies report that older adults tolerate chemotherapy as well as younger patients; however, these results are not generalizable because of a decreased number of patients older than 80 years participating in the trials and the selection bias toward healthier patients (NCCN, 2005a). Other studies have demonstrated that older patients are susceptible to myelotoxicity (NCCN, 2005a). However, the management of myelotoxicity by dose reductions or delays may lead to suboptimal patient outcomes (Dale, 2003). The need to better define the roles among age, drug toxicity, comorbidities, and the potential benefit of chemotherapy in common cancers is a national priority (Repetto, 2003).

Evaluation of the Older Adult With Cancer

The key decision is to properly select patients who will benefit from treatment with minimal risk of significant toxicity leading to decreased survival or quality of life. The initial assessment of patients includes determining who is expected to die of cancer or experience complications within their lifetime versus patients whose life expectancy is less than the probability of developing morbidity from cancer (Balducci, 2003c;

NCCN, 2005a). If the patient is felt to benefit from treatment, then further evaluation is needed to determine the potential for toxicity and the appropriate chemotherapy dose. These assessments are complex and require a multidisciplinary healthcare team of physicians, nurses, pharmacists, social workers, and physical therapists to provide an efficient but comprehensive assessment (Rao, Seo, & Cohen, 2004).

In preparation for chemotherapy, determining any disease or stress that can alter the delicate balance between functional reserve and physiologic functioning that exists in the older adult is important. This includes the evaluation of renal function, liver function, bone marrow reserves, and preexisting neurotoxicity (Extermann & Aapro, 2000). Comorbidity, functional status, depression, cognitive impairment, nutritional status, and insufficient social support affect the survival of older adults with cancer. A comprehensive geriatric assessment (CGA) (see Table 15-3) can help to determine candidates for life-prolonging treatment, as well as those candidates in which standard treatment may have greater risks than benefits (Balducci, 2003c; Extermann & Aapro). Various forms exist of the geriatric assessment; some can be time consuming and difficult to use in older patients. Ongoing work is being performed to construct an abbreviated CGA that would require less clinical time and act as a

Table 15-3. Comprehensive Geriatric Assessment

Parameter	Assessment
Function	Activities of daily living—Eating, dressing, continence, grooming, transferring, using the bathroom Instrumental activities of daily living—Use of transportation; management of money and medications; shopping; ability to provide own meals, do laundry, manage house, and use telephone Performance status
Comorbidity	Number of comorbid conditions Seriousness of comorbid conditions (comorbidity index)
Socioeconomic issues	Living conditions Presence and adequacy of caregiver Income Access to transportation
Geriatric syndromes	Dementia—Mini-Mental Status, other Depression—Geriatric Depression Scale Delirium—For minimal infection or medication Falls ($\geq$ 1 per month) Osteoporosis (spontaneous fractures) Neglect and abuse Failure to thrive Persistent dizziness
Polypharmacy	Number of medications Drug-to-drug interaction
Nutrition	Nutritional risk—Mini-Nutritional Assessment

Note. From "Clinical Practice Guidelines in Oncology: Senior Adult Oncology," by the National Comprehensive Cancer Network, 2005. Retrieved September 22, 2005, from http://www.nccn.org/professionals/physician_gls/PDF/senior.pdf. Copyright 2005 by the National Comprehensive Cancer Network. Reprinted with permission.

screening measure for patients who would benefit from the entire CGA (Overcash, Beckstead, & Cobb, 2004; Teret et al., 2004). Currently, the NCCN guidelines recommend some form of geriatric assessment in all patients 65 years of age or older, with brief screening tools to identify the patients who need a more comprehensive evaluation (NCCN, 2005a). The CGA evaluated key sections that influence treatment and toxicities, including functional status, comorbidities, socioeconomic issues, geriatric syndromes, polypharmacy, and nutrition.

Functional Status

Functional status measurement is very important and has been demonstrated to be a predictor of response to chemotherapy, treatment toxicities, as well as survival (Yancik et al., 1998). It measures the patient's ability to perform basic activities of daily living (ADL), instrumental ADL, and advanced ADL (ability to fulfill societal, community, and family roles) (Rao et al., 2004).

Comorbidities

Comorbidities are serious medical conditions unrelated to the cancer disease and affect the pulmonary, renal, hepatic, and/or cardiovascular system. They occur with increasing age, are viewed as negative prognostic factors, and are a major cause of mortality. Comorbidity can adversely affect the patient's functional status. However, a minimal direct correlation exists between these assessments (Extermann, Overcash, Lyman, Parr, & Balducci, 1998). Therefore, the two should be evaluated separately (Balducci, 2001).

Social Support

With the increasing number of older adults with cancer and the shift from inpatient to outpatient cancer treatment, the family caregiver has a critical role that may vary from providing minimal assistance in a highly functioning older patient with cancer to providing complete care to a highly debilitated patient. The caregiver also may need to provide transportation to and from appointments, administer medications, manage side effects, provide nutrition, and participate in end-of-life decisions. Research demonstrates that caregiver burden is an important factor in determining who uses formal services. The caregiver should be identified and the burden assessed as part of the CGA (Brown, Potter, & Foster, 1990; Haley, 2003).

Economic Assessment

Although many older adults with cancer may not be comfortable talking about their financial issues, they may be eligible for local or state benefits, as well as pharmaceutical drug plans and services for functional impairment. A social worker may help to identify patients who are eligible for assistance and begin the mobilization of resources to provide personal home attendants (Rao et al., 2004; Reuben, 1998).

Environmental Assessment

Hazards in the home can contribute to falls and physical disability, as well as provide information on sanitary conditions, medication use, nutrition use, and elder abuse/neglect. Hazards contributing to falls in the home include poor lighting, loose rugs, and inadequate bathroom grab rails, electric and telephone cords, and stairway banisters. The environmental assessment especially can be helpful in the frail older adult, who has difficulty navigating instrumental ADL as well as problems with mobility and balance (Rao et al., 2004).

Geriatric Syndrome

Mobility and Balance Disorders/Fall Risk

Older adults may be at high risk for falling and subsequent consequences. The assessment of fall risk for balance, gait, lower extremity strength, and a history of previous falls may identify patients at risk. The best assessment is to observe the patient performing tasks. Some simple assessments of balance and fall risk include testing the ability to maintain a tandem or semitandem stand for 10 seconds, resistance to a sternal nudge, and observation of a 360° turn (Reuben, 1998).

Visual and Hearing Impairment

The older adult with cancer is at risk for visual and hearing impairment that can be exacerbated by chemotherapy. Visual acuity can be tested using a Snellen eye chart. One way to assess hearing is to use the Welch Allyn Audioscope, a handheld otoscope with a built-in audiometer. Another test for hearing impairment is the whispered voice test, where three to six random words are whispered at a set distance (Reuben, 1998).

Urinary Incontinence

Urinary incontinence is a frequent problem in older adults and may occur in up to 30% of community-based older adults. Causes of urinary incontinence include delirium, medications, atrophic vaginitis, obstetric injury, stool impaction, and prior prostate surgery (Rao et al., 2004). It causes embarrassment to the patient and affects the patient's quality of life. To assess urinary incontinence, the healthcare provider should ask if the patient has lost his or her urine and gotten wet. If the answer is yes, then the patient should be asked if he or she has lost urine on at least six separate days. An affirmative answer should be followed by a formal urologic consultation (Rao et al.; Reuben, 1998).

Cognitive Assessment

Mental status affects the older adult's ability to comply with treatment, participate in end-of-life decisions, and give informed consent. Recent studies demonstrate that either emotional problems or cognitive impairment is associated with decreased survival rates (Callen, Vranas, Overcash, Boulware, & Extermann, 2004; Stommel, Given, & Given, 2002). Several factors can affect the mental status of the older adult with cancer. The incidence of dementia rises with age. Certain chemotherapies (e.g., high-dose cytarabine) and whole brain irradiation can cause significant neurotoxicities. Dehydration, malnutrition, corticosteroids, and electrolyte disturbances also can increase the risk of delirium. Simple screening tests can assess mental status and indicate if further testing should be undertaken. These screening tests include the Mini-Mental State Examination (Folstein, Folstein, & McHugh, 1975), the three-item recall, and the clock drawing test (Rao et al., 2004).

Cognitive deficits caused by stress, fatigue, acute illness, or depression are potentially reversible. However, impairment caused by Alzheimer disease is irreversible. Depression and mental impairment can mimic each other, and distinguishing between the two in order to prescribe the appropriate treatment is important. Depression is especially common in older adult patients with cancer and is an underdiagnosed disorder. Resolving depression through counseling and pharmacotherapy can produce significant improvement in the patient's ability to tolerate cancer treatment and can improve the patient's quality of life (Balducci, 2001).

Nutrition

Older patients often are malnourished, which can seriously affect patients' immune function and ability to tolerate chemotherapy. Because of a decreased thirst reflex and less social support, older patients are more likely than younger patients to suffer from dehydration caused by nausea, vomiting, or diarrhea (Extermann & Aapro, 2000). Distinguishing between correctable malnutrition and the irreversible wasting that may accompany terminal malignancy is important (Balducci, 2001).

Polypharmacy

Many older adults take multiple medications, with incidence cited from 5.7%–29% of older patients taking five or more medications (Extermann & Aapro, 2000). Mistakes of omission and substitution because of confusion are common. A thorough assessment of all medications is necessary of both prescriptive as well as over-the-counter medications.

Frail Older Adults

Frailty will become a major issue in oncology as the population ages (Repetto, Venturino, et al., 2003). Multiple criteria exist in the literature (see Figure 15-2) (Balducci, 2001; Chen, Kenefick, Tang, & McCorkle, 2004; Ferrucci et al., 2003).

Patient meets any of the following criteria:

- Cerebrovascular accident
- Chronic and disabling illness
- Confusion
- Dependence in activities of daily living
- Depression
- Dementia
- Falls
- Impaired mobility
- Incontinence
- Malnutrition
- Polypharmacy
- Pressure sore
- Prolonged bedrest
- Restraints
- Sensory impairment
- Socioeconomic/family problems

Figure 15-2. Criteria for Frailty

Note. From "Utilization of Comprehensive Geriatric Assessment in Cancer Patients," by C.C. Chen, A.L. Kenefick, S.T. Tang, and R. McCorkle, 2004, *Critical Reviews in Oncology/Hematology, 49,* p. 55. Copyright 2004 by Elsevier. Reprinted with permission.

Frailty is conceptualized as a pathologic condition, pictured as a constellation of signs and symptoms, and characterized by a high susceptibility to impending decline in physical function and a high risk of death (Ferrucci et al.). The implications of the frail older adult in life expectancy and treatment recommendations also differ in the literature. However, frailty appears to indicate conservative treatment measures.

Evidence Summary of the Comprehensive Geriatric Assessment

Multiple clinical trials demonstrate that geriatric interventions guided by the CGA have positive outcomes on health, functional status, and mortality. Although oncology researchers use the CGA to identify important health and functional problems, no randomized clinical trials are available to validate the CGA in older adults with cancer. More research is needed to investigate the effectiveness of the CGA in the care, management, and follow-up of older adult patients with cancer (Ferrucci et al., 2003).

Chemotherapy-Related Hematologic Toxicities

Patient assessment and cancer diagnostic evaluation provide information for clinical management of the patient. The decision to treat cancer in the older adult is based on all factors, including the type and stage of the disease, the patient's life expectancy to determine if the patient will live long enough to gain benefit from treatment, and the patient's physical and mental ability to tolerate treatment (Balducci, 2003c). One of the major toxicities of the patient undergoing treatment is CRHT secondary to decreased bone marrow reserve in the older adult. The risk of myelodepression increases substantially by the age of 65, with the incidence of neutropenic infection–related mortality varying between 5% and 30%. However, a classic study by Begg and Carbone (1983) using data from 19 studies by the Eastern Cooperative Oncology Group of advanced cancer in eight disease sites (lung, colorectal, gastric, sarcoma, head/neck, melanoma, renal, and ovarian) compared chemotherapy toxicities between patients younger than 70 years of age and patients 70 years of age or older. The results indicated that, in general, patients older than 70 years of age had comparable toxicities to their younger counterparts, except for a significantly higher rate of hematologic toxicity. Using a subset analysis of the same data, Begg, Elson, and Carbone (1989) further evaluated CRHT in solid tumors to determine which agents caused a greater risk of severe hematologic toxicity in the older adult. Hematologic toxicity was defined as a white blood count (WBC) of less than $2,000/mm^3$, platelet count less than $50,000/mm^3$, or a neutrophil count of less than $1,000/mm^3$ at any time during the chemotherapy course. Table 15-4 identifies the six drugs found to be most myelotoxic in the older adult. Except for methotrexate, the drugs causing the greatest hematologic toxicity in the older adult are primarily metabolized through the liver. Limitations of the study included possible drug interactions when using combination therapy and a limited patient population consisting primarily of those with solid tumors. The authors concluded that although it may be prudent to amend treatments to modify or exclude the myelotoxic drugs identified in this study, patients who are older than 70 years of age with normal renal and hepatic function and without serious comorbidities generally should not be denied effective chemotherapy.

Table 15-4. Increase in Risk of Severe Hematologic Toxicity in Older Adults

Drug	Adjusted Increase In Odds Compared With Control Group (< 60 years)	
	60–69 years (%)	≥ 70 years (%)
Actinomycin-D	94	319
Vinblastine	44	149
Methotrexate	25	119
Etoposide	91	155
Methyl CCNU	27	52
Doxorubicin	12	42

Note. From "A Study of Excess Hematologic Toxicity in Elderly Patients Treated on Cancer Chemotherapy Protocols" (p. 155), by C.B. Begg, P.J. Elson, and P.P. Carbone in R. Yancik and J.W. Yates (Eds.), *Cancer in the Elderly: Approaches to Early Detection and Treatment*, 1989, New York: Springer. Copyright 1989 by Springer. Reprinted with permission.

Since that time, clinical researchers have investigated CRHT in patients with NHL. Studies of older adults with NHL undergoing chemotherapy have demonstrated grade 4 neutropenia from 4%–50% and treatment-related mortality from 2%–19%, with the 19% mortality occurring in the 60–94 age group (Bastion et al., 1997; Gomez et al., 1998; Tirelli et al., 1998; Zinzani et al., 1997) (see Table 15-5). Bastion et al. also demonstrated that neutropenia may occur primarily in the first cycle.

Chemotherapy-Induced Neutropenia

Neutropenia is defined as an absolute neutrophil count (ANC) < 500 cells/mm³ or an ANC of 1,000 cells/mm³ expected to decrease to < 500 cells/mm³ (Fischer, Knobf, Durivage, & Beaulieu, 2003). Although the definition is numerical, neutropenia is a multidimensional experience resulting in vulnerability to infection, restrictions, fever and infection, and psychosocial alterations in quality of life (see Table 15-5) (Crighton, 2004). Chemotherapy-induced neutropenia is the major dose-limiting toxicity of systemic cancer chemotherapy. It is associated with substantial morbidity, mortality, and increased healthcare costs. It also can cause dose reductions or treatment delays, which may compromise treatment (NCCN, 2005). Clinical data suggest that the older adult is at a higher risk for first-cycle febrile neutropenia, particularly after 70 years of age (Lyman, Kuderer, Agboola, & Balducci, 2003).

The preventive or prophylactic use of granulocyte–colony-stimulating factors (G-CSFs) is associated with reduced length and severity of chemotherapy-related neutropenia. G-CSFs also may prevent life-threatening complications (NCCN, 2005). Several guidelines exist for the use of G-CSFs in chemotherapy. The American Society of Clinical Oncology's (ASCO's) guidelines for the use of G-CSFs recommended primary prophylaxis for patients expected to experience levels of febrile neutropenia at least comparable to or greater than those seen in control patients in randomized trials (expected incidence ≥ 40%) (Ozer et al.,

Table 15-5. Grade 4 Neutropenia and Treatment-Related Toxicity in Older Patients With Large Cell Non-Hodgkin Lymphoma Treated With CHOP and CHOP-Like Regimens

Author	Regimen (number of patients)	Patient Age (yrs.)	Grade 4 Neutropenia	Treatment-Related Mortality
Bastion et al., 1997	CVP (219)	≥ 70	4%[a,b]	12%
	CTVP (231)	≥ 70	15%[a,b]	15%
Gomez et al., 1998	CHOP (267)	60–69 (n = 126)	NR	12%
		70–79 (n = 115)	NR	13%
		80–94 (n = 26)	NR	19%
Tirelli et al., 1998	VMP (60)	≥ 70	50%	5%
	CHOP (60)	≥ 70	47%	2%
Zinzani et al., 1997	VNCOP B + G-CSF (77)	≥ 60	23%	NR
	VNCOP B (72)	–	55.5%	–

[a] Leukocyte count $< 0.5 \times 10^9$/L
[b] Absolute neutrophil count nadir $< 0.5 \times 10^9$/L

CHOP—cyclophosphamide, doxorubicin, vincristine, and prednisone; CTVP—cyclophosphamide, pirarubicin, teniposide, and prednisone; CVP—cyclophosphamide, teniposide, and prednisone; G-CSF—granulocyte–colony-stimulating factor; NR—not reported; VMP—etoposide, mitoxantrone, and prednisone; VNCOP-B—etoposide, mitoxantrone, cyclophosphamide, vincristine, prednisone, and bleomycin

Note. From "Increased Risk of Myelotoxicity in Elderly Patients With Non-Hodgkin Lymphoma," by L. Balducci and L. Repetto, 2004, *Cancer, 100,* p. 7. Copyright 2004 by Wiley. Adapted with permission.

2000). New NCCN (2005b) guidelines for myeloid growth factors recommended primary prophylactic use of colony-stimulating factors (CSFs) for high-risk patients. High risk was defined as 20% or higher probability of developing neutropenia or neutropenic events that result in compromising treatment (NCCN, 2005b). The NCCN (2005a) general guidelines for the management of the older adult with cancer recommended primary use of hematopoietic growth factors in people 65 years of age and older. The rationale based on patients treated with cyclophosphamide/vincristine/doxorubicin/prednisone (CHOP) chemotherapy for NHL is that the risk of myelosuppression increases substantially at age 70. In addition, data suggest that the use of prophylactic CSFs in older adult patients is associated with a lower risk of hospitalization and shorter hospital stays in patients treated for NHL (Ozer, 2003).

Evidence-Based Use of Colony-Stimulating Factors

A Working Party on the use of CSFs in older adults recently was established as part of an agreement between the European Organization for Research and Treatment of Cancer (EORTC) and the EORTC Cancer in the Elderly Task Force. The purpose of this group is to derive evidence-based conclusions on the value of prophylactic CSF administration in older adults receiving chemotherapy. A detailed literature search from 1992–2002 using Medline and Pre-Medline for clinical trials in patients 60 years of age or older produced 30 papers for review for evidence-based guidelines. The evidence demonstrates that G-CSF reduces the incidence of chemotherapy-induced neutropenia, febrile neutropenia, and infections in older adults receiving myelotoxic chemotherapy for NHL, small-cell lung cancer, or urothelial tumors (see Table 15-6). The authors concluded that because systematic dose reduction can affect outcome, all older adult patients receiving myelotoxic chemotherapy (CHOP or CHOP-like) should receive primary prophylactic G-CSF administration, and, as suggested by ASCO guidelines, a risk-adapted strategy with primary prophylactic use of G-CSF should be used in high-risk patients. Further evaluation of CSF with other chemotherapy regimens is needed, especially in regimens with a greater risk of severe myelosuppression, such as dose-intensification protocols. For example, the combination of methotrexate, vinblastine, doxorubicin, and cisplatin for bladder cancer appears to be excessively toxic, resulting in 23% of treatment-related deaths despite prophylactic G-CSF (Repetto, Biganzoli, et al., 2003).

Table 15-6. Guidelines for the Use of Colony-Stimulating Factors in Older Adult Patients With Cancer

Category/Disease	Evidence
Non-Hodgkin lymphoma	SE
Small cell lung cancer	SE
Urothelial tumors	SE
Granulocyte macrophage–colony-stimulating factor	IE
Toxic deaths	IE
Treatment efficacy in standard dose chemotherapy	NE

IE—insufficient evidence; NE—no evidence; SE—sufficient evidence

Note. Based on information from Repetto, Biganzoli, et al., 2003.

The Working Party found insufficient evidence to recommend use of granulocyte macrophage–colony-stimulating factor (GM-CSF) and evaluated the impact of prophylactic CSF on the incidence of toxic deaths in older adults with cancer. The Working Party noted a lack of evidence that the delivery of standard-dose chemotherapy on schedule improved treatment efficacy in older adults. The authors recommended future clinical trials to further define the use of G-CSF in older adults and to answer the critical question of the impact of CSF on older adult deaths from chemotherapy toxicity (Repetto, Biganzoli, et al., 2003).

Pegfilgrastim

A new drug, pegfilgrastim (Neulasta®, Amgen, Thousand Oaks, CA), simplifies hematopoietic support in patients receiving chemotherapy. Pegfilgrastim is a form of

G-CSF that is long acting because of the pegylation of the filgrastim molecule, which minimizes renal clearance. It is given once per chemotherapy cycle. Neutrophil-mediated clearance of the drug occurs as neutrophil levels return to normal (Holmes et al., 2002). Results from clinical trials have shown that a single dose of pegfilgrastim provides neutrophil support comparable to that of 11 daily injections of filgrastim in patients with breast cancer and is comparable to filgrastim in reducing neutropenic complications in patients with lymphoma. Recent data suggest that filgrastim and prophylactic antibiotics were more effective in preventing neutropenic infections compared to antibiotics alone. Multiple clinical trials also have demonstrated that the safety profile is similar to filgrastim (Crawford, 2003); however, some healthcare professionals are concerned that the combination of topoisomerase II inhibitors and growth factors is associated with an increased risk of acute leukemia (NCCN, 2005a). Despite these concerns, NCCN (2005a) guidelines recommended growth factors as the established strategy to improve treatment in older adults with cancer.

Anemia

Anemia is a significant problem in the older adult patient with cancer. Anemia is the most common hematologic abnormality seen with malignancies, occurring in more than 50% of patients with cancer. It is associated with debilitating symptoms, lower quality of life, and potentially poorer disease/treatment outcomes (Smith & Tchekmedyian, 2002). Multiple causes of malignancy-related anemia exist, including shortened red blood cell (RBC) life span because of hemorrhage, hemolysis, hemophagocytosis, and hypersplenism. Another cause of anemia is impaired erythropoietin production/bone marrow response triggered by the immune and inflammatory cytokines common to these conditions, such as tumor necrosis factor, interleukin-1, and the interferons. Although anemia in cancer generally is because of the disease and chemotherapy, a diagnostic evaluation should be conducted to prevent failure in correctly diagnosing the etiology. The diagnostic workup of anemia generally consists of the history of the anemia and cancer treatment, physical examination, and laboratory examination. In patients with anemia, several approaches are watch and wait, erythropoietic therapy, and/or a combination of the two approaches. Prior to the advent of erythropoietin, the patient generally received a transfusion with two or more units of packed RBCs when the hemoglobin level fell below 8 g/dl. Multiple transfusion reactions and marginal increases in quality of life led to a lack of enthusiasm by clinicians for transfusions.

In the 1990s, recombinant human erythropoietin (rHuEPO) was clinically developed and introduced into clinical trials as erythropoietin therapy. Since that time, multiple studies in patients with lung cancer have shown that treatment of anemia with epoetin alfa increases quality of life (Groopman & Itri, 1999). However, a multicenter, double-blind, randomized, placebo-controlled trial conducted in Germany with patients with head and neck cancer showed poorer survival with epoetin beta plus radiation therapy versus radiation therapy alone (Henke et al., 2003). One explanation by the authors of the study for the negative trial is that tumor cells use the erythropoietin system for growth and angiogenesis. Recently, preliminary data from the Radiation Therapy Oncology Group Study 99-03 showed similar findings. In this study, patients with squamous cell carcinoma of the head and neck receiving both epoetin alfa and radiation therapy with or without chemotherapy had a trend toward decreased survival compared with patients who received similar cancer treatment without epoetin alfa. The target hemoglobin for the study was higher than that seen in clinical practice (13.5–16 g/dl). However, the study recommendations called for further research involving tumor hypoxia, anemia, erythropoietin, and tumor biology to return to preclinical work (Machtay & Brown, 2004). The clinical ramifications from these new data have yet to be determined.

In the older adult, anemia may increase the risk of adverse drug reactions, risk of delirium, and complications of cytotoxic chemotherapy (Balducci, 2003a). NCCN (2005a) guidelines for the management of the older adult with cancer who is undergoing chemotherapy recommended maintaining hemoglobin levels ≥ 12 g/dl with an erythropoietin preparation for optimal relief of fatigue. However, further refinement of the guidelines may be necessary as more research investigates the use of erythropoietin in patients with cancer.

Two erythropoietic agents are approved for use in the United States for treatment of cancer chemotherapy anemia: epoetin alfa (Procrit®, Ortho Biotech, Bridgewater, NJ) and darbepoetin alfa (Aranesp®, Amgen). Currently, interesting data suggest that increased hemoglobin affects treatment outcomes and neurocognition of patients with cancer (Zinzani et al., 1999).

Minimizing Toxic Effects

If the decision is made to treat an older adult with chemotherapy, steps can minimize toxicities related to chemotherapy-induced bone marrow suppression, including referrals and preventing symptoms. First, all correctable conditions should be treated by promoting good nutrition, hydration, and hygiene. This can include referring the patient for well-fitting dentures, correcting dehydration and malnutrition, and eliminating polypharmacy. A question about the types and amounts of food the patient eats on an average day is a good screening tool to detect poor nutrition. Correcting problems and establishing a suitable dietary plan are simple interventions that can substantially impact the patient's quality of life and clinical outcome. Patient education about preventive hygiene can help to reduce the risk of infection because of chemotherapy-induced neutropenia. Oral rinses may help to prevent or relieve mucositis. Patients with visual and hearing impairment can be referred to specialists for further evaluation (Balducci, 2001).

Patient Education

Patient education about chemotherapy side effects is an important component to minimizing toxicities. Teaching should include a discussion that chemotherapy can cause myelosuppression leading to life-threatening infections, with an explanation of WBC count and the meaning of the WBC nadir. This instruction includes verifying that the patient knows how to take his or her temperature and is aware of the signs and symptoms of infection (see Figure 15-3) (Fischer et al., 2003).

A baseline educational needs assessment and use of adult learning principles, including use of past experiences as references for teaching, can help to focus educational material (Padberg & Padberg, 1997). Patients may have barriers to learning such as sight or hearing impairments, difficulty reading, difficulty understanding English, and limited healthcare experience. Including the family caregivers can enhance education. Patients may be overwhelmed with the new material, and

• Temperature greater than 100.4°F (38°C)	• Tenderness
• Chills	• Swelling
• Inflammation	• Headache
• Rash	• Inability to bend head forward
• Increased respiration	• Urinary frequency with or without pain
• General malaise	• Cough with or without sputum

Figure 15-3. Signs and Symptoms of Infection

Note. From *The Cancer Chemotherapy Handbook* (6th ed., p. 481), by D.S. Fischer, M.T. Knobf, J.J. Durivage, and N.J. Beaulieu, 2003, Philadelphia: Mosby. Copyright 2003 by Mosby. Reprinted with permission.

consistent repetition may be helpful for patient retention (Rutledge & McGuire, 2004). Educational tools should be judged on readability (Cooley et al., 1995) and cultural sensitivity.

Dose Adjustment

Another strategy to minimize chemotherapy toxicity is to modify the dosage to adjust for age-related declines in renal function without compromising treatment effectiveness. As previously discussed, pharmacokinetic parameters are highly variable for chemotherapy agents, especially in the older adult. Older adult patients often have a diminished volume of distribution and diminished renal function. Hepatic metabolism and excretion may be altered. Individual drugs differ in site of metabolism, and the effect of altered metabolism is secondary to the aging process. Therefore, individual assessment of the patient and the drug is needed, and, generally, the doses of chemotherapy drugs that undergo renal excretion should be adjusted according to the glomerular filtration rate (Balducci, 2003c; Lichtman, 2004).

Management of Febrile Neutropenia

The absence of neutrophils, the disruption of the skin and mucosal barriers, and inherent microbial flora shifts that accompany severe illness and antimicrobial usage predispose patients with neutropenia to infection. The development of a fever in a neutropenic patient is an urgent clinical problem. Although the definition may differ among healthcare facilities, neutropenic fever generally is defined as a single temperature over 101°F (38.3°C) or a persistent fever ≥ 100.4°F (38.0°C) (Fischer et al., 2003). Although uncommon, a patient with neutropenia and signs or symptoms of infection (e.g., severe mucositis, abdominal pain, perirectal pain) without fever also may be considered actively infected (NCCN, 2004) (see Figure 15-3). Febrile neutropenia in the older adult is even more of a serious clinical issue. A retrospective study of 267 older adults receiving CHOP chemotherapy for NHL revealed a 13% treatment-related mortality from neutropenic fever (Gomez et al., 1998).

Management of the older adult with febrile neutropenia is generally the same as for all populations. The primary intervention is to administer empiric antibiotics in patients with fever and neutropenia. This is necessary because currently available diagnostic therapies are not sufficiently specific, sensitive, or rapid enough to identify or exclude noninfectious versus infectious causes. The initial evaluation should focus on determining the causative organisms and potential sites of infection and assessing the patient's risk of developing an infection-associated comorbid medical disease. A healthcare professional should perform a history assessment and physical examination. Common sites of infection for patients with fever and neutropenia include the alimentary and urinary tracts, skin, lungs, sinus, and intravascular access devices. However, sometimes the signs and symptoms may be absent in these patients. Important aspects in the patient's history include recent antibiotic therapy and exposure to infections from household members. Laboratory evaluation should include a complete blood count, liver and renal function tests, oxygen saturation, and urinalysis. A chest radiograph should be considered, but initially, no (or minimal) significant findings may exist in patients with neutropenia. Blood cultures should be collected during or immediately after completion of examination and before the start of antibiotics (NCCN, 2004).

Before selecting an antibiotic, the patient should be stratified to high-risk or low-risk categories for developing infection-related complications during the course of neutropenia. The Multinational Association of Supportive Care in Cancer derived the criteria for risk assessment from a study at 20 institutions in 15 nations (NCCN, 2004) (see Figure 15-4). The selection of empiric antibiotic therapy is dependent upon multiple factors and institutional preference (see Figure 15-5). The following factors should be considered in the selection of an antibiotic in the setting of febrile neutropenia: most common potential infecting organism, comorbidity, potential sites of infection, antimicrobial susceptibilities of pathogens isolated locally, importance of broad-spectrum antibacterial activity, preexisting organ dysfunction, patient medication allergy, patient's infection risk assessment, and previous antibiotic therapy. In neutropenic older adults, the goal is to attempt coverage for gram-positive or gram-negative organisms according to the dominant organisms in that hospital's experience; in clinical practice, usually both organisms are covered with one broad-spectrum antibiotic or two drugs. Considerable debate exists about the addition of empiric vancomycin in febrile neutropenic patients. The major concern in the use of empiric vancomycin is the emergence of vancomycin-resistant organisms. However, clinical situations that may justify initial vancomycin therapy include serious, clinically apparent, catheter-related infections in patients; substantial mucosal damage and high risk for infection with penicillin-resistant viridans group streptococci; blood cultures positive for gram-positive bacteria before final identification and susceptibility testing; known colonization with beta-lactam–resistant pneumococci; previous prophylaxis with ciprofloxacin or trimethoprim/sulfamethoxazole; and hypotension or septic

---

- A burden of illness characterized by no or mild symptoms using a visual analog scale
- Lack of hypotension at the onset of the episode
- Absence of chronic obstructive pulmonary disease at the onset of the episode
- Solid tumor or hematologic malignancy with no prior fungal infection
- Absence of dehydration at the onset of the episode
- Outpatient status
- Age younger than 60 years

Figure 15-4. Multinational Association of Supportive Care in Cancer Factors for Low Risk of Developing Febrile Neutropenic Complications

---

Note. From "Clinical Practice Guidelines in Oncology: Fever and Neutropenia," by the National Comprehensive Cancer Network, 2004. Retrieved May 30, 2004, from http://www.nccn.org/professionals/physician_gls/PDF/fever.pdf. Copyright 2004 by the National Comprehensive Cancer Network. Reprinted with permission.

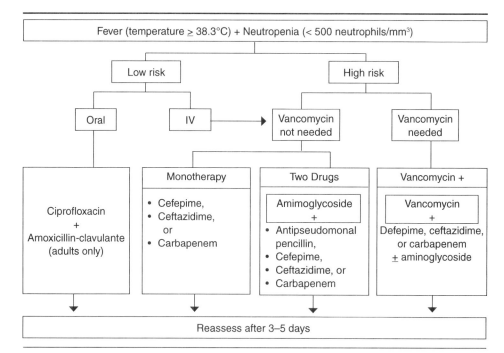

Figure 15-5. Algorithm for Initial Management of Febrile Neutropenia

Note. From "2002 Guidelines for the Use of Antimicrobial Agents in Neutropenic Patients With Cancer," by W.T. Hughes, D. Armstrong, G.P. Bodey, E.J. Bow, A.E. Brown, T. Calandra, et al., 2002, *Clinical Infectious Diseases, 34,* p. 735. Copyright 2002 by the University of Chicago Press. Reprinted with permission.

shock without a known pathogen. Patients who are considered low risk may be treated on an outpatient basis. However, patients 60 years of age or older are considered high risk and should be hospitalized (NCCN, 2004b).

According to ASCO guidelines, patients older than 65 years of age with febrile neutropenia are considered high risk for infection-associated complications (Ozer et al., 2000). In the clinical setting, with febrile neutropenia in older adults, the risk of fatality is so high that CSF should be initiated to decrease the duration of the neutropenia.

Nursing Care Issues

Nursing plays a key role in the care of the older patient experiencing chemotherapy-induced myelosuppression and anemia. Nurses often perform the initial patient assessment, identify patients at risk for treatment-related complications, provide essential patient education, and triage telephone calls from patients when complications occur. Nurses can improve patient outcomes and quality of life during chemotherapy treatment by knowing patient risk factors and interventions that can decrease the patient's susceptibility to infection and by performing appropriate and frequent patient education.

Case Study

Mr. Z is a 72-year-old male who recently had retired from his executive position at a large corporation. He enjoyed travel with his wife and his weekly golf game with former business associates. However, about one month ago, he started feeling fatigued, developed night sweats, noted that he had lost approximately 4 lbs in the last six months, and noticed a lump in his groin. He went to his primary clinician, who promptly referred him to a general surgeon. A biopsy showed diffuse large B-cell NHL, and Mr. Z was referred to an oncologist who recommended radiologic evaluation of the chest, abdomen, and pelvis, which showed increased lymphadenopathy in the retropelvic area and the right groin. The positron emission tomography scan confirmed these findings.

At the time of his visit with the oncologist, Mr. Z's lab work showed that his WBC was 7,750/mm³ with an ANC of 5,000/mm³, an Hgb of 13 mg/dl, and serum creatinine of 0.9. Using the Cockcroft-Gault measurement, his creatinine clearance was calculated to be 80 ml/min, which is within normal limits. The oncologist recommended a chemotherapy regimen of CHOP plus rituximab with full doses with growth factor support. At this time, Mr. Z met MaryAnn, the chemotherapy nurse clinician. She reviewed Mr. Z's laboratory data and his weight, which were normal for Mr. Z's height. She also evaluated Mr. Z for functional status, nutritional intake, eyesight, and hearing. She found that Mr. Z led an active life, had good nutritional intake, and good eyesight. However, Mr. Z was worried about the effect of his disease and treatment on his wife, who had insulin-dependent diabetes. Mr. Z was her main caregiver and drove her to her doctor's appointments. MaryAnn provided patient education materials about the chemotherapy and growth factors that Mr. Z easily could read and understand.

Because of the vesicant potential of the chemotherapy drugs, Mr. Z underwent placement of an indwelling vascular access device (VAD) and then returned to the office the next day to start his chemotherapy. Realizing that Mr. Z may be overwhelmed with the diagnosis and new information, MaryAnn again reviewed the information about the chemotherapy and growth factors, including the possible side effects. She instructed Mr. Z to call the office at any time of the day if he had a temperature $\geq 100.4°F$, shaking chills, and/or redness, swelling, or tenderness at the site of his VAD device. Mr. Z received his chemotherapy regimen in the office and felt well during and after the treatment. Two days after receiving his treatment, Mr. Z returned to the doctor's office and received an injection of pegfilgrastim. During this time, MaryAnn again repeated the instructions.

Mr. Z tolerated his chemotherapy well except for mild fatigue. After his fourth treatment, his hemoglobin fell to 9.5 mg/dl. The following laboratory studies were ordered: ferritin, iron studies, and reticulocyte count, and darbepoetin 200 mcg was prescribed every two weeks. Over the course of the next four weeks, Mr. Z's hemoglobin level increased to 12.2 mg/dl. Mr. Z continued receiving chemotherapy every three weeks on schedule, maintaining a WBC > 3,000 cells/mm³. After the eighth cycle, Mr. Z's groin lymphadenopathy had resolved, and computed tomography scans showed significant reduction of his lymphadenopathy. Mr. Z's night sweats had ceased, and his energy level gradually was increasing. He continued playing golf every week, helping his wife with her chronic disease, and began planning a cruise vacation.

Conclusion

Treating the older adult with chemotherapy is challenging because age-related changes of altered drug metabolism, decreased functional reserve, comorbidities, cognitive deficits, and altered social status make the older adult more susceptible to chemotherapy-related toxicities. This is especially true for the toxicity of myelosuppression, where the incidence of neutropenic infection-related mortality varies between 5% and 30% in people 70 years of age and older. Management of neutropenia by dose reduction may compromise treatment efficacy. CSFs decrease the risk of prolonged myelosuppression by 50%, do not appear to increase healthcare costs, and may be associated with cost savings if hospitalizations are prevented. However, limited data are available on the risks and benefits of treatment in the older population because of underrepresentation in clinical trials. More research is needed to better refine assessment tools, strategies, and symptom management to provide cost-effective, evidence-based health care in this population.

The author would like to thank James F. Holland, George Raptis, Fran Cartwright, M. Tish Knobf, and Ruth McCorkle for their careful review of the manuscript.

Ms. Van Cleave is supported, in part, by a predoctoral fellowship (T32NR008346) at the Yale University School of Nursing.

References

Balducci, L. (2000). Geriatric oncology: Challenges for the new century. *European Journal of Cancer, 36,* 1741–1754.

Balducci, L. (2001). Geriatric cancer patient: Equal benefit from equal treatment. *Cancer Control, 9*(Suppl. 2), 1–25.

Balducci, L. (2003a). Anemia, cancer, and aging. *Cancer Control, 10,* 478–486.

Balducci, L. (2003b). Myelosuppression and its consequences in elderly patients with cancer. *Oncology (Huntington), 17*(Suppl. 11), 27–32.

Balducci, L. (2003c). New paradigms for treating elderly patients with cancer: The comprehensive geriatric assessment and guidelines for supportive care. *Journal of Supportive Oncology, 1*(4 Suppl. 2), 30–37.

Balducci, L., & Corcoran, M.B. (2000). Antineoplastic chemotherapy of the older cancer patient. *Hematology/Oncology Clinics of North America, 14,* 193–211.

Bastion, Y., Blay, J., Divine, M., Brice, P., Bordessoule, D., Sebban, C., et al. (1997). Elderly patients with aggressive non-Hodgkin's lymphoma: Disease presentation, response to treatment, and survival. *Journal of Clinical Oncology, 15,* 2945–2953.

Begg, C.B., & Carbone, P.P. (1983). Clinical trials and drug toxicity in the elderly. *Cancer, 52,* 1986–1992.

Begg, C.B., Elson, P.J., & Carbone, P.P. (1989). A study of excess hematologic toxicity in cancer chemotherapy protocols. In R. Yancik & J.W. Yates (Eds.), *Cancer in the elderly: Approaches to early detection and treatment* (pp. 149–163). New York: Springer.

Brown, L.J., Potter, J.F., & Foster, B.G. (1990). Caregiver burden should be evaluated during geriatric assessment. *Journal of the American Geriatrics Society, 38,* 455–460.

Callen, L., Vranas, P., Overcash, J., Boulware, D., & Extermann, M. (2004, October). *Survival and patterns of care in older cancer patients with cognitive impairment.* Paper presented at the fifth meeting of the International Society of Geriatric Oncology, San Francisco, CA.

Carbone, P.P. (2000). Advances in the systemic treatment of cancers in the elderly. *Critical Reviews in Oncology/Hematology, 35,* 201–218.

Chen, C.C., Kenefick, A.L., Tang, S.T., & McCorkle, R. (2004). Utilization of comprehensive geriatric assessment in cancer patients. *Critical Reviews in Oncology/Hematology, 49,* 53–67.

Cockcroft, D.W., & Gault, M.H. (1976). Prediction of creatinine clearance from serum creatinine. *Nephron, 16,* 31–46.

Cooley, M.E., Moriarty, H.E., Berger, M.S., Selm-Orr, D., Coyle, B., & Short, T. (1995). Patient literacy and the readability of written cancer educational materials. *Oncology Nursing Forum, 22,* 1345–1351.

Crawford, J. (2003). Once-per-cycle pegfilgrastim (Neulasta) for the management of chemotherapy-induced neutropenia. *Seminars in Oncology, 30*(4 Suppl. 3), 24–30.

Crighton, M.H. (2004). Dimensions of neutropenia in adult cancer patients. *Cancer Nursing, 27,* 275–284.

Dale, D.C. (2003). Poor prognosis in elderly patients with cancer: The role of bias and undertreatment. *Journal of Supportive Oncology, 1*(4 Suppl. 2), 11–17.

Denduluri, N., & Ershler, W.B. (2004). Aging biology and cancer. *Seminars in Oncology, 31,* 137–148.

Earle, C.C., Neville, B.A., Landrum, M.B., Ayanian, J.Z., Block, S.D., & Weeks, J.C. (2004). Trends in the aggressiveness of cancer care near the end of life. *Journal of Clinical Oncology, 22,* 315–321.

Extermann, M., & Aapro, M. (2000). Assessment of the older cancer patient. *Hematology/Oncology Clinics of North America, 14,* 63–77.

Extermann, M., Overcash, J., Lyman, G.H., Parr, J., & Balducci, L. (1998). Comorbidity and functional status are independent in older cancer patients. *Journal of Clinical Oncology, 16,* 1582–1587.

Ferrucci, L., Guralnik, J.M., Cavazzini, C., Bandinelli, S., Lauretani, F., Bartali, B., et al. (2003). The frailty syndrome: A critical issue in geriatric oncology. *Critical Reviews in Oncology/Hematology, 46,* 127–137.

Fischer, D.S., Knobf, M.T., Durivage, H.J., & Beaulieu, N.J. (2003). *The cancer chemotherapy handbook* (6th ed.). Philadelphia: Mosby.

Folstein, M.F., Folstein, S.E., & McHugh, P.R. (1975). Mini-Mental State: A practical method of grading the cognitive states of patients for the clinician. *Journal of Psychiatric Research, 12,* 189–198.

Gelman, R.S., & Taylor, S.G. (1984). Cyclophosphamide, methotrexate and 5-fluorouracil chemotherapy in women more than 65 years old with advanced breast cancer. The elimination of age trends in toxicity by using doses based on creatinine clearance. *Journal of Clinical Oncology, 2,* 1406–1414.

Gomez, H., Hidalgo, M., Casanova, L., Colomer, R., Pen, D.L.K., Otero, J., et al. (1998). Risk factors for treatment-related death in elderly patients with aggressive non-Hodgkin's lymphoma: Results of a multivariate analysis. *Journal of Clinical Oncology, 16,* 2065–2069.

Groopman, J.E., & Itri, L.M. (1999). Chemotherapy-induced anemia in adults: Incidence and treatment. *Journal of the National Cancer Institute, 91,* 1616–1634.

Haley, W.E. (2003). Family caregivers of elderly patients with cancer: Understanding and minimizing the burden of care. *Journal of Supportive Oncology, 1*(4 Suppl. 2), 25–29.

Harrison, D.E. (1979). Proliferative capacity of erythropoietic stem cell lines and aging: An overview. *Mechanisms of Ageing and Development, 9,* 409–426.

Harrison, D.E., Astle, C.M., & Stone, M. (1989). Numbers and functions of transplantable primitive immunohematopoietic stem cells. Effects of age. *Journal of Immunology, 142,* 3833–3840.

Henke, M., Laszig, R., Rube, C., Schafer, U., Haase, K.D., Schilcher, B., et al. (2003). Erythropoietin to treat head and neck cancer patients with anaemia undergoing radiotherapy: Randomized, double-blind, placebo-controlled trial. *Lancet, 362,* 1255–1260.

Holmes, F.A., O'Shaughnessy, J.A., Vukelja, S., Jones, S.E., Shogan, J., Savin, M., et al. (2002). Blinded, randomized, multicenter study to evaluate single administration pegfilgrastim once per cycle versus daily filgrastim as an adjunct to chemotherapy in patients with high-risk stage II or stage III/IV breast cancer. *Journal of Clinical Oncology, 20,* 727–731.

Hutchins, L.F., Unger, J.M., Crowley, J.J., Coltman, C.A.J., & Albain, K.S. (1999). Underrepresentation of patients 65 years of age or older in cancer treatment trials. *New England Journal of Medicine, 341,* 2061–2067.

Lewis, J.H., Kilgore, M.L., Goldman, D.P., Trimble, E.L., Kaplan, R., Montello, M.J., et al. (2003). Participation of patients 65 years of age or older in cancer clinical trials. *Journal of Clinical Oncology, 21,* 1383–1389.

Lichtman, S.M. (2004). Chemotherapy in the elderly. *Seminars in Oncology, 31,* 160–174.

Lichtman, S.M., Skirvin, J.A., & Vemulapalli, S. (2003). Pharmacology of antineoplastic agents in older cancer patients. *Critical Reviews in Oncology/Hematology, 46,* 101–114.

Lyman, G.H., Kuderer, N., Agboola, O., & Balducci, L. (2003). Evidence-based use of colony-stimulating factors in elderly cancer patients. *Cancer Control, 10,* 487–499.

Machtay, M., & Brown, J.M. (2004, October). *Definitive radiotherapy +/- erythropoietin for squamous cell carcinoma of the head and neck: Preliminary report of RTOG 99-03*. Paper presented at the meeting of the American Society for Therapeutic Radiology and Oncology, Atlanta, GA.

National Comprehensive Cancer Network. (2004). *NCCN practice guidelines in oncology: Fever and neutropenia*. Retrieved May 30, 2004, from http://www.nccn.org/professionals/physician_gls/PDF/fever/pdf

National Comprehensive Cancer Network. (2005a). *Clinical practice guidelines in oncology: Senior adult oncology*. Retrieved September 22, 2005, from http://www.nccn.org/professionals/physician_gls/PDF/senior.pdf

National Comprehensive Cancer Network. (2005b). *Myeloid growth factors in cancer treatment*. Retrieved August 14, 2005, from http://www.nccn.org/professionals/physicians_pdf/myeloid_growth.pdf

Overcash, J., Beckstead, J., & Cobb, S. (2004, October). *The abbreviated geriatric assessment*. Paper presented at the fifth meeting of the International Society of Geriatric Oncology, San Francisco, CA.

Ozer, H. (2003). New directions in the management of chemotherapy-induced neutropenia: Risk models, special populations and quality of life. *Seminars in Oncology, 30*, 18–23.

Ozer, H., Armitage, J.O., Bennett, C.L., Crawford, J., Demetri, G.D., Pizzo, P.A., et al. (2000). 2000 update of recommendations for the use of hematopoietic colony-stimulating factors: Evidence-based, clinical practice guidelines. *Journal of Clinical Oncology, 18*, 3558–3585.

Padberg, R.M., & Padberg, L.F. (1997). Patient education and support. In S.L. Groenwald, M.H. Frogge, M. Goodman, & C.H. Yarbro (Eds.), *Cancer nursing: Principles and practice* (3rd ed., pp. 1642–1665). Sudbury, MA: Jones and Bartlett.

Pietropaolo, M., Gianni, W., Siliscavalli, A., Marigliano, V., & Repetto, L. (2003). The use of colony stimulating factors in elderly patients with cancer. *Critical Reviews in Oncology/Hematology, 48*(Suppl.), S33–S37.

Rao, A.V., Seo, P.H., & Cohen, H.J. (2004). Geriatric assessment and comorbidity. *Seminars in Oncology, 31*, 149–159.

Repetto, L. (2003). Greater risks of chemotherapy toxicity in elderly patients with cancer. *Journal of Supportive Oncology, 1*(4 Suppl. 2), 18–24.

Repetto, L., Biganzoli, L., Koehne, C.H., Luebbe, A.S., Soubeyran, P., Tjan-Heijnen, V.C.G., et al. (2003). EORTC in the Elderly Task Force guidelines for the use of colony-stimulating factors in elderly patients with cancer. *European Journal of Cancer, 39*, 2264–2272.

Repetto, L., Venturino, A., Fratino, L., Serraino, D., Troisi, G., Gianni, W., et al. (2003). Geriatric oncology: A clinical approach to the older patient with cancer. *European Journal of Cancer, 39*, 870–880.

Reuben, D.B. (1998). Geriatric assessment in oncology. *Cancer, 80*, 1311–1316.

Rutledge, D.N., & McGuire, C. (2004). Evidence-based symptom management. In C.H. Yarbro, M.H. Frogge, & M. Goodman (Eds.), *Cancer symptom management* (3rd ed., pp. 3–14). Sudbury, MA: Jones and Bartlett.

Smith, R.E., & Tchekmedyian, S. (2002). Practitioners' practical model of managing cancer-related anemia. *Oncology, 16*, 55–63.

Stommel, M., Given, B.A., & Given, C.W. (2002). Depression and functional status as predictors of death among cancer patients. *Cancer, 94*, 2719–2727.

Talarico, L., Chen, G., & Pazdur, R. (2004). Enrollment of elderly patients in clinical trials for cancer drug registration: A 7-year experience by the U.S. Food and Drug Administration. *Journal of Clinical Oncology, 22*, 4626–4631.

Teret, C., Albrand, G., & Droz, J. (2004, October). *Multidimensional geriatric assessment reveals unknown medical problems in elderly cancer patients*. Paper presented at the fifth meeting of the International Society of Geriatric Oncology, San Francisco, CA.

Tirelli, U., Errante, D., Van Glabbeke, M., Teodorovic, I., Kluin-Nelemans, J.C., Thomas, J., et al. (1998). CHOP is the standard regimen in patients > 70 years of age with intermediate-grade and high-grade non-Hodgkin's lymphoma: Results of a randomized study of the European Organization for Research and Treatment of Cancer Lymphoma Cooperative Study Group. *Journal of Clinical Oncology, 16*, 27–34.

Yancik, R., & Ries, L.A.G. (2004). Cancer in older persons: An international issue in an aging world. *Seminars in Oncology, 31*, 128–136.

Yancik, R., Wesley, M.N., Ries, L.A.G., Havlik, R.J., Long, S., Edwards, B.K., et al. (1998). Comorbidity and age as predictors of risk for early mortality of male and female colon carcinoma patients: A population-based study. *Cancer, 82*, 2123–2134.

Zinzani, P.L., Pavone, E., Storti, S., Moretti, L., Fattori, P.P., Guardini, L., et al. (1997). Randomized trial with or without granulocyte colony-stimulating factor as adjunct to induction VNCOP-B treatment of elderly high-grade non-Hodgkin's lymphoma. *Blood, 89,* 3974–3979.

Zinzani, P.L., Storti, S., Zaccariz, A., Moretti, L., Magagnoli, M., & Pavone, E. (1999). Elderly aggressive-histology non-Hodgkin's lymphoma: First line VNCOP-B regimen experience on 350 patients. *Blood, 94,* 33–38.

CHAPTER 16

Symptom Management of Mucositis

Stewart M. Bond, RN, MSN, AOCN®

Introduction

Mucositis is a general term for the injury of the mucosal lining of the entire alimentary and gastrointestinal (GI) tract, including the mouth, pharynx, esophagus, stomach, intestines, colon, rectum, and anus. Specific terms have been used to refer to mucositis in different regions. For example, stomatitis refers to oropharyngeal mucositis, gastritis is in the stomach, enteritis is in the bowel, and proctitis is in the rectum.

Mucositis is a common and serious side effect of cancer treatment associated with adverse clinical and economic outcomes. It is a primary dose-limiting effect of cancer therapy and contributes to significant morbidity and mortality and impaired quality of life. Additionally, mucositis has been associated with prolonged hospitalization and increased costs of care (Elting et al., 2003). A number of factors place older adult patients with cancer at increased risk for mucositis and its complications. This chapter provides an overview of mucositis as a side effect of cancer treatment. Special considerations in the care of older adults receiving oncologic treatment will be addressed.

Incidence

Accurate estimation of the incidence and prevalence of oral and GI mucositis is difficult because of the lack of standardized assessment and the difficulty assessing GI mucositis. In addition, patterns of mucositis vary with different cytotoxic regimens, and individual responses to cancer treatments are variable, with some patients with cancer never experiencing mucositis during their treatment. Oral mucositis incidence ranges from 40% in patients receiving standard chemotherapy up to 80% in patients receiving high-dose regimens associated with bone marrow and stem cell transplantation. Furthermore, up to 100% of patients receiving radiation therapy to fields involving the oral cavity will experience oral complications (National Cancer Institute [NCI], 2004).

GI mucositis occurs in 5%–10% of patients receiving standard-dose chemotherapy regimens. More than 20% of patients receiving certain doses and regimens of irinotecan develop severe GI mucositis (Rubenstein et al., 2004). Up to 100% of patients receiving high-dose chemotherapy regimens or radiation therapy with accelerated fractionation involving some regions of the head and neck or the chest, abdomen, or pelvis will experience GI mucositis (Sonis et al., 2004).

Risk Factors

A number of patient-related and treatment-related factors contribute to the frequency and severity of mucositis. Patient-related factors, including age, gender, oral health and hygiene, poor nutritional status, smoking history, baseline neutrophil level, genetic expression of cytokines, and prior cancer treatment, have been associated with the development of mucositis (Avritscher, Cooksley, & Elting, 2004; Beck, 2004; Knox, Puodziunas, & Feld, 2000). Treatment-related factors include the type, dosage, and schedule of chemotherapy, radiation fractionation, and the concomitant use of chemotherapy and radiation (Avritscher et al.; Kostler, Hejna, Wenzel, & Zielinski, 2001).

The classes of chemotherapy agents most commonly associated with oral mucositis are antimetabolites (e.g., 5-fluorouracil [FU], methotrexate, capecitabine, cytarabine), antitumor antibiotics (e.g., actinomycin D, bleomycin, etoposide, mitoxantrone), anthracyclines (e.g., daunorubicin, doxorubicin), taxanes (e.g., paclitaxel, docetaxel), vinca alkaloids (e.g., vinblastine, vinorelbine, vincristine), and high-dose therapy with alkylating agents (e.g., busulfan, cyclophosphamide, thiotepa, melphalan) (Beck, 2004; Camp-Sorrell, 2000; Dodd, 2004). Chemotherapy agents that cause GI mucositis include 5-FU, methotrexate, docetaxel, actinomycin D, doxorubicin, trimetrexate, and irinotecan (Camp-Sorrell).

Older adults with cancer are at increased risk for developing mucositis. In a retrospective analysis, Stein et al. (1995) found that those age 70 and older had increased toxicity and treatment-related mortality from 5-FU–based chemotherapy. In a more recent pooled analysis of 1,748 patients, Jacobson et al. (2001) found that older age (65 and older) was an independent risk factor for more severe oral and GI mucositis induced by various 5-FU–based regimens. Similarly, age predicted more frequent and severe diarrhea and stomatitis in 5-FU–containing regimens for colorectal cancer (Popescu, Norman, Ross, Parikh, & Cunningham, 1999) and in cyclophosphamide, methotrexate, and 5-FU (CMF) regimens for breast cancer (Crivellari, Bonetti, Castiglione-Gertsch, Gelber, & Rudenstam, 2000).

Age-related changes in the oral and GI mucosa, including decreased salivary flow, diminished keratinization of the mucosa, and an increased prevalence of gingivitis and other dental problems, may contribute to the increased risk of mucositis in older adults (Balducci & Corcoran, 2000; Beck, 2004). Decreased renal function associated with aging also may increase the risk of mucositis and other systemic toxicities in older patients with cancer. Additionally, decreased hematopoietic reserve may delay recovery of mucositis in older adults (Balducci & Corcoran; Balducci & Extermann, 2000).

Pathophysiology

Previously, it was thought that mucositis resulted from the direct effect of chemotherapy or radiation therapy on the rapidly dividing epithelial cells lining the oral cavity and GI tract. Recent scientific and clinical evidence has provided an improved understanding of the development of mucositis. Mucositis involves a multiphase process of biologic and genetic mechanisms occurring simultaneously in multiple cells and tissues of the mucosa and submucosa. Sonis (1998) first described a four-phase process that included the inflammatory or vascular phase, the epithelial phase, the ulcerative phase, and the healing phase. The four-phased model has been expanded to include five phases because of an improved understanding of the biologic and genetic mechanisms involved. The five phases are initiation, upregulation and generation of messengers, signaling and amplification, ulceration with inflammation, and healing (Sonis et al., 2004).

The initiation phase begins soon after administration of chemotherapy or radiation therapy. The initial insult results in the generation of oxidative stress and reactive oxygen species (ROS). ROS directly damages epithelial cells and tissues of the submucosa, including blood vessels. For example, damage to the DNA of epithelial cells results in apoptosis, or cell death (Sonis, 2004). Tissue damage caused by ROS and the stimulation of a number of transcription factors lead to a cascade of other biologic events.

The upregulation and messenger generation phase is characterized by the activation of transcription factors such as nuclear factor-kappa B (NF-κB) and the upregulation of genes that control the production of proinflammatory cytokines, including tumor necrosis factor-alpha (TNF-α), interleukin-1 beta (IL-1β), and IL-6 (Sonis, 2004; Sonis et al., 2004). These cytokines are biologically active messenger proteins that target and injure epithelial, endothelial, and connective tissues. In addition, other messenger molecules activate enzymes that increase cell death and cause further tissue damage.

In the signaling and amplification phase, the proinflammatory cytokines not only damage tissues directly but also amplify the process. For example, elevated levels of TNF-α in the submucosa cause tissue damage and activate the ceramide and caspase pathways and the transcription pathway mediated by NF-κB. The activation of these signaling pathways results in the further production of proinflammatory cytokines and cytokine-mediated tissue damage (Sonis et al., 2004). Much of the tissue damage up to this point has occurred beneath the mucosal surface. This submucosal injury continues after radiation therapy and chemotherapy have been completed (Sonis, 2004).

The ulceration phase of mucositis is the most clinically significant. During the ulceration phase, local mucosal injury is widespread. The integrity of the mucosal barrier is broken (Sonis, 2004). Nerve endings are exposed, causing significant pain. The microbial flora of the oral cavity colonizes the ulcerated mucosal surface. The bacterial colonization and subsequent release of cell wall products stimulate an immune response that results in further cytokine production, inflammation, and tissue destruction (Sonis, 2004; Sonis et al., 2004). The risk for secondary infection increases (Dodd, 2004). Bacteria may invade the submucosa and penetrate the vascular walls, placing neutropenic patients at increased risk for bacteremia and sepsis.

The healing phase is marked by epithelial cell proliferation and differentiation, the restoration of normal microbial flora, and the recovery of peripheral white blood cells (Dodd, 2004; Knox et al., 2000). Symptoms typically resolve soon after the ulcerated mucosa has healed. Although the tissues of the oral cavity may appear normal at this point, they are not. The mucosal environment is significantly altered because of persistent molecular and cellular changes that occurred in the previous phases. These changes may place the patient at increased risk for mucositis with subsequent therapies and the development of other oral complications (Sonis et al., 2004).

Mucositis of the oral cavity and the GI tract likely share similar mechanisms (Sonis et al., 2004), but the processes involved in GI mucositis may be more complex. The morphologic and functional differences in the GI tract account for the functional and symptomatic differences between oral and GI mucositis (Rubenstein et al., 2004). Chemotherapeutic agents act at different levels of the intestinal crypt cells, but all drugs cause crypt cell death followed by crypt hypoplasia and villous atrophy and then rebound hyperplasia before returning to normal (Keefe, Brealey, Goland, & Cummins, 2000; Rubenstein et al.). Mucositis in the small intestine is more common than in the colon. However, irinotecan causes significant colonic damage, and taxanes produce more cecal damage (Keefe, Gibson, & Hauer-Jensen, 2004).

Clinical Presentation

Oral mucositis is a progressive process characterized by the development of erythematous and erosive and ulcerative lesions in the oral cavity. In patients receiving chemotherapy, the most commonly affected sites include the labial, buccal, and soft palate mucosa, as well as the floor of the mouth and the ventral and lateral surfaces of the tongue. In patients receiving head and neck radiation therapy, the affected areas are primarily within the direct fields of the radiation (Peterson, 1999). Oral mucositis usually develops within five to seven days after the administration of chemotherapy and peaks around day 14 (Keefe et al., 2004). Oral mucositis is associated with pain, dysphagia, decreased oral intake, salivary gland dysfunction, speech alterations, and risk of bleeding and infection.

The clinical manifestations of chemotherapy-induced esophagitis and acute radiation esophagitis include dysphagia, odynophagia or painful swallowing, and substernal chest pain. Esophagitis associated with chemotherapy begins soon after the initiation of treatment, whereas acute radiation esophagitis begins near the end of the second week of treatment (Keefe et al., 2004). Mucosal injury in the stomach is associated with gastritis and dyspepsia. These manifestations usually are temporary and less problematic than other GI effects. Small intestine injury results in nausea, abdominal pain, and diarrhea. Malabsorption of nutrients in the small intestine may cause transient malnutrition. GI symptoms associated with chemotherapy usually peak three days post-treatment. The manifestations of radiation-induced small bowel injury occur two to three weeks into therapy and resolve two to four weeks after treatment (Keefe et al., 2004). Colonic injury from radiation results in diarrhea and crampy abdominal pain. Rectal injury is common with pelvic radiation. Acute radiation proctitis is associated with diarrhea, tenesmus, and bloody stools (Keefe et al., 2004).

Assessment

Systematic assessment of the mouth is a critical component in monitoring oral mucositis. A number of scales or instruments have been developed to evaluate mucositis (see Table 16-1). The majority of scales measure oral mucositis. Only a few measure GI mucositis. Many of the scales exhibit similar features, but they vary considerably in their complexity and have undergone different degrees of validation. These instruments have been reviewed elsewhere (Eilers & Epstein, 2004; Sonis et al., 2004).

The World Health Organization, NCI, and collaborative research groups such as the Eastern Cooperative Oncology Group and the Radiation Therapy Oncology Group (RTOG) have developed cancer treatment toxicity scales, which have been widely used in clinical trials and in clinical practice. These scales address a number of common toxicities associated with cancer treatment, including oral mucositis. In evaluating oral mucositis, the scales use a combination of objective, functional, and symptomatic variables, including mucosal appearance, severity of pain, and functional capabilities (e.g., ability to eat). The severity of mucositis is graded using a 0–4 or 0–5 point scale.

Additional oral assessment guides and objective rating scales have been developed as nursing management and clinical research tools. Scales in this category include the Oral Exam Guide (Beck, 1979), the Oral Assessment Guide (Eilers, Berger, & Petersen, 1988), the Oral Mucosa Rating Scale (OMRS) (Kolbinson, Schubert, Flournoy, & Truelove, 1988), the 34-item Oral Mucositis Index (Schubert, Williams, Lloid, Donaldson, & Chapko, 1992), the 20-item Oral Mucositis Index (McGuire et al., 2002), and the Oral Mucositis Assessment Scale (OMAS) (Sonis et al., 1999). Similar to the previous scales, these scales address objective, functional, and symptomatic variables but apply them to different oral anatomic sites. Individual variables or items on the scales are scored and then used to derive a composite oral mucositis score. Most of the scales are clinician-rated and require different levels of training and experience. The OMRS and OMAS also include visual analog scales to capture the patient's subjective complaints.

Table 16-1. Mucositis Assessment Tools

Assessment Tools	References
Toxicity Scales	
• World Health Organization (WHO)	WHO, 1979
• National Cancer Institute (NCI) Common Terminology Criteria for Adverse Events	NCI, 2003
• Eastern Cooperative Oncology Group Common Toxicity Criteria	Oken et al., 1982
• Radiation Therapy Oncology Group (RTOG)	RTOG, 1989, 2004a, 2004b
Oral Exam Guide	Beck, 1979
Oral Assessment Guide	Eilers et al., 1988
Oral Mucosa Rating Scale	Kolbinson et al., 1988
34-Item Oral Mucositis Index	Schubert et al., 1992
20-Item Oral Mucositis Index	McGuire et al., 2002
Oral Mucositis Assessment Scale	Sonis et al., 1999

Healthcare professionals must accurately monitor and document the extent and severity of GI mucositis. Currently, no instruments exist to specifically measure GI mucosal tissue injury. The measurement of GI mucositis relies on the presence and degree of nonspecific symptoms such as pain, diarrhea, nausea, vomiting, and bleeding. The cancer treatment toxicity scales include these symptoms. Therefore, these scales can be used to roughly assess and monitor the severity of GI mucositis. The RTOG scales are site specific (e.g., pharynx and esophagus, upper GI, lower GI) and address the acute and late effects of radiation therapy (RTOG, 1989, 2004a, 2004b). The NCI Common Terminology Criteria for Adverse Events also addresses site-specific GI complications associated with chemotherapy and radiation therapy (NCI, 2003).

Complications Associated With Mucositis

Infection

Infection is one of the most common and severe consequences of mucositis. Elting et al. (2003) found that patients with oral and GI mucositis were more likely to develop infection. When the protective barrier of the oral and GI mucosa is broken, microorganisms, especially the patient's own microbial flora, may enter the body and blood stream. Sepsis and bacteremia in neutropenic patients and others who are immunocompromised can be life-threatening. It is estimated that up to one-half of patients who become septic die (Brown & Wingard, 2004).

Infections associated with mucositis can be bacterial, fungal, or viral in origin. The most common pathogens in each category include *Streptococcus* species and gram-negative bacteria and *Candida* species and herpes simplex virus (HSV) (Camp-Sorrell, 2000). Although controversial, prophylactic antimicrobial therapy targeting these organisms is recommended in neutropenic patients. Otherwise, antimicrobial therapy should be based on the infectious agent. Oral *Candida* infections are treated topically with nystatin suspensions or clotrimazole troches. Ketoconazole or fluconazole are used to treat infections that are refractory to topical treatment and infections that are more widely disseminated. HSV infections are treated with topical or systemic acyclovir therapy.

Pain

Pain is likely the most distressing complication associated with mucositis. Oral pain negatively affects quality of life because it can interfere with eating and drinking, oral hygiene, wearing dentures and other dental appliances, talking, and taking medications (Epstein & Schubert, 2003). Healthcare professionals should assess pain intensity on an ongoing basis. Cella et al. (2003) found that oral pain scores are closely related to the degree of mucositis.

Pain associated with mucositis can be treated with topical anesthetics, coating agents, and systemic analgesics. Topical anesthetics such as viscous lidocaine, benzocaine, dyclonine hydrochloride, and mixtures containing these agents provide temporary pain relief. However, these agents often sting and may be irritating when applied to ulcerated mucosa. They also have negative effects such as loss of taste and diminished oral sensitivity, resulting in difficulty with eating and swallowing. Oral capsaicin in a taffy candy base reduced oral discomfort associated with chemotherapy and radiation-induced mucositis

(Berger et al., 1995). Benzocaine gel, hydroxypropyl cellulose film, and polyvinylpyr-rolidone/sodium hyaluronate are coating agents that provide a protective barrier. Pain relief with these agents occurs relatively quickly and lasts up to six hours.

Systemic analgesics often are required to provide adequate pain relief. If mucositis and its pain are mild or moderate and the patient is able to swallow, nonopioids or nonopioid/opioid combinations such as acetaminophen and oxycodone can be given orally as needed or on an around-the-clock schedule. More severe mucositis and pain may require long-acting opioids or continuous IV opioid infusions. Studies have shown that patient-controlled analgesia (PCA) and continuous opioid infusion provide similar levels of pain relief. However, patients with PCA used less opioids per hour, and their duration of pain was shorter (Worthington, Clarkson, & Eden, 2004). Adjuvant medications and complementary psychotherapeutic therapies, such as relaxation and imagery, may enhance pain relief (Epstein & Schubert, 2003).

Bleeding

Patients with mucositis, particularly those with chemotherapy-induced thrombocy-topenia, may experience oral and GI bleeding. Oral bleeding often results when the ulcerated tissues of the oral cavity are traumatized. Bleeding may occur anywhere in the mouth, but the lips, tongue, and gingiva are the most common sites (Camp-Sorrell, 2000). Rinsing the mouth with ice water may control oral bleeding. If the bleeding is localized, pressure can be applied using a piece of gauze soaked in ice water or a wet tea bag that has been frozen (Beck, 2004). Topical application of thrombin or aminocaproic acid may be used to promote clotting. Bleeding also is a common complication of chemotherapy-induced GI mucositis (Elting et al., 2003). GI bleeding should be monitored closely. Platelet transfusions may be necessary.

Nutritional Impairment

Patients with oral and GI mucositis are at high risk for nutritional impairment because of decreased oral intake and altered absorption of nutrients from the GI tract. Strategies to promote oral hydration and nutritional intake must be implemented early. Patients should be encouraged to increase their liquid intake and to make the dietary changes previously discussed. Nutritional and caloric supplements may be used. If patients have significant dysphagia, oral intake may need to be supplemented with enteral or parenteral nutrition. Total enteral or parenteral nutrition may be necessary in severe cases. If severe mucositis is anticipated, discussions about nutritional alternatives should be conducted, and a gastrostomy tube should be inserted prior to initiating therapy (Maher, 2000).

Dehydration

Decreased oral intake, nausea and vomiting, and frequent diarrhea associated with mucositis may lead to dehydration. Older patients with cancer are at risk for dehydration. They should be monitored closely for signs of dehydration, including rapid weight loss, orthostatic changes in blood pressure, dizziness, dry mucous membranes, and poor skin turgor (Maher, 2000). Some patients may require hospitalization and IV hydration.

Late Effects

Cancer treatment, particularly radiation therapy, can irreversibly injure the mucosa and supporting tissues and structures of the oral cavity and GI tract. In fact, the long-term effects of mucositis on the oral cavity and GI tract can be as devastating and debilitating as the acute effects (Avritscher et al., 2004). Late effects on the oral cavity include thinning of the oral mucosa that can result in chronic nonhealing ulceration. In severe cases, soft tissue necrosis and bone necrosis can occur. Other long-term effects on the oral cavity include xerostomia, taste alterations, dental caries, trismus, and secondary fungal and bacterial infections (NCI, 2004). Late effects of radiation therapy on the esophagus are rare. However, esophageal strictures requiring intermittent dilation may occur (Keefe et al., 2004). Late effects in the lower GI tract may result in intermittent constipation and diarrhea and nutritional impairment. More severe complications may include GI obstruction, ulceration, bowel ischemia and necrosis, perforation, and fistula formation (Keefe et al., 2004). Chronic radiation proctitis is common in patients following pelvic radiation therapy. The symptoms associated with chronic radiation proctitis may include frequent or clustered bowel movements, anal discharge, ulceration, rectal wall fibrosis and strictures, fistulas, rectal pain, urgency, tenesmus, incontinence, and bleeding (Keefe et al., 2004).

Nursing Care Issues

A number of nursing practices have been used to prevent and manage oral mucositis. Practices are highly variable among institutions, and the systematic use of oral care standards or protocols is rare (McGuire, 2003). In some cases, unproven and even harmful interventions continue to be used (Fulton, Middleton, & McPhail, 2002). Routine nursing care practices associated with the prevention and management of mucositis are identified in Table 16-2.

Patients should receive a thorough dental examination and cleaning and other corrective dental procedures prior to beginning cancer treatment (Brown & Wingard, 2004). Oral care protocols have been developed and are commonly used. General components of an oral care protocol include patient and family education, ongoing oral cavity assessment, daily oral hygiene measures, and pain assessment and management (Larson et al., 1998). Patients should be instructed to examine their mouth, including the lips, gums, buccal mucosa, and tongue, at least daily for redness, white patches, blisters, pimples, spots, sores, ulcers, lesions, or bleeding (Eilers, 2004). Furthermore, they should be instructed to contact their healthcare provider if they observe or experience any of the previous conditions, pain, or difficulty eating or drinking (Eilers; Larson et al.). Oral hygiene measures should include proper brushing with a soft-bristled toothbrush and fluoridated toothpaste, flossing, swishing with a bland mouthwash, and using lip and oral moisturizers (Beck, 2004; Yeager, Webster, Crain, Kasow, & McGuire, 2000). Patients should brush at least twice a day and floss at least daily. Other oral hygiene measures are recommended every two to four hours or more frequently if indicated. Patients also should maintain good oral hygiene during the night (Beck, 2004).

Healthcare providers should instruct denture wearers to remove their dentures when performing oral care, to soak their dentures daily in an antimicrobial solution and to rinse dentures with clean water before wearing them again, to clean and

Table 16-2. Nursing Care for Mucositis

General Areas	Care Strategies
Patient education	Provide information about mucositis. Perform an oral assessment. Perform oral hygiene. Note dietary changes. Eliminate alcohol and tobacco use. Monitor pain management. Monitor complications associated with mucositis. Explain when to notify provider.
Oral assessment	Inspect mouth at least daily. Look at lips, buccal mucosa, soft palate, tongue, and floor of mouth. Look for redness, white patches, blisters, pimples, sores, ulcers, lesions, or bleeding.
Oral hygiene	Brush with soft-bristled toothbrush at least twice a day. Floss at least daily. Rinse with bland mouthwash every two to four hours and more frequently if needed; rinse during the night. Apply oral moisturizer to lips and oral cavity. Provide instructions on denture care, if appropriate.
Dietary changes	Increase fluid intake. Eat a soft, bland diet. Avoid hot, spicy, salty, and acidic foods. Avoid foods with high sugar concentrations. Avoid dry, rough, and hard foods. Use nutritional and caloric supplements.
Nutrition assessment	Monitor dietary intake. Monitor weight. Assess for signs of dehydration.
Pain management	Perform pain assessment. Prescribe the following as needed: • Topical anesthetics • Nonopioids • Nonopioid/opioid combinations • Opioids (oral or parenteral) • Adjuvant medications • Complementary therapies.

brush dentures before soaking, and to wear dentures only when eating if mucosal breakdown is present (Eilers, 2004; Larson et al., 1998). Ill-fitting dentures should not be worn before, during, or right after treatment (Eilers). Patients with a partial plate should follow the mouth care protocol and denture care protocol.

Patients at risk for mucositis should minimize tissue irritation. Dietary guidelines have been recommended (Wohlschlaeger, 2004). Dietary recommendations include eating a soft, bland diet, drinking cool liquids to prevent dehydration, and avoiding hot, spicy, salty, acidic, or high sugar concentration foods. Nutritional and caloric supplements may help to maintain adequate nutritional intake. Patients also should avoid dry, rough, and hard foods because dry foods will decrease oral moisture, and rough and hard foods may cause irritation and abrasive injuries. Patients should eliminate the use of tobacco and alcohol (Epstein & Schubert, 2003).

Evidence-Based Clinical Practice Guidelines for the Prevention and Management of Oral and Gastrointestinal Mucositis

A number of authors have written reviews examining the literature associated with the prevention and management of chemotherapy- and radiation-induced mucositis (Epstein & Schubert, 2003; Knox et al., 2000; Kostler et al., 2001; Kwong, 2004; Miller & Kearney, 2001; Peterson, 1999; Shih, Miaskowski, Dodd, Stotts, & MacPhail, 2002). More recently and significantly, two international groups, the Cochrane Collaboration and the Multinational Association of Supportive Care in Cancer and International Society for Oral Oncology (MASCC/ISOO), have produced evidence-based guidelines for preventing and managing mucositis. The Cochrane Collaboration guidelines focus specifically on oral mucositis (Clarkson, Worthington, & Eden, 2003; Worthington et al., 2004). The MASCC/ISOO guidelines provide recommendations for both oral and GI mucositis (Rubenstein et al., 2004). The National Comprehensive Cancer Network (NCCN, 2005) has proposed evidence-based guidelines for the care of older adults receiving cancer treatment. The NCCN guidelines include mucositis as a treatment-related side effect affecting older patients with cancer. Together, these guidelines offer a significant improvement in how clinicians can approach the prevention and management of mucositis, in general, and the care of older adults receiving oncologic treatment, specifically.

Cochrane Collaboration Guidelines

The Cochrane Collaboration has established evidence-based guidelines for the prevention and management of oral mucositis (see Figure 16-1). Clarkson et al. (2003) reviewed 52 randomized clinical trials that evaluated the effectiveness of 21 interventions for preventing or reducing the severity of oral mucositis. The interventions were acyclovir, allopurinol mouth rinse, amifostine, antibiotic pastille or paste, benzydamine, chamomile, chlorhexidine, clarithromycin, folinic acid, glutamine, granulocyte macrophage–colony-stimulating factor (GM-CSF), hydrolytic enzymes, ice chips, oral care, pentoxifylline, povidone iodine, prednisone, propantheline, prostaglandin, sucralfate, and Traumeel. Nine of the 21 interventions showed some evidence to support their use. Allopurinol mouthwash possibly reduced the severity of mucositis. Amifostine provided a small benefit in preventing mucositis. Similarly, weak evidence showed the potential benefit of benzydamine, oral care protocols, and povidone iodine in preventing mucositis. Antibiotic pastille or paste, GM-CSF, and ice chips demonstrated moderate benefits in preventing mucositis. Hydrolytic enzymes provided a moderate reduction in the severity of mucositis.

More recently, Worthington et al. (2004) conducted a systematic review of randomized clinical trials to evaluate the effectiveness of interventions for treating oral mucositis. The authors reviewed 25 trials involving 1,292 patients. Weak evidence supported the effectiveness of allopurinol mouthwash, immunoglobulin, and human placental extract in treating oral mucositis. Other agents, including benzydamine,

Cochrane Collaboration
- Prevention of Oral Mucositis
  - Amifostine
  - Antibiotic paste or pastille
  - Granulocyte macrophage–colony-stimulating factor (GM-CSF)
  - Oral cryotherapy
  - Benzydamine
  - Oral care protocols
  - Povidine
- Improvement or Reduction in Oral Mucositis
  - Allopurinol
  - Hydrolytic enzymes
  - Immunoglobulin
  - Human placental extract
- Reduce Healing Time for Oral Mucositis
  - GM-CSF
  - Allopurinol

Multinational Association of Supportive Care in Cancer/International Society for Oral Oncology
- Prevention and Treatment of Oral Mucositis
  - Oral care protocols including patient education
  - Use of midline radiation blocks and three-dimensional treatment delivery
  - Topical benzydamine
  - Oral cryotherapy with 5-fluorouracil and edatrexate
  - Acyclovir should not be used to prevent oral mucositis.
  - Chlorhexidine should not be used to prevent or treat oral mucositis.
- Prevention and Treatment of Gastrointestinal Mucositis
  - Ranitidine or omeprazole to prevent epigastric pain
  - Octreotide to treat persistent diarrhea
  - Sulfasalazine to prevent or reduce enteritis and proctitis
  - Amifostine to prevent esophagitis with chemoradiation for lung cancer
  - Sucralfate enemas to treat chronic radiation-induced proctitis

Figure 16-1. Evidence-Based Practice Guidelines for the Prevention and Treatment of Mucositis

Note. Based on information from Clarkson et al., 2003; Rubenstein et al., 2004; Worthington et al., 2004.

sucralfate, tetrachlorodecaoxide, chlorhexidine, and magic mouthwash were found to be ineffective. GM-CSF compared to povidone iodine and allopurinol compared to placebo were found to significantly reduce the healing time for oral mucositis.

Multinational Association of Supportive Care in Cancer and International Society for Oral Oncology Guidelines

In 2000, MASCC/ISOO convened an interdisciplinary panel of 36 experts to create evidence-based guidelines for preventing and treating mucositis (see Figure 16-1). The panel reviewed the literature published between January 1966 and May 2002. The panel proposed either recommendations or suggestions for interventions to prevent and treat oral and GI mucositis based on the strength of the evidence. The guidelines include interventions that should be used for all patients receiving mucotoxic cancer treatment as well as interventions that are population and treatment specific (McGuire, Rubenstein, & Peterson, 2004; Rubenstein et al., 2004).

Basic oral care, though not explicitly defined, is suggested as a foundation of care for all patients. The panel found that no sufficient scientific evidence existed to provide a guideline for basic oral care. However, its importance in promoting and maintaining oral health generally is established. The panel suggested the use of oral care protocols, including patient education for all patients receiving chemotherapy and radiation therapy.

The panel also recognized the importance of pain control as a foundation of care for all patients with oral mucositis. Recommendations included the use of PCA morphine to control pain in patients undergoing hematopoietic stem cell transplantation. Additionally, the use of benzydamine and morphine as single-agent topical analgesics was suggested. The lack of evidence prevented the panel from recommending the use of compounded mixtures containing anesthetics and other agents such as lidocaine, benzocaine, milk of magnesia, kaolin, pectin, chlorhexidine, and diphenhydramine.

The panel provided several recommendations for the prevention of oral mucositis in patients undergoing radiation therapy for head and neck cancer. First, it recommended the use of midline radiation blocks and three-dimensional treatment delivery. It also recommended the use of topical benzydamine hydrochloride in patients receiving moderate-dose therapy. Finally, it recommended that chlorhexidine should not be used to prevent oral mucositis but suggested that it may be used for its hygienic and antimicrobial properties as part of an oral care protocol.

A number of strategies have been used to prevent and treat oral mucositis in patients receiving mucotoxic chemotherapy regimens. In general, the panel found insufficient evidence to support recommendations for or against their use. However, the panel provided positive and negative recommendations or suggestions for several strategies. It recommended using 30 minutes of oral cryotherapy with bolus doses of 5-FU and using 20–30 minutes of oral cryotherapy with bolus doses of edatrexate to prevent oral mucositis. The panel recommended that acyclovir should not be used to prevent mucositis, and chlorhexidine should not be used to treat established mucositis.

The panel provided two positive recommendations regarding the prevention and treatment of chemotherapy-induced GI mucositis. First, either ranitidine or omeprazole should be used to prevent epigastric pain following treatments with CMF and other 5-FU–containing regimens. Also, octreotide can be used to treat uncontrolled diarrhea. The panel recommended against the use of oral sucralfate and 5-aminosalicylic acid in the prevention of radiation-induced GI mucositis, specifically acute radiation proctitis.

Three positive suggestions were given for preventing and treating radiation-induced GI mucositis. The panel suggested the use of sulfasalazine to prevent and reduce the severity of enteritis and proctitis associated with external-beam pelvic radiation. Sucralfate enemas should be used to treat chronic radiation-induced proctitis with rectal bleeding. Finally, amifostine should be used to prevent esophagitis associated with combined chemoradiation in patients with non-small cell lung cancer.

National Comprehensive Cancer Network Guidelines

The NCCN Senior Adult Oncology Panel developed guidelines to address specific issues related to the management of older adults with cancer (Balducci & Yates, 2000; NCCN, 2005). The guidelines focus on appropriate treatment selection based on geriatric screening and assessment and on the prevention and management of treatment-related complications that are most common in older patients with cancer. The guidelines are from a uniform consensus of an expert panel based on low-level evidence, including clinical experience. Figure 16-2 presents the NCCN guidelines related to mucositis. The guidelines recommend the use of amifostine to prevent mucositis associated with head and neck radiation therapy. In general, chemotherapy dosages should be adjusted for glomerular filtration rate to reduce systemic toxicity. The use of capecitabine instead of IV fluorinated pyrimidines is recommended to prevent chemotherapy-induced mucositis. Additionally, the provider should consider giving patients a rest if the treatment includes prolonged infusional therapy. When mucositis is complicated by dysphagia and diarrhea, patients should be hospitalized, if necessary, to provide IV hydration and nutritional support.

- Amifostine to prevent mucositis in head and neck radiation therapy
- Chemotherapy dosage adjustment for glomerular filtration rate
- Give rest period with prolonged infusion.
- Use capecitabine instead of 5-fluorouracil.
- Oral care protocol
- Nutritional support
- Pain management
- Early hospitalization for IV hydration in patients with dysphagia or diarrhea

Figure 16-2. National Comprehensive Cancer Network Senior Adult Oncology Guidelines for Mucositis

---

Note. Based on information from National Comprehensive Cancer Network, 2005.

New Investigational Treatments

An improved understanding of the pathobiology of mucositis has led to the identification of potential treatment strategies for mucositis. Two interventions that have shown promising results include keratinocyte growth factors (KGFs) and L-glutamine drug delivery systems (AES-14).

Recombinant human KGFs may enhance wound healing in mucositis by promoting the growth of basal epithelial cells in the oral and GI mucosa (Eilers, 2004; Peterson, Beck, & Keefe, 2004). Spielberger et al. (2001) evaluated the efficacy of KGF in patients undergoing autologous peripheral blood cell transplantation with total body irradiation and high-dose chemotherapy. The duration of severe oral mucositis was significantly shorter in patients who received KGF. Patients also reported less mouth and throat soreness and improvements in swallowing, drinking, eating, talking, and sleeping. Furthermore, patients receiving KGF required IV opioid analgesics and total parenteral nutrition for a shorter period of time. KGF was well tolerated with few side effects.

L-glutamine is an essential amino acid that has important tissue functions (Peterson et al., 2004). AES-14 delivers L-glutamine directly to the oral mucosa. In a phase III study of patients receiving high-dose chemotherapy, daily topical administration of AES-14 provided a 20% reduction in the incidence of moderate-severe oral mucositis and a 10% increase in grade 0 mucositis (Peterson & Petit, 2003). AES-14 was well tolerated without side effects.

Areas for Future Research

Although research focusing on mucositis has increased and much has been learned, significant gaps in knowledge and practice exist in many areas. A number of research needs and opportunities have been identified (Avritscher et al., 2004; McGuire, 2002; Worthington et al., 2004). Additional research should focus on the pathobiology of mucositis to identify targets for prevention and treatment. Many potential strategies have been identified and used to prevent and manage mucositis, but the evidence supporting their use is limited. Well-designed clinical trials of interventions that may be effective in preventing and managing mucositis are needed. Risk factors for developing mucositis should be studied more thoroughly. The effects of aging on mucosal tissue and the relationship between aging and mucositis must be better understood.

The assessment and measurement of mucositis in research and clinical practice should be standardized to promote comparability. A variety of instruments have been developed to assess and measure mucositis. Standard assessment parameters should be defined. Instruments need to be refined and tested in different patient populations and settings. Furthermore, the instruments should have well-established psychometric properties. Instruments for measuring GI mucositis need to be developed and validated.

Studies of mucositis should include well-defined clinical and patient-based outcome measures. The severity of mucositis and the impact of mucositis on patients' well-being and quality of life are important outcomes. Additional outcomes should include oral functioning, complications such as pain, infection rates, nutritional impairment, and bleeding, as well as resource utilization and costs. Studies focusing specifically on mucositis in older patients with cancer and other high-risk populations are needed.

Research and quality improvement studies should focus on the development, implementation, and evaluation of oral care protocols and standards. Stricker and Sullivan (2003) described the process used to develop and implement evidence-based oncology oral care standards in a tertiary care hospital. Smink and Gosselin-Acomb (2004) described the development and evaluation of patient educational materials to enhance oral care in patients receiving radiation for head and neck cancer. The evaluation should examine the relationship between the protocols and outcomes of care. Healthcare professionals should identify barriers to the implementation of protocols and standards and strategies to reduce them (McGuire, 2002).

Conclusion

Mucositis is a common and potentially devastating side effect of cancer treatment. Only a few evidence-based interventions to prevent and manage mucositis currently exist. However, recent improvements in understanding the biologic and genetic mechanisms involved in the development of mucositis have led to promising interventions. The prevention and management of mucositis will improve quality of life, reduce costs, and enhance the use of more intensive cancer treatments that may produce better results.

Older patients with cancer are at increased risk for experiencing mucositis and its complications. Continual monitoring and assessment are necessary to effectively manage mucositis in older patients and to prevent sequelae that contribute to increased morbidity, impaired function, and diminished quality of life.

References

Avritscher, E.B.C., Cooksley, C.D., & Elting, L.S. (2004). Scope and epidemiology of cancer therapy-induced oral and gastrointestinal mucositis. *Seminars in Oncology Nursing, 20,* 3–10.

Balducci, L., & Corcoran, M.B. (2000). Antineoplastic chemotherapy of the older cancer patient. *Hematology/Oncology Clinics of North America, 1,* 193–212.

Balducci, L., & Extermann, M. (2000). Management of cancer in the older person: A practical approach. *Oncologist, 5,* 224–237.

Balducci, L., & Yates, J.W. (2000). General guidelines for the management of older patients with cancer. *Oncology, 14,* 221–227.

Beck, S. (1979). Impact of a systematic oral care protocol on stomatitis after chemotherapy. *Cancer Nursing, 2,* 185–199.

Beck, S. (2004). Mucositis. In C.H. Yarbro, M.H. Frogge, & M. Goodman (Eds.), *Cancer symptom management* (3rd ed., pp. 276–287). Sudbury, MA: Jones and Bartlett.

Berger, A., Henderson, M., Nadoolman, W., Duffy, V., Cooper, D., Saberski, L., et al. (1995). Oral capsaicin provides temporary relief for oral mucositis pain secondary to chemotherapy/radiation therapy. *Journal of Pain and Symptom Management, 10,* 243–248.

Brown, C.G., & Wingard, J. (2004). Clinical consequences of oral mucositis. *Seminars in Oncology Nursing, 20,* 16–21.

Camp-Sorrell, D. (2000). Chemotherapy: Toxicity management. In C.H. Yarbro, M.H. Frogge, M. Goodman, & S.L. Groenwald (Eds.), *Cancer nursing: Principles and practice* (5th ed., pp. 444–486). Sudbury, MA: Jones and Bartlett.

Cella, D., Pulliam, J., Fuchs, H., Miller, C., Hurd, D., Wingard, J.R., et al. (2003). Evaluation of pain associated with oral mucositis during the acute period after administration of high-dose chemotherapy. *Cancer, 98,* 406–412.

Clarkson, J.E., Worthington, H.V., & Eden, O.B. (2003). Interventions for preventing oral mucositis for patients with cancer receiving treatment. *Cochrane Database of Systematic Reviews, 3,* CD000978. Retrieved September 15, 2004, from http://www.update-software.com/publications/cochrane

Crivellari, D., Bonetti, M., Castiglione-Gertsch, M., Gelber, R.D., & Rudenstam, C. (2000). Burdens and benefits of adjuvant cyclophosphamide, methotrexate, and fluorouracil and tamoxifen for elderly patients with breast cancer: The International Breast Cancer Study Group Trial VII. *Journal of Clinical Oncology, 18,* 1412–1422.

Dodd, M. (2004). The pathogenesis and characterization of oral mucositis associated with cancer therapy. *Oncology Nursing Forum, 31*(Suppl.), 5–11.

Eilers, J. (2004). Nursing interventions and supportive care for the prevention and treatment of oral mucositis associated with cancer treatment. *Oncology Nursing Forum, 31*(Suppl.), 13–23, 37–39.

Eilers, J., Berger, A.M., & Petersen, M.C. (1988). Development, testing, and application of the oral assessment guide. *Oncology Nursing Forum, 15,* 325–330.

Eilers, J., & Epstein, J.B. (2004). Assessment and measurement of oral mucositis. *Seminars in Oncology Nursing, 20,* 22–29.

Elting, L.S., Cooksley, C., Chambers, M., Cantor, S.B., Manzullo, E., & Rubenstein, E.B. (2003). The burdens of cancer therapy: Clinical and economic outcomes of chemotherapy-induced mucositis. *Cancer, 98,* 1531–1539.

Epstein, J.B., & Schubert, M.M. (2003). Oropharyngeal mucositis in cancer therapy: Review of pathogenesis, diagnosis, and management. *Oncology, 17,* 1767–1779.

Fulton, J.S., Middleton, G.J., & McPhail, J.T. (2002). Management of oral complications. *Seminars in Oncology Nursing, 18,* 28–35.

Jacobson, S.D., Cha, S., Sargent, D.J., O'Connell, M.J., Poon, M., Buroker, T., et al. (2001). Tolerability, dose intensity, and benefit of 5FU-based chemotherapy for advanced colorectal cancer (CRC) in the elderly: A North Central Cancer Treatment Group (NCCTG) Study [Abstract 1534]. *Proceedings of the American Society of Clinical Oncology, 20,* 384A.

Keefe, D.M.K., Brealey, J., Goland, G.J., & Cummins, A.G. (2000). Chemotherapy for cancer causes apoptosis that precedes hypoplasia in crypts of the small intestine in humans. *Gut, 47,* 632–637.

Keefe, D.M.K., Gibson, R.J., & Hauer-Jensen, M. (2004). Gastrointestinal mucositis. *Seminars in Oncology Nursing, 20,* 38–47.

Knox, J.J., Puodziunas, A.L.V., & Feld, R. (2000). Chemotherapy-induced oral mucositis: Prevention and management. *Drugs & Aging, 17,* 257–267.

Kolbinson, D.A., Schubert, M.M., Flournoy, N., & Truelove, E.L. (1988). Early oral changes following bone marrow transplantation. *Oral Surgery, Oral Medicine and Oral Pathology, 66,* 130–138.

Kostler, W.J., Hejna, M., Wenzel, C., & Zielinski, C.C. (2001). Oral mucositis complicating chemotherapy and/or radiotherapy: Options for prevention and treatment. *CA: A Cancer Journal for Clinicians, 51,* 290–315.

Kwong, K.K.F. (2004). Prevention and treatment of oropharyngeal mucositis following cancer therapy: Are there new approaches? *Cancer Nursing, 27,* 183–205.

Larson, P.J., Miaskowski, C., MacPhail, L., Dodd, M.J., Greenspan, D., Dibble, S.L., et al. (1998). The PRO-SELF Mouth Aware program: An effective approach for reducing chemotherapy-induced mucositis. *Cancer Nursing, 21,* 263–268.

Maher, K.E. (2000). Radiation therapy: Toxicities and management. In C.H. Yarbro, M.H. Frogge, M. Goodman, & S.L. Groenwald (Eds.), *Cancer nursing: Principles and practice* (5th ed., pp. 323–351). Sudbury, MA: Jones and Bartlett.

McGuire, D.B. (2002). Mucosal tissue injury in cancer therapy: More than mucositis and mouthwash. *Cancer Practice, 4,* 179–191.

McGuire, D.B. (2003). Barriers and strategies in implementation of oral care standards for cancer patients. *Supportive Care in Cancer, 11,* 435–441.

McGuire, D.B., Peterson, D.E., Muller, S., Owen, D.C., Slemmons, M.F., & Schubert, M.M. (2002). The 20 item oral mucositis index: Reliability and validity in bone marrow and stem cell transplant patients. *Cancer Investigation, 20,* 893–903.

McGuire, D.B., Rubenstein, E.B., & Peterson, D.E. (2004). Evidence-based guidelines for managing mucositis. *Seminars in Oncology Nursing, 20,* 59–66.

Miller, J., & Kearney, N. (2001). Oral care for patients with cancer: A review of the literature. *Cancer Nursing, 24,* 241–254.

National Cancer Institute. (2003). *Common terminology criteria for adverse events.* Retrieved October 4, 2004, from http://ctep.info.nih.gov/reporting/ctc.html

National Cancer Institute. (2004). *Oral complications of chemotherapy and head/neck radiation.* Retrieved September 15, 2004, from http://www.cancer.gov/cancertopics/pdq/supportivecare/oralcomplications

National Comprehensive Cancer Network. (2005). *Clinical practice guidelines in oncology: Senior adult oncology.* Retrieved September 22, 2005, from http://www.nccn.org/professionals/physician_gls/PDF/senior.pdf

Oken, M.M., Creech, R.H., Tormey, D.C., Horton, J., Davis, T.E., McFadden, E.T., et al. (1982). Toxicity and response criteria of the Eastern Cooperative Oncology Group. *American Journal of Clinical Oncology, 5,* 649–655.

Peterson, D.E. (1999). Research advances in oral mucositis. *Current Opinion in Oncology, 11,* 261–266.

Peterson, D.E., Beck, S.L., & Keefe, D.M.K. (2004). Novel therapies. *Seminars in Oncology Nursing, 20,* 53–58.

Peterson, D.E., & Petit, R.G. (2003). Phase III study: AES-14 in chemotherapy patients at risk for mucositis [Abstract 2917]. *Proceedings of the American Society of Clinical Oncology, 22,* 725A.

Popescu, R.A., Norman, A., Ross, P.J., Parikh, B., & Cunningham, D. (1999). Adjuvant or palliative chemotherapy for colorectal cancer in patients 70 years or older. *Journal of Clinical Oncology, 17,* 2412–2418.

Radiation Therapy Oncology Group. (1989). *Cooperative group common toxicity criteria.* Retrieved October 14, 2004, from http://www.rtog.org/members/toxicity/tox.html

Radiation Therapy Oncology Group. (2004a). *Acute radiation morbidity scoring criteria.* Retrieved October 14, 2004, from http://www.rtog.org/members/toxicity/acute.html

Radiation Therapy Oncology Group. (2004b). *Chronic radiation morbidity scoring criteria.* Retrieved October 14, 2004, from http://www.rtog.org/members/toxicity/late.html

Rubenstein, E.B., Peterson, D.E., Schubert, M., Keefe, D., McGuire, D., Epstein, J., et al. (2004). Clinical practice guidelines for the prevention and treatment of cancer therapy-induced oral and gastrointestinal mucositis. *Cancer, 100*(Suppl. 9), 2026–2046.

Schubert, M.M., Williams, B.E., Lloid, M.E., Donaldson, G., & Chapko, M.K. (1992). Clinical assessment scale for the rating of oral mucosal changes associated with bone marrow transplantation. Development of an oral mucositis index. *Cancer, 69,* 2469–2477.

Shih, A., Miaskowski, C., Dodd, M.J., Stotts, N.A., & MacPhail, L. (2002). A research review of the current treatments for radiation-induced oral mucositis in patients with head and neck cancer. *Oncology Nursing Forum, 29,* 1063–1078.

Smink, K.A., & Gosselin-Acomb, T.K. (2004). Evaluation of an education tool to enhance outcomes for patients with head and neck cancer. *Clinical Journal of Oncology Nursing, 8,* 490–494.

Sonis, S.T. (1998). Mucositis as a biological process: A new hypothesis for the development of chemotherapy-induced stomatotoxicity. *Oral Oncology, 34,* 39–43.

Sonis, S.T. (2004). Pathobiology of mucositis. *Seminars in Oncology Nursing, 20,* 11–15.

Sonis, S.T., Eilers, J.P., Epstein, J.B., LeVeque, F.G., Liggett, W.H., Mulagha, M.T., et al. (1999). Validation of a new scoring system for the assessment of clinical trial research of oral mucositis induced by radiation or chemotherapy. Mucositis Study Group. *Cancer, 85,* 2103–2113.

Sonis, S.T., Elting, L.S., Keefe, D., Peterson, D.E., Schubert, M., Hauer-Jensen, M., et al. (2004). Perspectives on cancer therapy-induced mucosal injury: Pathogenesis, measurement, epidemiology, and consequences for patients. *Cancer, 100*(Suppl. 9), 1995–2025.

Spielberger, R.T., Stiff, P., Emmanouilides, C., Yanovich, S., Bensinger, W., Hedrick, E., et al. (2001). Efficacy of recombinant human keratinocyte growth factor (rHuKGF) in reducing mucositis in patients with hematologic malignancies undergoing autologous peripheral blood progenitor cell transplantation (auto-PBPCT) after radiation-based conditioning—Results of a phase 2 trial [Abstract 25]. *Proceedings of the American Society of Clinical Oncology, 20,* 7A.

Stein, B.N., Petrelli, N.J., Douglass, H.O., Driscoll, D.L., Arcangeli, G., & Meropol, N.J. (1995). Age and sex are independent predictors of 5-fluorouracil toxicity: Analysis of a large scale phase III trial. *Cancer, 75,* 11–17.

Stricker, C.T., & Sullivan, J. (2003). Evidence-based oncology oral care clinical practice guidelines: Development, implementation, and evaluation. *Clinical Journal of Oncology Nursing, 7,* 222–227.

Wohlschlaeger, A. (2004). Prevention and treatment of mucositis: A guide for nurses. *Journal of Pediatric Oncology Nursing, 21,* 281–287.

World Health Organization. (1979). *WHO handbook for reporting results of cancer treatment.* Geneva, Switzerland: Author.

Worthington, H.V., Clarkson, J.E., & Eden, O.B. (2004). Interventions for treating oral mucositis for patients with cancer receiving treatment. *Cochrane Database of Systematic Reviews, 2,* CD001973. Retrieved September 15, 2004, from http://www.update-software.com/publications/cochrane

Yeager, K.A., Webster, J., Crain, M., Kasow, J., & McGuire, D.B. (2000). Implementation of an oral care standard for leukemia and transplantation patients. *Cancer Nursing, 23,* 40–47.

CHAPTER 17

Symptom Management of Diarrhea and Constipation

Nancy M. Gardner, PhD, and
Diane G. Cope, PhD, ARNP, BC, AOCNP

Introduction

Gastrointestinal (GI) complications such as diarrhea and constipation, caused by cancer and its related treatment, negatively impact quality of life (QOL) and are associated with increased mortality and morbidity in the older adult. Although older adults do not have a greater risk for diarrhea in comparison to younger individuals, the older adult with cancer is at an increased risk for complications related to diarrhea such as dehydration, confusion, alteration of drug metabolism, and cardiovascular compromise. Research exploring constipation and the older adult with cancer is limited and, in general, focuses on patients with advanced cancer receiving palliative and hospice care and pain medication. The physiologic changes associated with aging in combination with other factors such as comorbidities, alterations in dietary and fluid intake, polypharmacy, and changes in physical activity predispose older adults to significant bowel alterations. By 2030, one in five Americans will be older than 65 years of age, and more than 60% of all malignancies will occur in people within this age group (U.S. Census Bureau, 1996; Yancik & Ries, 2000). Furthermore, colorectal cancer is one of the five most common cancers in the older adult and is associated with greater risk for bowel alterations. Greater attention is needed for assessment and evidence-based care and treatment of diarrhea and constipation in the older adult with cancer. This chapter will present the incidence, pathophysiology, risk factors, and treatment of diarrhea and constipation. Nursing care and research issues regarding diarrhea and constipation in the older adult with cancer will be highlighted.

Diarrhea

Incidence

Rutledge and Engelking (1998) explored all age incidence of diarrhea as a toxicity related to treatment and found that 31%–87% of patients undergoing chemotherapy, 18%–20% undergoing pelvic radiation, and up to 35% of those on combination chemotherapy and radiation experience diarrhea. In a retrospective study of 100 patients of all age groups receiving chemotherapy for colon cancer, Arbuckle, Huber, and Zacker (2000) explored all grades of diarrhea to determine clinical treatment decisions and economic impact. Approximately 50% of the patients required modifications in their chemotherapy treatment, such as dose reductions, treatment delays, or discontinuation of therapy. Thirty-seven percent required aggressive treatment, such as hospitalization or IV fluid hydration.

A pooled analysis of 3,351 patients involving seven trials comparing incidence of diarrhea in patients older than 65 to those younger than 65 years of age found no significant interaction between age and incidence of diarrhea related to cancer treatment (Sargent et al., 2001). However optimistic these findings are for older adults, the National Cancer Institute (NCI, 2004) emphasized awareness and aggressive control of diarrhea in all patients.

Physiology of the Gastrointestinal Tract Related to Diarrhea

Two key aspects exist of GI physiology in relation to diarrhea: GI motility and fluid secretion/absorption. GI motility involves processes that promote the absorption of nutrients, including fluid and electrolytes. Movement of material through the GI tract occurs via coordination of intraluminal pressures and smooth muscle contractions controlled by the enteric nervous system and peptide hormonal release. On average, 9 L/day of fluid is processed by the GI tract in 24 hours. The small intestine absorbs approximately 8 L/day of fluid. The colon absorbs the remaining fluid. Under normal physiologic conditions, individuals excrete no more than 200 ml/day of fluid in feces.

Pathophysiology of Diarrhea

Diarrhea is caused by an imbalance in the physiologic mechanisms of the GI tract. In radiation- and chemotherapy-induced diarrhea, acute damage occurs to the epithelial crypt cells. This damage causes necrosis, inflammation, and ulceration of the intestinal mucosa. Over time, atrophy and fibrosis of the lining occurs, with decreased absorption of water and electrolytes producing diarrhea (Gwede, 2003). Decreased fluid and electrolyte absorption also may occur as a result of either osmotically active substances in the lumen or increased intestinal motility. Endogenous secretagogues or exogenous toxins cause an increase of fluid and secretion.

Regardless of the cause, the loss of fluids and electrolytes caused by severe diarrhea can cause weakness, lethargy, orthostatic hypotension, dry mouth, and weight loss (Hogan, 1998).

Absorption, secretion, and intestinal motility are the three central mechanisms that are responsible for diarrhea associated with cancer therapy. Assessment of other potential causes of diarrhea is very important to determine the specific cause and subsequent treatment of the diarrhea. For example, refractory diarrhea often is caused by multiple factors such as medications, chemotherapy, and comorbidities (e.g., irritable bowel syndrome). Determination of the specific cause and proper classification of diarrhea based on pathophysiology is necessary for selecting the appropriate treatment regimen (Hogan, 1998).

Etiology

Although chemotherapy is the most common cause of diarrhea in patients undergoing cancer treatment, other etiologies may include surgical procedures, radiation therapy, bone marrow transplantation, drug reactions, comorbidities, infection, constipation, diet, and stress (see Table 17-1) (NCI, 2004).

Another method of classifying the etiology of diarrhea is by the underlying mechanism. These classifications include osmotic, secretory, exudative, malabsorptive, dysmotility-associated, and chemotherapy-induced diarrhea.

Table 17-1. Possible Causes of Diarrhea in Cancer

Etiologies	Examples
Cancer related	Carcinoid syndrome Colon cancer Lymphoma Medullary carcinoma of the thyroid Pancreatic cancer, particularly islet cell tumors (Zollinger-Ellison syndrome) Pheochromocytoma
Surgery or procedure related	Celiac plexus block Cholecystectomy, esophagogastrectomy Gastrectomy, pancreaticoduodenectomy (Whipple) Intestinal resection (malabsorption because of short bowel syndrome) Vagotomy
Chemotherapy related	Capecitabine, cisplatin, cytosine arabinoside, cyclophosphamide, daunorubicin, docetaxel, doxorubicin, 5-fluorouracil, interferon, irinotecan, leucovorin, methotrexate, oxaliplatin, paclitaxel, topotecan
Radiation therapy related	Irradiation to the abdomen, para-aortics, lumbar area, and pelvis
Bone marrow transplantation related	Conditioning chemotherapy, total body irradiation, graft-versus-host disease after allogeneic bone marrow or peripheral blood stem cell transplants
Drug adverse effects	Antibiotics, magnesium-containing antacids, antihypertensives, colchicine, digoxin, iron, lactulose, laxatives, methyldopa, metoclopramide, misoprostol, potassium supplements, propanolol, theophylline
Concurrent disease	Diabetes, hyperthyroidism, inflammatory bowel disease (Crohn disease, diverticulitis, gastroenteritis, HIV/AIDS, ulcerative colitis), obstruction (tumor related)

(Continued on next page)

Table 17-1. Possible Causes of Diarrhea in Cancer *(Continued)*

Etiologies	Examples
Infection	*Clostridium difficile, Clostridium perfringens, Bacillus cereus, Giardia lamblia, Cryptosporidium, Salmonella, Shigella, Campylobacter, Rotavirus*
Fecal impaction	Constipation leading to obstruction
Diet	Alcohol, milk, and dairy products (particularly in patients with lactose intolerance)
	Caffeine-containing products (coffee, tea, chocolate), specific fruit juices (prune juice, unfiltered apple juice, sauerkraut juice)
	High-fiber foods (raw fruits and vegetables, nuts, seeds, whole-grain products, dried legumes); high-fat foods (deep-fried foods, high fat–containing foods)
	Lactulose intolerance or food allergies
	Sorbitol-containing foods (candy and chewing gum); hot and spicy foods; gas-forming foods and beverages (cruciferous vegetables, dried legumes, melons, carbonated beverages)
Psychological factors	Stress

Note. Based on information from National Cancer Institute, 2004.

Osmotic diarrhea is caused by mechanical disturbances resulting from ingestion of hyperosmolar substances, such as nonabsorbable solutes in sorbitol or enteral feeding solutions. Intestinal hemorrhage also causes osmotic diarrhea. The large volume of fluid and electrolytes that enters the intestinal lumen overwhelms the absorptive capacity of the bowel. Diarrhea resolves when the causative agent is eliminated.

Secretory-type diarrhea is caused by a biochemical disturbance. The principal producers of the biochemical disturbance are enterotoxin-producing pathogens, such as *Clostridium difficile*, and endocrine tumors. The pathogens irritate and damage the epithelial cells of the bowel wall, while the endocrine or carcinoid tumors produce large quantities of peptides and secretagogues. Clinically, the diarrhea is watery, voluminous, and persistent despite fasting.

Exudative diarrhea is often a result of radiation to bowel mucosa causing depletion of crypt stem cells, mucosal atrophy, and fibrosis. The stool is characterized by mucus, serum protein, and blood. The volume of diarrhea varies, although it is less than 1,000 cc/day. Frequency, however, is high at more than six stools daily (Rutledge & Engelking, 1998).

Malabsorptive diarrhea is caused by mechanical and biochemical disturbances. Factors such as enzyme deficiencies alter mucosal integrity or membrane permeability and lead to abnormal enterohepatic circulation of bile salts. Consequently, osmotically active substances enter the colon and directly stimulate the bowel. Potential factors that cause malabsorptive diarrhea include enzyme deficiencies such as lactose and pancreatic enzyme deficiency and surgical resection of the intestines such as a right hemicolectomy. Malabsorptive diarrhea usually is frequent and voluminous and may be classified as steatorrhea or foul smelling.

Dysmotility-associated diarrhea may be a result of mechanical disturbance with abnormal intestinal motility or peristaltic dysfunction secondary to alterations in mechanical stretch or neural stimuli. The causes for these disturbances include irritable bowel syndrome, narcotic withdrawal syndrome, stress, anxiety, fear, and ingestion of peristaltic stimulants. The stools are often small and have a semi-solid/liquid consistency with variable volume and frequency.

Chemotherapy-induced diarrhea is a result of a cascade of events. Mitotic arrest of intestinal epithelial crypt cells leads to superficial necrosis and bowel wall inflammation that produces mucosal and submucosal factors such as leukotrienes, cytokines that cause an oversecretion of intestinal water and electrolytes. Fluoropyrimidines and topoisomerase inhibitors are the most common chemotherapeutic agents associated with diarrhea. Chemotherapy diarrhea is watery to semi-solid and begins 24–96 hours following chemotherapy administration.

Cancer Therapy and Diarrhea

Diarrhea from cancer therapy may directly affect the patient's treatment program. Patients may be unable to comply with their prescribed treatment, require dose modifications, or require delay in their treatment schedule. Cost of care also is negatively affected. Treatment costs increase significantly because of the need for additional medical treatment and for possible hospitalization to manage the diarrhea (Kornblau et al., 2000). Chemotherapy and radiation therapy both can cause diarrhea.

Chemotherapy

The exact incidence of chemotherapy-induced diarrhea has not been established. Anticancer agents commonly associated with diarrhea include 5-fluorouracil (5-FU)/leucovorin, irinotecan (CPT-11), cisplatin, cytosine arabinoside, methotrexate, doxorubicin, hydroxyurea, and interferon. Various studies involving a variety of chemotherapeutic options have reported diarrhea as a dose-limiting adverse event (Barbounis, Koumakis, Vassilomanolakis, Demiri, & Efremidis, 2001; Cunningham et al., 1998; Ito et al., 1999; Leichman et al., 1995; Van Cutsem et al., 1998). Studies investigating regimens with single-agent 5-FU, single-agent irinotecan, or combination 5-FU and irinotecan suggest that approximately 50%–80% of patients experience some grade of chemotherapy-induced diarrhea (Conti et al., 1996; Leichman et al.; Rothenberg et al., 1996; Wadler, Haynes, & Wiernik, 1995). More specifically, 31%–66% of patients treated with 5-FU, 74%–87% of those on irinotecan, and 43% of those on cisplatin-based therapy have experienced chemotherapy-induced diarrhea. Table 17-2 provides a review of chemotherapy regimens and incidence of grades 3 and 4 diarrhea. Diarrhea also may differ depending on dose, frequency, and duration of therapy (Rutledge & Engelking, 1998; Wadler et al., 1998).

Severe diarrhea can have a significant physical impact. Often debilitating, severe diarrhea can be life threatening, as suggested by reported increased morbidity and mortality rates in a clinical trial of 343 patients with metastatic colorectal carcinoma (Petrelli et al., 1989). Diarrhea caused by the combination of 5-FU with leucovorin accounted for 11 (5%) treatment-related deaths. More recently, a review of two NCI-sponsored cooperative group clinical trials investigating CPT-11 plus bolus 5-FU/leucovorin (IFL) regimens was conducted to evaluate reported early toxic deaths (Rothenberg, Meropol, Poplin, Van Cutsem, & Wadler, 2001). In the North

Table 17-2. Chemotherapy Regimens and Incidence of Severe Diarrhea

Chemotherapy Regimen	Incidence: Grade 3–4	References
Irinotecan + 5-FU + leucovorin (IFL)	24%–61%	Barbounis et al., 2001; Van Cutsem et al., 1998
Irinotecan	22%–31%	Cancerconsultants.com, 1998–2004
Fluoropyrimidines	30% or greater	Cancerconsultants.com, 1998–2004
Capecitabine + oxaliplatin	22%	Scheithauer et al., 2002
Oxaliplatin + 5-FU + leucovorin	11%	Sanofi Aventis, 2002
Floxuridine	30% or greater	Cancerconsultants.com, 1998–2004
High-dose chemotherapy with epirubicin	76%	Ito et al., 1999
5-FU	6%–14%	Leichman et al., 1995; O'Connell et al., 1994
IFL + bevacizumab	33%	Hurwitz et al., 2004
Oxaliplatin + 5-FU + leucovorin + bevacizumab	20%	Giantonio et al., 2004
Pelvic and abdominal radiation	15%–70%	Baillie-Johnson, 1996; Yavuz et al., 2002

Note. From *Cancer Treatment-Induced Diarrhea: Interventions to Minimize the Roller Coaster Ride* (p. 11), by W. Vogel and J. Stern, 2004, Pittsburgh, PA: Oncology Education Services. Copyright 2004 by Oncology Education Services. Reprinted with permission.

Central Cancer Treatment Group trial involving patients with metastatic colorectal cancer, 14 deaths (4.8%) occurred in patients treated in the IFL arm. In the Cancer and Leukemia Group B trial involving adjuvant therapy for stage III colon cancer, 14 deaths (2.2%) occurred in patients treated in the IFL arm. Findings of the review suggested that the majority of deaths resulted from GI toxicity and cardiovascular events. The GI toxicity was defined as a GI syndrome that included symptoms of severe diarrhea, nausea, vomiting, anorexia, and abdominal cramping and was associated with severe dehydration, neutropenia, fever, and electrolyte imbalances. As a result of this review, vigilant monitoring and weekly assessment of GI toxicities was recommended, especially in the older adult.

Radiation Therapy

The incidence of radiation-induced diarrhea is dependent upon the site and dose of radiation (Gwede, 2003). Approximately 70% of patients experience diarrhea of any grade, and 20% experience grade 3 or 4 with pelvic radiation. With combination radiation/chemotherapy, the incidence of diarrhea increases to 40%–80% for any grade and approximately 20%–35% for grade 3 or 4 (Miller et al., 2002; Rutledge & Engelking, 1998; Tepper et al., 1997).

In addition to the medical complications of diarrhea, the QOL of the patient with cancer is negatively affected. Prolonged or frequent stools can cause fatigue, anxiety, and sleep disturbances and limit travel, decrease sexual activity, and impair work performance.

Clinical Manifestations

For the older adult with cancer experiencing diarrhea, numerous presenting signs and symptoms can occur that necessitate immediate attention to prevent morbidity and mortality. The older adult may present with weight loss, weakness, lethargy, confusion, lightheadedness, orthostatic hypotension, dehydration, hypovolemia, and electrolyte imbalances that can rapidly progress to life-threatening cardiac compromise and arrhythmias. Furthermore, the older adult is at increased risk for falls with frequent trips to the bathroom or, if bed-bound, is at increased risk of skin breakdown involving the rectal area.

Assessment

The persistent loss of fluid and electrolytes associated with diarrhea can cause life-threatening dehydration, renal insufficiency, electrolyte imbalances, and cardiac complications, especially in the older adult. Prompt assessment and treatment are critical to prevent the morbidity and mortality associated with diarrhea. Few standardized assessment tools are available, and, therefore, healthcare professionals perform standardized assessment of diarrhea infrequently in the clinical setting (Rutledge & Engelking, 1998). Assessment of a patient with diarrhea involves a comprehensive health history, physical examination, and laboratory tests with emphasis on the patient's cancer treatment, comorbidities, coexisting symptoms, and a complete description of the diarrhea.

Health History

The baseline history should include the primary disease and treatments, previous history of diarrhea, onset of current diarrhea, frequency defined by the NCI Common Toxicity Criteria, characteristics that include consistency, color, bloody, odorous, and duration of diarrhea, other associated symptoms such as fever, pain, bleeding, skin integrity, dizziness, lethargy, cramping, abdominal pain, nausea, vomiting, and other contributing factors such as diet, medications, comorbid conditions, recent travel, and measures taken to control the diarrhea. The NCI Common Toxicity Criteria for Grading Severity of Diarrhea is the most commonly used assessment tool and is a scale that classifies diarrhea into four different grades (1–4) depending on the number of stools per day, the need for parenteral support or intensive care, and the presence of nocturnal stools (see Table 17-3). Separate criteria are given for patients without colostomy, patients with colostomy, patients with bone marrow transplant (BMT), and pediatric patients with BMT (NCI, 2004; Wadler et al., 1998).

Stool Characteristics

Color of stool is an indicator of what foods have been ingested, bleeding in the GI tract, and malabsorptive disorder. High-fat diets result in larger amounts of bile produced by the liver to aid in the digestion of fats. When bile is excreted from the

Table 17-3. National Cancer Institute Common Toxicity Criteria for Grading Severity of Diarrhea

Toxicity	0	1	2	3	4
Patients without a colostomy	None	Increase of < 4 stools/day over pretreatment	Increase of 4–6 stools/day or nocturnal stools	Increase of ≥ 7 stools/day	> 10 stools/day
	None	None	Moderate cramping, not interfering with normal activity	Severe cramping and incontinence, interfering with daily activities	Grossly bloody diarrhea and need for parenteral support
Patients with a colostomy	None	Mild increase in loose, watery colostomy output compared with pretreatment	Moderate increase in loose, watery colostomy output compared with pretreatment, but not interfering with normal activity	Severe increase in loose, watery colostomy output compared with pretreatment, interfering with normal activity	Physiologic consequences requiring intensive care; hemodynamic collapse
For patients undergoing bone marrow transplant (BMT)	None	> 500 ml to ≤ 1,000 ml of diarrhea/day	> 1,000 ml to ≤ 1,500 ml of diarrhea/day	> 1,500 ml of diarrhea/day	Severe abdominal pain with or without ileus
For children undergoing BMT	None	> 5 ml/kg to ≤ 10 ml/kg of diarrhea/day	> 10 ml/kg to ≤ 15 ml/kg of diarrhea/day	> 15 ml/kg of diarrhea/day	Severe abdominal pain with or without ileus

Note. From *Gastrointestinal Complications: Diarrhea*, by the National Cancer Institute, 2005. Retrieved June 1, 2005, from http://www.nci.nih.gov/cancertopics/pdq/supportivecare/gastrointestinalcomplications/HealthProfessional/page5#Section_129

liver, it is yellow-green in color. This color becomes altered as digestive enzymes in the GI tract mix with the bile to digest food. Therefore, green stool indicates food is moving too quickly through the intestine. Possible dietary causes include green, leafy vegetables with food coloring (green). A pale or clay-colored stool is associated with a lack of bile, often caused by obstruction of the bile duct or by medications such as Kaopectate® (Pfizer, New York, NY). Yellow, greasy, foul-smelling stool is an indication of excess fat because of high dietary intake and malabsorption. Black stool is caused by bleeds in the upper GI tract caused by blood mixing with hydrochloric acid in the stomach and the ingestion of iron, Pepto-Bismol® (Procter & Gamble, Cincinnati, OH), or black licorice. Bright red stool indicates a lower GI bleed located in the lower intestines or rectum. Ingestion of beets, gelatin, or products containing red food coloring also can cause bright red stools (Rutledge & Engelking, 1998).

Physical Examination and Diagnostic Studies

The physical evaluation of a patient complaining of diarrhea should include vital signs; assessment of postural hypotension; hydration status evaluated by buccal membrane moisture and skin turgor; skin integrity of anal area or stoma; and an abdominal examination to evaluate for hypoactive or hyperactive bowel sounds, tympany, distention, tenderness, guarding, and rebound tenderness. Baseline laboratory testing should include a complete chemistry profile to evaluate renal function, electrolytes, and serum albumin, and a complete blood count should note any elevations of the white blood count to suggest infection. Stool samples also should be obtained for *C. difficile*, ova and parasites, and cultures to rule out infection. If a bowel obstruction is suspected, radiographic tests may be indicated.

Treatment

Evidence-based guidelines for the assessment and management of chemotherapy-induced diarrhea were originally published in 1998 and recently have been updated (see Figure 17-1) (Benson et al., 2004). The treatment of radiation-induced diarrhea is similar. The overall goals of treatment include elimination of potential causative factors when possible, patient education, dietary management, fluid and electrolyte replacement, and antidiarrheal therapy.

Patient Education

Patient education should include when to start antidiarrhea treatment, how to treat—in writing, and when to seek help (red flags). Patients should be advised of symptoms considered red flags that require immediate attention, including fever, excessive thirst, dizziness, palpitations, abdominal cramps, watery stool, bloody stool, and refractory diarrhea for more than 24 hours.

Patient education regarding dietary modifications to manage diarrhea is also important. Foods greatly affect the presence of diarrhea, particularly in patients who are at risk because of chemotherapy and radiation therapy. Management of diarrhea includes careful individualized dietary planning, preferably with guidance from a dietitian. Healthcare providers should instruct patients to avoid foods and beverages that contain lactose, spices, high levels of fiber or fat, caffeine, and alcohol. Oral hydration should include daily consumption of 8–10 large glasses of clear fluids, such as broth or Gatorade®, to replace lost fluids and electrolytes. Ginger tea, glutamine, and peeled apples are useful homeopathic remedies for diarrhea. Patients should be instructed to eat small, frequent meals that include potassium-rich, bland foods such as bananas, rice, applesauce or peeled apples, dry white toast, or plain pasta (Benson et al., 2004). Because of increased transit time and decreased absorption, patients may become deficient in certain vitamins, particularly those that are fat soluble. Vitamin supplementation should be considered (Engelking, 2004). Once the diarrhea has resolved, patients slowly may add solid foods to their diet.

Antidiarrheal therapy always must be individualized based on the needs of the patient, particularly for the older adult. Recommended treatment for the first report of diarrhea is loperamide, which acts to decrease peristalsis in the small and large bowels. Standard loperamide doses often are ineffective in managing grade 2 or higher diarrhea (Kornblau et al., 2000). Current recommendations are for loperamide 4 mg initial dose followed by 2 mg every four hours or after every unformed stool for patients with grade 1 or 2 uncomplicated diarrhea. For persistent grades 1 and 2 diarrhea, loperamide 2 mg every two hours should be administered in addition to

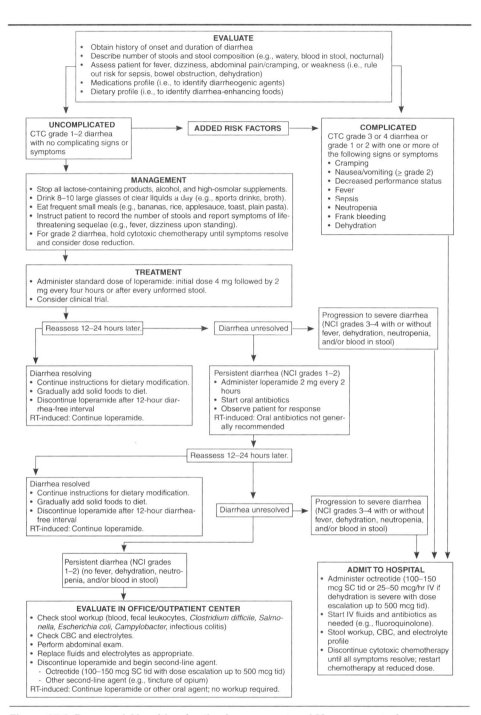

Figure 17-1. Proposed Algorithm for the Assessment and Management of Chemotherapy-Induced Diarrhea

Note. From "Recommended Guidelines for the Treatment of Cancer Treatment-Induced Diarrhea," by A.B. Benson, J.A. Ajani, R.B. Catalano, C. Engelking, S.M. Kornblau, J.A. Martenson, et al., 2004, *Journal of Clinical Oncology, 22,* p. 2923. Copyright 2004 by the American Society of Clinical Oncology. Reprinted with permission.

oral antibiotics. Loperamide may be discontinued following a 12-hour diarrhea-free period.

If the diarrhea progresses to grades 3 or 4, more aggressive approaches with octreotide are recommended (Benson et al., 2004). Octreotide acts to improve diarrhea associated with cancer therapy through a number of understood and proposed mechanisms. Octreotide inhibits pancreatic and GI hormones, such as insulin, gastrin, secretin, and pancreatic polypeptide. Through this inhibition, octreotide is theorized to influence various GI functions (Fuessl, Carolan, Williams, & Bloom, 1987). In conjunction with its inhibitory hormonal effects, octreotide is hypothesized to reduce diarrhea as a result of its interaction with epithelial cells. The interaction causes decreased luminal fluid in the upper jejunum with subsequent inhibition of chloride secretion and stimulation of sodium and chloride absorption (Yavuz, Yavuz, Aydin, Can, & Kavgaci, 2002). Octreotide also prolongs mouth-to-cecum transit time, thereby increasing the contact time between luminal contents and the GI mucosal surface. If the diarrhea remains unresolved with persistent grade 3 or 4 toxicity with or without fever, neutropenia, dehydration, and/or blood in the stool, patients should be hospitalized for continued treatment and supportive care.

Nursing Care Issues

Treatment goals include the prevention of diarrhea, enhanced recovery of intestinal mucosa from the effects of chemotherapy or radiation therapy, elimination/reduction of diarrhea-associated morbidity and mortality, prevention of cancer treatment delays or regimen modifications, improvement of cancer treatment outcomes, protection of skin integrity, preservation of nutrition and electrolyte status, and optimization of QOL by decreasing patient discomfort and inconvenience (Kornblau et al., 2000; Rutledge & Engelking, 1998; Wadler et al., 1998). Oncology nurses can take an active role in achieving these goals through patient education and assessment.

Patient education should begin before the first cycle of chemotherapy or first radiation treatment and include verbal and written information regarding diet, medication use, and healthcare provider notification of persistent problems. This is particulary important for the older adult who may have sensory impairments and require additional time and instruction. If a family member or caregiver is available, he or she should be encouraged to participate in patient education sessions.

Patient assessment is critical in preventing diarrhea. Assessment should be ongoing and continous with each patient contact and may be facilitated by a standard tool that will enhance documentation and communication among healthcare providers. Initiating prompt, early treatment also is critical to prevent progression to more severe diarrhea that can lead to possible life-threatening complications. Assessment of diarrhea treatment is equally important to establish treatment effectiveness and should be ongoing, especially in the older adult. Effectiveness of treatment only can be accurately determined if a baseline initial clinical assessment has been completed prior to initiation of therapy. Follow-up should begin within 24 hours of treatment and may require phone contact with the patient to evaluate severity of the diarrhea and response to treatment. If the diarrhea fails to resolve, further clinical evaluation of the patient should be performed. Once a patient has been identified to be at high risk for diarrhea, careful monitoring and patient education for early detection and treatment of diarrhea should occur prior to any additional therapy.

Constipation

Constipation, similar to diarrhea, is a symptom that can negatively affect a patient's QOL and can cause other complications, such as nausea and vomiting and bowel obstruction. Constipation is a common symptom of older adults because of the physiologic changes in the GI tract with aging, altered nutritional intake, and decreased activity levels. However, older adults with cancer are at even greater risk for the development of constipation because of cancer treatment and pain medication. Historically, constipation is an understudied clinical problem, and no well-validated guidelines are available to provide evidence-based care for the prevention and management of constipation. One issue that presents challenges in studying constipation is the lack of a uniform definition because of individual variation in frequency of bowel movements. In general, a normal bowel pattern is considered to be at least three stools per week and no more than three stools per day (NCI, 2004). McMillan (2004) suggested that constipation may be defined as "a decrease in the frequency of passage of formed stools and characterized by stools that are hard and difficult to pass" (p. 4).

Incidence

The exact incidence of constipation in patients with cancer is unknown. In general, studies exploring constipation have involved older adults in long-term care facilities and patients with advanced cancer requiring narcotic pain medication. In the general population, the incidence of constipation is approximately 2% in individuals younger than 65 years of age (McMillan, 2004; Schaefer & Cheskin, 1998). For community-dwelling older adults older than 65 years of age, constipation affects 26% of men and 34% of women (Schaefer & Cheskin), with approximately a 40%–50% incidence for older adults in long-term care facilities (Bosshard, Dreher, Schnegg, & Bula, 2004; McMillan, 2004). For patients with cancer, studies suggest that constipation incidence in hospitalized patients receiving cancer treatment ranges from 70%–100% (McMillan & Tittle, 1995; McMillan & Williams, 1989; Tittle & McMillan, 1994). In patients with advanced cancer receiving hospice care, constipation incidence ranges between 40%–64% (McMillan, 2002; McMillan & Weitzner, 2000; Weitzner, Moody, & McMillan, 1997).

Physiology of the Gastrointestinal Tract Related to Constipation

Under normal conditions, peristalsis moves stool through the small bowel by both voluntary and involuntary muscular movements. Increased stool volume and stimulation of stretched bowel walls cause peristalsis on a regular, ongoing basis. When stool enters the rectum, the internal sphincter, composed of visceral smooth muscle, relaxes, and stool is passed through the external sphincter. The external sphincter contracts with rectal distention to maintain continence (Cope, 2001). Stool collection in the rectum stimulates anal stretch receptors and causes the urge to defecate.

Pathophysiology of Constipation

When stool transit time, or the amount of time it takes for stools to pass through the colon, increases, greater fluid absorption occurs, and the stool becomes dry, hard, and difficult to pass. If the urge to defecate is ignored, the rectal nerve sensitivity is decreased, additional fluid is absorbed from the stool in the rectal vault, and stool becomes even drier and harder.

Etiology

Although narcotic use is a major contributor to constipation in patients with cancer, constipation can result from extrinsic factors, pathologic disorders, and pharmacologic agents. Constipation can be classified as primary, secondary, or iatrogenically induced (see Figure 17-2). Primary constipation is caused by extrinsic factors that produce decreased bowel motility and increased fecal transit time, causing stools to be dry and hard. Examples of extrinsic factors are decreased fluid intake, decreased activity level, and decreased dietary fiber intake. Secondary constipation is caused by pathologic disorders. Iatrogenically induced constipation is caused by certain drug therapies. For older adults, constipation can be caused by multiple factors such as decreased mobility, decreased fiber intake, failure to respond to the urge to defecate if mobility is compromised, depression, and increased laxative use (Schaefer & Cheskin, 1998).

Primary	Secondary	Iatrogenically Induced
Lack of fiber	Parkinson disease	Antacids
Lack of exercise	Intestinal obstruction	Anticholinergics
Lack of fluid intake	Volvulus	Antihistamines
	Adhesions	Barium sulfate
	Stroke	Calcium channel blockers
	Hypercalcemia	Diuretics
	Hypokalemia	Ganglionic blockers
	Diverticulosis	Hypotensives
	Spinal cord compression	Iron supplements
	Rectocele	Monoamine oxidase inhibitors
	Multiple sclerosis	Opiates
	Diabetes	Psychotherapeutic drugs
	Hypothyroidism	Tricyclic antidepressants
	Chronic renal failure	

Figure 17-2. Etiologies of Constipation

Note. From "Assessing and Managing Opiate-Induced Constipation in Adults With Cancer," by S.C. McMillan, 2004, *Cancer Control, 11*(Suppl. 3), p. 5. Copyright 2004 by the Moffitt Cancer Center. Adapted with permission.

Cancer Therapy and Constipation

Constipation can be a presenting symptom of cancer, or it can occur later in the disease trajectory. Contributing factors include the tumor itself, cancer treatments, pharmacologic agents for cancer pain, organ failure, decreased physical activity, altered nutrition with decreased dietary fiber and fluid intake, or dehydration.

Chemotherapy

Several chemotherapeutic agents are associated with greater incidence of constipation (see Figure 17-3). These chemotherapeutic agents produce neurotoxic effects by causing autonomic nerve dysfunction, affecting the smooth muscles of the bowel. As a result, there is a lack of stimulation and peristalsis and decreased transit time of the stool that leads to decreased frequency of defecation and constipation (Cope, 2001).

- Oxaliplatins
- Taxanes
- Thalidomide
- Vinca alkaloids
- $5HT_3$ antagonists

Figure 17-3. Cancer Treatment Agents Associated With Constipation

Note. From *Gastrointestinal Complications: Constipation*, by the National Cancer Institute, 2005. Retrieved June 1, 2005, from http://www.nci.nih.gov/cancertopics/pdq/supportivecare/gastrointestinalcomplications/HealthProfessional/page2

Analgesics

Patients with cancer frequently experience pain at some point during their illness and require pain medication, such as opiates. Opiates act to delay gastric emptying and cause gastroparesis and increased stool transit time. As a result, the stool becomes hard and dry, causing constipation. Constipation from opiate use is immediate and dose-related (McMillan, 2004).

Radiation Therapy

Radiation to the abdomen and pelvis also may contribute to constipation. Radiation therapy can produce scarring, thus narrowing the lumen of the colon and making it difficult to pass stool.

Clinical Manifestations

The older adult with cancer experiencing constipation may present with numerous symptoms, including passage of hard, dry stools, straining to defecate, absence of bowel movements, abdominal pain or cramping, rectal pain, or abdominal distention. The older adult also may report rectal bleeding that would necessitate immediate assessment and management.

Assessment

Constipation is a subjective symptom and often is overlooked as an important assessment piece in the patient with cancer. Patients may be attempting to self-medicate with over-the-counter preparations to resolve their constipation and associated symptoms and may forget to discuss this with the healthcare provider. Currently, no well-defined assessment tools are available. However, a complete assessment is critical to understand the etiology of the constipation and provide specific management. Assessment of the patient with constipation is similar to that of diarrhea and should include a comprehensive health history, physical examination, and laboratory tests with emphasis on the patient's cancer treatment, comorbidities, coexisting symptoms, and a complete description of the constipation.

Health History

The baseline history should include the primary disease and treatments; previous history of constipation; a complete evaluation of the patient's dietary intake, highlighting fluid and fiber intake; daily activity level; current prescription and over-the-counter medications, including patterns of laxative use; and bowel habits, highlighting any recent changes in stool characteristics, any measures taken to control the constipation, and any associated symptoms such as fever, abdominal pain or cramping, nausea, vomiting, or diarrhea alternating with constipation. In the older adult, elevated temperature, incontinence, unexplained falls, or changes in mental status may be the only presenting symptoms of constipation (McMillan, 2004).

Physical Examination

The physical examination should include an assessment of the patient's weight and a complete oral, abdominal, and rectal examination (McMillan, 2004; Schaefer & Cheskin, 1998). The oral exam should focus on dentition and chewing, noting any lesions or infections. The abdominal exam should evaluate for abdominal distention, tenderness, hypoactive, hyperactive, or absent bowel sounds, and palpable masses. Hyperactive, high-pitched, or absent bowel sounds are suggestive of a bowel obstruction. With deep palpation, a sausage-mass in the left colon may be suggestive of a feces-filled colon and constipation (McMillan, 2004). The rectal examination should evaluate for masses, hemorrhoids, and hard stool in the rectal vault. The stool should be screened for occult blood.

Diagnostic Studies

Diagnostic studies should include a complete metabolic panel to assess for hypokalemia, hypercalcemia, and renal function and hydration status. A thyroid profile also should be performed to assess thyroid function. Radiographic studies may include a plain abdominal film or a barium enema to evaluate for fecal retention, obstruction, or ileus. A radiographic transit study may be performed to evaluate for colonic dysmotility syndrome (Schaefer & Cheskin, 1998).

Treatment

Treatment strategies should focus on the etiology of the constipation in the older adult with cancer and should include nonpharmacologic and pharmacologic treatment. Based on the assessment and history, nonpharmacologic treatment would include increasing dietary fiber, increasing fluid intake, maintaining adequate exercise and activity level as appropriate for the older adult, and maintaining a regular toileting regimen (McMillan, 2004; Schaefer & Cheskin, 1998).

When developing a pharmacologic treatment plan for the older adult with constipation, a thorough review of current medications should be conducted to identify any medications that may be contributing to the problem of constipation. Eliminating the contributing factor may be the initial step, but this may be challenging or impossible with the older adult with cancer who requires narcotics for pain management or is receiving a chemotherapeutic agent associated with increased risk of constipation. In these situations, pain management and cancer treatment are critical, and, therefore, the focus is on prevention and treatment of constipation. For a discussion of opiate-induced constipation management, the reader is referred to Chapter 19 on pain in the older adult with cancer.

Several pharmacologic agents are available to treat constipation and include bulk, emollient, lubricant, osmotic, saline, and stimulant laxatives and prokinetic agents (see Table 17-4) (Avila, 2004). Each type of laxative can be classified according to the mechanism of action; therefore, it is important to understand the etiology of the patient's constipation, comorbidities, performance status, medication use, and cancer diagnosis and treatment to facilitate specific, appropriate constipation treatment. In the case of a suspected bowel obstruction, laxatives would not be indicated. Furthermore, advantages and disadvantages are associated with each type of laxative that should be incorporated in the treatment decision-making process (see Table 17-5). The following discussion will highlight the mechanism of action of each type of laxative and recommendations for practice.

Bulk-Forming Laxatives

Bulk-forming laxatives act by increasing absorption of water into the intestine, thereby increasing fecal bulk, increasing peristalsis, and reducing transit time (Avila, 2004; Hawkins, 2000; McMillan, 2004; Schaefer & Cheskin, 1998). The onset of action is 12 hours and may take up to three days for its maximum effect. Bulk-forming laxatives are recommended for mild constipation or for patients with cancer who possess a good performance status because they require mixing with at least eight ounces of fluid. As a result, this class of agents should not be recommended for patients who cannot meet these fluid requirements, such as some older adults and patients with advanced cancer (Avila).

Emollient and Lubricant Laxatives

Emollient laxatives act by lubricating and softening the stool by facilitating the mixture of fat and water in the intestines (Avila, 2004; Schaefer & Cheskin, 1998). The onset of action is eight hours, with results usually in one to two days. Emollient laxatives also require increased fluid intake and, because peristalsis is not stimulated, should be given with stimulant laxatives to facilitate evacuation of the softer stool. This class of agents should not be recommended for patients with chronic constipation or for patients who cannot meet the fluid requirements. Mineral oil, a lubricant, should not be given with emollient laxatives because the combination of these drugs may increase risk of absorption and toxicity of mineral oil (Avila). In addition, excess use of mineral oil can result in malabsorption of fat-soluble vitamins.

Osmotic and Saline Laxatives

Osmotic laxatives are nonabsorbable sugars that act by retaining fluid in the bowel to soften stool. The onset of action is two hours, with effects ranging from 24–72 hours. Saline laxatives also cause water retention osmotically but further act to promote peristalsis. The onset of action of saline laxatives is 30 minutes, with maximum effects usually occurring within 12 hours. Osmotic and saline laxatives have limited use in the management of chronic constipation in the patient with cancer. The sweet taste of osmotic laxatives may discourage use in patients who are

Table 17-4. Laxative Dosage Information

Type of Laxative	Route(s)/Onset of Action	Dosage Forms	Usual Dosage
Bulk-Forming			
Methylcellulose	po: 12–72 hrs	Powder	1 tbsp up to tid mixed in 8 fl oz
Psyllium	po: 12–72 hrs	Powder	1 tsp–1 tbsp qd to qid mixed in 8 fl oz
Polycarbophil	po: 12–72 hrs	Powder	1 g qid or prn (no more than 6 g/24 hrs)
Emollient			
Docusate sodium	po: 12–72 hrs	Capsules/tablets	50–300 mg daily
Docusate calcium	po: 12–72 hrs	Syrup/capsules	240 mg daily until normal
Lubricant			
Mineral oil	po: 6–8 hrs Rectal: 5–15 min	Liquid Enema	15–45 ml at bedtime 118 ml (4–5 oz) in single daily dose
Osmotic			
Lactulose	po: 24–48 hrs	Solution	30–45 ml qd to qid
Sorbitol	po: 24–48 hrs Rectal: 15 min–1 hr	Solution Enema	30 ml at bedtime 120 ml as 25%–30% solution
Glycerin	Rectal: 15 min–1 hr	Suppository	1 as needed, retain 15–30 min
PEG with electrolytes	po: 1–4 hrs (bowel-cleansing dose)	Powder (oral solution)	200–500 ml qd
PEG without electrolytes	po: 2–4 days (constipation dose)	Powder (oral solution)	17 g daily in 8 fl oz
Saline			
Magnesium hydroxide	po: 30 min–3 hrs	Suspension (400 mg/5 ml)	30–60 ml daily
Magnesium citrate	po: 30 min–3 hrs	Solution (1.75 g/30 ml)	5–10 fl oz daily
Sodium phosphate	po: 30 min–3 hrs Rectal: 2–5 min	Solution Enema	20–45 ml daily 118 ml qd
Stimulant			
Bisacodyl	po: 6–10 hrs Rectal: 15–60 min	Tablets Suppositories	5–15 mg qd at bedtime 10 mg qd
Senna	po: 6–12 hrs	Tablets Liquid	8.6 g sennosides: 1 bid to 2 qid 5–15 ml daily, preferably at bedtime
Cascara	po: 6–12 hrs	Tablets Liquid	325 mg per day 5 ml per day, preferably at bedtime
Castor oil (ricinoleic acid)	po: 2–6 hrs	Liquid, emulsion	15–60 ml per day
Casanthranol (with docusate)	po: 6–12 hrs	Capsule (combined with docusate)	1–4 capsules per day

(Continued on next page)

Table 17-4. Laxative Dosage Information *(Continued)*

Type of Laxative	Route(s)/Onset of Action	Dosage Forms	Usual Dosage
Prokinetic			
Metoclopramide	po: 15–60 min	Tablets	10 mg qid
	IV: 1–3 min	Syrup	10 mg qid
	IM: 10–15 min	Solution	10 mg qid

bid—twice daily; IM—internal medicine; PEG—polyethylene glycol; po—by mouth; prn—whenever necessary; qid—four times daily; qd—each day; tid—three times a day

Note. From "Pharmacologic Treatment of Constipation in Cancer Patients," by J.G. Avila, 2004, *Cancer Control, 11,* p. 12. Copyright 2004 by the Moffitt Cancer Center. Adapted with permission.

Table 17-5. Advantages, Disadvantages, and Therapeutic Role of Commonly Used Laxative Agents

Type of Laxative	Advantages	Disadvantages	Suggested Role in Therapy
Bulk-Forming Methylcellulose Psyllium Polycarbophil	Most closely mimics the physiologic mechanism in promoting evacuation; useful in patients with colostomies	May take up to three days for effect; increased gas and bloating during initiation of therapy; potential for drug-drug interaction when coadministered with other medication; significant hydration requirement; contraindicated in patients who have obstructive symptoms or fecal impaction	Ideal as first-line agents in cases of mild or transient constipation not associated with opioid-induced constipation
Emollient Docusate	Effective stool softener, particularly in cases where painful defecation and straining need to be avoided; available in tablets or liquid formulations	Increased fluid intake requirement; increased risk of absorption of poorly absorbed drugs when given concurrently; unpleasant taste of liquid formulation	First-line agent concomitantly with stimulant laxatives in the prevention of iatrogenic constipation; beneficial when given with bulk-forming agents to reduce straining
Lubricant Mineral oil	Useful in situations of excessive straining	Chronic use may lead to malabsorption of fat-soluble vitamins; risk of possible aspiration when given orally; enhanced toxicity when given with docusate	Not routinely recommended

(Continued on next page)

Table 17-5. Advantages, Disadvantages, and Therapeutic Role of Commonly Used Laxative Agents *(Continued)*

Type of Laxative	Advantages	Disadvantages	Suggested Role in Therapy
Osmotic Lactulose Sorbitol Glycerin PEG with electrolytes PEG without electrolytes	Useful in liquefying stools to allow for defecation; sorbitol less nauseating than lactulose	May cause abdominal pain and distention shortly after ingestion; excessive bloating and colic with larger doses of lactulose; sweet taste may exacerbate underlying nausea	Second-line therapy when a stimulant laxative and stool softener do not relieve constipation
Saline Magnesium hydroxide Magnesium citrate Sodium phosphate	Fewer doses needed of magnesium formulations for effect compared to phosphate formulations; magnesium citrate available in carbonated liquid	Can produce undesirably strong purgative actions; chronic use may lead to dehydration; use with caution in patients with comorbid conditions (e.g., cardiac disease, renal insufficiency); risk of accumulation of magnesium in renal failure	Indicated when acute evacuation of the bowel is desired; third-line treatment if previous therapy is ineffective in producing evacuation
Stimulant Bisacodyl Senna Cascara Castor oil (ricinoleic acid) Casanthranol (with docusate)	Stimulate the colon to contract	Long-term use associated with development of melanosis coli, cathartic colon, and potentially cancer; discoloration of urine; may need to titrate to higher doses (multiple daily tablets) for adequate control; may cause abdominal cramping and hypokalemia	First-line (senna) for prevention of opioid-induced constipation; may be used first-line in combination with stool softener; useful in iatrogenic constipation (vincas, 5-HT$_2$ antagonists)
Prokinetic Metoclopramide	Fairly rapid onset	Adverse effects including restlessness, drowsiness; potential for development of extrapyramidal symptoms	May be beneficial in refractory cases or when first- or second-line agents not tolerated
Opioid Antagonists Naloxone	Low bioavailability, thus concentrating antagonism or opioid receptors in the GI tract; can produce laxative effect without reversing analgesic effect	May induce withdrawal symptoms	Currently being investigated to reverse opioid-induced constipation only

GI—gastrointestinal; PEG—polyethylene glycol

Note. From "Pharmacologic Treatment of Constipation in Cancer Patients," by J.G. Avila, 2004, *Cancer Control, 11,* p. 15. Copyright 2004 by the Moffitt Cancer Center. Reprinted with permission.

experiencing nausea. The high sodium content and resulting hypomagnesium associated with saline laxatives do not make this class of agents appropriate for use in older adults with cardiac disorders or renal insufficiency (Avila, 2004). Both osmotic and saline laxatives should be used as second- or third-line therapy because of their acute evacuation properties.

Stimulant Laxatives

Stimulant laxatives alter electrolyte exchange by changing the permeability of the intestinal mucosa and stimulating intestinal motility. For oral administration, the onset of action is 6–12 hours and 15–60 minutes for rectal administration (Avila, 2004). Stimulant laxatives are recommended for patients receiving constipating antineoplastic agents and narcotics.

Prokinetic Agents

Prokinetic agents facilitate gastric emptying and act within 30–60 minutes of administration. This class of agents is recommended in patients who are refractory to emollient, osmotic, or saline laxatives (Avila, 2004).

Nursing Care Issues

Constipation in the older adult is a common ailment as a result of physiologic aging changes, a decline in physical activity, and changes in dietary intake with decreased fiber and fluid intake that usually occur in this age group. Constipation can be further accentuated in the older adult with cancer as a result of the disease, cancer treatment, and pain management. In addition to treatment of constipation, greater focus of nursing care should involve prevention of constipation. Awareness of antineoplastic agents that have an increased risk of constipation will facilitate proactive treatment with stimulant laxatives that are recommended for the patient with cancer who is undergoing this type of treatment. In addition, all patients receiving narcotic analgesics should be given laxatives to prevent opioid-induced constipation.

Assessment and early detection of constipation also are critical in the older adult with cancer. Nurses should perform assessments of bowel function with each patient contact and can stress, with the older adult and caregiver, key factors to monitor and report to the healthcare provider. Patient education of dietary fiber and fluid intake, how to maintain a bowel regimen with privacy (allowing adequate time), and awareness of defecation urges will supplement pharmacologic treatment. The selection of laxative, route, and dosage must be specific for the patient with cancer experiencing constipation. For the older adult, special considerations should include comorbidities, performance status, and laxative side effects.

Areas for Future Research

Numerous research issues exist for the older adult with cancer experiencing diarrhea or constipation. Development of assessment tools is of critical need for oncology clinical nursing practice. Currently, no well-defined assessment tools are available for diarrhea or constipation, especially a brief assessment that could be used with each patient contact. These tools should specifically focus on the older adult with cancer because of the special needs for this age group.

Another critical area for nursing research is in symptom management. The older adult with cancer experiencing diarrhea and constipation possesses a multitude of other factors that should be considered in making treatment decisions. These factors may include comorbidities, prior history of diarrhea or constipation, polypharmacy, availability of social support, nutritional status, and performance status. Research specifically exploring symptom management and symptom clusters is limited in the older adult with cancer.

In addition to nursing research issues related to the older adult with cancer experiencing diarrhea and constipation, healthcare professionals are exploring treatment options based on a better understanding of the pathophysiology and the enteric nervous system (Schiller, 2004). Phase III trials currently are under way evaluating prokinetic agents that stimulate the 5-HT_4 receptors, enhancing the peristaltic reflex, and peripheral opiate antagonists that do not affect the opiate receptors in the central nervous system. Further research and development are needed with these new agents, although possibilities exist for use in the older adult with bowel alterations in the oncology setting.

Conclusion

Diarrhea and constipation in the older adult with cancer can cause significant morbidity and mortality in addition to poor QOL. Nurses play a key role in patient assessment and education and can have a direct impact on patient care and prompt treatment. In the older adult with cancer, a team approach by members of the healthcare team with the patient and caregivers is essential. Ultimately, the overall goal should be prevention of diarrhea and constipation for the older adult to avoid life-threatening complications.

References

Arbuckle, R.B., Huber, S.L., & Zacker, C. (2000). The consequences of diarrhea occurring during chemotherapy for colorectal cancer: A retrospective study. *Oncologist, 5,* 250–259.

Avila, J.G. (2004). Pharmacologic treatment of constipation in cancer patients. *Cancer Control, 11,* 10–18.

Baillie-Johnson, H.R. (1996). Octreotide in the management of treatment-related diarrhea. *Anticancer Drugs, 7*(Suppl. 1), 11–15.

Barbounis, V., Koumakis, G., Vassilomanolakis, M., Demiri, M., & Efremidis, A.P. (2001). Control of irinotecan-induced diarrhea by octreotide after loperamide failure. *Supportive Care in Cancer, 9,* 258–260.

Benson, A.B., Ajani, J.A., Catalano, R.B., Engelking, C., Kornblau, S.M., Martenson, J.A., et al. (2004). Recommended guidelines for the treatment of cancer treatment-induced diarrhea. *Journal of Clinical Oncology, 22,* 2918–2926.

Bosshard, W., Dreher, R., Schnegg, J.F., & Bula, C.J. (2004). The treatment of chronic constipation in elderly people: An update. *Drugs and Aging, 21,* 911–930.

Cancerconsultants.com. (1998–2004). *Chemotherapy induced diarrhea.* Retrieved December 27, 2004, from http://www.cancerconsultants.com

Conti, J.A., Kemeny, N.E., Saltz, L.B., Huang, Y., Tong, W.P., Chou, T.C., et al. (1996). Irinotecan is an active agent in untreated patients with metastatic colorectal cancer. *Journal of Clinical Oncology, 14,* 709–715.

Cope, D. (2001). Management of chemotherapy-induced diarrhea and constipation. *Nursing Clinics of North America, 36,* 695–707.

Cunningham, D., Pyrhonen, S., James, R.D., Punt, C.J., Hickish, T.F., Heikkila, R., et al. (1998). Randomised trial of irinotecan plus supportive care versus supportive care alone after fluorouracil failure for patients with metastatic colorectal cancer. *Lancet, 352,* 1413–1418.

Engelking, C. (2004). Diarrhea. In C.H. Yarbro, M.H. Frogge, & M. Goodman (Eds.), *Cancer symptom management* (3rd ed., pp. 528–558). Sudbury, MA: Jones and Bartlett.

Fuessl, H.S., Carolan, G., Williams, G., & Bloom, S.R. (1987). Effect of a long-acting somatostatin analogue (SMS 201-995) on postprandial gastric emptying of 99mTc-tin colloid and mouth-to-cecum transit time in man. *Digestion, 36,* 101–107.

Giantonio, G.J., Catalano, P.J., Meropol, N.J., O'Dwyer, P.J., & Benson, A.B. (2004). *The addition of bevacizumab (anti-VEGF) to FOLFOX4 in previously treated advanced colorectal cancer (advCRC): An updated interim toxicity analysis of the Eastern Cooperative Oncology Group (ECOG) study E3200* [Abstract 241]. Retrieved December 27, 2004, from http://www.asco.org

Gwede, C.K. (2003). Overview of radiation- and chemoradiation-induced diarrhea. *Seminars in Oncology Nursing, 19*(4 Suppl. 3), 6–10.

Hawkins, R.A. (2000). Constipation. In D. Camp-Sorrell & R. Hawkins (Eds.), *Clinical manual for the oncology advanced practice nurse* (pp. 339–342). Pittsburgh, PA: Oncology Nursing Society.

Hogan, C.M. (1998). The nurse's role in diarrhea management. *Oncology Nursing Forum, 25,* 879–886.

Hurwitz, H., Fehrenbacher, L., Cartwright, T., Hainsworth, J., Heim, W., Berlin, J., et al. (2004). Bevacizumab plus irinotecan, fluorouracil, leucovorin for metastatic colorectal cancer. *New England Journal of Medicine, 350,* 2335–2342.

Ito, Y., Mukaiyama, T., Ogawa, M., Mizunuma, N., Takahashi, S., Aiba, K., et al. (1999). Epirubicin-containing high-dose chemotherapy followed by autologous hematopoietic progenitor cell transfusion for patients with chemotherapy sensitive metastatic breast cancer: Results of 5-year follow-up. *Cancer Chemotherapy and Pharmacology, 43,* 8–12.

Kornblau, S., Benson, A.B., Catalano, R., Champlin, R.E., Engelking, C., Field, M., et al. (2000). Management of cancer treatment-related diarrhea. Issues and therapeutic strategies. *Journal of Pain and Symptom Management, 19,* 118–129.

Leichman, C.G., Fleming, T.R., Muggia, F.M., Tangen, C.M., Ardalan, B., Doroshow, J.H., et al. (1995). Phase II study of fluorouracil and its modulation in advanced colorectal cancer: A Southwestern Oncology Group study. *Journal of Clinical Oncology, 13,* 1303–1311.

McMillan, S.C. (2002). Presence and severity of constipation in hospice patients with advanced cancer. *American Journal of Hospice and Palliative Care, 14,* 190–195.

McMillan, S.C. (2004). Assessing and managing opiate-induced constipation in adults with cancer. *Cancer Control, 11*(Suppl. 3), S3–S9.

McMillan, S.C., & Tittle, M. (1995). A descriptive study of the management of pain and pain-related side effects in a cancer center and a hospice. *Hospital Journal, 10,* 89–108.

McMillan, S.C., & Weitzner, M. (2000). How problematic are various aspects of quality of life in patients with cancer at the end of life? *Oncology Nursing Forum, 27,* 817–825.

McMillan, S.C., & Williams, F.A. (1989). Validity and reliability of the constipation assessment scale. *Cancer Nursing, 12,* 183–188.

Miller, R.C., Sargent, D.J., Martenson, J.A., Macdonald, J.S., Haller, D., Mayer, R.J., et al. (2002). Acute diarrhea during adjuvant therapy for rectal cancer: A detailed analysis from a randomized intergroup trial. *International Journal of Radiation Oncology, Biology, Physics, 54,* 409–413.

National Cancer Institute. (2004). *Gastrointestinal complications.* Retrieved December 20, 2004, from http://www.cancer.gov/cancertopics/pdq/supportivecare/gastrointestinalcomplications/healthprofessional

O'Connell, M.J., Martenson, J.A., Wieand, H.S., Krock, J.E., Macdonald, J.S., Haller, D.G., et al. (1994). Improving adjuvant therapy for rectal cancer by combining protracted-infusion fluorouracil with radiation therapy after curative surgery. *New England Journal of Medicine, 331,* 502–507.

Petrelli, N., Douglas, H.O., Jr., Herrera, L., Russell, D., Stablein, D.M., Bruckner, H.W., et al. (1989). The modulation of fluorouracil with leucovorin in metastatic colorectal carcinoma: A prospective randomized phase III trial. Gastrointestinal Tumor Study Group. *Journal of Clinical Oncology, 7,* 1419–1426.

Rothenberg, M.L., Eckardt, J.R., Kuhn, J.G., Burris, H.A., Nelson, J., Hilsenbeck, S.G., et al. (1996). Phase II trial of irinotecan inpatients with progressive or rapidly recurrent colorectal cancer. *Journal of Clinical Oncology, 14,* 1128–1135.

Rothenberg, M.L., Meropol, N.J., Poplin, E.A., Van Cutsem, E., & Wadler, S. (2001). Mortality associated with irinotecan plus bolus fluorouracil/leucovorin: Summary findings of an independent panel. *Journal of Clinical Oncology, 19,* 3801–3807.

Rutledge, D.N., & Engelking, C. (1998). Cancer-related diarrhea: Selected findings of a national survey of oncology nurse experiences. *Oncology Nursing Forum, 25,* 861–873.

Sanofi Aventis. (2002). Eloxatin [Package insert]. New York: Author.

Sargent, D.J., Goldberg, R.M., Jacobson, S.D., Macdonald, J.S., Labianca, R., Haller, D.G., et al. (2001). A pooled analysis of adjuvant chemotherapy for resected colon cancer in elderly patients. *New England Journal of Medicine, 345,* 1091–1097.

Schaefer, D.C., & Cheskin, L.J. (1998). Constipation in the elderly. *American Family Physician, 58,* 907–914.

Scheithauer, W., Kornek, G.V., Raderer, M., Schull, B., Schmid, K., Langle, F., et al. (2002). Intermittent weekly high-dose capecitabine in combination with oxaliplatin: A phase I/II study in first-line treatment of patients with advanced colorectal cancer. *Annals of Oncology, 13,* 1583–1589.

Schiller, L.A. (2004). New and emerging treatment options for chronic constipation. *Reviews in Gastroenterological Disorders, 4*(Suppl. 2), S43–S51.

Tittle, M., & McMillan, S.C. (1994). Pain and pain-related side effects in an ICU and on a surgical unit: Nurses' management. *American Journal of Critical Care, 3,* 25–30.

Tepper, J.E., O'Connell, M.J., Petroni, G.R., Hollis, D., Cooke, E., Benson, A.B., et al. (1997). Adjuvant post-operative fluorouracil-modulated chemotherapy combined with pelvic radiation therapy for rectal cancer: Initial results of intergroup 0114. *Journal of Clinical Oncology, 15,* 2030–2039.

U.S. Census Bureau. (1996). *Population projections of the United States by age, sex, race, and Hispanic origin: 1995 to 2050.* Washington, DC: U.S. Government Printing Office. Retrieved October 15, 2004, from http://www.census.gov/prod/1/pop/p25-1130/p251130a.pdf

Van Cutsem, E., Pozzo, C., Starkhammar, H., Dirix, L., Terzoli, E., & Cognetti, F. (1998). A phase II study of irinotecan alternated with five days of bolus of 5-fluorouracil and leucovorin in first-line chemotherapy of metastatic colorectal cancer. *Annals of Oncology, 9,* 1199–1204.

Wadler, S., Benson, A.B., Engelking, C., Catalano, R., Field, M., Kornblau, S.M., et al. (1998). Recommended guidelines for the treatment of chemotherapy-induced diarrhea. *Journal of Clinical Oncology, 16,* 3169–3178.

Wadler, S., Haynes, H., & Wiernik, P.H. (1995). Phase I trial of the somatostatin analog octreotide acetate in the treatment of fluoropyrimidine-induced diarrhea. *Journal of Clinical Oncology, 13,* 222–226.

Weitzner, M.A., Moody, L.N., & McMillan, S.C. (1997). Symptom management issues in hospice care. *American Journal of Hospice and Palliative Care, 14,* 190–195.

Yancik, R., & Ries, L.A. (2000). Aging and cancer in America: Demographic and epidemiologic perspectives. *Hematology/Oncology Clinics of North America, 14,* 17–23.

Yavuz, M.N., Yavuz, A.A., Aydin, F., Can, G., & Kavgaci, H. (2002). The efficacy of octreotide in the therapy of acute radiation-induced diarrhea: A randomized controlled study. *International Journal of Radiation Oncology, Biology, Physics, 54,* 195–202.

CHAPTER 18

Nutritional Care of the Older Adult With Cancer

Ronni Chernoff, PhD, RD

Introduction

Epidemiologic evidence supports the belief that cancer is a chronic condition of older people. Cancer could possibly be more prevalent in older adults because of the length of time (often 20 years or longer) it takes for cancer to develop after exposure to carcinogens, because the immune system is less efficient in old age, or because people are living longer because of advances in medical care, new drugs, and better treatment of other chronic disease (Chernoff & Ropka, 1988; Dreosti, 1998). This chapter will address diet and nutritional factors as they relate to the development of cancer as well as when the older adult with cancer has been diagnosed and is undergoing treatment.

Diet as a Cancer Etiology

Diet may be one of the most common contributing factors in the development of cancer. However, most studies of diet and cancer etiology are epidemiologic in nature, and very small differences in disease incidence yield highly significant effects with small interventions. Because cancer develops after many years of exposure, it is hard to link specific dietary components to disease development in later life. Diet, dietary patterns, and method of food preparation long have been linked to increased risk for various cancers. Although these factors introduce an enormous variety of variables, investigators have tended to focus on one factor at a time, thereby leading to discrepancies among research reports on the role of nutrition and cancer etiology (Rennert, 2003). One of the recent theories concerning cancer prevention is caloric restriction in early life. In animal species, caloric restriction in postweaning early life has been shown to prolong life and reduce the risk for cancer in later life. The applicability of this theory from animal models to humans is challenging but is being investigated (Frame, Hart, & Leakey, 1998; Hursting, Lavigne, Berrigan, Perkins, & Barrett, 2003).

Nutritional factors that have been linked with cancer etiology for breast, colon, and prostate cancers include high levels of dietary fat, inadequate dietary fiber, and obesity (Adderly-Kelly & Williams-Stephens, 2003; Asano & McLeod, 2002), although new evidence suggests that the link between diet and cancer may not be that compelling (Kushi & Giovannucci, 2002), and studies found that physical activity and weight control may be more important (Chlebowski, Aiello, & McTiernan, 2002; Moyad, 2002).

Conversely, high dietary intake levels of fruits and vegetables that are rich in beta-carotene, vitamin A, vitamin C, and antioxidant vitamins (Lee, Lee, Surh, & Lee, 2003; Riboli & Norat, 2003) have been linked to a reduction in cancer risk (Willet, 2003), particularly for epithelial cancers. However, in a review of reported studies, many confounding variables and challenges about the role of specific fruits and vegetables in anticancer actions are valid and reliable (Temple & Gladwin, 2002). Additionally, the interactions among micronutrients found in food may be the key to whether specific foods have anticancer properties (Temple & Gladwin).

Breast, colon, and prostate cancers are the most common among adults older than 75 years of age, so addressing the dietary risk issues in earlier life is an important health promotion message. Many new investigations are emerging that divert attention from epidemiologic dietary studies and offer promising new avenues for understanding what initiates abnormal cell growth leading to cancer. These include recent evidence of genetic triggers and genetic controls over cell growth cycles and elucidation of pathways that regulate cell growth and development (Milner, 2002).

Effects of Cancer on Nutritional Status

By the time cancer is diagnosed in older adults, their nutritional status may be compromised by a multitude of chronic diseases, including diabetes, cardiovascular disease, stroke, chronic obstructive pulmonary disease, hepatic or renal disease, gastrointestinal problems, or bone and joint disease. Compounding the effects of chronic disease for older adults are financial problems, disabilities, oral health challenges, social isolation, or restricted mobility.

For older adults, the ability to procure, prepare, and consume an adequate diet may confound the risks for poor nutrition associated with cancer. Many older adults have asymptomatic chronic undernutrition that becomes obvious when a physiologic challenge associated with an acute illness is introduced. Reserve capacity (the concept that, when challenged by a physiologic insult, the human body will respond rapidly with an appropriate response by mobilizing substrate to fight infection, make new tissue, heal wounds, or repair fractures) may be seriously compromised in chronically ill older adults (Bozzetti, 2003). The presence of cancer is a significant burden on the human body and may push older adults to a state of malnutrition (Guenter, Ferguson, Thrush, & Voss, 2002).

Weight loss may occur because of the hypermetabolic effects of cancer and the physiologic burden associated with cancer treatments. Both cachexia and anorexia are associated with the presence of cancer and cancer treatment. Cachexia is a syndrome that combines loss of appetite, weight loss, muscle wasting, early satiety, and alterations in energy metabolism (Inui, 2002; Strasser & Bruera, 2002). Loss of appetite and anorexia may occur for many reasons, including emotional stress, pain, discomfort, and treatment side effects (e.g., nausea, vomiting, enteritis, other gastrointestinal symptoms) (Laviano, Meguid, & Rossi-Fanelli, 2003). In older adults who may have a compromised reserve capacity, both cachexia and anorexia will lead to malnutrition that may be difficult to reverse (Lelli et al., 2003).

In addition to anorexia, another impediment to the maintenance of nutritional status may be the obstructive interference of a solid tumor that may occur with tumors of the esophagus, stomach, or small or large bowel (Echenique & Correia, 2003; Gupta & Ihmaidat, 2003). Head and neck cancers may interfere with chewing or swallowing, necessitating a change in food texture, food temperature, or type of food consumed. Patients who have head and neck cancer frequently alter their diet so that they are only consuming small volumes of liquids.

Surgery on the gastrointestinal tract (from mouth to anus) may lead to loss of access to normal absorptive surfaces and may necessitate alternative feeding options. Postsurgical complications may include the development of adhesions in the gastrointestinal tract that may cause pain and obstruction. Surgery also will increase nutritional demands for healing and fighting infection.

Radiation therapy directed toward the gastrointestinal tract or to nearby tissue may cause serious enteritis or damage. Damaged tissue may leak serous fluids and create a nutritional deficit of lost protein. The effects of radiation therapy may occur years after the cancer has been treated when damaged tissue becomes friable, breaks down, and fistulas form. The result may be malabsorption of needed nutrients, and a loss of fluids and electrolytes is associated with damaged tissues with damaged cell membranes that are unable to perform their function. In older adult patients with cancer, this may be particularly risky because these individuals may not have the intact mechanisms to compensate. Older adults lose thirst sensitivity and will be less efficient at replenishing fluids, thereby potentially becoming dehydrated. Dehydration is a consequence of altered drug distribution, and dehydrated individuals may be getting concentrated doses of medication because the drug is not appropriately distributed or flushed through excretory organs, such as the kidney.

Chemotherapy may cause serious nutritional consequences because of its administration method (oral or IV) and, therefore, is systemic and generally toxic. Although older adults withstand aggressive chemotherapy, they must be carefully monitored to maintain hydration and prevent excess loss of lean body mass. As people get older, a decrease in total lean body mass and total body water occurs. Protein mass loss may become difficult to reverse, compromise organ function, and contribute to a decrease or concentration of chemotherapeutic drug distribution leading to increased toxicity. Often, drug dosages are calculated according to body weight so that changes in weight may affect the protocol for treatment.

In addition to nausea, vomiting, diarrhea, anorexia, and edema, the most common side effects of chemotherapeutic agents are changes in saliva production, taste perception, mucosal lesions such as mouth sores, and infections. Symptoms may be both site specific and unique among individuals. Nevertheless, overcoming these symptoms often requires higher levels of nutrients, particularly protein, which are needed to heal faster, fight infections, and provide nutritional substrate for normal body function.

Supporting Nutrition for Older Adult Patients With Cancer

Malnutrition is prevalent in patients with cancer because of the impact of the disease as well as the side effects of treatment protocols. Poor nutritional status can interfere with planned therapies by reducing response to therapy, increasing hospital stays, causing a poorer quality of life, and reducing survival rates (Holder, 2003). Nutrition interventions for older adults with cancer must be planned when the diagnosis is made and be started early in the treatment protocol. If nutrition interventions are delayed until 10% or more of body weight is lost, extraordinary measures may be required to prevent further loss or eventually restore nutritional status. The first option in nutrition planning should be to maximize oral intake.

Developing a nutrition strategy for older adults requires an assessment of nutritional status at the time of diagnosis to identify obvious deficits; to establish baseline information; to assess oral health status, including dentition, dentures, and swallowing capability; to review chronic conditions and associated medications and dietary modifications; and to evaluate socioeconomic and cognition status. Although no specific laboratory studies are recommended, serum albumin commonly is used, although not the most sensitive, to facilitate malnutrition assessment. Patients may be malnourished before their serum albumin level is low because albumin has a half-life of 20 days (Sargent, Murphy, & Shelton, 2002). Lower serum albumin levels may contribute to decreased immune function and poor wound healing (Sargent et al.). The National Comprehensive Cancer Network's (2005) senior adult oncology guidelines recommend the use of the Mini Nutritional Assessment. This screening test is sensitive in older adults and can be completed in less than 20 minutes (Guigoz, Vellas, & Garry, 1996). Direct discussions with patients and their caregivers are the best way to obtain needed information. Full knowledge of treatment protocols will help clinicians to plan for anticipated consequences of the treatment and how these will affect nutritional intake and how best to provide early intervention.

Feeding suggestions for patients who experience the more common side effects of cancer therapy are included in Figure 18-1.

Nausea/Vomiting
- Eat crackers or dry toast.
- Eat small, frequent meals.
- Eat slowly.
- Consume light, bland foods.
- Cold foods may be more appealing.
- Avoid foods with strong odors.
- Intake calorie-dense liquids throughout the day.
- Intake fluids through periods of nausea/vomiting, even in small amounts.
- Eat tart or sour foods unless mouth sores are present.

Anorexia
- Eat small, frequent meals and snacks.
- Keep snacks readily available.
- Try alternate meal patterns (e.g., breakfast foods for dinner).
- Add calories to foods whenever possible, but be careful of added milk if diarrhea is present.
- Use strong flavorings or seasonings.
- Try a variety of foods, including ones different in temperature, texture, and color.

Figure 18-1. Feeding Suggestions for Common Cancer Treatment Effects

When modifying diets for older adult patients with cancer, involve them in the process to get a good sense of what they like and what they may eat when they are not feeling well. Older adults have well-defined food preferences, and it may be easier to achieve success with dietary changes if they are involved in the planning process. Serious illness is associated with a loss of control over one's own body, medical decisions, and outcomes, so encouraging participation in menu or meal planning gives back some feeling of control to older adult patients.

If oral feeding is not adequate to meet the patient's needs, oral liquid supplements may be used as between-meal feedings. Encouraging dietary intake of nutrient-dense foods should not be abandoned in favor of liquid supplements if at all possible. When consuming oral nutrients becomes too stressful or not possible, enteral feeding is an option (Barrera, 2002). It provides access to the gastrointestinal tract, whether by nasogastric or gastrostomy tube, to ensure infusion of essential nutrients and fluids (Arbogast, 2002; Chandu, Smith, & Douglas, 2003; Schattner, 2003). This option also may decrease the pressure to eat and relieve the anxiety of not eating and making the condition worse.

If surgery, radiation, or chemotherapy has damaged the gastrointestinal tract and enteral feeding is not a good choice, parenteral nutrition may be considered. Peripheral parenteral feeding may be a good choice for short-term intervention; total parenteral nutrition may be selected when no other options are available but should be carefully considered in older adults (Sargent et al., 2002). Older adults may not be able to efficiently metabolize hypertonic glucose solutions and may not be proficient at clearing IV-infused lipid emulsions. Parenteral support must be managed carefully in older adults. Projections as to the length of time the nutrition intervention will be needed should be factored into the methodology selection.

Conclusion

Cancer is a common chronic condition in older adults because of the length of time it takes for most cancers to develop. Healthcare professionals can successfully and aggressively meet the nutritional needs of older adults with cancer by carefully considering other chronic conditions frequently seen in older adults and by accommodating physiologic changes associated with advanced age. Nutrition interventions should be assessed and planned early in the diagnosis and treatment decision stages. If older adult patients with cancer are recognized as unique and special and are cared for accordingly, achieving success in nutritional support is possible.

References

Adderly-Kelly, B., & Williams-Stephens, E. (2003). The relationship between obesity and breast cancer. *Journal of the Association of Black Nursing Faculty in Higher Education, 14*(3), 61–65.

Arbogast, D. (2002). Enteral feedings with comfort and safety. *Clinical Journal of Oncology Nursing, 6,* 275–280.

Asano, T., & McLeod, R.S. (2002). Dietary fiber for the prevention of colorectal adenomas and carcinomas. *Cochrane Database Systems Review, 2,* CD003430.

Barrera, R. (2002). Nutritional support in cancer patients. *Journal of Parenteral and Enteral Nutrition, 26*(Suppl. 5), S63–S71.

Bozzetti, F. (2003). Nutritional issues in the care of the elderly patient. *Critical Reviews in Oncology/Hematology, 48,* 113–121.

Chandu, A., Smith, A.C., & Douglas, M. (2003). Percutaneous endoscopic gastrostomy in patients undergoing resection for oral tumors: A retrospective review of complications and outcomes. *Journal of Oral and Maxillofacial Surgery, 61,* 1279–1284.

Chernoff, R., & Ropka, M. (1988). The unique nutritional needs of the elderly patient with cancer. *Seminars in Oncology Nursing, 4,* 189–197.

Chlebowski, R.T., Aiello, E., & McTiernan, A. (2002). Weight loss in breast cancer patient management. *Journal of Clinical Oncology, 20,* 1128–1143.

Dreosti, I.E. (1998). Nutrition, cancer, and aging. *Annals of the New York Academy of Sciences, 854,* 371–377.

Echenique, M., & Correia, M.I. (2003). Nutrition in advanced digestive cancer. *Current Opinion in Clinical Nutrition and Metabolic Care, 6,* 577–580.

Frame, L.T., Hart, R.W., & Leakey, J.E. (1998). Caloric restrictions as a mechanism mediating resistance to environmental disease. *Environmental Health Perspectives, 106*(Suppl. 1), 313–324.

Guenter, P., Ferguson, M., Thrush, K., & Voss, A.C. (2002). Understanding tumor-induced weight loss. *Medsurg Nursing, 11*(5), 215–225.

Guigoz, Y., Vellas, B., & Garry, P.J. (1996). Assessing the nutritional status of the elderly: The Mini Nutritional Assessment as part of the geriatric evaluation. *Nutrition Review, 54*(1 Pt. 2), S59–S65.

Gupta, R., & Ihmaidat, H. (2003). Nutritional effects of oesophageal, gastric and pancreatic carcinoma. *European Journal of Surgical Oncology, 29,* 634–643.

Holder, H. (2003). Nursing management of nutrition in cancer and palliative care. *British Journal of Nursing, 12,* 667–668, 670, 672–674.

Hursting, S.D., Lavigne, J.A., Berrigan, D., Perkins, S.N., & Barrett, J.C. (2003). Calorie restriction, aging, and cancer prevention: Mechanisms of action and applicability to humans. *Annual Review of Medicine, 54,* 131–152.

Inui, A. (2002). Cancer anorexia-cachexia syndrome: Current issues in research and management. *CA: A Cancer Journal for Clinicians, 52,* 72–91.

Kushi, L., & Giovannucci, E. (2002). Dietary fat and cancer. *American Journal of Medicine, 113*(Suppl. 9B), 63S–70S.

Laviano, A., Meguid, M.M., & Rossi-Fanelli, F. (2003). Improving food intake in anorectic cancer patients. *Current Opinion in Clinical Nutrition and Metabolic Care, 6,* 421–426.

Lee, K.W., Lee, H.J., Surh, Y.J., & Lee, C.Y. (2003). Vitamin C and cancer chemoprevention: Reappraisal. *American Journal of Clinical Nutrition, 78,* 1074–1078.

Lelli, G., Montanari, M., Gilli, G., Scapoli, D., Antonietti, C., & Scapoli, D. (2003). Treatment of cancer anorexia-cachexia syndrome: A critical reappraisal. *Journal of Chemotherapy, 15,* 220–225.

Milner, J.A. (2002). Strategies for cancer prevention: The role of the diet. *British Journal of Nutrition, 87*(Suppl. 2), S265–S272.

Moyad, M.A. (2002). Is obesity a risk factor for prostate cancer, and does it even matter? A hypothesis and different perspective. *Urology, 59*(Suppl. 4), 41–50.

National Comprehensive Cancer Network. (2005). *Clinical practice guidelines in oncology: Senior adult oncology.* Retrieved September 22, 2005, from http://www.nccn.org/professionals/physician_gls/PDF/senior.pdf

Rennert, G. (2003). Diet and cancer: Where are we and where are we going? *Proceedings of the Nutrition Society, 62*(1), 59–62.

Riboli, E., & Norat, T. (2003). Epidemiologic evidence of the protective effect of fruit and vegetables on cancer risk. *American Journal of Clinical Nutrition, 78*(Suppl. 3), 559S–569S.

Sargent, C., Murphy, D., & Shelton, B.K. (2002). Nutrition in critical care. *Clinical Journal of Oncology Nursing, 6,* 287–289.

Schattner, M. (2003). Enteral nutritional support of the patient with cancer: Route and role. *Journal of Clinical Gastroenterology, 36,* 297–302.

Strasser, F., & Bruera, E.D. (2002). Update on anorexia and cachexia. *Hematology/Oncology Clinics of North America, 16,* 589–617.

Temple, N.J., & Gladwin, K.K. (2002). Fruit, vegetable, and the prevention of cancer: Research challenges. *Nutrition, 19,* 467–470.

Willet, W. (2003). Lessons from dietary studies in Adventists and questions for the future. *American Journal of Clinical Nutrition, 78*(Suppl. 3), 539S–543S.

CHAPTER 19

Symptom Management of Pain

Nessa M. Coyle, PhD, NP, FAAN, and
Susan Derby, MA, CGNP, ACHPN

Introduction

Severe and uncontrolled pain is one of the most feared consequences of cancer, especially at the end of life (Coyle, 1995; Ferrell & Whiteman, 2003; Foley, 1991; Ng & von Gunten, 1998). For a variety of reasons, older adults have been identified as an "at risk group" for poorly managed or undertreated pain (Bernabei et al., 1998; Cleeland, Gonin, Baez, Loehrer, & Pandya, 1997; Feldt, Ryden, & Miles, 1998; Ferrell & Whiteman; Fine, 2001, 2004; Morrison & Sui, 2000). The intent of this chapter is to provide the oncology nurse with basic information on the prevalence of pain in the older patient with cancer, its pathophysiology, clinical assessment, barriers that prevent good pain management, and pharmacologic treatments used to provide pain relief. The reader is referred to other texts for in-depth discussion of nondrug measures for the management of pain in the older adult.

Although this chapter is focusing on one symptom—pain—pain management in the older person living with cancer is part of a more comprehensive approach—palliative care. Palliative care is not just end-of-life care but "is an approach to care which improves quality of life of patients and their families facing life threatening illness, through the prevention, assessment, and treatment of pain and other problems, physical, psychological and spiritual" (World Health Organization [WHO], 2002). The National Comprehensive Cancer Network (NCCN) has developed guidelines to facilitate the "appropriate integration of palliative care into anticancer therapy" (NCCN, 2004). This group also has developed guidelines for the management of cancer pain (NCCN). In addition, the American Geriatrics Society (2002) has developed clinical practice guidelines for the management of persistent pain in older adults.

Prevalence of Pain in the Older Adult With Cancer

Whether pain sensitivity changes across the life span is unclear, although some suggest that overall pain perception does not change much (Ferrell, B.A., 1996; Gibson & Helme, 2001). Significant pain in older adults living in the community varies from 25%–56% (Helme & Gibson, 2000), whereas pain experienced by those living in nursing homes is reported at being between 45%–80% (Ferrell, 1995). Arthritis and other muscular skeletal disorders are the most common causes of pain in this age group (Ferrell & Whiteman, 2003). A number of studies have suggested that pain often is under-recognized and undertreated in the older population as well as in women and minorities (Cleeland et al., 1994, 1997). Among the most vulnerable in this group are those with cancer pain in nursing homes (Bernabei et al., 1998), the cognitively impaired (Feldt et al., 1998; Morrison & Sui, 2000), those with postoperative pain (Feldt et al.; Morrison & Sui), and those with a history of substance abuse or major psychiatric disorders (Ferrell & Whiteman) (see Figure 19-1). Unrelieved pain affects every aspect of an older adult's quality of life; it is never benign (see Figure 19-2).

In general, approximately one-third of people who are receiving active therapy for their cancer and two-thirds of those with advanced disease experience pain (Meuser et al., 2001; Morita, Ichiki, Tsunoda, Inoue, & Chihara, 1998; Wells, 2000). The type of cancer, stage of cancer, site(s) of metastatic spread, and other factors influence the prevalence of pain. Cancer pain coexists with other symptoms and frequently occurs

---

- Those in long-term care facilities
- Those who are 85 years old and older
- Those with severe cognitive impairment
- Those with postoperative pain
- Those with chronic pain being cared for in a setting where the staff is only familiar with acute pain presentation
- Those with a history of substance abuse or a major psychiatric disorder
- Those whose language and form of communication is not understood
- Those who are minorities or are culturally "different"

Figure 19-1. Older Patients With Cancer Most at Risk for Under-Recognition and Undertreatment of Pain

Note. Based on information from Bernabei et al., 1998; Cleeland et al., 1997; Feldt et al., 1998; Ferrell, B.A., 1996; Ferrell & Whiteman, 2003; Ferrell, B.R., et al., 1991; Fine, 2001, 2004; Miaskowski, 2000; Morrison & Sui, 2000.

- Depression
- Decreased socialization
- Sleep disturbances
- Impaired ambulation and overall function
- Increased burden on caregivers
- Loss of hope and desire for death
- Increased healthcare utilization and costs

Figure 19-2. Consequences of Unrelieved Pain in the Older Adult With Cancer

Note. Based on information from Cherny & Coyle, 1994, 1999; Cherny & Portenoy, 1994a; Coyle, 1995; Foley, 1991; Saunders, 1967; Stiefel, 1993.

as part of a "symptom cluster" (Miaskowski, 2002; National Institutes of Health, 2002; Portenoy et al., 1994). Pain can cause or exacerbate other non–pain-related symptoms (e.g., insomnia, depression). Pain assessment and management in the older adult is made more difficult because these individuals frequently under-report their pain (Ferrell, B.A., 1996; Ferrell, B.R., 1996; Miaskowski, 2000) and present with concurrent medical illnesses, multiple problems, and a variety of painful muscular skeletal disorders unrelated to the cancer or its treatment. In addition, older individuals have a higher incidence of cognitive impairment, hearing and visual deficits, and medication side effects than a younger age group (Ferrell & Whiteman, 2003). Despite these challenges, most pain in the older adult with cancer can be managed.

Pathophysiology of Pain in the Older Adult

The older adult has multiple potential sources of pain unrelated to cancer or its treatment. In general, as previously mentioned, the most common causes of pain in this age group are those related to musculoskeletal disorders such as back pain, arthritis, or other degenerative diseases. Neuralgia or neuropathic pain also is common, stemming from such diseases as diabetes and herpes zoster. Nighttime leg cramps or restless legs also can be a source of distress in the older adult (Ferrell & Whiteman, 2003). Pain associated with cancer and its treatment may be superimposed on these underlying chronic pain states, making management in the older population more complex and underscoring the importance of a comprehensive pain history (Helme & Gibson, 2000; Herr & Mobily, 1991). A growing understanding of the pathophysiology of cancer pain has helped to target pain management strategies more effectively.

Types of Pain

Two major types or classifications of pain, *nociceptive pain* (including somatic, visceral pain) and *neuropathic pain,* have been described in patients with cancer based on their inferred neurophysiologic mechanisms (Payne & Gonzales, 2004) (see Figure 19-3). Understanding these basic mechanisms of pain is a necessary background for the nurse to arrive at a reasoned analgesic pain management approach for the patient.

Somatic or nociceptive pain occurs as a result of activating pain-sensitive structures or nociceptors in the cutaneous and deep muscular skeletal structures. The pain typically is well localized and may be felt in the superficial cutaneous or deeper musculoskeletal structures. Examples of somatic pain include bone metastases, postsurgical incisional pain, and pain accompanying myofascial or musculoskeletal inflammation or spasm (Payne & Gonzales, 2004). Somatic pain is responsive to nonsteroidal anti-inflammatory drugs (NSAIDs), opioid drugs, and steroids.

Visceral pain results from infiltration, compression, or stretching of thoracic or abdominal viscera (e.g., liver metastases, pancreatic cancer). This type of pain is poorly localized, often described as deep, squeezing, pressure, and may be associated with nausea, vomiting, and diaphoresis (especially when acute). Visceral pain often refers to cutaneous sites, which may be remote from the site of the lesion (e.g., shoulder pain associated with diaphragmatic irritation). Tenderness and pain on touching the referral cutaneous site may occur. Visceral pain is responsive to NSAIDs and to opioid drugs (Payne & Gonzales, 2004).

- Nociceptive pain
  - Somatic (injury to cutaneous or deep tissue, may be acute or chronic; typically well localized, described as aching or throbbing)
  - Visceral (originates from stretching or distention of thoracic or abdominal viscera; poorly localized and can be referred to distant cutaneous sites; described as cramping, deep aching, squeezing pressure)
- Neuropathic pain
  - Occurs after injury to the peripheral or central nervous system (described as sharp, shooting, electric shock–like, aching, burning)
- Psychological pain (suffering and existential distress)
- Mixed pain syndromes

Figure 19-3. Classification of Pain—Inferred Pain Mechanism

Note. Based on information from American Pain Society, 2003; Foley, 2004; Hanks et al., 2004; Payne & Gonzales, 2004.

Neuropathic pain results from injury to the peripheral and/or central nervous system (CNS). In the patient with cancer, neuropathic pain most commonly occurs as a consequence of a tumor compressing or infiltrating peripheral nerves, nerve roots, or the spinal cord. In addition, surgical trauma, chemical- or radiation-induced injury to peripheral nerves or the spinal cord from cancer therapies, may result in this type of pain. Examples of common neuropathic pain include plexopathies, epidural spinal cord and/or cauda-equina compression, postherpetic neuralgia, and painful chemotherapy-induced neuropathy.

Neuropathic pain often is described as having sharp, shooting, electric shock-like qualities that are unfamiliar to the patient. The pain also can be described as a constant dull ache, sometimes with a pressure or vice-like quality, with episodic paroxysms of burning and/or electric shock–like sensations. Neuropathic pain often is severe, very distressing to the patient, and sometimes difficult to control. Although partially responsive to NSAIDs and to opioid drugs (higher doses often are needed), neuropathic pain also is responsive to adjuvant drugs, such as anticonvulsants, antidepressants, local anesthetics, and steroids (Foley, 2004).

Temporal Pattern of Pain

Pain also can be defined on a temporal basis (e.g., acute pain, chronic pain, breakthrough pain). The older patient with cancer frequently has a combination of all three types of pain (see Figure 19-4).

Acute pain is characterized by a well-defined pattern of onset. Generally, the cause of pain can be identified, and, frequently, the pain is accompanied by physiologic signs of hyperactivity of the CNS, such as a rapid pulse and elevated blood pressure. Acute pain usually has a precipitating cause (e.g., small bowel obstruction, a painful dressing change, a pathologic fracture). The pain tends to be time limited and responds to analgesic drug therapy and, where possible, treatment of the underlying cause. Acute pain can be further subdivided into *subacute pain* and *intermittent* or *episodic* types of acute pain (Foley, 2004). *Subacute pain* describes pain that comes on over several days, often with increasing intensity, and may be associated with a variety of causes such as a progressive pathologic process or an analgesic regimen that has not been titrated upward to accommodate for a progressive, painful disease process. *Episodic pain* refers to

- Acute pain (characterized by a well-defined pattern of onset; cause usually can be identified; may be accompanied by physiologic signs of hyperactivity of the central nervous system (CNS); tends to be time limited and responds to analgesic therapy)
  - Subacute
  - Intermittent or episodic
- Chronic pain (pain that persists for longer than three months; hyperactivity of the CNS not seen; patient may not look as though he or she is in pain, therefore at risk for undertreatment)
- Breakthrough pain
  - Incident pain (occurs during or following certain activity, such as a dressing change or movement)
  - End-of-dose failure (pain recurs before the next dose of medication is scheduled)

Figure 19-4. Temporal Patterns of Pain

Note. Based on information from American Pain Society, 2003; Foley, 2004.

pain that occurs during defined periods of time, on a regular or irregular basis (Foley, 2004). *Intermittent pain* is an alternative way to describe episodic pain. Such pain may be associated with movement, dressing changes, or other activities. Because the trigger for intermittent pain often can be identified, the nurse, through appropriate use of analgesics or other modalities prior to the pain-provoking event, can have a significant impact on decreasing these painful episodes for the patient. The fear of pain associated with these activities therefore is lessened for the older adult.

Chronic pain differs from acute pain in its representation. These differences are essential for the nurse to be aware of, as patients with chronic pain are at risk to have their pain unrecognized, untreated, or undertreated. Chronic pain is defined as pain that persists for greater than three months (Foley, 2004). Adaptation of the autonomic nervous system occurs, and the patient does not exhibit the objective signs of pain found frequently in those with acute pain (e.g., there is no rapid pulse or elevated blood pressure). Poorly relieved chronic pain in older patients with cancer contributes to their experience of fatigue, depression, insomnia, general despair, withdrawal from interactions with others, and in some a desire for death (Cherny & Coyle, 1994; Coyle, 2004; Foley, 1991).

Breakthrough pain is a more recent classification within the various types of pain. Breakthrough pain is defined as a transient increase in pain to greater than moderate intensity, occurring on a baseline pain of moderate intensity or less (American Pain Society, 2003; Foley, 2004). Breakthrough pain has a diversity of characteristics. In some patients, for example, it is identified by marked worsening of pain at the end of the dosing interval of regularly scheduled analgesics. In other patients, it is induced by an action of the patient or nurse; for example, when the patient is turning or having a dressing change. This is referred to as *incident* pain. Older patients frequently have a combination of these different types of pain. Noting the patterns of pain in a particular individual is an essential component of pain assessment, and attention to such details is the essence of pain management. A pain diary or log, kept by the patient or family, can help to identify the pattern of pain for the individual.

Clinical Assessment of Pain

The previously described mechanisms of pain, types of pain, and patterns of pain provide background information from which to start a clinical pain assessment. The clinical pain assessment in the older adult is based on a process of both observation and interview and can present many unique challenges (see Figure 19-5). Because the older adult may have hearing and visual deficits and take longer to process information than a younger age group, enough time must be built into the system to allow for effective communication. If this is not done, both parties will be left feeling frustrated. Environmental distractions should be kept to a minimum, speech should be clear and unhurried, words and questions should be rephrased to be sure that they are understood by both parties, and the patient should be allowed plenty of time to ask and respond to questions (Taylor & Herr, 2003). The basic principles of a pain assessment in the older adult are outlined in Figure 19-6. Taking a history of the pain complaint in the older adult as in any other patient involves the following parameters (Foley, 2004).

Onset—When did the pain begin? Was it associated with a particular activity or known medical event? Did other symptoms, such as nausea or vomiting, accompany the onset of pain?

Sites(s)—Where is the site of pain? Frequently, older adults will have multiple sites and sources of pain. Each site of pain needs to be assessed, as the management approach may differ depending on the etiology of the pain.

Quality—What is the quality of the pain? Does the pain radiate? Have the patients describe the quality of the pain in their own words. Word descriptors used by patients to describe their pain and its impact on them will help the nurse to understand the inferred pain mechanism. That, in turn, influences the choice of pharmacotherapy. For example, if patients use word descriptors to describe their pain that suggest a neuropathic component, such as sharp, shooting, electric shock–like, or burning, then adjuvant drugs as well as the opioids and/or anti-inflammatory drugs might be suggested as an important component of their drug regimen.

Severity of the pain—What is the severity of the patient's pain? Have the individual describe the severity of his or her pain using a standardized tool (Taylor & Herr, 2003). A variety of tools are available for use by older adults. For those with mild cognitive impairment, standard scales can be used (see Figure 19-7). For those with severe cognitive impairment, selecting a tool where behavioral observations are made, such as breathing pattern, vocalization, facial expression, body language, restlessness, or

---

- Multiple concurrent medical problems
- Multiple symptoms (symptom clusters)
- Cognitive impairment, including poor memory
- Language of pain foreign to the individual
- Sensory losses (visual hearing)
- Depression
- Under-reported pain (fear pain means disease progression; fear of hospitalization if they report escalating pain; see pain as a natural part of aging)
- Fearful of using opioids (addiction; side effects, especially constipation and confusion)
- Not use to "complaining"
- Require more time than younger age groups
- Become easily overwhelmed if they feel rushed
- Can become self-blaming and demoralized if they feel not "heard"

Figure 19-5. Pain Assessment in the Older Adult With Cancer: Unique Challenges

---

Note. Based on information from Coyle, 2004; Ferrell, B.A., 1996; Ferrell, B.R., 1996; Ferrell & Whiteman, 2003; Miaskowski, 2000; Paice et al., 1998; Taylor & Herr, 2003; Ward et al., 1993; Weiner & Rudy, 2002.

(Must allow sufficient time to communicate effectively with the older adult—60–90 minutes may be required for an initial assessment, with 30 minutes for a follow-up visit.)
- Pain history—identify words patients use to describe their pain.
- Past medical history—identify coexisting disease and previous experience with pain and analgesic use (e.g., opioid use, side effects, outcomes).
- Review systems with special focus on musculoskeletal system.
- Ask about falls.
- Assess functional status—can be used as an important outcome measure for overall pain management.
- Evaluate cognitive status, psychological status, and social situation (depression, anxiety, social isolation).
- Evaluate sleep patterns, eating, daily activities, and impact of pain on these parameters.
- Provide a focused physical examination, with careful attention to the painful site(s).

Figure 19-6. Pain History and Physical Examination in the Older Adult

Note. Based on information from Ferrell & Whiteman, 2003; Foley, 2004; Taylor & Herr, 2003.

(Standard scales can be used for those with mild cognitive impairment. Behavioral observation should be used for those with severe cognitive impairment.)
- Descriptive words
  – None, slight, moderate, severe
- Numerical estimates
  – 0–10
- Visual analog scales
- Happy/sad faces
- Behavioral observation for the severely cognitively impaired

Figure 19-7. Pain Assessment Scales

Note. Based on information from Ahles et al., 1983; Fishman et al., 1987; Jacox et al., 1994; Taylor & Herr, 2003; Wong & Baker, 1988, 1995.

combative behavior and consolability, is suggested. Herr, Decker, and Bjoro (2004) compiled a summary of a state-of-the-art review of tools for assessment of pain in nonverbal older adults (see Table 19-1). Noting changes in behavior is extremely important in the severely cognitively impaired. A general rule is that if a patient is in a situation that would be painful in a cognitively intact individual, assume pain is present, and take the appropriate steps. Some cognitively impaired individuals may become agitated and combative when they are uncomfortable because they have a full bladder, are wet, have been sitting in one position for too long, are hungry or thirsty, or just want to be touched or held. Paying attention to these basic needs of the older patient with cancer is part of pain management in the broadest sense.

In pain associated with cancer, the nurse must recognize the significance of escalating pain within the background of this particular patient's disease process, past treatments and present treatment options, value system, goals of care, and nearness to death. The impact of the pain on the individual's day-to-day functions, including ability to sleep, and quality of life also must be assessed. The staff should be consistent in using a particular assessment tool with an individual patient so that communication regarding that patient's pain management can be enhanced.

Pain severity should be assessed at rest, during movement, and in relation to daily activity and the patient's analgesic regimen. Asking questions such as "How

Table 19-1. State-of-the-Art Review of Tools for Assessment of Pain in Nonverbal Older Adults

American Geriatrics Society Guideline	FLACC* (Merkel et al., 1997)	NOPPAIN* (Snow et al., 2004)	PADE (Villanueva et al., 2003)	PAINAD* (Warden et al., 2003)	PACSLAC (Fuchs-Lacelle & Hadjistavropoulos, 2004)
Facial expressions Slight frown; sad, frightened face; Grimacing, wrinkled forehead, closed or tightened eyes; Any distorted expression; Rapid blinking	No particular expression or smile; Occasional grimace or frown; Withdrawn; Disinterested	Pain faces (grimaces, furrowed brow, winces)	Frowning; Sad facial expression; Anxious/frightened facial expression	Facial expression	Facial expressions: Grimacing, sad look, tighter face, dirty look; Change in eyes, frowning; Pain expression, grim face, clenching teeth, wincing, opening mouth, creasing forehead, screwing up nose
Verbalizations, vocalizations Sighing, moaning, groaning; Grunting, chanting, calling out; Noisy breathing; Asking for help; Verbally abusive	Cry: • No cry (awake or asleep) • Moans or whimpers • Occasional complaint; Frequent or constant quivering chin; Crying steadily, screams or sobs, frequent complaints	Pain words ("That hurts!", "Ouch!", "Stop that!", cursing); Pain noises (moans, groans, grunts, cries, gasps, sighs)	Moaning/groaning, breathing rapidly or hyperventilating; Breathing sounds, loud gasping, etc.; Speech or other vocalizations sound distressed	Negative vocalization; Breathing	Screaming/yelling, calling out (i.e., for help), a specific sound or vocalization for pain, such as "ou", "ouch", moaning and groaning, mumbling, grunting, verbal aggression
Body movements Rigid, tense body posture, guarding; Fidgeting; Increased pacing, rocking; Restricted movement; Gait or mobility changes	Legs: Normal position or relaxed; Uneasy, restless, tense, kicking, legs drawn up; Activity: Lying quietly, normal position, moves easily; Squirming, shifting back and forth; Tense; Arched, rigid, or jerking	Rubbing (massaging the affected area); Restlessness (frequent shifting, rocking, inability to stay still)	Tense body language; Guarding the affected area; Restless; Fidgeting; Pacing	Body language 0—Relaxed 1—Tense, distressed pacing, fidgeting 2—Rigid, fists clenched, knees pulled up, pulling or pushing away, striking out	Activity/body movement: Fidgeting, pulling away, flinching, restless, pacing, refusing to move, thrashing, decreased activity, moving slowly, impulsive behavior (repetitive movements), guarding sore area, touching/holding sore area, limping, clenched fist, going into fetal position, stiff/rigid

(Continued on next page)

Table 19-1. State-of-the-Art Review of Tools for Assessment of Pain in Nonverbal Older Adults (Continued)

American Geriatrics Society Guideline	FLACC* (Merkel et al., 1997)	NOPPAIN* (Snow et al., 2004)	PADE (Villanueva et al., 2003)	PAINAD* (Warden et al., 2003)	PACSLAC (Fuchs-Lacelle & Hadjistavropoulos, 2004)
Changes in interpersonal interactions Aggressive, combative, resisting care Decreased social interactions Socially inappropriate, disruptive Withdrawn	—	—	Language coherence and complexity Pattern of social interaction Pattern of cooperation	—	Social/personality/mood Physical aggression Not wanting to be touched Not allowing people near Angry/mad, throwing things
Changes in activity patterns or routines Refusing food, appetite changes Increase in rest periods Sleep, rest pattern changes Sudden cessation of common routines Increased wandering	—	—	Eating pattern Sleep/wake pattern Pattern of wandering	—	Changes in sleep Changes in appetite Trying to leave
Mental status changes Crying or tears Increased confusion Irritability or distress	—	—	—	—	Increased confusion

(Continued on next page)

Table 19-1. State-of-the-Art Review of Tools for Assessment of Pain in Nonverbal Older Adults (Continued)

American Geriatrics Society Guideline	Abbey Scale* (Abbey et al., 2004)	ADD (Kovach et al., 1999)	CNPI (Feldt, 2000)	DS-DAT (Hurley et al., 1992)	Doloplus 2 (Doloplus Group, 2001)
Facial expressions Slight frown; sad, frightened face Grimacing, wrinkled forehead, closed or tightened eyes Any distorted expression Rapid blinking	Frowning, grimacing, looking frightened, looking tense	Sad or frightened facial expression	Facial grimacing or wincing (clenched teeth, furrowed brow, tightened lips, narrowed eyes)	Frown Sad facial expression Frightened facial expression Content of facial expressions	Expression • Showing pain • Unusually blank look (voiceless, staring, blank looks)
Verbalizations, vocalizations Sighing, moaning, groaning Grunting, chanting, calling out Noisy breathing Asking for help Verbally abusive	Whimpering, groaning	Intense, repetitive verbalization Verbal outburst toward another person Noisy breathing	Vocal complaints: "That hurts," "Ouch," "Stop" Nonverbal vocalization: sighs, gasps, moans, cries	Negative vocalization Noisy breathing	Somatic complaints • Expressed upon enquiry only • Occasional involuntary • Continuous involuntary
Body movements Rigid, tense body posture, guarding Fidgeting Increased pacing, rocking Restricted movement Gait or mobility changes	Guarding part of body Fidgeting Rocking	Tense body language Fidgeting Tense, repetitive movement During transfers: grimaces, braces himself or herself, groans	Massaging the affected area Restlessness: shifting, rocking, inability to sit still Bracing behavior: clutching or holding affected area during movement	Tense body language Fidgeting Relaxed body language	Somatic reactions • Protective body postures at rest • Avoiding certain positions • Protective postures • Protection of sore areas Mobility • Usual activities reduced • Resistive to movement

(Continued on next page)

Table 19-1. State-of-the-Art Review of Tools for Assessment of Pain in Nonverbal Older Adults (Continued)

American Geriatrics Society Guideline	Abbey Scale* (Abbey et al., 2004)	ADD (Kovach et al., 1999)	CNPI (Feldt, 2000)	DS-DAT (Hurley et al., 1992)	Doloplus 2 (Doloplus Group, 2001)
Changes in interpersonal interactions Aggressive, combative, resisting care Decreased social interactions Socially inappropriate, disruptive Withdrawn	Withdrawn	Physical aggression Withdrawn behavior	—	—	Communication • Heightened, demanding attention and lessened, absence/refusal of any form of communication Social life • Participation in activities: normal, only when asked to do so, sometimes refuses, refuses to participate in anything Behavioral problems
Changes in activity patterns or routines Refuses food, appetite changes Increase in rest periods Sleep, rest pattern changes Sudden cessation of common routines Increased wandering	Alteration in usual patterns Refusing to eat	Wandering requiring intervention Repetitive waking during the night	—	—	Psychomotor reactions • Changes in ability to wash and/or dress Somatic reactions • Sleep pattern changes with waking and restlessness or insomnia
Mental status changes Crying or tears Increased confusion Irritability or distress	Increased confusion Crying	Tearfulness Delusions Phobias or fears Hallucinations	—	—	—

* In addition to the behavioral indicators listed, the Abbey Scale includes two nonbehavioral categories: Physiologic change (e.g., temperature, pulse, or blood pressure outside of normal limits, perspiring, flushing, pallor) and a category for etiologic factors: Physical changes (e.g., skin tears, pressure areas, contractures, previous injuries). FLACC includes a category called "consolability." PACSLAC includes physiologic items (pale face, flushed red face, teary eyed, sweating, shaking/trembling, cold and clammy). PADE includes an item called "consolability." NOPPAIN includes a pain thermometer for global assessment of pain.

Note. Table courtesy of K. Herr, S. Decker, and K. Bjoro, 2004. Used with permission. *State of the Art Review of Tools for Assessment of Pain in Nonverbal Older Adults.* City of Hope Beckman Research Institute Web page http://www.cityofhope.org/prc/elderly.asp

much pain is relieved when you take the pain medication?" "How long does the relief last?" "Does the pain come back before your next dose of pain medication is due?" "Are you having any side effects from the medication?" helps to establish if the appropriate drug has been selected for the patient, if the dose the patient is receiving is too much, too little, or just right, and if the dosing time interval is the correct one. For the nonverbal severely cognitively impaired patient, asking the nurse, nursing aide, or family to observe for behavioral changes that would indicate the answer to each of the previous questions can be used as a proxy for the patient's verbal response. A more global 24-hour assessment of the adequacy of their pain management in general includes asking the patients their pain score (e.g., "right now," "at its best," "at its worst," "on average") (Daut, Cleeland, & Flanery, 1983).

Exacerbating and relieving factors—Identifying factors that increase or relieve the older adult's pain can be helpful both in arriving at a pain diagnosis and in providing the nurse the opportunity to reinforce techniques that the patient has found useful in the past to relieve pain. A patient with cancer who reports rapidly escalating back pain, with a band-like quality that is worse when lying in bed and better when standing, is considered to have a cord compression unless proved otherwise (Foley, 2004). Early recognition of cord compression and treatment, frequently with steroids and/or radiation therapy, may prevent paraplegia in the last few weeks to months of a patient's life. Escalating back pain may be the only sign of impending cord compression.

Impact of pain on the patient's psychological state—The interface between pain and suffering is well known (Cherny & Coyle, 1994, 1999; Cherny & Portenoy, 1994a; Coyle, 1995; Foley, 1991; Saunders, 1967; Stiefel, 1993). When an older patient with cancer is asked, "What does this pain mean to you?" or "What do you think is causing the pain?", a flood of suffering and fear often is expressed. Patients are fearful that their disease is getting worse; they are dying; their pain will continue to escalate without the possibility of relief; they will burden and financially drain their family; and the use of opioid drugs will dull their minds and cause addiction. All of these worries and fears must be addressed if pain is to be relieved (Coyle, 2004; Paice, Toy, & Shott, 1998; Ward et al., 1993; Weiner & Rudy, 2002).

Pain Treatment History and Responses to Previous and Current Analgesic Regimens

The patient needs to be asked specific questions about what approaches have been used to manage pain in the past, both pharmacologic (including over-the-counter medications) and nonpharmacologic, and how effective those approaches have been. Included should be analgesics that have been previously prescribed, dosages, time intervals, routes of drug administration, efficacy in providing pain relief, side effects, and the reason why a particular approach was discontinued. Fear of recurrence of previously experienced side effects such as sedation, nausea, mental haziness, and constipation may make an older adult reluctant to start a new analgesic regimen. Healthcare professionals should focus their attention on the older adults' concerns, provide a clear explanation of how side effects will be managed if they occur, and know that "starting low and going slow" can allay these fears. However, this is a commitment that will require the nurse to closely monitor the patient's response to therapy and a rapid response to the management of any adverse side effects should they occur.

Examining the Site of the Pain

Examining the site of the pain and possible referral sites may help to identify the source of the patient's pain (Foley, 2004). This is always performed within knowledge of the patient's disease process, extent of disease, treatment history, possible referral sites, and goals of care. The source of pain may be obvious, including a distended abdomen associated with a full bladder, bowel obstruction, or liver distention, a prior skin eruption with postherpetic neuralgia, a bony deformity or inability to use a limb because of a pathologic fracture, or an open fungating infected wound. In other instances, pain may be reproduced (e.g., when palpating the abdomen, moving an extremity).

Pain as a Multifactorial Phenomenon and Multidimensional Experience

In the older adult with advanced cancer, the cause of pain frequently is multifactorial and multidimensional, requiring a multimodal approach. Whenever possible, an attempt is made to treat the cause of the pain as well as the pain itself. The extent of the diagnostic workup depends on the goals of care and the likely impact of the results of the diagnostic workup on the patient's treatment plan and overall quality of life. The benefit to burden ratio to the patient is of uppermost concern.

Pain as a multidimensional experience involves sensory, affective, cognitive, behavioral, and sociocultural components (Ahles, Blanchard, & Ruckdeschel, 1983; Bates, 1987; Ferrell, Rhiner, Cohen, & Grant, 1991; Foley, 2004; McGuire, 1995). Although pharmacotherapy is the foundation of cancer pain management, pharmacotherapy alone will not be an effective approach to the management of pain in the patient with cancer. A multimodal approach usually is required, including attention to the suffering component of the patient's pain. In addition, the needs of the family must be met (Ferrell et al., 1991; Ferrell, Ferrell, Ahn, & Tran, 1994; Ferrell, Grant, Chan, Ahn, & Ferrell, 1995). This concept of "total pain" (Ferrell et al., 1991; Saunders, 1967; Twycross & Wilcock, 2001), including the physical, psychological, social, spiritual, and existential domains, is a critical one. Unless the suffering associated with each of these domains is addressed, pain is unlikely to be adequately controlled.

Pharmacologic Management of Pain

Inadequate knowledge of analgesic pharmacotherapy is one of the most commonly cited reasons for undertreatment of pain (Fine, 2001; Jacox et al., 1994; Lasch et al., 2002; O'Brien, Dalton, Konsler, & Carlson, 1996; Weinstein et al., 2000). Developing expertise in the use of analgesic drugs is an integral part of oncology nursing care.

More than a decade ago, the cancer unit of WHO convened an expert committee and developed a three-step analgesic ladder approach to the selection of drugs for the treatment of cancer pain (WHO, 1986). Three categories of analgesic drugs are included in the three-step analgesic ladder: NSAIDs, opioids, and adjuvant analgesics. With a focus on pain management in the older adult, discussion around these groups of drugs will include rationale for selection, dose titration, routes of administration, and side-effect management (Hanks, Cherny, & Fallon, 2004; Hewitt & Foley, 1997; Hofmann, Farnon, Javed, & Posner, 1998).

Nonsteroidal Anti-Inflammatory Drugs

NSAIDs include many subclasses, are frequently used in all steps of the "analgesic ladder" (McQuay & Moore, 2004), and are analgesic, antipyretic, and anti-inflammatory (see Table 19-2). Aspirin is the prototype of NSAIDs. Acetaminophen, although lacking in significant anti-inflammatory effects and with a different side-effect profile, often is classified within this group. NSAIDs are most effective in treating mild to moderate pain when an inflammatory component is present and are used in step 1 of the analgesic ladder. When greater relief is needed, they are continued along with the opioid drugs in steps 2 and 3. NSAIDs can be extremely effective when combined with an opioid drug in treating bone pain in patients with cancer (prostaglandins, which are rich in the periosteum of the bone, are implicated in pain modulation) (Paice, 1999). Unlike opioid drugs, NSAIDs have a ceiling effect (a dose beyond which added analgesia is not obtained) (American Pain Society, 2003). These drugs do not produce tolerance or physical dependence and are not associated with psychological dependence (addiction). This class of drugs also may have an opioid-sparing effect in some patients. Ketorolac is the only NSAID that is available parenterally in the United States.

Mechanism of Action

NSAIDs affect pain perception in three ways. First, they inhibit the conversion of arachidonic acid to prostaglandin G2 by inhibiting the enzyme cyclooxygenase (COX) (American Pain Society, 2003; Jenkins & Bruera, 1999). Two types of COX enzymes exist: COX-1, which is part of normal cells, and COX-2, which is induced in the inflammatory process. Inhibition of COX-2 is responsible for the anti-inflammatory processes of NSAIDs, whereas COX-1 inhibition is responsible for many of the side effects of NSAIDs (American Pain Society; Jenkins & Bruera). A new group of NSAIDs have been developed that selectively inhibit COX-2 enzymes, while leaving the more protective COX-1 enzyme intact (McQuay & Moore, 2004). The second way in which NSAIDs affect pain perception is through their action on the cell membranes of neutrophils to inhibit the release of inflammatory mediators. These two mechanisms reduce inflammation in tissues and thus decrease the release of substance P and pain-producing cytokines, thereby reducing nociception (Jenkins & Bruera). A third way in which NSAIDs may impact pain perception is through mechanisms at the brain and spinal cord level (Yaksh, Dirig, & Malmberg, 1998).

Acetaminophen, although lacking in significant anti-inflammatory effects, often is classified with NSAIDs. Its mechanism of action is not known (American Pain Society, 2003). Acetaminophen has fewer adverse effects than NSAIDs. Gastrointestinal toxicity is rare, and no adverse effects are present on platelet function or cross-reactivity in patients with aspirin hypersensitivity (American Pain Society). Hepatic toxicity can occur, however, and patients with chronic alcoholism and liver disease can develop severe hepatotoxicity even when the drug is taken in usual therapeutic doses (Whitcomb & Block, 1994). Acetaminophen is one of the safest analgesics for long-term use in the older adult and should be used for mild to moderate pain. The compound

Table 19-2. Examples of Selected Nonopioid Analgesics*

Drug	Average Analgesic Dose (mg)	Dosing Interval (hours)	Comments
Acetaminophen (Tylenol®)	500–1,000 (Maximum daily dose 4,000 mg)	4–6	Use for mild to moderate pain. Adjust dose by 50% in patients with impaired hepatic function.
Aspirin	500–1,000	4–6	Prototype, nonselective COX-2 inhibitor. Anti-inflammatory, antipyretic. Gastrointestinal (GI), renal, and central nervous system toxicities. Platelet inhibition.
Celecoxib (Celebrex®)	200–400 (Maximum daily dose 400 mg)	12–24	Selective COX-2 inhibition. Analgesic effects similar to naproxen. Less GI toxicity. Growing evidence of cardiac toxicities in this class of drugs.
Nabumetone (Relafen®)	1,000 initial, 500–750 subsequent (Maximum daily dose 2,000)	8–12	Pain relief similar to aspirin, indomethacin, naproxen, and sulindac. Fewer side effects.
Ibuprofen (Motrin® by prescription; Advil®, Nuprin®, and other over-the-counter medication)	200–400 (Maximum daily dose 2,000)	–	Gastric, renal, and abnormal platelet function may be dose dependent; constipation, confusion, and headaches may be more common in older adults.
Naproxen (Naprosyn® by prescription, Aleve®, and other over-the-counter drugs)	500 initial, 250 subsequent	6–8	Dose may need downward adjustment for older adults or frail older adults.
Diflunisal (Dolobid®)	1,000 initial, 500 subsequent (Maximum daily dose in older adults is 500–1,000)	8–12	Dose in older adults is 500–1,000 mg per day.
Ketorolac (Toradol®)	Only nonsteroidal anti-inflammatory drugs approved for IM administration. 120 qd (30–60 mg loading dose, followed by half the loading dose, 15–30 mg q6h, limited to not more than five days). PO 60 mg qd (q6h dosing limited to not more than 14 days)	6	Substantial GI toxicity as well as renal and platelet dysfunction. Duration of treatment limited because of high toxicities. Reduce dose by half for those > 65 years of age. Average dose in older adults 10–15 mg IM/IV q6h. May precipitate renal failure in dehydrated patients.

* This table is to be used as a guide only and not to replace a more comprehensive review.

Starting doses should be one-half to two-thirds recommended dose in older adults, those on multiple drugs, or those with renal insufficiency.

h—hour; IM—intramuscular; IV—intravenous; q—every

Note. From "Principles of Analgesic Use in the Treatment of Acute Pain and Cancer Pain" (5th ed., p. 216), by B. Ferrell and J.E. Whiteman in R.S. Morrison and D.E. Meier (Eds.), *Geriatric Palliative Care*, 2003, New York: Oxford University Press. Copyright 2003 by Oxford University Press. Adapted with permission.

is particularly helpful in the management of musculoskeletal pain and often is used in combination with opioids.

Adverse Effects and Their Management

Older adults are more susceptible to adverse side effects of pharmacotherapy than is the younger age group. A careful balance is needed between achieving the desired effect of the selected drug for the patient and the potential for adverse effects (Drage & Schug, 1996; Shimp, 1998). This is particularly important in this group of drugs. Unlike opioids where the adverse effects usually are dose dependent and controllable, NSAIDs have a largely "hidden" side-effect profile (Jenkins & Bruera, 1999). These adverse effects often are "silent," not producing symptoms until a major event occurs, such as gastrointestinal bleeding without prior warning. The nurse is an active participant in assessing the risk/benefit ratio for the older adult and needs to become familiar with the relative side-effect profile for each of the drugs within this category. The potential adverse effects of NSAIDs (excluding acetaminophen, which was described earlier) include those affecting the CNS and hematologic, gastrointestinal, and renal systems. COX-2 inhibitors differ in their side-effect profile from other NSAIDs in relation to potential for gastric irritation and interference with platelet aggregation. However, selective COX-2 inhibitors have similar renal effects (sodium retention, edema, hypertension) as with traditional NSAIDs.

Principles of Administration of Nonsteroidal Anti-Inflammatory Drugs

Drug Selection. A careful medical and pain history provides the nurse with information about potential benefits and risks for a patient about to receive an NSAID. An analgesic history should illuminate the patient's prior exposure to NSAIDs, including frequency of administration and both analgesic effects and side effects. Information regarding the timing interval of other analgesics is important so that a prescribed NSAID regimen fits with the patient's total analgesic plan. For example, if a patient is on an 8- or 12-hour dosing regimen of a controlled-release morphine preparation, an NSAID with a similar dosing profile would be appropriate. This may aid the older adult with compliance and cut down on the feeling of having to constantly take medication.

Choice of a Starting Dose and Dose Titration. An NSAID is combined with an opioid drug in steps 2 and 3 of the analgesic ladder. Doses often are started at the lower end of the recommended scale in the medically fragile and older adult. Although several weeks are needed to evaluate the efficacy of a dose when NSAIDs are used in the treatment of grossly inflammatory conditions such as arthritis, clinical observation suggests that a shorter time period, usually a week, is adequate for pain relief in a patient with cancer pain. Pain and other symptoms should be monitored before and after starting NSAIDs in the older patient with cancer to document any improvement or adverse effects. If no benefit is seen or if adverse effects are noted, consideration should be given to discontinuing the drug or switching to an alternate NSAID, as marked variability has been noted in patients' response to different NSAIDs. Indicators of an effective response would be either a significant improvement in pain or a significant decrease in opioid use, with a subsequent reduction in opioid-related side effects. The degree of monitoring for adverse effects from NSAIDs should be individualized to the patient. Figure 19-8 gives key points to consider when administering NSAIDs to the older adult.

- The older adult is more susceptible to adverse side effects of pharmacotherapy; therefore, start low and go slow.
- Unlike with opioids, the adverse effects of NSAIDs often do not produce obvious symptoms until a major event such as a gastrointestinal bleed occurs.
- Selective COX-2 inhibitors differ in their side-effect profile from other NSAIDs in relation to gastric irritation and interference with platelet aggregation.
- However, selective COX-2 inhibitors have similar renal adverse effects (e.g., sodium retention, edema, hypertension) as traditional NSAIDs.
- NSAIDs should not be used concomitantly with other drugs that have the potential to cause gastric erosion (e.g., corticosteroids).
- Older adults with chronic heart failure, renal insufficiency, cirrhosis with ascites, significant athero-sclerotic disease, or multiple myeloma are at risk for NSAID-induced renal failure.

Figure 19-8. Nonsteroidal Anti-Inflammatory Drugs and the Older Adult

---

Note. Based on information from American Pain Society, 2003; Drage & Schug, 1996; Jenkins & Bruera, 1999; McQuay & Moore, 2004; Shimp, 1998; and authors' clinical experience.

Opioid Drugs

Opioid analgesics are the mainstay of cancer pain treatment (see Table 19-3). These drugs are used for moderate to severe pain in steps 2 and 3 of the analgesic ladder. They frequently are used in combination with an NSAID (American Pain Society, 2003). When formulated in combination with an NSAID, dose escalation is limited by reaching the maximum recommended daily dose of the NSAID. When used as a single agent, however, no ceiling effect appears to be present. Adverse effects such as sedation, confusion, nausea and vomiting, myoclonus, and (rarely) respiratory depression may limit dose escalation (Hanks et al., 2004). The balance between pain relief and intolerable and unmanageable side effects governs dose escalation. This balance only can be determined by ongoing assessment and documentation of the effects and side effects produced by the opioid. Older adults are more sensitive to the therapeutic and toxic effects of opioids than is the younger age group.

A clear understanding of the clinical significance of tolerance, physical dependence, and psychological dependence, as these terms relate to the use of opioid drugs, is essential if nurses are to break down the pervasive barriers that surround the use of these drugs and contribute to inadequate pain relief and much unnecessary suffering in the older adult.

Tolerance is the phenomenon characterized by the need to increase the dose to maintain the same drug effect (American Pain Society, 2003). Usually the reason for dose escalation at the end of life occurs in the setting of increasing pain associated with progressive disease (Foley, 1993). Patients with stable disease usually do not require increasing opioid doses (Foley, 1993). This observation, integrated with the knowledge that no "ceiling" effect occurs to opioid drugs, implies the following: (a) concern about tolerance to analgesic effects should not impede the use of opioids early in the course of the disease; and (b) worsening pain in a patient on a stable dose

Table 19-3. Equianalgesic Dose Table: Relative Potencies, Half-Lives, and Duration of Action of Commonly Used Opioids for Cancer Pain*,**

Drug	Half-Life	Equianalgesic Intramuscular Dose (mg)***	Intramuscular Oral Potency (mg)	Starting Oral Dose (mg)	Comment
Morphine-like Agonists Morphine	2–3	10	3 (repeated dose)	15–30 (q4h)	Standard of comparison for opioid analgesics. Available in liquid, tablet, suppositories. Controlled-release available. Morphine-6-glucuronide and morphine-3-glucuronide accumulation in patients with renal failure. Use with caution in older adults. Do not use if elevated creatinine levels. Delirium is a common sign of toxicity in older adults.
Oxymorphone	–	1	–	1	Available in suppository form as Numorphan® 5 mg and 10 mg
Hydromorphone	2–3	1.5	5	2 (q4h)	Useful alternative for morphine. Active metabolite hydromorphone-3-glucuronide. Available in liquid, tablet, suppositories. Controlled release is available.
Methadone	15–190	10****	2	2.5 (q12–8h)	Accumulates with repetitive dosing. Available in liquid and tablet form. Can be formulated into suppositories. Monitor patient closely for increased sedation during titration phase.
Meperidine	2–3	75	4	Not recommended	Central nervous system excitatory toxic metabolite normeperidine accumulates with repetitive dosing. Contraindicated for management of chronic pain or in patients with renal failure or those who are receiving monoamine oxidase inhibitors

(Continued on next page)

Table 19-3. Equianalgesic Dose Table: Relative Potencies, Half-Lives, and Duration of Action of Commonly Used Opioids for Cancer Pain*,** *(Continued)*

Drug	Half-Life	Equianalgesic Intramuscular Dose (mg)***	Intramuscular Oral Potency (mg)	Starting Oral Dose (mg)	Comment
Fentanyl	4–7	–	–	–	Short half-life when used acutely. Parenteral use via infusion. Clinical experience suggests 4 mg IV morphine sulfate/hr = 100 mg transdermal patch. Patches available to deliver 12.5, 25, 50, 75, and 100 mcg/hr. Transmucosal delivery system available in 200–1,600 mcg oralets. Only to be used in opioid-tolerant patients.
Oxycodone	2–3	–	2	5 (q4h)	Available in liquid or tablet preparation. Also in combination with a nonopioid. Controlled-release available.
Codeine	2–3	130	1.5	30–60	Used orally for less severe pain. Usually combined with a nonopioid; limits titration. Constipation limits usefulness.
Hydrocodone	4	–	–	5 (q4h)	Usually combined with nonopioid; limits titration

* This table is to be used as a guide only and is not to replace a more comprehensive review.

** Starting doses based on opioid naive older adults; dose titration usually will be required.

*** Dose that provides analgesia equivalent to 10 mg intramuscular (IM) morphine. These ratios are useful guides when switching drugs or routes of administration. In clinical practice, the potency of the IM route is considered to be identical to the IV and subcutaneous routes. IM route is to be avoided if possible.

**** When switching from another opioid to methadone, the potency of methadone is much greater than indicated on this table. Frequently, 5%–10% of the equianalgesic dose is used.

Note. Based on information from American Pain Society, 2003; Cherny & Portenoy, 1994a; Coyle & Portenoy, 1995; Hanks et al., 2004; Hewitt & Foley, 1997; Jacox et al., 1994.

of opioids is assumed to be evidence of disease progression until proved otherwise (Coyle & Portenoy, 1995; Foley, 1993).

Physical dependence is an altered physiologic state that occurs in patients who use opioids on a long-term basis. If the drug is stopped abruptly or an antagonist is given, the patient exhibits signs of withdrawal. Signs of opioid withdrawal include anxiety, alternating hot flashes and cold chills, salivation, rhinorrhea, diaphoresis, piloerection, nausea, vomiting, abdominal cramping, and insomnia (American Pain Society, 2003). The time frame of the withdrawal syndrome depends on the half-life of the drug. For example, abstinence from drugs with a short half-life, such as morphine and hydromorphone, may occur within 6–12 hours of stopping the drug and may be most severe after 24–72 hours. After withdrawal of drugs with a long half-life, such as methadone, the symptoms may not occur for a day or longer (Hanks et al., 2004). Gradual reduction of the opioid dose in the physically dependent patient who no longer has pain will prevent the withdrawal syndrome (American Pain Society). Clinical experience suggests that administering 25% of the previous analgesic dose will prevent the withdrawal syndrome (Hanks et al.). Healthcare professionals must closely monitor patients during the tapering process to be sure they are not experiencing symptoms of withdrawal, as patients' responses to the tapering process may vary.

The use of an antagonist such as naloxone in the physically dependent patient will precipitate acute withdrawal symptoms unless carefully titrated (Manfredi, Ribeiro, & Payne, 1996). If a drug overdose manifested by respiratory depression is suspected in a patient who has received opioids for more than a few days, a dilute solution of naloxone can be used (0.4 mg in 10 ml of normal saline solution) (American Pain Society, 2003). This may be administered in 1 ml bolus injections every one to three minutes until the patient becomes responsive. As the half-life of naloxone is considerably shorter than that of the majority of opioid drugs, an IV infusion of naloxone carefully titrated to respirations and level of pain occasionally may be necessary.

Psychological dependence (addiction) is defined as a pattern of compulsive drug use characterized by a continued craving for an opioid, loss of control, and continued use despite harm. Clinical experience and limited studies suggest that addiction is extremely uncommon in patients without a history of drug abuse who are receiving opioids for pain (Passik, Portenoy, & Ricketts, 1998; Perry & Heidrich, 1982; Porter & Jick, 1980; Schug et al., 1992). In patients who have a history of drug abuse, the data are scant. Concerns about this outcome, however, continue to be a reason for undertreatment of pain (Cleeland, 1989; Hanks et al., 2004). In the setting of poorly relieved pain, "aberrant" drug-seeking behavior such as "clock watching" requires careful nursing assessment. The term *pseudo-addiction* has been used to describe drug-seeking behavior, reminiscent of addiction, that occurs in the setting of inadequate pain relief and is eliminated by improved analgesia (Weissman, Burchman, Dinndorf, & Dahl, 1990). For the most part, this behavior signifies inadequate pain relief.

Older adults and their families need to be reassured that use of opioid drugs in the amount that is needed to control pain, regardless of that amount, is extremely unlikely to result in psychological dependence in someone without a history of drug abuse. In the patient who has a history of previous drug abuse, whether remote or recent, pain still can be managed using this class of drugs. Frequently, a higher level of opioid is required to control the pain because of the development of tolerance. In these situations, the nurse must be knowledgeable about both pain medicine and addiction medicine or access appropriate resources if this knowledge is lacking (Gonzales & Coyle, 1992; Passik et al., 1998; Portenoy et al., 1997). A team approach is essential.

Mechanism of Action

Opioids produce their effects through binding to receptors in the brain and spinal cord to prevent the release of neurotransmitters involved in pain transmission (Paice,

1999). Opioids also can have a peripheral site of action in the presence of inflammation (Stein, 1995). Opioids can be divided into agonist, agonist-antagonist, and antagonist classes based on their interactions with the receptor types. Pure opioid agonists (e.g., morphine, hydromorphone, oxycodone, fentanyl, methadone) bind primarily to the mu receptors.

Partial agonists and mixed agonist-antagonists either block or remain neutral at the mu opioid receptors while activating kappa opioid receptors (Jaffe & Martin, 1990). Partial agonists (e.g., butorphanol, pentazocine) have limited use in the older adult with cancer experiencing pain. Their pharmacology is characterized by a ceiling effect to analgesia and the ability to precipitate withdrawal symptoms in patients who are physically dependent on pure agonist drugs (e.g., morphine) (Hanks et al., 2004). Opioid antagonist drugs include naloxone and naltrexone. These drugs bind to opioid receptors and block the effect of morphine-like agonists. The most commonly used opioids in the older patient with cancer are reviewed here.

Morphine is the prototype opioid agonist. WHO placed morphine on the essential drug list and requested that it be made available throughout the world for cancer pain relief (WHO, 1986). Morphine is available in tablet, elixir, suppository, and parenteral forms. Various controlled-release oral preparations provide analgesia with a duration of 8–24 hours depending on the preparation. Alternate routes of drug administration are available for patients who are unable to use the oral route.

Patients with severe pain initially usually are titrated with immediate-release morphine tablets, and once the pain is stabilized, they are converted to a controlled-release preparation. To manage breakthrough pain or incident pain, immediate-release morphine should be made available to all patients receiving controlled-release preparations. Absorption of morphine after oral administration occurs mostly in the upper small bowel. The average bioavailability for oral morphine is 20%–30% (Gourlay, Plummer, Cherry, & Purser, 1991). This explains the need to increase the patient's opioid dose when changing from the parenteral to the oral route of drug administration. In patients with normal renal function, the average plasma half-life is two to three hours, whereas the average duration of analgesia is approximately four hours (Hanks et al., 2004). Morphine-6-glucuronide, an active metabolite of morphine and a powerful analgesic (Portenoy, Thaler, Inturrisi, Friedlander-Klar, & Foley, 1992), may accumulate in the older patient with impaired renal function. This accumulation may lead to signs of opioid toxicity, which will be described later in the chapter. Morphine-3-glucuronide also is an active metabolite of morphine and may contribute to myoclonus, seizures, and hyperalgesia in the older adult with renal impairment (Anderson, Jensen, Christrup, Hansen, & Sjogren, 2002; Smith, 2000). Because of these as well as other factors, the nurse must be aware of the patient's renal status when administering morphine and monitor accordingly for signs of opioid toxicity.

If an older adult has signs of renal failure or if new and unexplained confusion, cognitive changes, or sedation are present, morphine may not be the appropriate drug for this patient, and the opioid should be changed. Fentanyl or methadone (in the hands of a skilled practitioner) may be better choices. In general, morphine clearance decreases with age, and the older adult should be monitored closely for adverse side effects when this drug is used.

Hydromorphone and oxycodone are synthetic, short half-life opioids that are a useful alternative for older patients who tolerate morphine poorly. Hydromorphone is five times more potent than morphine and can be administered by the oral, rectal, parenteral, and intraspinal routes (Hanks et al., 2004). The half-life of hydromorphone (one and one-half to three hours) is slightly shorter than that of morphine, and it has an oral bioavailability of 30%–40% (Houde, 1986). The comparative potency of the opioid drugs and bioavailability are dependent on route of administration and underscore the need for nurses to be competent in the use of the equianalgesic table. The main metabolite of hydromorphone, hydromorphone-3-glucuronide, may lead to CNS toxicity, including myoclonus, hyperalgesia, and seizures, especially in the setting of renal failure (Fainsinger, Schoeller, Boiskin, & Bruera, 1993; Lee, Leng, & Tierman, 2001; Smith, 2000; Wright, Mather, & Smith, 2001). These adverse effects usually occur in the setting of high parenteral doses being administered by continuous infusion.

Oxycodone is a synthetic opioid with a better oral absorption than that of morphine (Kalso & Vainio, 1990; Poyhia, Vainio, & Kalso, 1993). The equianalgesic ratio to that of morphine is 20–30:30. It has a half-life of two to four hours and mainly is excreted by the kidneys. Oxycodone is available in combination with aspirin (Percodan®, Endo Pharmaceuticals, Chadds Ford, PA) or acetaminophen (Percocet®, Endo Pharmaceuticals) or as a single immediate-release or controlled-release tablet. The controlled-release tablet (OxyContin®, Purdue Pharma, Stamford, CT) provides the patient with analgesia for 8–12 hours. Oxycodone is used in steps 2 and 3 of the analgesic ladder. Oxycodone is not available in parenteral form.

Fentanyl is a potent, short, half-life semisynthetic opioid that is being used with increasing frequency in palliative care and cancer pain management. Fentanyl comes in transdermal, transmucosal, and parenteral forms. The transdermal fentanyl delivery system consists of a drug reservoir in the form of a patch that is separated from the skin by a copolymer membrane that controls the rate of drug delivery to the skin surface. This approach provides the means to continuously infuse an opioid drug. Empirical observations with patients with cancer suggest that a 100 mcg fentanyl patch is equianalgesic to 4 mg of parenteral morphine. Transdermal fentanyl has only been approved for chronic cancer pain and not for acute pain.

Although most patients maintain satisfactory pain control with a patch change every 72 hours, some patients require the patch to be changed after 48 hours (Payne, Chandler, & Einhaus, 1995). Careful monitoring of adequacy of pain relief and evidence of end-of-dose failure will guide the nurse in the needs of the particular patient. The nurse also must be aware of the lag in absorbing fentanyl through the skin. It takes 12–16 hours for the patient to see a substantial therapeutic effect. Availability of a different route of drug administration therefore is necessary during the 12–16 hours following the initial patch placement. An alternate route of drug administration also is required for breakthrough pain medication. Significant concentrations of fentanyl remain in the plasma for approximately 24 hours after removal of the patch because of delayed release from the tissues and subcutaneous depots. Drug side effects (if present) may persist for that length of time. Although the fentanyl patch can be used safely in older adults, frail older adults who have experienced multiple side effects from a variety of opioids may not do well with this route of administration. Fever, cachexia, obesity, and ascites all may have a significant effect on absorption predictability of blood levels and clinical effect (Menten, Desmedt, Lossignol, & Mullie, 2002; Radbruch et al., 2001).

Oral transmucosal fentanyl citrate (OTFC) provides a useful mode of delivering a potent, short–half-life opioid to a patient who requires a potent drug with a rapid onset of action and short duration of effect for severe breakthrough pain. OTFC is recommended only to be used in patients who are opioid tolerant and who are receiving the equivalent of no less than 60 mg of oral morphine a day or transdermal fentanyl 50 mcg every three days. OTFC differs from other breakthrough pain medication in that no relationship exists between the baseline dose of the patient's pain medication and the microgram dose of OTFC required to relieve breakthrough pain (American Pain Society, 2003; Christie et al., 1998; Streisand et al., 1998). In all other opioid drugs, a relation exists between the two. With OTFC, the smallest available dose is initially chosen (200 mcg) and titrated up, depending on the patient's response (available strengths range from 200–1,600 mcg per unit). The author's personal clinical experience with the use of OTFC has indicated its benefit for patients with acute, predictable, breakthrough pain, such as a fungating chest wall dressing change.

Methadone is another useful synthetic opioid for the management of pain in the older adult but mandates careful patient monitoring for signs of drug accumulation (Davis, & Walsh, 2001). Clinical experience suggests that administering this opioid is more difficult than other morphine-like opioids because of its variable long half-life (13–100 hours) (Hanks et al., 2004) and a discrepancy between drug half-life and the duration of analgesic effect (6–8 hours). Patients are at increased risk for drug accumulation and subsequent toxicity when treatment is initiated, the dose is increased, or multiple organ failure develops. Older as well as younger patients may become confused, increasingly sedated, and progress to a respiratory arrest if not closely monitored, especially during the titration period (Fainsinger, Schoeller, & Bruera, 1993; Hunt & Bruera, 1995). Because of this risk, methadone currently is considered a second-line drug in the treatment of pain. The risk of delayed toxicity from methadone accumulation can be reduced if the initial period of dosing is accomplished with "as needed" administration. The patient should be closely monitored for the first 7–10 days of treatment for signs of drug accumulation and toxicity. When a steady state has been approached, a fixed dosing schedule of every 6–8 hours can be substituted for most patients, although some individuals require a shorter time interval between doses. An opioid with a short half-life, such as morphine or hydromorphone, frequently is used for supplementary or "rescue" dosing, although methadone also can be used.

Knowledge of the long half-life of methadone has a special relevance for the nurse if severe respiratory depression associated with drug accumulation occurs and the use of naloxone is felt to be appropriate. Because of the short half-life of naloxone in comparison with methadone, either repeated doses or an infusion of naloxone may be required to prevent recurrence of respiratory depression as the effects of the naloxone decline and the methadone rebinds to the opioid binding sites. The need to reverse the respiratory effects of an opioid drug in patients who have been exposed to opioid drugs over time is extremely uncommon. Most patients become tolerant to the respiratory depressant effects of these drugs.

The equianalgesic dose ratio of morphine to methadone has been a matter of controversy and uncertainty for clinicians. Early studies suggested that the ratio was 1:1, and this still appears to hold true for opioid-naive patients or in acute pain situations. However, data from recent studies indicate that the ratio correlates with the total opioid dose administered before switching to methadone, and the ratio increases (methadone is much more potent) as the previous dose of oral opioid increases (Moryl et al., 2002; Santiago-Palma et al., 2001; Watanabe, Tarumi, Oneschuk, & Lawlor, 2002).

For example, among patients receiving low doses of morphine before switching to methadone, the ratio is 4:1. In contrast, for patients receiving more than 300 mg of oral morphine, the ratio is approximately 10:1 or 12:1 (Ripamonti et al., 1998). In addition, recent studies suggest high doses of parenteral methadone may lead to a prolonged QT wave interval (Kornick et al., 2003; Kranz, Kutinsky, Robertson, & Mehler, 2003). This is thought to be associated with the preservative.

Methadone has activity at the N-methyl–D-aspartate receptors, which may be useful in the management of neuropathic pain (Morley et al., 2003). From a cost perspective, methadone is one of the least costly opioids, making it very appealing to some patients on limited incomes.

Meperidine, with rare exceptions, should not be used for the management of chronic pain. Meperidine has an active metabolite, normeperidine, that is twice as potent as a convulsant and one-half as potent as an analgesic as its parent compound (Kaiko, 1983). The half-life of normeperidine is three to four times that of meperidine, and accumulation of the metabolite with repetitive dosing can result in CNS excitability characterized by tremor, myoclonus, agitated delirium, and seizures (Szeto et al., 1977). Naloxone does not reverse meperidine-induced seizures and potentially could precipitate seizures by blocking the depressant effects of meperidine and allowing the convulsant effects of normeperidine to become manifest (Kaiko; Umans & Inturrisi, 1982).

Case Study

Mr. AB is an 84-year-old attorney with a diagnosis of prostate cancer and chronic leukemia, for which he receives chronic blood transfusions. He is fairly active, totally alert and oriented, and lives with his daughter. He slipped while getting up from a chair and was taken to the emergency room with severe pain in his back. An x-ray revealed a fracture of the symphysis pubis, and he was given intermittent boluses of morphine sulfate 2 mg IV, which relieved his pain. He became mildly agitated and confused and was given one dose of lorazepam 0.5 mg IV.

About 12 hours after admission, Mr. AB was started on a morphine patient-controlled analgesic pump at 0.5 mg/hr. During the next 24 hours, his cognitive function declined, he developed an agitated delirium alternating with sedation, and a psychiatry consult was called. After three initial bolus doses of haloperidol IV, he was started on a regimen of around-the-clock Haldol® (Ortho McNeil, Raritan, NJ) 2 mg IV q 6 hours + 2 mg IV q 2 hours prn.

A pain and palliative care consult was called two days after the patient's admission. When seen, the patient was in bed, one hand had a mitten on it, and he had around-the-clock supervision. Mr. AB was agitated, delirious, and sedated. Laboratory studies revealed BUN 65 and serum creatinine 1.5. The morphine infusion was discontinued, and the patient was given fentanyl 20 mcg IV boluses prn for his pain. During the next six hours, his mental status improved dramatically, and during the next 48 hours, he became clear-headed.

Assessment

Although delirium in this patient probably was multifactorial (advanced age, low-grade fever, and abnormal renal function), the most probable precipitating cause was toxicity from accumulation of two active morphine metabolites—morphine-3- and morphine-6-glucuronide. Both can accumulate in the setting of renal insufficiency in an older adult and lead to CNS toxicity.

Key Point

In older adults with impaired renal function, the use of morphine should be avoided because of potential opioid toxicity from accumulation of active metabolites. If morphine is used, patients require careful monitoring. If any signs of mental status changes (e.g., sedation, delirium, hallucinations) occur, morphine should be discontinued and an equianalgesic dose of a new opioid started.

Principles of Opioid Administration in the Older Patient With Cancer

Numerous factors, both patient-related and drug-related, must be considered in the selection of an appropriate opioid for a patient (Hanks et al., 2004) (see Figure 19-9). The opioid should be compatible with the patient's pain severity, age,

---

- The older adult is more susceptible to the adverse side effects of pharmacotherapy; therefore, start low and go slow.
- Select a drug from step 2 or 3 of the analgesic ladder that is appropriate to the patient's level of pain and analgesic history.
- Take into consideration the patient's age, metabolic state, presence of major organ failure (renal, hepatic, or respiratory), and presence of coexisting disease.
- Consider pharmacologic issues (e.g., potential accumulation of active metabolites, possible drug interactions).
- Know the drug class (e.g., agonist, agonist-antagonist), duration of analgesic effects, and pharmacokinetic properties.
- Be knowledgeable about the various drug formulations (e.g., controlled release, immediate release, liquid, transmucosal).
- Be aware of the available routes of administration (e.g., oral, rectal, transdermal, subcutaneous, IV, epidural, intrathecal).
- Select the least invasive route appropriate to the patient's needs.
- Consider issues in patient compliance (e.g., convenience, ease for home management, cost).
- Administer the analgesic on an around-the-clock basis for chronic pain. Make sure that rescue doses are available for breakthrough pain.
- If appropriate, use drug combinations such as nonsteroidal anti-inflammatory drugs and adjuvant analgesics.
- Avoid drug combinations that increase sedation without enhancing analgesia.
- Anticipate and treat side effects (most commonly occur when drug is initiated or dose is increased).
- Prevent precipitating an acute withdrawal syndrome in patients who are physically dependent; never abruptly stop opioids, always taper the dose.
- Systemically evaluate the effectiveness of an analgesic regimen (e.g., amount of relief, duration of relief, frequency of breakthrough pain, frequency and pattern of rescue use, presence of adverse effects, satisfaction with mode of therapy).
- Teach the patient and family the principles of analgesic therapy. Address their fears about addiction, opioid side effects, and tolerance.

Figure 19-9. Opioid Administration in the Older Adult

Note. Based on information from Coyle, 2001; Ferrell, B.A., 1996; Ferrell & Whiteman, 2003; Ferrell et al., 1994; Fine, 2004; Jacox et al., 1994; Paice et al., 1998; Walsh, 1990; Ward et al., 1993.

dosing and route requirements, underlying illness, and metabolic state. Selection of an opioid that is available as a controlled-release formulation (e.g., morphine, oxycodone) may be an important consideration for some patients. For the older adult or those who have major organ dysfunction, an opioid with a short half-life, such as morphine, hydromorphone, or oxycodone, may be preferable. However, patients with marked renal impairment must be monitored closely for the accumulation of active metabolites and resultant toxicities.

The nurse must recognize the potential for additive side effects and serious toxicities from drug combinations in the older adult each time a new drug is added to the patient's regimen. Patients frequently have many distressing symptoms and are receiving multiple drugs. For example, it is not unusual for a patient with advanced cancer to be receiving an opioid, an NSAID, a tricyclic antidepressant, an anxiolytic, an H_2 blocker, or a neuroleptic, as well as a variety of other drugs for comorbidities. In these circumstances, additive side effects, especially those of sedation, are frequent, yet the opioid drug tends to get blamed in isolation for these side effects.

Opioid Rotation

Sequential trials of opioid drugs ("opioid rotation") may be needed in the older adult to find the most favorable balance between pain relief and adverse effects (Hanks et al., 2004). The patient and family should be warned that this is a possibility so that they do not become discouraged during the process. Usually if one or two side effects are present and pain control is good, an attempt is made to treat the side effects and maintain the current opioid. If more than two side effects are present, opioid rotation probably is warranted. Figure 19-10 gives the nurse guidelines when changing from one opioid to another. In all instances, when an opioid dose is decreased or the drug is changed because of large interpatient variability, the nurse must closely monitor the patient for adequacy of pain relief or presence of adverse side effects.

- If one or two side effects present and pain control is good, attempt to treat the side effects and maintain the current opioid.
- If more than two side effects are present, refer to the equianalgesic dose table (see Table 19-3) prior to switching the opioid.
- In a minority of patients, two or three different opioids will need to be tried before a balance is obtained between adequate pain relief and manageable side effects.
- A large interpatient variability is present in the way opioids are metabolized.
- If the pain control is good but significant side effects are present, reduce the equianalgesic dose of the new opioid by 50% (accommodates for cross tolerance). Continue to monitor the patient for adverse side effects and adequacy of pain relief. Provide for rescue doses as needed.
- If pain control is poor and significant side effects are present, reduce the equianalgesic dose by 25%–50%. Continue to monitor closely for reduction of adverse side effects and adequacy of pain relief. Provide for frequent rescue doses.
- If converting to methadone, decrease equianalgesic dose by 90% and monitor closely, especially during the first 10 days of methadone use, for signs of drug accumulation (e.g., sedation).
- In all situations of opioid rotation, monitor the patient closely for adequacy of pain relief and gradual clearing of adverse side effects.

Figure 19-10. Guidelines When Switching From One Opioid to Another

---

Note. Based on information from Davis & Walsh, 2001; De Stoutz et al., 1995; Hanks et al., 2004; Moryl et al., 2002; Ripamonti et al., 1998; and authors' clinical experience.

Selecting a Route and Dosing Intervals

The Route

Opioids should be administered by the least invasive and safest route capable of producing adequate analgesia. Clinical experience indicates that the majority of patients can use the oral route of drug administration throughout the course of most of their disease. However, at times, some patients become unable to use this route and require an alternate approach (Coyle, Adelhardt, Foley, & Portenoy, 1990). Nurses must be skilled in selecting among the alternate routes to meet the needs of a particular patient. The most commonly used alternate routes include rectal, sublingual, transmucosal, transdermal, subcutaneous, IV, epidural, and intrathecal.

Patient-controlled analgesia (PCA) is a method that refers to parenteral drug administration (IV or subcutaneous) in which the patient controls a pump that delivers analgesics according to parameters set by the nurse and/or physician. These parameters include concentration of the drug, basal infusion rate, and bolus or rescue doses that the patient can access for breakthrough pain. Use of a PCA device is fairly common in patients requiring a parenteral route of drug administration. This technique can be managed safely at home for most patients, provided that a system of education, monitoring, and support is in place (Coyle, Cherny, & Portenoy, 1994). The device could be a problem for older adults who are unfamiliar with this type of technology, are made nervous by it, or want no part of it. PCA is contraindicated in a patient who is confused or delirious.

The Dosing Interval

Patients with continuous or frequently occurring pain generally benefit from scheduled around-the-clock analgesic dosing (Jacox et al., 1994). This provides a more stable plasma level of the drug and helps to prevent pain from recurring. A rescue dose is offered on an as-needed basis and provides a means to treat pain that breaks through the fixed analgesic schedule. The drug used for breakthrough pain usually is the same as that administered on a regular basis. An alternative short half-life drug usually is recommended when using methadone or transdermal fentanyl (Hanks et al., 2004). Clinical guidelines suggest that the oral rescue dose in the older adult should be calculated as approximately 5%–15% of the 24-hour baseline dose (Jacox et al.).

Choice of a Starting Dose and Dose Titration

A patient who is relatively opioid naive generally should begin treatment at an opioid dose equivalent to 5–10 mg of parenteral morphine every four hours (Cherny & Portenoy, 1994b; NCCN, 2004). An older adult or frail patient with cancer may need to start at the lower end of the scale. Titration of the opioid dose usually is necessary at the start of pain therapy and at different points during the disease course. At all times, inadequate relief should be addressed with dose escalation until relief is reported or until intolerable and unmanageable side effects occur. Integration of around-the-clock dosing with supplemental rescue doses provides a rational stepwise approach to dose escalation and is appropriate to all routes of drug administration. Patients who require more than four to six rescue doses per day generally should undergo escalation of the baseline dose. In all cases, escalation of the baseline dose should be accompanied by a proportional increase in the rescue dose so that the size of the supplemental dose remains a constant percentage of the fixed dose (NCCN). Nursing assessment of the patient's pattern of pain, rescue use, and level of pain relief is essential for appropriate dose titration (see Figure 19-11).

- Three choices are available in titrating an opioid dose to a higher dose.
  - Increase the basal or around-the-clock (ATC) dose (oral, transdermal, subcutaneous, IV).
  - Increase the rescue dose.
  - Increase both the basal (ATC) dose and the rescue dose.
- Most patients will require an increase in both the basal (ATC) and rescue dose.
  - Calculate the number of rescue doses the patient has used in the past 24 hours.
  - Increase the basal (ATC) dose by that amount or by 25%–50%.
  - Then increase the rescue dose by 5%–15% of the new 24-hour dose.
- Monitor closely for effectiveness of new dose and presence of adverse effects, such as sedation and/or confusion.

Figure 19-11. Adjusting the Opioid Dose

Note. Based on clinical experience of the authors.

In patients who do not respond to opioid titration or who develop intolerable side effects, the following adjuvants should be considered: (a) a parenteral NSAID (e.g., ketorolac) for no longer than five days. During this period, other more long-term approaches for pain relief should be considered; (b) a parenteral steroid (e.g., dexamethasone), the dose gradually tapered down to the lowest effective dose for the patient. Anecdotal experience has shown the use of parenteral NSAIDs or steroids to be effective in a pain crisis associated with bone pain or neuropathic pain (Lussier & Portenoy, 2004). If the pain is predominantly neuropathic, IV ketamine or lidocaine can be helpful for some patients (Fine, 2000; Lussier & Portenoy). The pain and palliative care team must carefully weigh the risk/benefit ratio of these approaches for the older adult. The efficacy of a nerve block or spinal delivery system of drug administration for this particular clinical situation should be considered (Swarm, Karanikolas, & Cousins, 2004).

A proportion of patients with cancer will experience refractory symptoms at the end of life, including pain, that are not possible to control in the absence of sedation. The number of patients involved is not clear. Palliative sedation at the end of life is always an option for the patient (Chater, Viola, Paterson, & Jarvis, 1998; Cherny & Portenoy, 1994b; Morita, Inoue, & Chihara, 1996).

Opioid Side Effects and Their Management

Constipation

Older adults are particularly susceptible to opioid-induced constipation. Constipation can be life threatening in the debilitated older adult, especially if it is unrecognized and untreated. The initial presentation of opioid-induced constipation may be confusion in the older adult. Abdominal signs and symptoms, including pain, distention, and nausea, may be absent, and patients may present with confusion, depressed mood, and loss of appetite. Assessment of the older adult should include all medications, such as over-the-counter drugs—iron preparations, antacids, and drugs with anticholinergic properties—that may contribute to the constipation. A healthcare professional should routinely prescribe a bowel regimen (e.g., senna, stool softeners) for any patients receiving opioid analgesics (Hanks et al., 2004; Walsh, 1990). Rule of thumb: "The hand that writes the opioid prescription should also write the laxative prescription" (original source unknown). Fluids should be encouraged, although older patients may have difficulty taking in adequate amounts of oral fluids. Of note is that in the frail older adult, an increased intake of fluids may further worsen other symptoms, including peripheral edema, dyspnea, and ascites.

In cases of refractory opioid-induced constipation, naloxone, an opioid antagonist with an oral bioavailability of only 3%, can be given orally to produce "bowel withdrawal" through local action on opioid receptors in the gut without causing systemic opioid withdrawal. Because of individual variability, however, nurses must watch patients in whom this therapy is administered for symptoms indicative of systemic opioid withdrawal, such as abdominal cramping, diarrhea, rhinorrhea, muscle cramps, and feeling shivery or with "goose flesh" (Sykes, 1996; Yuan et al., 1997). Treatment always should start with a low dose, such as 0.4 mg by mouth once or twice daily, followed by dose escalation every few days. Clinical experience suggests oral doses such as 12–18 mg a day or higher may be needed to reverse opioid-induced constipation. Much-needed research continues in this area, as constipation is the one opioid side effect to which tolerance does not develop.

Sedation

Older patients may experience some level of sedation at the initiation of opioid therapy and during significant dose escalation. Patients usually develop tolerance to this effect in days or weeks (Bruera, Macmillan, & MacDonald, 1989; Bruera, Miller, McCallion, Macmillan, & Hanson, 1992; Hanks et al., 2004; Portenoy, 1994). Should sedation persist at a level that is unacceptable to the patient, the nurse should perform a careful assessment. Confounding factors such as other sedating drugs, metabolic disturbances, sleep deprivation, and the somnolence that may occur at end of life must be identified. Management steps include eliminating nonessential drugs with CNS depressant effects, reducing the opioid dose, if feasible, changing to an alternate opioid drug, and, if necessary, adding a psychostimulant (e.g., modafinil, methylphenidate) (Portenoy; Webster, Andrews, & Stoddard, 2003).

Confusion

Similar to sedation, mild cognitive impairment may occur after initiation of opioid therapy in the older adult (Bruera et al., 1989, 1992; Portenoy, 1994). Patients may express this as feeling "mentally hazy" or "not as sharp as before." Patients should be reassured that these effects are transient in most individuals and last from a few days to a week or two. If persistent, a change in opioid may be indicated. Persistent confusion attributable to opioids alone is uncommon. More commonly, confusion in the older adult is multifactorial, including electrolyte disorders, neoplastic involvement of the

CNS, sepsis, vital organ failure, and hypoxia (De Stoutz, Bruera, & Suarez-Almazor, 1995; Portenoy).

Nausea and Vomiting

Nausea and vomiting are common at the start of opioid therapy (Hanks et al., 2004; Portenoy, 1994). Tolerance to this effect typically develops within weeks. Both peripheral and central mechanisms are thought to be involved. Opioids stimulate the medullary chemoreceptor trigger zone and increase vestibular sensitivity. Direct effects on the gastrointestinal tract include increased gastric antral tone, diminished motility, and delayed gastric emptying (Hanks et al.; Portenoy). Constipation also may be a contributing factor. Establishing the pattern of nausea may clarify the etiology of the symptom and guide management approaches. For nausea associated with early satiation and bloating, metoclopramide often is the initial pharmacologic approach. If vertigo or movement-induced nausea is the predominant feature, the patient may benefit from an antivertiginous drug, such as scopolamine (transdermal) or meclizine. However, scopolamine may cause confusion in the older adult. Other options include trials of alternative opioids, treatment with an antihistamine (e.g., hydroxyzine, diphenhydramine), a neuroleptic (e.g., haloperidol, chlorpromazine), benzodiazepine (e.g., lorazepam), or a steroid (e.g., dexamethasone). The nurse should monitor the older patient for confusion and/or sedation when any new drugs are added to the regimen. The role of serotonin antagonists (e.g., ondansetron) has not been established in opioid-induced nausea and vomiting (Hanks et al.; Portenoy).

Multifocal Myoclonus

Mild and infrequent multifocal myoclonus can occur with all opioids (Hanks et al., 2004). The effect is dose-related, and the mechanism is unclear. Pronounced myoclonus is extremely distressing to the patient. The uncontrolled, abrupt, jerking movements of the patient's limbs and/or torso can increase already existing pain. Myoclonus can be a sign of opioid toxicity and is a reason to switch to an alternate opioid. In addition, a benzodiazepine (e.g., clonazepam) can be used to treat the symptom (Portenoy, 1994).

Urinary Retention

Urinary retention can occur in patients receiving opioid drugs, especially in those who require rapid escalation of the drug, are receiving other drugs with anticholinergic effects such as the tricyclic antidepressants, or have compromised bladder function. Older men with an enlarged prostate are particularly at risk. Opioids increase smooth muscle tone and infrequently cause bladder spasm or an increase in sphincter tone, which may lead to urinary retention (Hanks et al., 2004).

Pruritus

Pruritus can occur with any of the opioids, is associated with histamine release, and is seen most commonly with morphine use. Fentanyl and oxymorphone may be associated with less histamine release (American Pain Society, 2003). Ondansetron has been reported to relieve opioid-related pruritus (Larijani, Goldberg, & Rogers,

1996). Antihistamines often are a first-line approach if pruritus is troublesome to the patient. However, sedation may be a problem for the older adult.

Respiratory Depression

Fear of respiratory depression is a frequently cited concern among medical and nursing staff when initiating opioid therapy or when rapidly increasing opioid drugs to control pain in a debilitated older adult. Clinically significant respiratory depression always is accompanied by other signs of CNS depression such as sedation and mental clouding and is unusual in the patient receiving chronic opioid therapy unless other contributing factors are present. Pain antagonizes CNS depression, and respiratory effects are unlikely to occur in the presence of severe pain. With repeated administration of an opioid, tolerance develops rapidly to the respiratory depressant effects of the drug (Foley, 1991). Unwarranted fears of respiratory depression should not interfere with appropriate upward titration of opioid drugs for pain relief (American Pain Society, 2003; Brescia, Portenoy, Ryan, Drasnoff, & Gray, 1992). Opioid-induced respiratory depression, however, can occur if the patient's pain is abruptly eliminated (e.g., after a neurolytic or neuroablative procedure) and the opioid drug is not reduced.

Adjuvant Analgesia

Adjuvant analgesics are those drugs that have a primary indication other than pain but are analgesic in certain pain states (see Table 19-4). These drugs can be used at any step of the analgesic ladder. As with the institution of any analgesic regimen, their use is based on a careful assessment of the pain, inferred pain mechanism(s), and analgesic history. Adjuvant drugs in the palliative care setting typically are used to enhance the effects of the opioid drugs or to allow for dose reduction because of adverse opioid side effects (Lussier & Portenoy, 2004). It is useful to classify the adjuvant analgesics into three broad groups: multipurpose adjuvant analgesics, adjuvant analgesics used primarily for neuropathic pain, and adjuvant analgesics used for bone pain (see Figure 19-12). As a general principle, in the older patient with cancer, low initial doses with dose titration should be administered until symptom relief is achieved (see Figure 19-13).

Bone Pain

Bone pain can be an extremely troublesome problem for patients with advanced disease. As previously described, NSAIDs can be helpful in combination with opioid drugs (steps 2 and 3 of the analgesic ladder). Parenteral NSAIDs as well as corticosteroids can produce dramatic relief for the patient with bone pain who presents in a pain crisis. They should not be given simultaneously. Bisphosphonates inhibit osteoclast-mediated bone resorption and help to alleviate pain related to metastatic bone disease and multiple myeloma (Berenson, Lichtenstein, & Porter, 1996; Walker et al., 2002; Wong & Wiffen, 2002).

Radiation therapy is extremely helpful in relieving painful bone lesions (Janjan, 2001). In some instances, single fraction external beam therapy can be used (Jeremic, 2001). Onset of relief can be fairly rapid, often within days of treatment, and may be a helpful intervention when patients are having inadequate relief from opioid

Table 19-4. Adjuvants: Co-Analgesics for Pain That Also Are Used for Treatment of Some Opioid-Related Side Effects*

Drug	Description	Comments
Tricyclic antidepressants Adjunct to other therapies for pain (amitriptyline, desipramine, nortriptyline)	Used for burning neuropathic pain. Additional benefits are antidepressant properties and aid to sleep.	Anticholinergic effects may outweigh benefits in the older adult; desipramine or nortriptyline is a better choice than amitriptyline in this age group. Start low and increase slowly.
Anticonvulsants (gabapentin, carbamazepine)	Used for lancinating neuropathic pain	Start low and increase slowly. Gabapentin may cause dizziness in older adults, increasing the risk for falls.
Local anesthetics (lidocaine, IV or transdermal patch, EMLA® cream)	Used for neuropathic pain	IV lidocaine is associated with delirium. Trial in refractory neuropathic pain.
Oral local anesthetics (mexiletine)	Used for neuropathic pain	Common side effects include tremor, dizziness, paresthesias; rarely may cause blood dyscrasias and hepatic damage. Avoid use in patients with preexisting heart disease. Start low and titrate slowly. Not considered first-line drug. Monitor electrocardiograms.
Muscle relaxants (baclofen, chlorzoxazone, cyclobenzaprine)	Antispasmodic agents	Monitor for sedation and anticholinergic effects. Taper baclofen if to be discontinued. Abrupt withdrawal may cause central nervous system irritability. Baclofen can be administered orally or intrathecally.
Capsaicin—topical	Substance P inhibitor. Is an enzyme found in all hot peppers	Must be applied three to four times daily to affected area. Initially causes local burning sensation and limits acceptability to many patients. Tolerance develops to this sensation. May take two to three weeks for maximum analgesic response. Can be partially removed with vegetable oil.
Alpha-2 adrenergic agonists (clonidine)	Clonidine is useful for difficult-to-control pain.	Can be used in combination with an opioid epidurally
N-methyl–D-aspartate (NMDA) receptor antagonists (dextromethorphan, ketamine, amantadine)	NMDA antagonists Ketamine potent anesthetic in higher doses Parenteral ketamine in lower doses useful for refractory neuropathic pain	Use with caution because of psychomimetic effects. Can be given IV, subcutaneous, or po. Consult with anesthesia colleagues.

(Continued on next page)

Table 19-4. Adjuvants: Co-Analgesics for Pain That Also Are Used for Treatment of Some Opioid-Related Side Effects* *(Continued)*

Drug	Description	Comments
Corticosteroids (dexamethasone, prednisone)	Powerful anti-inflammatory, reduces edema Higher doses used in cord compression	Useful for pain from infiltration of neural structures; bone pain, pain crisis. May cause delirium.
Neuroleptics (haloperidol)	Commonly used for side effects associated with opioids (e.g., delirium and pain complicated by delirium or nausea)	Can be given po or IV Available in concentrated liquid form for oral use
Analeptics (methylphenidate, modafinil)	Useful to treat opioid-related sedation	Methylphenidate also used as a rapid onset antidepressant. May be used in combination with a standard antidepressant while awaiting antidepressant effects
Bisphosphonates (pamidronate)	Used for bone pain. Inhibits osteoclast activity	Monitor calcium, phosphate, magnesium, and potassium blood levels.
Bowel obstruction (octreotide)	Reduces secretions. Useful for conservative management of bowel obstruction causing abdominal pain and nausea	–

* This table is to be used as a guide only and is not to replace a more comprehensive review.

Note. From "Principles of Analgesic Use in the Treatment of Acute Pain and Cancer Pain" (5th ed., p. 221), by B. Ferrell and J.E. Whiteman in R.S. Morrison and D.E. Meier (Eds.), *Geriatric Palliative Care*, 2003, New York: Oxford University Press. Copyright 2003 by Oxford University Press. Adapted with permission.

Multipurpose adjuvants
- Corticosteroids (neuropathic pain, bone pain, liver capsule pain)
- Benzodiazepines (lancinating neuropathic pain, muscle spasms)

Adjuvants used primarily for neuropathic pain
- Antidepressants (e.g., nortriptyline or desipramine for continuous dysesthesias)
- Anticonvulsants (e.g., gabapentin for sharp, shooting, stabbing component)
- GABA (gamma-aminobutyric acid) agonists (e.g., baclofen for lancinating and paroxysmal pain)
- Alpha-2 adrenergic antagonists (e.g., clonidine for pain refractory to opioids)
- Local anesthetics (second-line drugs for patients who have not responded to antidepressants and anticonvulsant adjuvants; route can be oral or epidural combined with an opioid)
- Topical local anesthetic (e.g., EMLA® cream, Lidoderm® patch)
- Topical capsaicin (unpleasant burning sensation limits patient acceptability)
- N-methyl–D-aspartate receptor agonists (e.g., dextromethorphan). Ketamine (for refractory neuropathic pain)—use with caution because of psychomimetic effects.

Figure 19-12. Adjuvant Analgesics Commonly Used for Pain

Note. Based on information from Fine, 2004; Lussier & Portenoy, 2004; McQuay & Moore, 2004.

- The older adult is more susceptible to adverse side effects of pharmacotherapy (e.g., sedation, orthostatic hypotension, constipation, dry mouth, dizziness); therefore, start low and go slow.
- Side effects make the older adult more susceptible to falls.
- If a tricyclic antidepressant is the adjuvant drug of choice for the older adult, choose one with less potent anticholinergic effects, such as nortriptyline or desipramine.
- Start low and increase the dose every few days.

Figure 19-13. Adjuvant Analgesics Used Primarily for Neuropathic Pain in the Older Adult—Key Points

Note. Based on clinical experience of the authors.

and adjuvant therapy alone. Patients should be warned, however, that a transitory pain flare may occur at the start of radiation therapy, and analgesics may need to be titrated if that occurs. Radionuclide therapy also may be helpful when widespread bony metastatic disease is present that cannot be easily targeted with localized radiotherapy (Serafini, 2001).

Invasive Approaches

Anesthetic and neurosurgical approaches are indicated when conservative measures using opioids and adjuvant analgesics have failed to provide adequate analgesia or when the patient is experiencing intolerable side effects from systemic opioids (Saberski, 1998; Swarm et al., 2004). The use of these approaches is not contraindicated in the older adult. These procedures include regional analgesia, sympathetic blockade and neurolytic procedures, or pathway ablation procedures (e.g., chemical or surgical rhizotomy, cordotomy). These approaches may be useful in some older patients who have intractable pain that cannot be managed with systemic treatment.

Complementary and Alternative Therapies in the Management of Pain in the Older Adult

As with pain control in general, a variety of factors promote or inhibit the use of nondrug techniques (Decker, 2000; Loscalzo, 1996). Patients independently initiate nondrug interventions such as applying heat, cold, or vibration. The different methods patients choose frequently are based on previous use or word of mouth. Compared to the extensive studies that support the use of pharmacologic techniques, no strong evidence base supports the efficacy of many of these techniques. However, patients report using them and finding them extremely helpful (Johansson, Dahl, Jannert, Melin, & Anderson, 1998; Kwekkeboom, Kneip, & Pearson, 2003; Magill, 2001; Meek, 1993; Post-White et al., 2003; Rhiner, Ferrell, Ferrell, & Grant, 1993; Spiegel & Moore, 1997; Stephenson, Dalton, & Carlson, 2003; Syrjala, Donaldson, Davis, Kippes, & Carr, 1995; Weinrich & Weinrich, 1990; Zappa & Cassileth, 2003). The five main categories of nondrug approaches to pain management are psychological interventions, physiatric interventions, neurostimulatory interventions, invasive interventions, and integrative interventions. The reader is referred to more specific texts for detailed discussion of these approaches.

Discharge Planning and Follow-Up

Discharge planning and follow-up are extraordinarily important in the care of the older adult with pain (Ferrell, B.R., 1996; Ferrell et al., 1994). The older adult may live alone or with an elderly spouse and frequently has limited financial resources. In addition, the older adult's ability to independently self-medicate and participate in the pain management plan may be affected by functional factors such as impaired vision, impaired fine motor skill of the hands, memory problems, and cognitive impairments. The older adult may run into other difficulties when trying to put a pain management regimen into place at home. These include being unable to obtain the prescribed medications either because they are not available from their community pharmacist or they have no prescription plan and are financially burdened; having difficulty in cognitively processing information and tailoring the prescribed regimen to their home routine and individual needs; and managing side effects and multiple symptoms simultaneously.

Paying attention to certain pain management details before the older adult is discharged home can make a huge difference to his or her well-being and will help to facilitate continued pain control during the transition from hospital to home. For example, prior to discharge, the healthcare professional should establish if the prescribed analgesics are available in the patient's community pharmacy and if the patient has an outpatient prescription plan or is able to pay for the pain medication out of pocket. In addition, older adults must be given sufficient medication at time of discharge to continue their pain management regimen until they are able to have their prescription filled at a community pharmacy (Coyle, 2001).

Conclusion

Nurses, as core members of an interdisciplinary pain team, play a huge role in the management of pain in the older adult with cancer across all care settings, both as expert clinician and patient/family advocate. Poorly controlled pain in the older adult can lead to cognitive failure, insomnia, depression, and mood disturbances, all factors that negatively affect quality of life. Barriers to effective analgesic use frequently stem from misconceptions, lack of education, and financial concerns. In addition, aging causes physiologic changes that alter the pharmacokinetics and pharmacodynamics of analgesics, thus making the older adult more susceptible to the toxicities of polypharmacy.

Because of the central role of oncology nurses in the care of older patients with cancer throughout the course of their disease and because of the prevalence of pain in this population, knowledge in the basic principles of pain assessment and management in the older patient with cancer is imperative for competent, safe, and compassionate practice.

References

Abbey, J.A., Piller, N., De Bellis, A., Esterman, A., Parker, D., Giles, L., et al. (2004). The Abbey pain scale: A 1-minute numerical indicator for people with end-stage dementia. *International Journal of Palliative Nursing, 10,* 6–13.

Ahles, T.A., Blanchard, E.B., & Ruckdeschel, J.C. (1983). The multidimensional nature of cancer-related pain. *Pain, 17,* 277–288.

American Geriatrics Society. (2002). The management of persistent pain in older persons. *Journal of the American Geriatrics Society, 50*(Suppl. 6), S205–S224.

American Pain Society. (2003). *Principles of analgesic use in the treatment of acute pain and cancer pain* (5th ed.). Glenview, IL: Author.

Anderson, G., Jensen, N.H., Christrup, L., Hansen, S.H., & Sjogren, P. (2002). Pain, sedation and morphine metabolism in cancer patients during long term treatment with sustained–release morphine. *Palliative Medicine, 16,* 107–114.

Bates, M.S. (1987). Ethnicity and pain: A bicultural model. *Social Science and Medicine, 25,* 47–50.

Berenson, J.R., Lichtenstein, A., & Porter, L. (1996). Efficacy of pamidronate in reduction of skeletal events in patients with advanced multiple myeloma. *New England Journal of Medicine, 334,* 488–493.

Bernabei, R., Bambassi, G., Lapane, K., Landi, F., Gatsonis, C., Dunlop, R., et al. (1998). Management of pain in elderly patients with cancer. *JAMA, 279,* 1877–1882.

Brescia, F., Portenoy, R.K., Ryan, M., Drasnoff, L., & Gray, G. (1992). Pain, opioid use and survival in hospitalized patients with advanced cancer. *Journal of Clinical Oncology, 10,* 149–155.

Bruera, E., Macmillan, K., & MacDonald, N. (1989). The cognitive effects of the administration of narcotic analgesics in patients with cancer pain. *Pain, 39,* 13–26.

Bruera, E., Miller, L., McCallion, J., Macmillan, K., & Hanson, J. (1992). Cognitive failure in patients with terminal cancer, a prospective study. *Journal of Pain and Symptom Management, 7,* 192–195.

Chater, S., Viola, R., Paterson, J., & Jarvis, V. (1998). Sedation for intractable distress in the dying. A survey of experts. *Palliative Medicine, 12,* 255–269.

Cherny, N., & Coyle, N. (1994). Suffering in the advanced cancer patient: A definition and taxonomy. *Journal of Palliative Care, 10,* 57–70.

Cherny, N., & Coyle, N. (1999). Ethical principles in the management of cancer pain. In G.M. Aronoff (Ed.), *Evaluation and treatment of chronic pain* (3rd ed., pp. 643–654). Baltimore: Williams & Wilkins.

Cherny, N., & Portenoy, R.K. (1994a). The management of cancer pain. *CA: A Cancer Journal for Clinicians, 44,* 262–303.

Cherny, N., & Portenoy, R.K. (1994b). Sedation in the management of refractory symptoms: Guidelines for evaluation and treatment. *Journal of Palliative Care, 10,* 31–38.

Christie, J.M., Simmonds, M., Patt, R., Coluzzi, P., Busch, M.A., Nordbrock, E., et al. (1998). Dose titration: A multicenter study of oral transmucosal fentanyl citrate for the treatment of breakthrough pain in cancer patients using transdermal fentanyl for persistent pain. *Journal of Clinical Oncology, 16,* 3238–3245.

Cleeland, C.E. (1989). Pain control: Public and physicians' attitudes. In C.S. Hill & W.S. Fields (Eds.), *Drug treatment of cancer pain in a drug-oriented society. Advances in pain research and therapy* (pp. 81–89). New York: Raven.

Cleeland, C.S., Gonin, R., Baez, L., Loehrer, P., & Pandya, K.J. (1997). Pain and treatment of pain in minority patients with cancer. The Eastern Cooperative Oncology Group Minority Outpatient Study. *Annals of Internal Medicine, 127,* 813–816.

Cleeland, C.S., Gonin, R., Hatfield, A.K., Edmonson, J.H., Blum, R.H., Stewart, J.A., et al. (1994). Pain and its treatment in outpatients with metastatic cancer. *New England Journal of Medicine, 330,* 592–596.

Coyle, N. (1995). Suffering in the first person. In B.R. Ferrell (Ed.), *Suffering* (pp. 29–64). Sudbury, MA: Jones and Bartlett.

Coyle, N. (2001). Facilitating pain management in the home: Opioid-related issues. *Current Pain and Headaches Reports, 5,* 217–226.

Coyle, N. (2004). In their own words: Seven advanced cancer patients describe their experience with pain and the use of opioid drugs. *Journal of Pain and Symptom Management, 27,* 300–309.

Coyle, N., Adelhardt, J., Foley, K.M., & Portenoy, R.K. (1990). Character of terminal illness in the advanced cancer patient: Pain and other symptoms in the last four weeks of life. *Journal of Pain and Symptom Management, 5,* 83–93.

Coyle, N., Cherny, N.I., & Portenoy, R.K. (1994). Subcutaneous infusions at home. *Oncology, 8,* 21–32.

Coyle, N., & Portenoy, R.K. (1995). Pharmacologic management of cancer pain. In D.B. McGuire, C.H. Yarbro, & B.R. Ferrell (Eds.), *Cancer pain management* (2nd ed., pp. 89–130). Sudbury, MA: Jones and Bartlett.

Daut, R.L., Cleeland, C.S., & Flanery, R.C. (1983). Development of the Wisconsin Brief Pain Questionnaire to assess pain in cancer and other diseases. *Pain, 17,* 197–210.

Davis, M.P., & Walsh, D. (2001). Methadone for the relief of cancer pain: A review of pharmaco-kinetics, pharmacodynamics, drug interactions and protocols of administration. *Supportive Care in Cancer, 9,* 73–83.

De Stoutz, N., Bruera, E., & Suarez-Almazor, M.E. (1995). Opioid rotation for toxicity reduction in terminal cancer patients. *Journal of Pain and Symptom Management, 10,* 378–384.

Decker, G.M. (2000). An overview of complementary and alternative therapies. *Clinical Journal of Oncology Nursing, 4,* 49–52.

Doloplus Group. (2001). *Doloplus 2 Scale.* Retrieved July 1, 2004, from http://www.doloplus.com/versiongb/index.htm

Drage, M.P., & Schug, S.A. (1996). Analgesia in the elderly. Practical treatment recommendations. *Drugs and Aging, 9,* 311–318.

Fainsinger, R., Schoeller, T., Boiskin, M., & Bruera, E. (1993). Palliative care round: Cognitive failure and coma after renal failure in a patient receiving captopril and hydromorphone. *Journal of Palliative Care, 9,* 53–55.

Fainsinger, R., Schoeller, T., & Bruera, E. (1993). Methadone in the management of cancer pain: A review. *Pain, 52,* 137–147.

Feldt, K.S. (2000). Improving assessment and treatment of pain in cognitively impaired nursing home residents. *Annals of Long-Term Care, 8*(9), 36–42.

Feldt, K.S., Ryden, M.B., & Miles, S. (1998). Treatment of pain in cognitively impaired compared to cognitively intact older adults with hip fracture. *Journal of the American Geriatrics Society, 46,* 1079–1085.

Ferrell, B.A. (1995). Pain evaluation and management in the nursing home. *Annals of Internal Medicine, 123,* 681–687.

Ferrell, B.A. (1996). Overview of aging and pain. In B.R. Ferrell & B.A. Ferrell (Eds.), *Pain in the elderly* (pp. 1–10). Seattle, WA: IASP Press.

Ferrell, B.A., & Whiteman, J.E. (2003). Pain. In R.S. Morrison & D.E. Meier (Eds.), *Geriatric palliative care* (pp. 205–229). New York: Oxford University Press.

Ferrell, B.R. (1996). Patient education and non-drug interventions. In B.R. Ferrell & B.A. Ferrell (Eds.), *Pain in the elderly* (pp. 35–44). Seattle, WA: IASP Press.

Ferrell, B.R., Ferrell, B.A., Ahn, C., & Tran, K. (1994). Pain management for elderly patients with cancer at home. *Cancer, 74*(Suppl. 7), 2139–2146.

Ferrell, B.R., Grant, M., Chan, J., Ahn, C., & Ferrell, B.A. (1995). The impact of cancer pain education on family caregivers of elderly patients. *Oncology Nursing Forum, 22,* 1211–1218.

Ferrell, B.R., Rhiner, M., Cohen, M.Z., & Grant, M. (1991). Pain as a metaphor for illness. Part 1: Impact of pain on family caregivers. *Oncology Nursing Forum, 18,* 1303–1309.

Fine, P.G. (2000). Low-dose ketamine in the management of opioid non-responsive terminal cancer pain. *Journal of Pain and Symptom Management, 17,* 296–300.

Fine, P.G. (2001). Opioid analgesic drugs in older people. *Clinical Geriatric Medicine, 17,* 479–487.

Fine, P.G. (2004). Pharmacological management of persistent pain in older patients. *Clinical Journal of Pain, 20,* 220–226.

Fishman, B., Pasternak, S., Wallenstein, S.L., Houde, R.W., Holland, J.C., & Foley, K.M. (1987). The Memorial Pain Assessment Card. A valid instrument for the evaluation of cancer pain. *Cancer, 60,* 1151–1158.

Foley, K.M. (1991). The relationship of pain and symptom management to patient requests for physician-assisted suicide. *Journal of Pain and Symptom Management, 6,* 289–297.

Foley, K.M. (1993). Changing concepts of tolerance to opioids: What the cancer patient has taught us. In C.R. Chapman & K.M. Foley (Eds.), *Current and emerging issues in cancer pain: Research and practice* (pp. 331–350). New York: Raven.

Foley, K.M. (2004). Acute and chronic pain syndromes. In D. Doyle, G. Hanks, N. Cherny, & K. Calman (Eds.), *Oxford textbook of palliative medicine* (3rd ed., pp. 298–316). Oxford, United Kingdom: Oxford University Press.

Fuchs-Lacelle, S., & Hadjistavropoulos, T. (2004). Development and preliminary validation of the Pain Assessment Checklist for Seniors with Limited Ability to Communicate (PACSLAC). *Pain Management Nursing, 5,* 37–49.

Gibson, S.J., & Helme, R.D. (2001). Age related differences in pain perception and report. *Clinical Geriatric Medicine, 17,* 433–456.

Gonzales, G.R., & Coyle, N. (1992). Treatment of cancer pain in a former opioid abuser: Fears of the patient and staff and their influence on care. *Journal of Pain and Symptom Management, 7,* 246–249.

Gourlay, G.K., Plummer, J.L., Cherry, D.A., & Purser, T. (1991). The reproducibility of bioavailability of oral morphine under fed and fasted conditions. *Journal of Pain and Symptom Management, 6,* 431–436.

Hanks, G.W., Cherny, N.I., & Fallon, M. (2004). Opioid analgesic therapy. In D. Doyle, G. Hanks, N. Cherny, & K. Calman (Eds.), *Oxford textbook of palliative medicine* (3rd ed., pp. 316–341). Oxford, United Kingdom: Oxford University Press.

Helme, R.D., & Gibson, S.J. (2000). Pain in older people. In I.K. Cronbie, R. Croft, S.J. Linton, L. Leresche, & M. Von Dorff (Eds.), *Epidemiology of pain* (pp. 103–112). Seattle, WA: IASP Press.

Herr, K., Decker, S., & Bjoro, K. (2004). *State of the art review of tools for assessment of pain in nonverbal adults.* Retrieved July 1, 2004, from http://www.cityofhope.org/prc

Herr, K.A., & Mobily, P.R. (1991). Pain assessment in the elderly. *Journal of Gerontological Nursing, 17,* 12–19.

Hewitt, D.J., & Foley, K.M. (1997). Pain and pain management. In C.K. Cassel, H.J. Cohen, E.B. Larson, D.E. Meier, N.M. Resnick, L.Z. Rubenstein, et al. (Eds.), *Geriatric medicine* (3rd ed., pp. 865–882). New York: Springer-Verlag.

Hofmann, M.T., Farnon, C.U., Javed, A., & Posner, J.D. (1998). Pain in the elderly hospice patient. *American Journal of Hospice and Palliative Care, 15,* 259–265.

Houde, R.W. (1986). Clinical analgesic studies of hydromorphone. In K.M. Foley & C.E. Inturrisi (Eds.), *Advances in pain research and therapy* (pp. 129–136). New York: Raven.

Hunt, G., & Bruera, E. (1995). Respiratory depression in a patient receiving oral methadone for cancer pain. *Journal of Pain and Symptom Management, 10,* 401–404.

Hurley, A.C., Volicer, B.J., Hanrahan, P.A., Houde, S., & Volicer, L. (1992). Assessment of discomfort in advanced Alzheimer patients. *Research in Nursing and Health, 15,* 369–377.

Jacox, A., Carr, D.B., Payne, R., Berde, C.B., Breitbart, W., & Cain, I.M. (1994). *Management of cancer pain. Clinical practice guideline No. 9.* AHCPR Publication No. 94–0592. Rockville, MD: Agency for Health Care Policy and Research, U.S. Department of Health and Human Services, Public Health Services.

Jaffe, J.H., & Martin, W.R. (1990). Opioid analgesics and antagonists. In A.G. Gilman, T.W. Rall, A.S. Nies, & P. Taylor (Eds.), *Goodman and Gilman's the pharmacological basis of therapeutics* (8th ed., pp. 485–521). New York: Pergamon Press.

Janjan, N. (2001). Bone metastasis: approaches to management. *Seminars in Oncology, 28*(Suppl. 11), 28–34.

Jenkins, C.A., & Bruera, E. (1999). Nonsteroidal anti-inflammatory drugs as adjuvant analgesics in cancer patients. *Palliative Medicine, 13,* 183–196.

Jeremic, B. (2001). Single fraction external beam radiation therapy in the treatment of localized metastatic bone pain. A review. *Journal of Pain and Symptom Management, 22,* 1048–1058.

Johansson, C., Dahl, J., Jannert, M., Melin, L., & Anderson, G. (1998). Effects of a cognitive behavioral pain-management program. *Behavior Research and Therapy, 36,* 915–930.

Kaiko, R.F. (1983). Central nervous system excitatory effects of meperidine in cancer patients. *Annals of Neurology, 13,* 180–185.

Kalso, E., & Vainio, A. (1990). Morphine and oxycodone hydrochloride in the management of cancer pain. *Clinical Pharmacology and Therapeutics, 47,* 639–646.

Kornick, C.A., Kilborn, M.J., Santiago-Palma, J., Schulman, G., Thaler, H.T., Keefe, D.L., et al. (2003). QT interval prolongation associated with intravenous methadone. *Pain, 105,* 499–506.

Kovach, C.R., Weissman, D.E., Griffie, J., Matson, S., & Muchka, S. (1999). Assessment and treatment of discomfort for people with late-stage dementia. *Journal of Pain and Symptom Management, 18,* 412–419.

Kranz, M.J., Kutinsky, I.B., Robertson, A.D., & Mehler, P.S. (2003). Dose-related effects of methadone on QT prolongation in a series of patients with torsade de pointes. *Pharmacotherapy, 23,* 802–805.

Kwekkeboom, K.L., Kneip, J., & Pearson, L. (2003). A pilot study to predict success with guided imagery for cancer pain. *Pain Management Nursing, 4,* 112–123.

Larijani, G.E., Goldberg, M.E., & Rogers, K.H. (1996). Treatment of opioid-induced pruritus with ondansetron: Report of four patients. *Pharmacotherapy, 16,* 958–960.

Lasch, K., Greenhill, A., Wilkes, G., Carr, D., Lee, M., & Blanchard, R. (2002). Why study pain? A qualitative analysis of medical and nursing faculty and student's knowledge of and attitudes to cancer pain management. *Journal of Palliative Medicine, 5,* 57–71.

Lee, M.A., Leng, M.E., & Tierman, E.J. (2001). Retrospective study of the use of hydromorphone in palliative care patients with normal and abnormal urea and creatinine. *Journal of Palliative Medicine, 15,* 26–34.

Loscalzo, M. (1996). Psychological approaches to the management of pain in patients with advanced cancer. *Hematology/Oncology Clinics of North America, 10,* 139–155.

Lussier, D., & Portenoy, R.K. (2004). Adjuvant analgesics in pain management. In D. Doyle, G. Hanks, N. Cherny, & K. Calman (Eds.), *Oxford textbook of palliative medicine* (3rd ed., pp. 349–377). Oxford, United Kingdom: Oxford University Press.

Magill, L. (2001). The use of music therapy to address suffering in advanced cancer pain. *Journal of Palliative Care, 17*, 167–172.

Manfredi, P.L., Ribeiro, S.W., & Payne, R. (1996). Inappropriate use of naloxone in cancer patients with pain. *Journal of Pain and Symptom Management, 11*, 131–134.

McGuire, D.B. (1995). The multiple dimensions of cancer pain: A framework for assessment and management. In D.B. McGuire, C.H. Yarbro, & B.R. Ferrell (Eds.), *Cancer pain management* (2nd ed., pp. 1–17). Sudbury, MA: Jones and Bartlett.

McQuay, H.J., & Moore, A. (2004). Non-opioid analgesics. In D. Doyle, G. Hanks, N. Cherny, & K. Calman (Eds.), *Oxford textbook of palliative medicine* (3rd ed., pp. 342–349). Oxford, United Kingdom: Oxford University Press.

Meek, S.S. (1993). Effects of slow stroke back massage on relaxation in hospice clients. *Image: The Journal of Nursing Scholarship, 25*, 17–21.

Menten, J., Desmedt, M., Lossignol, D., & Mullie, A. (2002). Longitudinal follow-up of TTS-fentanyl use in patients with cancer-related pain: Results of a compassionate-use study with special focus on elderly patients. *Current Medical Research and Opinion, 18*, 488–498.

Merkel, S.I., Voepel-Lewis, T., Shayevitz, J.R., & Malviya, S. (1997). The FLACC: A behavioral scale for scoring postoperative pain in young children. *Pediatric Nursing, 23*, 293–297.

Meuser, T., Pietruck, C., Radbruch, L., Stute, P., Lehmann, K.A., & Grond, S. (2001). Symptoms during cancer treatment following WHO-guidelines: A longitudinal follow-up study of symptom prevalence, severity and etiology. *Pain, 93*, 247–257.

Miaskowski, C. (2000). The impact of age on a patient's perception of pain and ways it can be managed. *Pain Management Nursing, 1*(Suppl. 1), 2–7.

Miaskowski, C. (2002). The need to assess multiple symptoms. *Pain Management Nursing, 3*, 115.

Morita, T., Ichiki, T., Tsunoda, J., Inoue, S., & Chihara, S. (1998). A prospective study on the dying process in terminally ill cancer patients. *American Journal of Hospice and Palliative Care, 15*, 217–222.

Morita, T., Inoue, S., & Chihara, S. (1996). Sedation for symptom control in Japan: The importance of intermittent use and communication with family members. *Journal of Pain and Symptom Management, 12*, 32–38.

Morley, J.S., Bridson, J., Nash, T.P., Miles, J.B., White, S., & Makin, M.K. (2003). Low-dose methadone has an analgesic effect in neuropathic pain: A double-blind randomized controlled crossover trial. *Palliative Medicine, 17*, 576–587.

Morrison, R.S., & Sui, A.L. (2000). A comparison of pain and its treatment in advanced dementia and cognitively intact patients with hip fracture. *Journal of Pain and Symptom Management, 19*, 240–248.

Moryl, N., Santiago-Palma, J., Kornick, C., Derby, S., Fishberg, D., Payne, R., et al. (2002). Pitfalls of opioid rotation: Substituting another opioid for methadone in patients with cancer pain. *Pain, 96*, 325–328.

National Comprehensive Cancer Network. (2004). *Clinical practice guidelines in oncology*. Retrieved July 10, 2004, from http://www.nccn.org

National Institutes of Health. (2002, July). *NIH state-of-the-science statement on symptom management in cancer: Pain, depression, and fatigue*. Retrieved July 10, 2004, from http://consensus.nih.gov/ta/022/022_intro.htm

Ng, K., & von Gunten, C.F. (1998). Symptoms and attitudes of 100 consecutive patients admitted to an acute hospice/palliative care unit. *Journal of Pain and Symptom Management, 16*, 307–316.

O'Brien, S., Dalton, J.A., Konsler, G., & Carlson, J. (1996). The knowledge and attitudes of experienced oncology nurses regarding the management of cancer-related pain. *Oncology Nursing Forum, 23*, 515–521.

Paice, J.A. (1999). Symptom management. In C. Miaskowski & P. Buchscl (Eds.), *Oncology nursing: Assessment and clinical care*. St. Louis, MO: Mosby.

Paice, J.A., Toy, C., & Shott, S. (1998). Barriers to cancer pain relief: Fear of tolerance and addiction. *Journal of Pain and Symptom Management, 16*, 1–9.

Passik, S.D., Portenoy, R.K., & Ricketts, P.L. (1998). Substance abuse issues in cancer patients. Part 1: Prevalence and diagnosis. *Oncology, 12*, 517–521.

Payne, R., Chandler, S.W., & Einhaus, E. (1995). Guidelines for the clinical use of transdermal fentanyl. *Anti-Cancer Drugs, 6*, 50–53.

Payne, R., & Gonzales, R.G. (2004). Pathophysiology of pain in cancer and other terminal diseases. In D. Doyle, G. Hanks, N. Cherny, & K. Calman (Eds.), *Oxford textbook of palliative medicine* (3rd ed., pp. 288–298). Oxford, United Kingdom: Oxford University Press.

Perry, S., & Heidrich, G. (1982). Management of pain during debridement: A survey of U.S. burn units. *Pain, 13,* 267–280.

Portenoy, R.K. (1994). Management of common opioid side effects during long-term therapy of cancer pain. *Annals of the Academy of Medicine, Singapore, 23,* 160–170.

Portenoy, R.K., Dole, V., Joseph, H., Lowinson, J., Rice, C., Segal, S., et al. (1997). Pain management and chemical dependency: Evolving perspectives. *Journal of the American Academy of Medicine, 278,* 592–593.

Portenoy, R.K., Thaler, H.T., Inturrisi, C.E., Friedlander-Klar, H., & Foley, K.M. (1992). The metabolite morphine-6-glucuronide contributes to the analgesia produced by morphine infusion in patients with pain and normal renal function. *Clinical Pharmacology and Therapeutics, 51,* 422–431.

Portenoy, R.K., Thaler, H.T., Kornblith, A.B., Lepore, J.M., Friedlander, K.H., & Coyle, N. (1994). Symptom prevalence, characteristics and distress in a cancer population. *Quality of Life Research, 3,* 183–189.

Porter, J., & Jick, H. (1980). Addiction rare in patients treated with narcotics. *New England Journal of Medicine, 302,* 123.

Post-White, J., Kinney, M.E., Savik, K., Gau, J.B., Wilcox, C., & Lerner, I. (2003). Therapeutic massage and healing touch improve symptoms in cancer. *Integrative Cancer Therapeutics, 2,* 332–344.

Poyhia, R., Vainio, A., & Kalso, E. (1993). A review of oxycodone's clinical pharmacokinetics and pharmacodynamics. *Journal of Pain and Symptom Management, 8,* 63–67.

Radbruch, L., Sabatowski, R., Petzke, F., Brunsch-Radbruch, A., Grond, S., & Lehmann, K.A. (2001). Transdermal fentanyl for the management of cancer pain: A survey of 1,005 patients. *Palliative Medicine, 15,* 309–321.

Rhiner, M., Ferrell, B.R., Ferrell, B.A., & Grant, M.M. (1993). A structured nondrug intervention program for cancer pain. *Cancer Practice, 1,* 137–143.

Ripamonti, C., Groff, L., Brunelli, C., Polastri, D., Stravrakis, A., & DeConno, F. (1998). Switching from oral morphine to oral methadone in treating cancer pain: What is the equianalgesic dose ratio? *Journal of Clinical Oncology, 16,* 3216–3221.

Saberski, L.R. (1998). Interventional approaches in oncologic pain management. In A. Berger, R.K. Portenoy, & D.E. Weissman (Eds.), *Principles and practice of supportive oncology* (pp. 93–107). Philadelphia: Lippincott-Raven.

Santiago-Palma, J., Khojainova, N., Kornick, C., Fishberg, D.J., Primavera, L.H., Payne, R., et al. (2001). Intravenous methadone in the management of chronic cancer pain: Safe and effective starting doses when substituting methadone for fentanyl. *Cancer, 92,* 1919–1925.

Saunders, C.M. (1967). *The management of terminal illness.* London: Hospital Medicine Publications.

Schug, S.A., Zech, D., Grond, S., Jung, H., Meuser, T., & Stobbe, B. (1992). A long-term survey of morphine in cancer pain patients. *Journal of Pain and Symptom Management, 7,* 259–266.

Serafini, A.N. (2001). Therapy of metastatic bone pain. *Journal of Nuclear Medicine, 42,* 895–906.

Shimp, L.A. (1998). Safety issues in the pharmacologic management of chronic pain in the elderly. *Pharmacotherapy, 18,* 1313–1322.

Smith, M.T. (2000). Neuroexcitatory effects of morphine and hydromorphone: Evidence implicating the 3-glucuronide metabolites. *Clinical and Experimental Pharmacology and Physiology, 27,* 524–528.

Snow, A.L., Weber, J.B., O'Malley, K.J., Cody, M., Beck, C., Bruera, E., et al. (2004). NOPPAIN: A nursing assistant-administered pain assessment instrument for use in dementia. *Dementia and Geriatric Cognitive Disorders, 17,* 240–246.

Spiegel, D., & Moore, R. (1997). Imagery and hypnosis in the treatment of cancer patients. *Oncology (Huntington), 11,* 1179–1189.

Stein, C. (1995). The control of pain in peripheral tissues by opioids. *New England Journal of Medicine, 332,* 1685–1690.

Stephenson, S.L., Dalton, J.A., & Carlson, J. (2003). The effect of reflexology on pain in patients with metastatic cancer. *Applied Nursing Research, 16,* 284–286.

Stiefel, F. (1993). Psychosocial aspects of cancer pain. *Supportive Care in Cancer, 1,* 130–134.

Streisand, J., Busch, M.A., Egan, T.D., Gaylord Smith, B., Gay, M., & Pace, N.L. (1998). Dose proportionality and pharmacokinetics of oral transmucosal fentanyl citrate. *Anesthesiology, 88,* 305–309.

Swarm, R.A., Karanikolas, M., & Cousins, M.J. (2004). Anaesthetic techniques for pain control. In D. Doyle, G. Hanks, N. Cherny, & K. Calman (Eds.), *Oxford textbook of palliative medicine* (3rd ed., pp. 378–396). Oxford, United Kingdom: Oxford University Press.

Sykes, N.P. (1996). An investigation of the ability of oral naloxone to correct opioid-related constipation in patients with advanced cancer. *Palliative Medicine, 10,* 135–144.

Syrjala, K.L., Donaldson, G.W., Davis, M.W., Kippes, M.E., & Carr, J.E. (1995). Relaxation and imagery and cognitive-behavioral training reduce pain during cancer treatment: A controlled clinical trial. *Pain, 63,* 189–198.

Szeto, H.H., Inturrisi, C.E., Houde, R., Saal, R., Cheigh, J., & Reidenberg, M.M. (1977). Accumulation of normeperidine, an active metabolite of meperidine, in patients with renal failure or cancer. *Annals of Internal Medicine, 86,* 738–741.

Taylor, L.J., & Herr, K. (2003). Pain intensity assessment: A comparison of selected pain intensity scales for use in cognitively intact and cognitively impaired African American older adults. *Pain Management Nursing, 4,* 87–95.

Twycross, R., & Wilcock, A. (2001). *Symptom management in advanced cancer* (3rd ed.). Oxford, United Kingdom: Radcliffe Medical Press.

Umans, J.G., & Inturrisi, C.E. (1982). Antinociceptive activity and toxicity of meperidine and normeperidine in mice. *Journal of Pharmacology and Experimental Therapeutics, 223,* 203–206.

Villanueva, M.R., Smith, T.L., Erickson, J.S., Lee, A.C., & Singer, C.M. (2003). Pain Assessment for the Dementing Elderly (PADE): Reliability and validity of a new measure. *Journal of the American Medical Directors Association, 4,* 1–8.

Walker, K., Medhurst, S.J., Kidd, B.L., Glatt, M., Bowes, M., Patel, S., et al. (2002). Disease modifying and anti-nociceptive effects of bisphosphonate, zoledronic acid in a model of bone cancer pain. *Pain, 100,* 219–229.

Walsh, T.D. (1990). Prevention of opioid side effects. *Journal of Pain and Symptom Management, 5,* 363–367.

Ward, S.E., Goldberg, N., Miller-McCauley, V., Mueller, C., Nolan, A., Pawlik-Plank, D., et al. (1993). Patient related barriers to management of cancer pain. *Pain, 52,* 319–324.

Warden, V., Hurley, A.C., & Volicer, L. (2003). Development and psychometric evaluation of the Pain Assessment in Advanced Dementia (PAINAD) scale. *Journal of the American Medical Directors Association, 4,* 9–15.

Watanabe, S., Tarumi, Y., Oneschuk, D., & Lawlor, P. (2002). Opioid rotation to methadone: Proceed with caution. *Journal of Clinical Oncology, 20,* 2409–2410.

Webster, L., Andrews, M., & Stoddard, G. (2003). Modafinil treatment of opioid-induced sedation. *Pain Medicine, 4,* 135–140.

Weiner, D.K., & Rudy, T.E. (2002). Attitudinal barriers to effective treatment of persistent pain in nursing home residents. *Journal of the American Geriatrics Society, 50,* 2035–2040.

Weinrich, S.P., & Weinrich, M.C. (1990). The effect of massage on pain in cancer patients. *Applied Nursing Research, 3,* 140–145.

Weinstein, S.M., Laux, L.F., Thornby, J.L., Lorimor, R.J., Hill, C.S., Thorpe, D.M., et al. (2000). Physicians' attitudes towards pain and the use of opioid analgesics: Results of a survey from the Texas Cancer Pain Initiative. *Southern Medical Journal, 93,* 479–487.

Weissman, D.E., Burchman, S.L., Dinndorf, P., & Dahl, J.L. (1990). *Handbook of cancer pain management* (2nd ed.). Milwaukee, WI: Wisconsin Cancer Pain Initiative.

Wells, N. (2000). Pain intensity and pain interference in hospitalized patients with cancer. *Oncology Nursing Forum, 27,* 985–991.

Whitcomb, D.C., & Block, G.D. (1994). Association of acetaminophen toxicity with fasting and ethanol use. *JAMA, 272,* 1845–1850.

Wong, D., & Baker, C. (1988). Pain in children: Comparison of assessment scales. *Pediatric Nurse, 14,* 9–17.

Wong, D., & Baker, C. (1995). *Reference manual for the Wong-Baker FACES pain rating scale.* Tulsa, OK: Wong and Baker.

Wong, R., & Wiffen, P.J. (2002). Bisphosphonates for the relief of pain secondary to bone metastases. *Cochrane Database Systematic Review, 2,* CD002068. Retrieved July 10, 2004, from http://www.cochrane.org/cochrane/revabstr/AB002068.htm

World Health Organization. (1986). *Cancer pain relief and palliative care. Report of a WHO expert committee* (WHO Technical Support Series, No. 804). Geneva, Switzerland: Author.

World Health Organization. (2002). *Palliative care.* Retrieved July 1, 2004, from http://www.who.int/hiv/topics/palliative/care/en/

Wright, A.W., Mather, L.E., & Smith, M.T. (2001). Hydromorphone-3-glucoronide: A more potent neuro-excitant than its structural analogue, morphine-3-glucoronide. *Life Science, 69,* 409–420.

Yaksh, T.L., Dirig, D.M., & Malmberg, A.B. (1998). Mechanism of action of non-steroidal anti-inflammatory drugs. *Cancer Investigation, 16,* 509–527.

Yuan, C.S., Foss, J.F., O'Connor, M., Osinski, J., Roizen, M.F., & Moss, J. (1997). The safety and efficacy of oral methylnaltrexone in preventing morphine-induced oral-cecal transit time. *Clinical Pharmacology and Therapeutics, 4,* 467–475.

Zappa, S.B., & Cassileth, B.R. (2003). Complementary approaches to palliative oncological care. *Journal of Nursing Care Quality, 18,* 22–26.

CHAPTER 20

Sexuality Care of the Older Adult With Cancer

Judith A. Shell, PhD, LMFT, RN

Introduction

The youth-oriented culture is glorified by the cosmetic and clothing industries, by movies and television, and of course, the "beautiful people" molded by plastic surgery. According to society today, superheated sex characterizes romantic love, and this usually precludes anyone older than 50 years of age indulging in any type of sexual playfulness, pleasure, or relationship. Stereotypes such as these do little to honor humankind or the changes in wisdom and beauty that come with age. Society tends to hold the opinion that sexuality stops or is definitely not as exciting as it was before the age of retirement. Masters, Johnson, and Kolodny (1994) explained, "A tremendous taboo surrounds the subject of sex in the geriatric years. It combines with general negative attitudes toward aging that create an unfortunate set of stereotypes: older individuals are widely believed to be rigid and incapable of growth or change; they are also commonly seen as hypochondriacs who are especially prone to depression; and they are often considered to be not only old-fashioned and unproductive but disengaged and more or less senile. Given the preceding stereotypes, it is little wonder that the elderly are seen as sexless" (p. 463). Although physical changes may take place over the years, affection, sensuality, and passion do not have to decline.

Jim and Mary H., who had been married 53 years, were together at the doctor's office where Jim was being examined. He complained to the physician, "Doctor, I'm losing my sex urge." The doctor replied, "That's understandable at age 84. When did you first notice this?" The patient said, "Last night and again this morning." Most people have difficulty imagining their parents or grandparents as sexual beings; however, younger generations must respect the decisions made by this population in regard to privacy, dating, cohabitation, or remarriage. Even though culture, in general, remains rather disapproving, a trend is being made toward acceptance of the sexual nature of people who are older than age 55. This new attitude is appreciated as we watch Jack Nicholson and Diane Keaton romp their way through the 2003 movie *Something's Gotta Give*. Their characters dispel some myths about older couples and display the physical capability and the feelings that create a pleasurable sexual and, in the end, meaningful relationship.

This chapter will introduce sexuality in later life to the reader by emphasizing normal physical changes that occur with age and how a focus on sexual health can enhance quality of life. Recent research with the aging population, sociocultural issues, normal life cycle changes, nontraditional relationships, some myths and realities, and theories of development and aging will enhance the knowledge of and enlighten the geriatric caregiver. Healthcare professionals should emphasize sexual problems induced by cancer in this ever-increasing population and suggest interventions to promote the adaptation to the changes induced by age and illness.

Focus on Sexual Health

By 2030, approximately 70 million Americans will be age 65 or older. The trend toward better health is redefining the image of aging in America (Sharpe, 2004) (see Figure 20-1). People in their 50s, 60s, and 70s generally are more healthy and active than their parents were at a similar age; however, because about 20% of Americans will be 65 or older in 2030, this population also is at a greater risk of developing

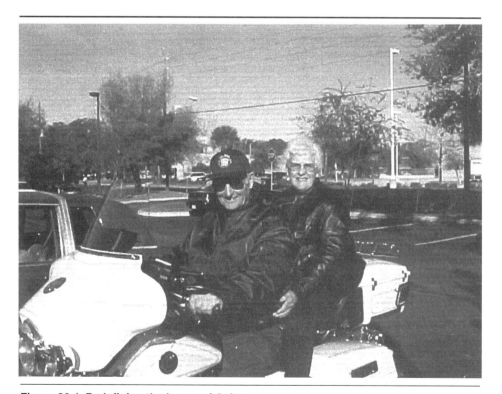

Figure 20-1. Redefining the Image of Aging

cancer (Balducci, 2003). During a cancer crisis, healthcare professionals can focus on the individuals' or couples' strengths and resilience and promote and encourage the concept of sexual health.

NANDA International stated its definition of sexual dysfunction as "the state in which problems with sexual function exist" (Korb, 1996, p. 777). Authors and healthcare providers tend to focus on sexual *dysfunction*; however, this chapter will focus on how best to help the older adult with cancer to attain sexual *function*. Sexual function could be defined as the ability to express one's sexuality in a manner that is consistent with personal needs and preferences (Hughes, 1996).

Physical sexual performance embraces sexual drive and draws people together for biologic reproduction and physical satisfaction, and it often brings people together to share an expression of passion and devotion (Shell, 2001). Although the medical model of sexuality tends to focus on genital sex, expression of sexuality among seniors may not always center around intercourse. They may be more interested in touching and cuddling and the companionship that comes with this kind of closeness. The sexual experience may take on a different quality; it may become more intimate and more selfless. AARP (1999b) studied 1,384 Americans who were 45 years of age and older and found that during a six-month period of time, men and women with partners engaged about once a week in kissing and hugging (85% and 86%, respectively), sexual touching or caressing (76% and 73%, respectively), and sexual intercourse (52% and 55%, respectively).

Although sexual touching and intercourse are important forms of intimacy, for many people, this is not the desired form of closeness or perhaps is not available to them. A grandparent-grandchild relationship or close friendship may be an alternate form of intimacy that is just as rewarding. Leiblum and Segraves (2000) explained that many older couples grew up in traditional families where "sex is sanctioned primarily for procreation; sexual behaviors other than intercourse, such as oral-genital sex, are considered unnatural; sexual relations outside marriage are forbidden; and masturbation is sinful . . . the opportunity to 'retire' from an active sexual life may be ardently anticipated and easily accepted" (p. 426). The key is what each couple desires and what they can establish with one another.

The Aging Population and Recent Research

Many baby boomers who were part of the sexual revolution have taken the posture that they are not going to grow old as gracefully as their predecessors. They do not merely want to exist, but rather they want to enjoy what they always have enjoyed; they will not allow their sex life to go calmly away (Richard, 2001). Enter Bob Dole, whose new job is to be the spokesman for Viagra® (Pfizer, New York, NY), and we witness how attitudes have begun to change about "senior sexuality."

Sexuality Mid- to Late-Life

The Sexuality, Information, and Education Council of the United States (SIECUS) provides research reports on sexuality in middle and later life. This information furnishes insight for healthcare providers regarding "sexual behavior, health, attitudes, values, and beliefs of individuals from their forties through their eighties and older" (SIECUS, 2001/2002, p. 1). The National Council on Aging (NCOA) and AARP surveyed 1,000 men and women older than 50 years of age and found that 60% were satisfied with their sex lives; 70% had sex about once a week; and 61% proclaimed that sex was as good as or better than when they were younger (AARP, 1999a). Thirty-four percent reported a bland or nonexistent sexual relationship, but this was usually because of illness, loss of a partner, medication, or treatments for cancer or kidney failure. These predicaments often preclude sexual activity because of a lack of energy or motivation. NCOA (1998) conducted another study that found 30% of women and more than half of men age 70 years and older engaged in sexual activity once a month or more during the past year. Finally, AARP (1999b) acknowledged that a satisfying sexual relationship is important to quality of life for 44% of women and half of men 75 years and older.

Relationships and Physical Health

Research on the association between relationships and physical health indicates that married people are healthier than nonmarried people (Snyder & Whisman, 2004). In addition, the *quality* of relationships has been found to impact perceived physical health. Ren (1997) reported on global health perceptions in 12,000 married and nonmarried adults and found that perceived health was related to relationship distress. Rodrigue and Park (1996) investigated adults with cancer regarding relationship distress and its effect on patient psychological adjustment. They found more depression, anxiety, and illness-induced family dilemmas if a high relationship disorder was present. If a major health crisis exists, people have more problems dealing with the illness if they are unhappy in their relationships.

Sociocultural Issues

Developmental Theories and Tasks of Aging

The process of aging is depicted through developmental theory. From the age of 65 until death, Erik Erikson's theory affirms that integrity versus despair portrays the last state of human development (Bornestein, 1986). *Integrity* consists of the following conditions (Shell & Smith, 1994).
- Personal acceptance of how one has lived his or her life
- Acceptance of one's choices made in a given situation
- Recognition that these choices were the best possible for that moment in time
- Subjective review of his or her life and acceptance of how it has been lived to date
- Continuing to live with self-respect and an acceptance of death

Despair is distinguished by (Shell & Smith)
- Feelings of disappointment or failure about how one has lived life
- Feelings of self-absorption, passing on few insights gained throughout their life experience
- Perception of little control over life events and fear of death
- Negativism and withdrawal from others.

Resolution of this developmental stage can occur if the individual can balance the acceptance of how one has lived life with the reality that change is part of life, and change may occur up to the end of life.

Another focus of developmental theory is that of "disengagement," which portrays older adults cultivating new roles and relationships as they withdraw from the activities of middle age. When the developmental tasks of later life are successfully accomplished, a more positive attitude will most likely be fostered regarding sexuality (see Figure 20-2). If an older individual is occupied with living life to the fullest and remains active within a social circle of friends, a better opportunity exists to develop and nurture an intimate relationship and continue or develop an interest in a satisfactory sexual connection.

Individual Adjustments
- Adjusting to decreased physical strength and health
- Adjusting to retirement and reduced income
- Adjusting to a spouse's death
- Establishing satisfactory physical living arrangements

Social Adjustments
- Establishing an explicit affiliation with one's age group
- Adjusting to social roles in a flexible manner

Figure 20-2. Developmental Tasks of Later Life

Note. Based on information from Jones, 1988.

Nontraditional Relationships

When cancer interferes in the relationships of aging men and women, they experience many difficulties. When the couple is gay or lesbian, they face particular problems that heterosexual people do not experience. One of these is "heterosexism." Fields and Scout (2001) explained, "Heterosexism, a term that is replacing homophobia, describes a societal condition in which the expectation exists that all individuals are heterosexual. This pervasive assumption in healthcare settings can be overt or subtle, but its impact is nonetheless damaging. The assumption of straightness that permeates healthcare assessment and sexual history forms perpetuates lesbian invisibility and marginalizes lesbian health needs" (p. 185).

Many myths also exist concerning older gay men and women; these may include more isolation, loneliness, fearfulness, and depression. Older gay men generally are not lonely any more than the younger generation, but as with heterosexual men, a decrease in sexual frequency usually occurs as they get older, and more gay men live alone (Leiblum & Segraves, 2000). Cities with a high gay/lesbian population have organizations that provide support for seniors, including the Senior Action in a Gay Environment in New York and the Gay and Lesbian Outreach to Elders in San Francisco (Leiblum & Segraves).

Healthcare provider discrimination, including disrespectful comments, belligerence toward the patient and/or partner, unnecessary roughness during physical examinations, or other perversions, can impact the care and treatment of gays and lesbians with cancer (Fields & Scout, 2001; Matthews, 1998). A more agreeable milieu can be created by "displaying a nondiscrimination statement which includes sexual orientation; using inclusive language on all intake and sexual history forms; including partners in all decision-making; ensuring confidentiality of patient information; making lesbian health information and resources available to patients; and displaying symbols of diversity, such as rainbow flags, pink triangles, or signs designating the space as safe for discussing sexual orientation issues" (Fields & Scout, p. 186).

Holistic care, inclusive of sexuality issues, is essential for all patient populations irrespective of age or gender identity, and although many of these comments are focused on the lesbian with cancer, they apply to gay men as well. To review a copy of The Lesbian Cancer Patient's Bill of Rights, please see Fields and Scout (2001).

Although older adults already are occupied with managing normal age-related activities, cancer can bring on new and challenging complications. People who must manage these complications face emotional, spiritual, and physical changes that will impact their feelings of sexuality. Cancer and its treatment "can have an impact on overall physical strength and elicit a heightened preoccupation with mortality. In addition, social relationships may be limited because of the reduced energy that is available to invest in such relationships" (Shell & Smith, 1994, p. 554). The older adult faces life events and deviations that can impact well-being and transform relationships.

Life Cycle Changes

Life cycle experiences may comprise unexpected relationship alterations, retirement, chronic illnesses, and considerations related to long-term care facilities. Any of these concerns is difficult to encounter and manage, especially if a person has aged, has few resources, and has no partner with whom to share the emotional burden.

Marriage, Divorce, and Death

Currently, approximately 50% of first marriages end in divorce, and this rate is no different in the cancer population (Holland & Lewis, 2000). If a relationship is strong to begin with, a couple most likely will weather an illness, such as cancer; if it is troubled, the relationship probably will not get better (Holland & Lewis; Schover, 2000). Although divorce is difficult at any age, it is particularly problematic for older women because they usually are not as financially secure as men, and they are not as likely to be working outside of the home, which affords the opportunity for diverse relationships. Because fewer older men are in the population, it may be troublesome for women to find an acceptable companion if remarriage is conceivable. Divorce also can affect self-esteem and a woman's image that she is sexually desirable. "In addition, despite greater acceptance of nontraditional relationships, such as bisexual, gay, or lesbian relationships, many older people, particularly older women, do not accept these as alternatives" (Shell & Smith, 1994, p. 556).

Relationships end not only with divorce but also through the death of the partner. Because cancer can be a lengthy illness, a partner may experience "anticipatory grief" before death. "Although such grieving may result in a closer relationship with the ill partner, there are instances when the grieving person may close himself or herself off, as though the partner were already dead" (Butler & Lewis, 2002, pp. 247–248). Finding a new partner is difficult, and forming new relationships may be intimidating. Many older adults who have lost their spouse either remarry or choose to cohabit, which may create moral conflict for the couple and for their children. If a parent remarries later in life, children may feel betrayed or that their parent is being disloyal, and they also may have concerns about their inheritance and position in the family (Shell & Smith, 1994).

Although marriage or partnered relationships are valued for many reasons, including their potential to meet intimacy needs, the unmarried or unpartnered person can find ways to be intimate with others. People who are not immediate family also are very important to most people. Neighbors, store clerks, and members of a church congregation all provide individuals with a sense of belonging. This sense of community is larger than the immediate family and can give a sense of intimacy. Most patients have had or will have some periods in their lives when a loving partner is not available for sexual activity. What does this mean to the sense of self and well-being? Sometimes people are alone because their capacity to be in intimate relationships is either damaged or taken away from them. These people can enjoy solitary activities or find ways to relate with others that are less intimate but still meaningful, such as the pleasant interactions many have at work.

Most people accept that intense sexual fulfillment is a sometimes thing, even for those who are married. For those who are not currently married, the sense of fulfillment varies. Many single people take opportunities to give and receive sexual pleasure. However, these opportunities are mostly available to the young and early middle-aged. Older people, especially women, may not have the same opportunities. What effect does this have on their sense of fulfillment? Those who have the capacity to be alone turn to the resources within themselves for completion and satisfaction. Those who are older may look back on the enthusiasms of their youth and take up interests and solitary activities long-abandoned during the busy period of early and middle adulthood. One can accept the single life as well as life with a partner, and the inner world of the spirit as well as the external world of family and community.

Retirement

Retirement may cause some concern because a couple may move to a warmer climate, and their regular support system—children and other relatives—may not be nearby to help. Conversely, retirement has some advantages that may be particularly important for the couple with a cancer diagnosis. More time can be dedicated to caregiving and therapeutic support (e.g., going to doctors' and treatment visits, participating in support groups). This ability to have a flexible schedule to sustain a loved one in time of crisis may entice a couple to become closer to each other and enhance intimacy, whether it be sexual, emotional, or both. When couples are truly enjoying companionship, their struggles with challenges are minimized, and they create a strong emotional bond.

Chronic Illness

Chronic illness presents in many forms, and because of this, patients often are taking care of patients. The incidence of chronic illnesses such as diabetes, hypertension, and heart disease increases as a person ages; consequently, cancer caregivers frequently are managing their own ailments along with the patient's. Although they start out being concerned and willing to take on nursing duties, as the illness progresses, they may find that they also are angry and resentful because they feel overworked and exhausted. Butler and Lewis (2002) reported that "it is important that you do not feel guilty about resentments and a sense of burden in the care giving role. Face your feelings frankly and secure outside help whenever possible from your relatives, neighbors, friends, or professional homemakers to reduce your burden" (p. 240). The fear that the loved one may be lost because of death is an imminent threat to the relationship; however, the couple may experience a new closeness and be able to treasure precious moments together that also may enhance a sexual closeness.

Assisted Living Facilities

When older people must live in long-term care facilities, limited privacy may be an issue if the individual or the couple wishes to be sexually intimate (this may mean touching, holding and kissing, or other sexual expression such as self-stimulation or intercourse). Usually the doors are not locked, the rooms are semiprivate where visitors can be seen and heard by other residents, and only single beds are provided. Patients often are confined to single-sex environments, and staff members often consider their patients to be devoid of any sexual needs. Single older people who have lost a spouse certainly do not abandon sexual desire or capacity (Richardson & Lazur, 1995). Facilities should provide for an environment that allows sexual expression for its residents. For example, if a couple is living there together, they could bring their own double bed from home and room together. A sign could be placed on the door when privacy is desired, whether this is for married residents or for others who are not married but who wish to engage in sexual activity with other residents or with an outside guest (Butler & Lewis, 2002; Shell & Smith, 1994). If a nursing home is a Medicare and Medicaid participant, federal regulations instituted in 1978 require some privacy rights, but only for those who are married. Information about these regulations can be obtained from the Health Standards and Quality Bureau (Butler & Lewis).

Myths and Realities

One prominent misperception is that older people, especially after the age of 65, no longer engage in sexual activity. The Association of Reproductive Health Professionals refuted this myth after reporting that 36% of men and 18% of women age 70 years and older considered themselves sexually active (SIECUS, 2001/2002).

Sexual desire and activity in later years depends largely upon the enjoyment and fulfillment that sex provided for individuals in their younger years (Leiblum & Segraves, 2000; Masters et al., 1994). Two other important factors that enable rewarding and gratifying sex and sexuality later in life are relatively good health and a cooperative, interested, and interesting partner (Butler & Lewis, 2002; Masters et al.). Alternative sexual expression may have to be entertained if disability or serious illness occurs, but sharing an intimate moment can promote an "alive" feeling.

Changes occur with age in both physical and physiologic expressions of sex. Another myth that these changes foster is that the physical capacity for sex deteriorates. Older women generally retain the capacity for sexual activity, and most changes are attributed to a decrease of female hormones as menopause takes place. Although menopause affects sexual function, it does not mark the end of sexuality. Men who are older than 50 often are believed to be sexually impaired, when, in reality, they do not lose their ability to have erections and ejaculate. The process slows down, and some define this as "andropause" (Butler & Lewis, 2002). However, in a study of more than 300 people who were 50 years or older, 38% of the men and 28% of the women 60–69 years of age reported that they considered themselves better lovers than they were in the past (SIECUS, 2001/2002).

Although sex in youth often is a way of asserting independence or power, it also involves exploring one's sexuality. A fulfilling sexual relationship as an older adult provides pleasure, release, communication, and shared intimacy. The effect of aging on sex often is positive, because as people have more experience with sex, more knowledge is gained about their bodies and what pleases them. A "second language of sex" also is developed that is emotional and communicative and more than just the physical. This is important to a couple who must endure cancer because this second language provides recognition and shared feelings in words, actions, and unspoken perceptions. The couple can achieve a mutual tenderness and a particular thoughtfulness between the two that grows and is nurtured. Although emotion and communication are essential factors, the status of a person's physical state also makes a significant contribution to a sexual relationship.

Normal Psychosexual Development in Later Adulthood

What are the obstacles to a healthy sex life? Sex is something that always has been taken for granted and now suddenly may be "iffy" at 60. Noted sex therapist Barry McCarthy (2002) provided guidelines for heterosexual couples older than 60 that can be shared with patients and partners. In addition, although sex does not necessarily require the stamina of a marathoner, it requires reasonably good health, and nurses can promote a healthy attitude in the cancer population (see Table 20-1).

Table 20-1. Healthy Lifestyles for the Older Adult

Health	Sexuality
Healthful eating	Follow a balanced, low-fat diet; increase bulk. Avoid routine laxative intake. Small, frequent meals may be better than one or two large ones. Moderate weight loss can sometimes reverse impotence.
Exercise	Exercise improves motivation and social enrichment; physical fitness helps to control weak and flabby musculature and enhances self-image.
Smoking cessation	Men who smoke heavily are more likely to be impotent; smokers are at increased risk of arteriosclerosis, which can cause impotence.
Limited alcohol intake	Chronic alcohol and drug abuse can cause psychological and neurologic problems related to impotence and decreased arousal and orgasmic ability in both sexes.
Protection against HIV and sexually transmitted diseases	A monogamous relationship is the best protection; a condom is second best.

Note. Based on information from the National Institute on Aging, 2000.

Age-Related Changes in Women and Men

Although menopause does not eradicate a woman's sexuality, she may feel threatened by the changes in body shape and firmness that signal the aging process. She now must contend with hot flashes and night sweats, but the cessation of menstruation may be a welcome deletion (Demeter, 1998). Other changes occur physically in the sexual response cycle that may affect sexual function (see Table 20-2). Physical

Table 20-2. Normal Psychosexual Developmental Changes in Older Women and Men

Sexual Focus	Physiologic Response
Normal Sexuality Changes in Women	
Menopause	Hot flashes, night sweats, difficulty sleeping, fatigue, memory problems, stress incontinence, thinning pubic hair, osteoporosis, emotional instability
Vaginal changes	The vaginal mucosa becomes thinner, appearance changes to a paler color, length is shortened, lubrication is reduced, and vaginal expansion decreases in degree and speed. Vaginal secretions become less acidic, and the number of infections often increases.
Clitoris	Labia skin folds can shrink and become thinner, exposing the clitoris; this can lead to reduced sensitivity or an unpleasant tingling or prickling when touched. The clitoris may reduce in size because of decreased estrogen.
Desire	Sex drive is partially determined by emotional and social factors; hormones such as estrogen and testosterone play an important role; decreased or absent testosterone affects libido.
Orgasm	Orgasm remains possible throughout life; a diminished or slower response may occur and with less intensity.
Normal Sexuality Changes in Men	
Erectile response	By age 60, more stimulation may be required to get and maintain an erection; erections will be less firm and take longer to occur (faster does not equal better). The erect penis may be less sensitive than at a younger age, and the testicles will decrease in size and firmness.
Arousal	More direct genital stimulation may be needed, as this phase is extended as men get older.
Ejaculation	Ejaculation amount and intensity decrease. Men, however, usually remain fertile.
Orgasm	A decrease in the intensity of the orgasm may occur. Aging increases the length of time that must pass after an ejaculation and before stimulation to another climax. This interval may be as much as 48 hours by the age of 70.
Refractory period	This period increases with age and can extend from 12–24 hours.

changes in men's sexual response parallel those seen in postmenopausal women, except for the menopausal process. Their hormone levels do not seem to drop as drastically as those in women, and men continue to have nocturnal penile tumescence as they age. These nocturnal erections are not as firm after age 50, but they usually remain constant as long as no medical problems are present (Leiblum & Segraves, 2000; Masters et al., 1994).

Sexual Changes Because of Illness Other Than Cancer

Other illnesses and disabilities can interfere with how a person responds sexually, but even very serious illness rarely justifies stopping sexual activity completely (Badeau, 1995). Many of the chronic illnesses can be corrected or at least controlled.

The following maladies often may need to be managed by both the patients and their partners in addition to cancer.

Heart disease—The fear of a heart attack or recurrence of one (sometimes called "death by orgasm") will impact sexual behavior and may lead many older people to give up sex altogether (Butler & Lewis, 2002; Steinke & Patterson-Midgley, 1996). Even though heart rate, respiratory rate, and blood pressure rise during intercourse, they return to normal within minutes, and the risk of death during sexual intercourse is rare; usually sex may be resumed about 12–16 weeks after a heart attack following the doctor's advice (Masters et al., 1994; Muller, Mittleman, Maclure, Sherwood, & Tofler, 1996). Heart performance can be augmented by exercise programs, changing positions during intercourse to conserve energy, and reducing food and alcohol intake before intercourse (Tremethick, Tornabene, & Eibes, 2002).

Diabetes—Although sexual function in both men and women can be affected by diabetes, women seem to be less handicapped, possibly because they have been studied less extensively and less is known about the effects (Sharpe, 2004). Women can experience frequent vaginal and urinary tract infections, secondary anorgasmia, reduced vaginal lubrication, and sexual desire problems, which may be indirectly caused by neuropathy in the pelvic region (Masters et al., 1994). Approximately 50% of men with diabetes suffer some kind of potency problem because it can cause either a diabetic neuropathy that creates nerve damage, or fatty deposits can collect in blood vessels and restrict the flow of blood to the penis (Masters et al.; Tallis, Fillit, & Brocklehurst, 1998). If neuropathy is severe, penile implants may be considered. Despite these adverse effects, sexual desire, genital sensations, and ejaculation remain normal.

Stroke—Sexual desire will remain the same after a stroke unless severe damage occurs to the brain. If a man has erectile or ejaculatory problems, a woman has difficulty with vaginal lubrication, and/or the person is paralyzed, a sexual relationship is possible if consideration is given to restoring sexual function. Sexual intimacy does not have to be forfeited, and the following patient clearly emphasizes that he wanted his doctors and nurses to help him to regain his sense of self, but to no avail. "After I had the stroke, I began asking doctors and nurses about how it would affect my sexuality. Many of them were embarrassed, some laughed, and all shrugged their shoulders and said they didn't know. I got the message that nobody wanted to talk about it, except me. I did have erections. I told everybody about it. Again, the responses were mostly perfunctory and/or embarrassed. I asked about achieving orgasm, and again they shrugged. While everybody was willing to talk to me about what I might expect with rehabilitation and movement on my right side, and about speech improvement, nobody wanted to talk about sex or my sexual organs" (Matola, 2000, pp. 90–91).

Depression—If people are depressed, they will most likely experience a reduction in their sex drive, especially if this has been a chronic condition. Clinical depression occurs approximately 20%–30% of the time in patients with cancer (Massie & Popkin, 1998). Depression can cause withdrawal from social interaction, which can cause a couple's intimacy to suffer (McDaniel, Musselman, Porter, Reed, & Nemeroff, 1995; Shell & Kirsch, 2001). Ironically, many of the medications used to relieve depression can themselves cause sexual side effects, such as decreased sexual desire and a delay, a reduction, or an inability to reach orgasm (Masters et al., 1994). Some of the drugs reported to cause adverse sexual side effects include fluoxetine, sertraline, paroxetine, venlafaxine, fluvoxamine, and escitalopram oxalate (Spratto & Woods, 2003). Those that may cause fewer problems include nefazodone, bupropion, and mirtazapine (Spratto & Woods). For people with cancer, an often welcome side effect of mirtazapine is weight gain. Butler and Lewis (2002) detailed suggestions from physicians that may help to decrease the problems associated with medications; measures include dose reduction, a change in the antidepressant drug, a drug holiday for a weekend, or use of a different medication as an antidote (e.g., methylphenidate hydrochloride, ginkgo biloba, dextroamphetamine, caffeine). Along with antidepressants, another very important component in treatment for depression includes cognitive behavioral psychotherapy (Massie & Popkin; Shell & Kirsch). In this psychotherapeutic intervention, the therapist intervenes to influence thinking, acting, feeling, and bodily reaction patterns. An example may be when the nurse helps a patient to reduce negative self-talk, reframe obstacles as challenges, and expand possibilities to prevent anxiety or reduce negative self-talk (Shell & Kirsch). When both medication and therapy are applied and the symptoms of depression (decreased energy, appetite and weight loss, difficulty sleeping, feelings of worthlessness and hopelessness) begin to subside, a person's sexual interest frequently recovers (Masters et al.).

Sexual Problems Induced by Cancer: Sexual Desire, Arousal, Orgasm Impairment

Although insufficient research has been conducted that documents interventions to promote sexual function in the patient with cancer (and particularly in the older adult with cancer), sexual dysfunction in this population exists anywhere from 20% to 100% of the time (Ganz, Rowland, Desmond, Meyerowitz, & Wyatt, 1998; Monga, 1995; Rowland & Massie, 1996; Shell, 2001, 2002). Some forms of cancer can cause anemia, loss of appetite, muscle wasting, or neurologic impairment that leads to weakness, and this may affect sexual function indirectly, whereas other forms of cancer may cause direct damage to sexual organs. Cancer treatments frequently lead to physically altering surgery or other physiologic side effects that also directly impact sexuality, sexual desire, and pleasure in all age groups. However, in the older adult with cancer, various other circumstances intensify these treatment outcomes, such as other chronic illnesses; sensory, motor, and cognitive changes; and a lack of social support (Shell & Smith, 1994).

Sexual Desire and Interest in Sex

Although aging itself does not precipitate the abrupt loss of desire, the motivation to remain sexually active can be stifled because of the process of becoming ill and entering active treatment for cancer (Holland & Lewis, 2000; Schover, 2000; Shell & Smith, 1994). The diagnosis, disruption in one's schedule to attend to doctor appointments, x-rays, and laboratory tests, the treatments themselves, and the possible threat of losing a partner can cause anxiety.

Prostate Cancer

Cancer of the prostate is a common diagnosis in older men, and approximately 80% of cases occur in men 65 years and older (Monga, 1995). Treatment for this cancer frequently causes some form of sexual dysfunction, particularly if radical surgery is employed (Stanford et al., 2000). When men sustain lowered levels of testosterone because of androgen reduction therapy, their level of sexual desire decreases as well (Shell, 2001; Wilmoth & Bruner, 2002). When either radiation alone or radiation with hormonal therapy is employed, a decrease in desire has been reported. Sixty-two men with localized prostate cancer (mean age 67.6 years) who were treated with radiation therapy participated in a quality-of-life study to describe their sexual function before and after treatment. Complete responses were received from 40 of the subjects; 35% were sexually active before treatment, 37.5% were active at completion of radiotherapy, and 40% were active long term. During the study period, no significant change was seen in satisfaction with sexual activity; in fact, activity increased. However, more patients reported a decrease in sexual interest and desire after treatment completion and long-term follow-up than before treatment (Monga, Kerrigan, Garber, & Monga, 2001). In an exploratory study, 67 men with localized prostate cancer (ages 50–65) were treated using radiation therapy with or without hormonal therapy. Researchers assessed the men's sexual function after treatment and compared it to age-matched controls (N = 48). Mean follow-up was 2.6 years. The group treated with hormone therapy had significantly inferior sexual function (functions included desire along with arousal, frequency, function, and enjoyment) than both the radiotherapy-only group and the control group (Bruner, Hanlon, Nicolaou, & Hanks, 1997).

Breast Cancer

Women have problems with low sexual desire during cancer treatment. Older women who have undergone menopause already have realized some normal changes, such as a general slowing and a decrease in the intensity of the sexual response cycle; however, because of hormone replacement therapy (HRT), these women have been able to continue to experience normal sexual libido (Anderson & Cyranowski, 1995). Even more than estrogen, androgens are a stimulant for desire in the female. When cancer treatments such as chemotherapy create a hormone-deficient state with associated symptoms of hot flashes and poor vaginal lubrication, women often experience decreased sexual desire (Davis, 2000; Ganz et al., 1998; Leiblum & Segraves, 2000). Young-McCaughan (1996) compared sexual functioning in women with breast cancer who were treated with no pharmacologic manipulation to those treated either with chemotherapy or endocrine therapy. This descriptive study included a sample of 67 women with local or regional disease (stages I, II, and III). Young-McCaughan found that women were three times more likely to complain of decreased sexual desire if they were treated with chemotherapy. Those treated with endocrine therapy did not experience sexual dysfunction symptoms significantly different from those not treated (Young-McCaughan). Another recent survey (N = 864) compared breast cancer survivors to healthy, age-matched women in regard to sexual functioning after breast cancer. The investigators were surprised to find that women 50 years and older who were taking tamoxifen did not encounter worsened sexual functioning, whereas those women in all age groups who had received chemotherapy experienced increased sexual dysfunction (Ganz et al.). Although the breast cancer survivors reported more physical and menopausal symptoms than their healthy cohorts, their sexual functioning was comparable.

In summary, both men and women can experience desire issues if they suffer with fatigue, from the cancer itself, or from the anemia associated with cancer. Those who experience depression also may experience problems with low sexual desire (Holland & Lewis, 2000).

Arousal Problems Related to Surgery, Radiation, and Chemotherapy

Surgery—Male

An inability to achieve and maintain an erection is a common complaint in men who have had treatment for testicular, prostate, colorectal, bladder, and even head and neck cancers (Bertero, 2001; Monga, 1995; Monga et al., 2001; Siston, List, Schleser, & Vokes, 1997; Talcott et al., 1998). Although treatment for head and neck cancer does not directly affect the genital area, Monga reported that in a study of 20 patients with head and neck cancer, 60% of the men had erectile dysfunction (ED), and 40% had stopped having intercourse. Although little research has been done in this population, Monga, Tan, Ostermann, and Monga (1997) conducted a descriptive, self-report study in a convenience sample of 55 patients (54 were men) with head and neck cancer following radiation therapy (with or without surgery). The purpose of the study was to ascertain sexual functioning and its relationship with age, extent of disfigurement, performance status, and psychological functioning. Although the majority reported arousal and orgasmic problems and did not participate in sexual intercourse, they also reported that they were satisfied with their current partner, and 49% said they were satisfied with their current sexual functioning. The authors emphasized that "despite experiencing sexual problems, sexuality continues to be a priority in the majority of patients studied" (p. 302).

Surgical procedures can disrupt parasympathetic innervation during prostate or bladder surgery and sympathetic innervation during retroperitoneal lymph node dissection for testicular cancer. Further, abdominoperineal resection can damage the autonomic nervous system following colorectal surgery (Monga, 1995; Stanford et al., 2000; Wilmoth & Bruner, 2002). Although nerve-sparing procedures have been able to achieve moderate results, men with prostate cancer still complain about ED about 80% of the time, and 45% of men with colorectal cancer complain about ED (Talcott et al., 1997; Wilmoth & Bruner).

Radiation Therapy—Male

Radiation therapy causes approximately a 40% risk for ED in patients with prostate cancer, and although the exact mechanism is not clear, it is most likely because of vascular scarring from the radiation treatment. The premise is that vascular insufficiency is caused by accelerated atherosclerotic disease, where blood can no longer get to the penis for an adequate erection (Ofman, 1995; Schover, 2000; Talcott et al., 1996).

Chemotherapy—Male

ED can occur secondarily because of administration of many chemotherapy products, particularly alkylating agents; endocrine dysfunction is induced, with a resulting decrease in sexual desire and ED (Monga, 1995). However, chemotherapy causes the most problems for men in relation to testicular function and spermatogenesis. Alkylating agents can cause functional impairment because of depletion of the germinal epithelial lining of the seminiferous tubules. Testicular atrophy then can occur because luteinizing hormone-releasing hormone (LHRH), luteinizing hormone, and follicle-stimulating hormone are increased with a consequent decrease in serum testosterone (Monga). The effects of these agents appear to be dose-related.

Surgery—Female

Surgical procedures that may affect the arousal phase of the female response cycle include all gynecologic cancer surgeries (hysterectomy, oophorectomy, vulvectomy, pelvic exenteration), as well as surgery for breast, colorectal, bladder, and head and neck cancers (Butler, Banfield, Sveinson, & Allen, 1998). After hysterectomy, the woman may be anxious and worried that her vagina will not expand or lubricate properly or be adequate for intercourse (Anderson, Woods, & Copeland, 1997). If the vagina must be removed, the total reconstruction process may be a concern. Cancer of the vulva occurs more frequently in older women, and they often present with advanced disease because they tend to be more reluctant or unable to examine themselves on a regular basis and/or to seek medical treatment if they find something wrong (Shell, 2001). Consequently, vulvectomy may be the treatment of choice, and that necessitates removal of the clitoris with resulting problems in arousal and possibly with orgasm (Monga, 1995).

If a woman has had mastectomy with reconstruction for breast cancer, she often reports difficulty in accepting the loss of sensation in the reconstructed breast (Fleming & Kleinbart, 2001; Wilmoth & Ross, 1997). This loss of sensation often is unexpected because of the lack of education patients receive and can produce a harmful effect on sexual arousal. Initially, the surgeon is responsible for informing the patient of the expected results; however, because this is not always the case, the nurse should be aware of this unexpected experience and ensure that part of the educational process includes information regarding the frequent loss of sensation. Monga (1995) reported that women who have had reconstruction also are faced with limitations of the procedure, which include operative risks, infection potential, and some scarring. However, the benefit is that many patients who have undergone reconstruction report an improved body image. Monga said that "one's self-image and view of sexuality is critical for sexual arousal and responsiveness. In general, a young woman's psychological and sexual adaptation is more negatively affected by breast cancer surgery than an older woman's. However, the older woman may feel equal distress, but may be too self-conscious to express it" (p. 424).

Radiation Therapy—Female

Radiation therapy can have a dramatic effect on the vagina because vascular damage and fibrosis will occur, and this leads to decreased blood flow, vaginal dryness, and stenosis (Schover, 2000). Fibrosis is one of radiotherapy's most often-mentioned gynecologic side effects that influences sexuality and often results in the need to use vaginal dilation to maintain comfortable intercourse. Pain can end sexual arousal (Butler et al., 1998; Holland & Lewis, 2000). Suggested intervention for vaginal stenosis includes encouragement of frequent vaginal intercourse with water-soluble lubricants. For women who are not sexually active, use of vaginal dilators is encouraged for 5–10 minutes twice a day immediately postradiation for about two months and less frequently thereafter (three times per week for the next year) (Shell, 1991).

Chemotherapy—Female

Chemotherapy does not have an effect on ovarian function in postmenopausal women; however, it has been reported that women still may endure problems with libido, reduced vaginal lubrication, and dyspareunia (Young-McCaughan, 1996). These outcomes will, in turn, affect arousal and combine with fatigue and potential weight gain to decrease sexual desirability even further (Schover, 2000).

Orgasmic Impairment

Male

Men treated for cancer rarely experience a complete inability to achieve orgasm (Schover, 2000). They may undergo a decreased intensity in their orgasm because of radiation for testicular cancer, or dry orgasm (without ejaculation of semen) will occur if cystectomy, prostatectomy, or other radical pelvic surgery is employed (Arai, Kawakita, Okada, & Yoshida, 1997; Monga, 1995; Schover, 2000). Schover (2000) explained, "The sensory nerves that control the muscular contractions of ejaculation as well as the sensation of orgasmic pleasure are protected near the side wall of the pelvis so that they are rarely damaged" (p. 406). Orgasm remains possible even if the penis must be amputated because of cancer. Although it seems reasonable that men treated for cancers in their pelvic region would be the most severely affected sexually, Monga reported in a study of 20 patients treated for head and neck cancer that 50% suffered anorgasmia. Hormonal therapy with LHRH antagonists and combination chemotherapies also can impact systemic sexual function and create difficulty in achieving male orgasm (Monga; Wilmoth & Bruner, 2002).

Female

Reaching orgasm for women usually is more adversely affected secondarily by disruption in sexual desire and arousal than by direct cause from the cancer and its treatment effects (Schover, 2000). Radical vulvectomy may directly affect orgasmic ability because a good deal of erogenous tissues, including the clitoris, may need to be removed. Monga (1995) reported on several studies with small subject numbers that a definite decline existed in sexual activity, with complaints of persistent numbness (some women could not sense penile penetration) and poor body image. They also regarded the information provided about the surgery as either absent or falsely reassuring. However, Monga reported one study where half of the patients (N = 10) were able to reach orgasm after radical vulvar surgery.

Although breast cancer treatment clearly should not have a direct effect on the sexual response cycle, reports have shown that mastectomy can cause decreased orgasm and coital frequency approximately 25% of the time (Monga, 1995; Schover et al., 1995).

Much of chemotherapy's impact on sexuality is because of side effects such as fatigue, alopecia, and changes in ovarian function in pre- and perimenopausal women (Wilmoth & Bruner, 2002). Effects of the chemotherapy drugs on the sexual response cycle include decreased desire and inhibited orgasm. These effects primarily are associated with alkylating agents (Wilmoth & Ross, 1997; Young-McCaughan, 1996). Hormonal therapy with antiestrogen preparations also can decrease orgasmic response. Although some women can use HRT to counteract some of the side effects, nonhormonal alternatives also must be considered. Graf and Geller (2003) provided excellent information relative to alternatives to HRT (e.g., megestrol acetate, soy, black cohosh, vitamin E, antihypertensives, antidepressants) for the treatment of hot flashes in women with breast cancer. Another recent randomized controlled study with 16,608 healthy postmenopausal women 50–79 years of age was undertaken to assess risks and benefits of commonly used combined hormone preparations. The risks outweighed the benefits when a combined estrogen and progestin regimen was administered. At the 5.2-year follow-up, more risk was evident for coronary heart disease, stroke, pulmonary embolism, and invasive breast cancer (Writing Group for the Women's Health Initiative Investigators, 2002).

Maintaining Patient Confidence in Their Sexuality

Assessment and Communication

It would be wonderful if healthcare professionals could communicate about sex and sexuality as naturally as they communicate about the other side effects of cancer and its treatment. However, this remains a delicate subject, especially with older adults. As public acceptance of sexuality in later life continues to increase and nurses begin to talk about it more freely with their patients, a better understanding and greater refinement of the diagnosis and treatment of sexual problems will evolve. More information must be provided about sexuality before, during, and after treatment commences so that patients can gain better mind and body self-awareness that will enhance the survivorship experience.

The key to better patient education is to ask the questions and to be ready for the answers. Although most nurses and physicians are not sexuality experts, they can be familiar with basic guidelines (see Figure 20-3), be prepared to ask three or four generic assessment questions (see Figure 20-4), and have some appropriate educational materials available for take-home reading. If professionals would take a few moments to review the American Cancer Society's materials on sexuality for men and women with cancer, it will increase their own knowledge and comfort level, and they will be able to address most of the questions that patients are prone to ask (Schover, 2001a, 2001b). If patients have more in-depth concerns, they can be referred to a sex therapist, preferably one with American Association of Sex Educators, Counselors, and Therapists credentials. Some recommendations to further increase comfort when speaking to patients and partners include (a) providing privacy, (b) assuring confidentiality, (c) obtaining a sexual history early, (d) avoiding verbal and nonverbal overreaction or boredom, (e) proceeding from less sensitive to more sensitive topics, (f) determining that goals are the patients' and not your goals, and (g) knowing when to refer (Shell, 2001).

1. You are a sexual person from the day you are born until the day you die. Aging does not cause sexuality to cease.
2. The key to maintaining a vital sexuality is to integrate intimacy, nondemand pleasuring, and erotic scenarios and techniques.
3. Contrary to popular myths about couples who stop being sexual, in more than 90% of cases, the man makes the decision because he finds sex frustrating and embarrassing.
4. Sexuality is more likely to remain functional and satisfying when both the man and woman value a variable, flexible, pleasure-oriented sexual style rather than a performance-oriented, pass-fail intercourse approach.
5. Medical interventions such as testosterone, hormone replacement therapy, and Viagra® (Pfizer, New York, NY) are not a "magic cure" but a valuable resource. The medical intervention needs to be integrated into the couple's sexual style.
6. With aging, the hormonal, vascular, and neurologic systems function less efficiently, so psychological, relational, and erotic skill factors become more important in maintaining a healthy sexuality.
7. The best aphrodisiac is an involved, aroused partner.
8. The "give to get" pleasuring guideline has particular value for the aging couple. This promotes mutual stimulation and multiple stimulation.
9. The major physiologic changes in male sexual response are that it takes longer and requires more direct penile stimulation to obtain an erection, the erection is not as firm, the erection is more likely to wane, and the need to ejaculate at each sexual opportunity is lessened.
10. The major physiologic changes in female sexual response are diminished vaginal lubrication, thinner vaginal walls, more time and stimulation are required for arousal and orgasm, and less intense orgasmic response.
11. Estrogen replacement for women, the use of Viagra by both men and women, and testosterone augmentation for both men and women can be positive resources to enhance sexual functioning. A physician should prescribe and monitor these interventions.
12. Positive and realistic expectations are crucial in maintaining a healthy sexual relationship. Do not compare sexuality at age 60 with sexuality at age 20. Focus on quality and pleasure, not quantity and performance.
13. Sexuality is more than genitals, intercourse, and orgasm. Sexuality involves affectionate, sensual, playful, erotic, and intercourse touch. Not all touching can or should result in intercourse.
14. A crucial factor, especially for women, is acceptance of her changing body image. Traditionally, female sexual desire and sense of attractiveness was contingent on everything being perfect. Self-acceptance, especially for older people, promotes partner acceptance.
15. Maintaining a regular rhythm of sexual contact is crucial—the guideline of "use it or lose it." The average sexual frequency is once a week. When couples are sexual less often than every two weeks, self-consciousness and anxiety replace comfort and positive anticipation. A key to satisfying sexuality is to maintain a pleasure-oriented connection.
16. Couples who cling to the traditional male-female double standard are vulnerable to inhibited sexual desire. Male-female equity and being an intimate sexual team facilitates a variable, flexible sexual style.
17. The couple can appreciate and enjoy the role reversal where female sexual response is easier and more predictable than male sexual response. Remember, sex is about sharing pleasure, not a competition or performance.
18. Most women use a lubricant to facilitate intercourse and reduce the likelihood of dyspareunia (painful intercourse). Additionally, if the woman guides intromission, male performance anxiety is reduced.
19. The man needs to accept his penis and its response rather than compare it to the easy, predictable, autonomous erections of his 20s. Individuals should enjoy their bodies, their partners' bodies, and the whole sexual experience rather than have a narrow focus on erection and intercourse.
20. Sex after age 60 is a more intimate, interactive, and involved sexuality than sex at age 20. Enjoy these new opportunities, feelings, and experiences.

Figure 20-3. Guidelines for Sex After 60

Note. Based on information from McCarthy, 2002.

1. Has having cancer (or its treatment) interfered with being a mother (father, partner)?
2. Has your cancer (or its treatment) changed the way you see yourself as a woman (man)?
3. Has your cancer (or its treatment) caused any change in your sexual functioning (sexual relationship)?
4. Do you expect your sexual functioning (sexual relationship) to be changed in any way after you leave the hospital (after you finish your treatment)?

Figure 20-4. Basic Sexual Assessment Questions

Note. Based on information from McPhetridge, 1968.

Discussion related to a patient's sexuality and how it will be affected by cancer treatment should take place all along the cancer continuum, but especially before treatment begins (Bertero, 2001). When this information is incorporated into the education process, it normalizes sexuality concerns for both the patient and partner as well as for the professional (Daniluk, 1998; Gallo-Silver, 2000). Oncology professionals familiar with some basic sexual rehabilitation techniques can be supportive and provide a sense of hope to those who wish to maintain a sense of physical intimacy at a most frightening time in their lives (Glass & Webb, 1995).

Rehabilitation Interventions

The way to achieve sexual happiness is by merging emotional needs with physical needs. Often older people with cancer may wonder how sex can survive amid tubes, pumps, and lubes that make them feel more like mechanics than romantics. In reality, many older adults discover that late-life sexuality survives in an increased diversity of expression: sometimes slow, tender, and affectionate and sometimes more intense and spontaneous. Middle- and late-life sex actually may be better than the more frantic pace of younger years. Biology finally puts sex in sync.

In younger years, patients probably were more driven by hormones and societal pressure. Now they may find that desire, arousal, and orgasm take longer and are not always a sure thing. Further, they may find that setting and mood are more important factors. Touch and extended foreplay may become just as satisfying as more urgent needs for arousal and release. They may feel more relaxed and less inhibited in later life and may be more confident to assert their sexual desires openly.

Although romance adds spice to any couple, true intimacy goes beyond a heart that skips a beat; good communication is essential in adapting a patient's sexuality to changes because of the aging process. To help patients and partners to achieve lasting intimacy and guide them down a path of increased closeness, nurses can provide both physical and emotional interventions. Couples who have been together for many years tend to fall into lovemaking patterns that have become fixed or perhaps insensitive. This may be a good time to give these couples permission to take a risk and to learn some new and different techniques; one way may be to refer them to the American Cancer Society's books on sexuality (Schover, 2001a, 2001b). The nurse also can provide suggestions specific to women and men, which may encourage reaffirmation or experimentation with new styles and techniques of intimacy between partners, whether in a new relationship or one that has lasted many loving years (see Figure 20-5). Physical intimacy brings comfort, closeness,

Women
- Use a water-based vaginal lubricant or suppository (e.g., Astroglide® [BioFilm, Vista, CA], Slippery Stuff® [Wal-Med, Inc., Puyallup, WA], Replens® [Lil' Drug Store Products, Cedar Rapids, IA], Lubrin® [Aurora Pharmaceuticals, North Ryde, Australia]). Flavored and/or warming lubricants may be more exciting. Do not use petroleum jelly, as this may obstruct the urethra.
- Increase foreplay time. Couples may wish to start somewhere other than the bedroom.
- Avoid direct stimulation of the clitoris if painful (clitoris may be exposed because of atrophy of the labia).
- Practice Kegel exercises (alternately contracting and relaxing the muscles in the pelvic area).
- Urinate immediately after coitus because of irritation to the urethra and bladder during sexual activity.
- Consult with a physician about the use of systemic estrogen therapy or topical estrogen cream to forestall and prevent the physiologic effects of aging (Masters et al., 1994). A safer alternative may be the Estring® (Pfizer, New York, NY), a 2-inch circle of estradiol surrounded by a silicon polymer that regulates release of estrogen; this is inserted in the vagina like a diaphragm and remains in for three months.
- Testosterone cream may be used to enhance desire if the testosterone level (free and bound) is low. A pea-sized amount of compounded cream of testosterone propionate 2% in petrolatum may be applied to the skin twice a week or prn (personal communication from Patricia Ganz, MD).
- For hot flashes, try venlafaxine 75 mg daily; a 61% reduction has been reported (Loprinzi et al., 2000). Other medications include paroxetine 10 mg daily (67% reduction) and fluoxetine 20 mg daily (50% reduction) (Loprinzi et al., 2002).

Men
- Have the female partner try a new coital position by bending her knees and placing a pillow under her hips to elevate the pelvis. This will more easily accommodate a partially erect penis.
- Massage the penis or have the partner massage the penis. Do not pull it up toward the abdomen where it will lose blood, but rather push down with pressure at the base of the penis. Pressure on the major blood vessels will hold blood in the penis.
- The female partner can place the partially erect penis into the vagina and flex the vaginal muscles that have been strengthened by the Kegel exercises to assist in a more full erection.
- If one of the partners has a protruding abdomen, the couple should find a position that allows the penis to reach the vagina. One technique (triangle) is to have the woman lie on her back with legs apart and knees sharply bent, while the man places himself over her with his hips under the angle formed by her raised knees. This may be difficult if the female is arthritic.
- Pharmacologic agents used for erectile dysfunction include Viagra® (Pfizer) and, a newer drug, Cialis® (Eli Lilly, Indianapolis, IN). These drugs do not improve desire but increase erectile response to sexual stimulation.
- Consult with a physician about penile implants. Several are available, including rigid, semi-rigid, and inflatable prostheses (Schover, 2001a).
- Consult with a physician about the use of penile self-injection with phentolamine/papaverine, which will elicit an erection that lasts for about one hour. Medication is injected into the base of the penis with a small-gauge needle. Effectiveness varies for diabetics.
- Consider vacuum therapy, which mimics the natural process of creating and maintaining an erection with a vacuum cylinder (e.g., ErecAid Systems® [Timm Medical Technologies, Eden Prairie, MN]).

General
- Use mood enhancers (e.g., candlelight, music, romantic thoughts).
- Use a double/queen size bed for lovemaking and talking. Place a single bed in the room if you must separate to sleep.
- Do not line up medications on the bedside stand; this is unattractive, dangerous if sleepy, and a constant reminder of illness.
- Plan for privacy: Nothing shatters romance like hearing visiting children fixing a midnight snack.
- Choose different times for lovemaking; in the evening, go to bed early before becoming overtired, then wake up in the middle of the night after having some good rest; morning may be best because enough time has been dedicated to rest and relaxation.
- Trade houses with another couple, and an instant vacation is created.
- A warm bath with candlelight, soft music, and wine may help to soothe away the day's aches and pains for both the patient and partner and creates closeness without the anxiety of performance.
- Eliminate guesswork. The couple should tell each other what they like the most about their sexual activity and be able to ask for what they want.

Figure 20-5. Gender-Specific and General Sexual Interventions

Note. From "Sexuality and the Older Person With Cancer," by J.A. Shell and C.K. Smith, 1994, *Oncology Nursing Forum, 21,* pp. 557–558. Copyright 1994 by the Oncology Nursing Society. Adapted with permission.

and a sense of security; however, cultivating some communication principles helps to secure the relationship (see Table 20-3). Finally, all patients may not have a partner with whom to communicate either emotionally or physically. Even if an active partner is present, some type of self-pleasuring activity may be explored with this population to provide a sexual outlet. Although most men and women have masturbated some time during their lives, this subject continues to be rather taboo and requires delicate and sensitive conversation. Gallo-Silver (2000) stated, "'Self-pleasuring' is a cognitive reframing of masturbation to make the activity more acceptable for the purpose of sexual rehabilitation. Self-pleasuring enables individuals to explore their body's response to sexual stimulation without the added pressure of performance anxiety and concerns about their partner's reactions, concerns, and fears" (p. 12).

Table 20-3. Communication Principles to Enhance Intimacy

Goal	Means
Accept each other.	Two people create a couple; different backgrounds, opinions, quirks, strengths, and weaknesses are involved. Respect the differences. Value the partner for the unique contribution he or she brings to the relationship. Do not put conditions on love, such as "I'll love you if/when . . ."
Show gratitude.	No one wants to be taken for granted. Express thanks and appreciation. Send a card. Give a foot massage. Use the manners taught to children; say please and thank you.
Affirm one another.	Praise and encourage unconditionally. Everyone likes to hear that he or she looks nice or did a good job. Remember, a partner does not have to *do* anything to deserve affirmation.
Show consideration.	Show respect or regard for a partner through careful thought and behavior. Do something meaningful and enjoyable, and expect nothing in return.
Establish healthy communication.	Take the risk of telling the other your needs, feelings, ideas, and fears. When conflict is present, do not place blame. Be ready to listen.
Demonstrate physical affection.	Tender touching is vital to an intimate and healthy physical relationship. Hold hands. Give big hugs. Touching and kissing are more than a prelude to intercourse; they are ways of communicating and of enhancing intimacy.

Areas for Future Research

Although the aforementioned interventions are and have been evident in the nursing literature for years, these are considered to be nonresearch-based and stem from expert opinion and case studies. For an in-depth examination of evidence-based research to manage sexual dysfunction in the patient with cancer with site-specific intervention (in all adults with cancer), please see Shell (2002). This article reveals that few high-level studies exist regarding sexuality and cancer. Eight research studies were found, and none of these were of the highest caliber of "levels of evidence." These studies included fewer than 100 subjects, and although some were randomized, they were not integrative reviews or meta-analyses, nor were they well-designed trials even without randomization (e.g., single group prepost, cohort, time series, meta-analysis of cohort studies). The other evidence included practice guidelines, expert opinion, and case studies (Shell, 2002).

Studies that examined the control of hot flashes in breast cancer survivors are some of the few randomized controlled intervention trials executed to address problems with sexual function in patients with cancer, and this does not necessarily speak to older adults with cancer (Loprinzi et al., 2000, 2002). One other randomized study consisted of 36 women with gynecologic cancer and examined the effect of a specialist nurse intervention (psychosexual) on sexual function. Maughan and Clarke (2001) found improved sexual function in the group that received the special psychosexual educational counseling. The challenge is to create intervention-based controlled trials for the purpose of enhancing and/or improving the sexual function of older adults with cancer, as well as all adults with cancer.

Although several adequate tools are available to assess for sexual distress, a lack of sufficient high-level, quality, evidence-based interventions exist for the cancer population. Further, the most appropriate time to provide interventions is not clear. Nurses can be proactive in discussion, assessment, and education of this significant concern, and that, in itself, can be an important intervention. In the author's experience, sexuality is one issue that is infrequently addressed, both by nurses and physicians; however, sexuality needs to be an important concern because patients continuously verbalize how validated they feel when discussion ensues. "Patients and their partners will continue to require intervention to employ all of their resources to retain a sense of sexual being and intimate relationship during and after the cancer experience" (Shell, 2002, p. 64).

Case Study

Mr. B, a 69-year-old Caucasian male, was newly diagnosed (via bronchoscopy) with non-small cell lung cancer and was being seen for the first time at the clinic. Mrs. B accompanied him, and both appeared very hesitant and frightened. The doctor talked to them at length about the plan of care and the type of chemotherapy that would be used for his type of cancer. The doctor answered general questions and then referred the couple to the clinical nurse specialist (CNS) for a more in-depth explanation of his treatment. As the CNS discussed the different drugs that he would be receiving, she also included that he would most likely experience some fatigue and that the couple would probably want to refrain from sexual intercourse until the fatigue subsided. This fact was mentioned right along with all of the other expected side effects; this normalized conversation about their intimate relationship as well as other medical concerns they may have related to the drugs.

The couple's demeanor changed immediately, and both seemed to give an audible sigh of relief. The CNS was curious and asked if they had questions regarding her comments thus far. Mr. B excitedly explained that he had recently, in the past year, had a penile implant placed because of impotence due to diabetes. The implant had worked very well for this couple, and they enjoyed an active sex life. Now that he had cancer, both of them had just assumed that they would no longer be able to engage in sexual relations, but now that the CNS had explained that they only had to postpone sexual relations, they were most pleased. Their intimate relationship always had been a meaningful part of their marriage, and they were mourning the fact that they thought this would no longer be a part of their loving relationship. They asked a few more questions regarding this issue, and the CNS then proceeded to finish their educational session and gave them the American Cancer Society's booklet *Sexuality and Cancer: For the Man Who Has Cancer and His Partner* (Schover, 2001a).

The CNS spoke to this couple periodically during the husband's treatment to see how things were going and to check if they had further concerns related to sexuality or other issues. She also kept in touch with them after completion of treatment. Because the CNS simply made sexuality a part of her educational sessions with this couple, they were able to verbalize their fears about their sexual relationship, whereas they had not been able to speak to the physician about these issues during his extensive treatment explanation because it had not been mentioned.

Conclusion

It takes determination to resist the "over-the-hill" mentality demonstrated by society toward sexuality. Age brings changes at age 17 the same as it does at age 70. People never outgrow the need for intimate love and affection, particularly in times of illness. Whether one seeks intimacy through nonsexual touching and companionship or through sexual activity, obstacles may be overcome. The sexual experience may become more intimate and more selfless. The foundation is caring, adapting, and communicating—something each person or couple desires and what they can establish with another. When nurses acknowledge the challenges that age- and disease-related change creates, they can embrace the older adults' values, ethics, and cultural mores and then provide information, support, and acceptance of the patient's and partner's choices of sexual expression.

As one older adult explained, "I live in senior housing and do volunteer work at other senior residences. What is this idea that you have to stop having sex when you reach a certain age? It can be even more fun when your arthritis acts up. Wow, it took us two hours to get all of our clothes off! Or, we had to do it twice when we couldn't get out of the tub. The urge is always there. Just like bicycle riding, we do not forget. In fact, as we get older, we may kick ourselves, regretting things we did not try earlier" (McDonald, 2000, p. 157).

References

AARP. (1999a). *Healthy sexuality and vital aging.* Washington, DC: Author.

AARP. (1999b). *Modern maturity sexuality study.* Washington DC: Author.

Anderson, B.L., & Cyranowski, J.M. (1995). Women's sexuality: Behaviors, responses, and individual differences. *Journal of Consulting and Clinical Psychology, 63,* 891–906.

Anderson, B.L., Woods, X.A., & Copeland, L.J. (1997). Sexual self-schema and sexual morbidity among gynecologic cancer survivors. *Journal of Consulting and Clinical Psychology, 65,* 221–229.

Arai, Y., Kawakita, M., Okada, Y., & Yoshida, O. (1997). Sexuality and fertility in long-term survivors of testicular cancer. *Journal of Clinical Oncology, 15,* 1444–1448.

Badeau, D. (1995). Illness, disability and sex in aging. *Sexuality and Disability, 13,* 219–237.

Balducci, L. (2003). The elderly patient with cancer: New approaches for improved outcomes. *Journal of Supportive Oncology, 1*(Suppl. 2), 3–4.

Bertero, C. (2001). Altered sexual patterns after treatment for prostate cancer. *Cancer Practice, 9,* 245–251.

Bornestein, R. (1986). Cognitive and psychosocial development of older adults. In C.S. Schuster & S.S. Ashburn (Eds.), *The process of human development: A holistic life span approach* (2nd ed., pp. 815–832). Boston: Little, Brown.

Bruner, D.W., Hanlon, A., Nicolaou, N., & Hanks, G. (1997). Sexual function after radiotherapy + androgen deprivation for clinically localized prostate cancer in younger men (age 50–65) [Abstract]. *Oncology Nursing Forum, 24,* 327.

Butler, L., Banfield, V., Sveinson, T., & Allen, K. (1998). Conceptualizing sexual health in cancer care. *Western Journal of Nursing Research, 20,* 683–699.

Butler, R.N., & Lewis, M.I. (2002). *The new love and sex after 60* (4th ed.). New York: Ballantine Publishing.

Daniluk, J.C. (1998). *Women's sexuality across the life span: Challenging myths, creating meanings.* New York: Guilford Press.

Davis, S. (2000). Testosterone and sexual desire in women. *Journal of Sex Education and Therapy, 25,* 25–32.

Demeter, D. (1998). *The human sexuality web: Sex and the elderly.* Retrieved March 23, 2004, from http://www.umkc.edu/sites/hsw/age/index.html

Fields, C.B., & Scout. (2001). Addressing the needs of lesbian patients. *Journal of Sex Education and Therapy, 26,* 182–188.

Fleming, M.P., & Kleinbart, E. (2001). Breast cancer and sexuality. *Journal of Sex Education and Therapy, 26,* 215–224.

Gallo-Silver, L. (2000). The sexual rehabilitation of persons with cancer. *Cancer Practice, 8,* 10–15.

Ganz, P.A., Rowland, J.H., Desmond, K., Meyerowitz, B.E., & Wyatt, G.E. (1998). Life after breast cancer: Understanding women's health-related quality of life and sexual functioning. *Journal of Clinical Oncology, 16,* 501–514.

Glass, J.C., & Webb, M.L. (1995). Health care educators' knowledge and attitudes regarding sexuality in the aged. *Educational Gerontology, 21,* 713–733.

Graf, M.C., & Geller, P.A. (2003). Treating hot flashes in breast cancer survivors: A review of alternative treatments to hormone replacement therapy. *Clinical Journal of Oncology Nursing, 7,* 637–640.

Holland, J.C., & Lewis, S. (2000). *The human side of cancer.* New York: HarperCollins.

Hughes, M.K. (1996). Sexuality issues: Keeping your cool. *Oncology Nursing Forum, 23,* 1597–1600.

Jones, A. (1988). Developmental changes. In M.O. Hogstel (Ed.), *Nursing care of the older adult* (2nd ed., pp. 33–62). Media, PA: Harwal.

Korb, C.S. (1996). Sexual dysfunction; altered sexuality patterns. In G.K. McFarland & E.A. McFarlane (Eds.), *Nursing diagnosis and intervewntion: Planning for patient care* (3rd ed., pp. 777–786). St. Louis, MO: Mosby.

Leiblum, S.R., & Segraves, R.T. (2000). Sex therapy with aging adults. In S.R. Leiblum & R.C. Rosen (Eds.), *Principles and practice of sex therapy* (3rd ed., pp. 423–448). New York: Guilford Press.

Loprinzi, C.L., Kugler, J.W., Sloan, J.A., Mailliard, J.A., LaVasseur, B.I., Barton, D.L., et al. (2000). Venlafaxine in management of hot flashes in survivors of breast cancer: A randomized controlled trial. *Lancet, 356,* 2059–2063.

Loprinzi, C.L., Sloan, J.A., Perez, E.A., Quella, S.K., Stella, P.J., Mailliard, J.A., et al. (2002). Phase III evaluation of fluoxetine for treatment of hot flashes. *Journal of Clinical Oncology, 20,* 1578–1583.

Massie, M.J., & Popkin, M.K. (1998). Depressive disorders. In J.C. Holland (Ed.), *Psycho-oncology* (pp. 518–540). New York: Oxford University Press.

Masters, W.H., Johnson, V.E., & Kolodny, R.C. (1994). *Heterosexuality.* New York: HarperPerennial.

Matola, T. (2000). Stroke. In J. Blank (Ed.), *Still doing it: Women and men over 60 write about their sexuality* (pp. 90–91). San Francisco: Down There Press.

Matthews, A.K. (1998). Lesbians and cancer support: Clinical issues for cancer patients. *Health Care for Women International, 19,* 193–203.

Maughan, K., & Clarke, C. (2001). The effect of a clinical nurse specialist in gynecological oncology on quality of life and sexuality. *Journal of Clinical Nursing, 10,* 221–229.

McCarthy, B.W. (2002). *Restoring and revitalizing marital sexuality.* Eau Claire, WI: Health Education Network.

McDaniel, J.S., Musselman, D.L., Porter, M.R., Reed, D.A., & Nemeroff, C.B. (1995). Depression in patients with cancer: Diagnosis, biology, and treatment. *Archives of General Psychiatry, 52,* 89–99.

McDonald, S. (2000). Clean old man. In J. Blank (Ed.), *Still doing it: Women and men over 60 write about their sexuality* (p. 157). San Francisco: Down There Press.

McPhetridge, L. (1968). Nursing history: One means to personalized care. *American Journal of Nursing, 68,* 68–75.

Monga, U. (1995). Sexuality in cancer patients. *Physical Medicine and Rehabilitation, 9,* 417–442.

Monga, U., Kerrigan, A.J., Garber, S., & Monga, T.N. (2001). Pre- and post-radiotherapy sexual functioning in prostate cancer patients. *Sexuality and Disability, 19,* 239–252.

Monga, U., Tan, G., Ostermann, H.J., & Monga, T.N. (1997). Sexuality in head and neck cancer patients. *Archives of Physical Medicine and Rehabilitation, 78,* 298–304.

Muller, J.E., Mittleman, A., Maclure, M., Sherwood, J.B., & Tofler, G.H. (1996). Triggering myocardial infarction by sexual activity. Low absolute risk and prevention by regular physical exertion. *JAMA, 275,* 1405–1409.

National Council on Aging. (1998). *Healthy sexuality and vital aging.* Washington, DC: Author.

National Institute on Aging. (2000). *Exercise: A guide from the National Institute on Aging* [49-minute video and 100-page book]. Bethesda, MD: Author.

Ofman, U.S. (1995). Preservation of function in genitourinary cancers: Psychosexual and psychosocial issues. In J. Klastersky, S.C. Schimpff, & H.J. Senn (Eds.), *Handbook of supportive care in cancer* (pp. 125–131). New York: Marcel Dekker.

Ren, X.S. (1997). Marital status and quality of relationships: The impact on health perception. *Social Science and Medicine, 44,* 241–249.

Richard, D. (2001). With age comes wisdom—with wisdom, new lessons. *Contemporary Sexuality, 35,* 1–12.

Richardson, J.P., & Lazur, D. (1995). Sexuality and the nursing home patient. *American Family Physician, 51,* 121.

Rodrigue, J.R., & Park, T.L. (1996). General and illness-specific adjustment to cancer: Relationship to marital status and marital quality. *Journal of Psychosomatic Research, 40,* 29–36.

Rowland, J.H., & Massie, M.J. (1996). Psychological reactions to breast cancer diagnosis, treatment, and survival. In J.R. Harris, M.E. Lippman, M. Morrow, & S. Hellman (Eds.), *Diseases of the breast* (pp. 919–938). Philadelphia: Lippincott-Raven.

Schover, L.R. (2000). Sexual problems in chronic illness. In S.R. Leiblum & R.C. Rosen (Eds.), *Principles and practice of sex therapy* (3rd ed., pp. 398–422). New York: Guilford Press.

Schover, L.R. (2001a). *Sexuality and cancer: For the man who has cancer and his partner.* Atlanta, GA: American Cancer Society.

Schover, L.R. (2001b). *Sexuality and cancer: For the woman who has cancer and her partner.* Atlanta, GA: American Cancer Society.

Schover, L.R., Yetman, R.J., Tuason, L.J., Meisler, E., Esselstyn, C.B., Hermann, R.E., et al. (1995). Comparison of partial mastectomy with breast reconstruction on psychosocial adjustment, body image, and sexuality. *Cancer, 75,* 54–64.

Sexuality Information and Education Council of the United States. (2001/2002). Fact sheet: Sexuality in middle and later life. *SIECUS Report, 30*(2), 1–9.

Sharpe, T.H. (2004). Introduction to sexuality in late life. *Family Journal: Counseling and Therapy for Couples and Families, 12,* 199–205.

Shell, J.A. (1991). Sexuality for patients with gynecologic cancer. In D. Lowdermilk (Ed.), *NAACOG's clinical issues in perinatal and women's health nursing* (pp. 479–495). Philadelphia: Lippincott.

Shell, J.A. (2001). Impact of cancer on sexuality. In S. Otto (Ed.), *Oncology nursing* (4th ed., pp. 973–999). St. Louis, MO: Mosby.

Shell, J.A. (2002). Evidence-based practice for symptom management in adults with cancer: Sexual dysfunction. *Oncology Nursing Forum, 29,* 53–66.

Shell, J.A., & Kirsch, S. (2001). Psychosocial issues, outcomes, and quality of life. In S. Otto (Ed.), *Oncology nursing* (4th ed., pp. 948–972). St. Louis, MO: Mosby.

Shell, J.A., & Smith, C.K. (1994). Sexuality and the older person with cancer. *Oncology Nursing Forum, 21,* 553–558.

Siston, A.K., List, M.A., Schleser, R., & Vokes, E. (1997). Sexual functioning and head and neck cancer. *Journal of Psychosocial Oncology, 15,* 107–122.

Snyder, D.S., & Whisman, M.A. (2004). Treating distressed couples with coexisting mental and physical disorders: Directions for clinical training and practice. *Journal of Marital and Family Therapy, 30,* 1–12.

Spratto, G.R., & Woods, A.L. (2003). *PDR: Nurse's drug handbook.* Clifton Park, NY: Thomson Delmar Learning.

Stanford, J.L., Feng, Z., Hamilton, A.S., Gillilland, F.D., Stephenson, R.A., Eley, J.W., et al. (2000). Urinary and sexual function after radical prostatectomy for clinically localized prostate cancer. *JAMA, 283,* 354–360.

Steinke, E., & Patterson-Midgley, P. (1996). Sexual counseling following acute myocardial infarction. *Clinical Nursing Research, 5,* 462–472.

Talcott, J.A., Rieker, P., Clark, J., Propert, K.J., Weeks, J.C., Beard, C.J., et al. (1996). Long-term complications of treatment for early prostate cancer: 2-year follow-up in a prospective, multi-institutional outcomes study [Abstract 644]. *Proceedings of the American Society of Clinical Oncology, 15,* 252.

Talcott, J.A., Rieker, P., Clark, J.A., Propert, K.J., Weeks, J.C., Beard, C.J., et al. (1997). Patient-reported impotence and incontinence after nerve-sparing radical prostatectomy. *Journal of the National Cancer Institute, 89,* 1117–1123.

Talcott, J.A., Rieker, P., Clark, J.A., Propert, K.J., Weeks, J.C., Beard, C.J., et al. (1998). Patient-reported symptoms after primary therapy for early prostate cancer: Results of a prospective cohort study. *Journal of Clinical Oncology, 16,* 275–283.

Tallis, R., Fillit, H., & Brocklehurst, R.C. (1998). *Brocklehurst's textbook of geriatric medicine and gerontology* (5th ed.). London: Churchill Livingstone.

Tremethick, M.J., Tornabene, L., & Eibes, C. (2002). Sexuality and older adults: A Web-based resource for health educators. *International Electronic Journal of Health Education.* Retrieved March 8, 2004, from http://www.aahperd.org/iejhe/template.cfm?template=current/tremethick.html

Wilmoth, M.C., & Bruner, D.W. (2002). Integrating sexuality into cancer nursing practice. *Oncology Nursing Updates, 9*(1), 1–14.

Wilmoth, M.C., & Ross, J.A. (1997). Women's perception: Breast cancer treatments and sexuality. *Cancer Practice, 5,* 353–359.

Writing Group for the Women's Health Initiative Investigators. (2002). Risks and benefits of estrogen plus progestin in healthy postmenopausal women. *JAMA, 288,* 321–333.

Young-McCaughan, S. (1996). Sexual functioning in women with breast cancer after treatment with adjuvant therapy. *Cancer Nursing, 19,* 308–319.

CHAPTER 21

Palliative Care of the Older Adult With Cancer

Kathleen Murphy-Ende, RN, PhD, AOCNP

Introduction

The focus of care for the older adult with advanced cancer throughout the course of the illness is on enhancing quality of life (QOL) through symptom management. The survival time for many has been extended as a result of more effective treatment and supportive care, resulting in a chronic illness trajectory. Many older adults living with cancer have coexisting medical problems that create additional physical limitations and symptoms. Attention to aggressive symptom management and advanced care planning is necessary to avoid physical distress, fragmented care, and caregiver burden. The special needs of the older adult population should be considered in planning healthcare services.

Hospice is a model of care for people facing a life-limiting illness, with a focus on caring not curing, provided by a multidisciplinary team (National Hospice and Palliative Care Organization, 2004). The mission of hospice is based on the understanding that dying is a part of the normal life cycle, with care directed at supporting the patient and family through the dying process and bereavement. The services include medical and supportive care in the home, inpatient units, residential facilities, nursing facilities, prisons, and other settings (Egan & Labyak, 2001). Historically, the term *hospice* has been used in three ways: the place where patients who are dying receive care; an organization providing services for dying patients and family members; and an approach to care for the dying (Committee on Care at the End of Life, 1997). Currently, hospice care is covered through the Medicare Hospice Benefit as well as through private insurance companies.

The definition of the specialty of palliative care is comprehensive care provided by an interdisciplinary team to patients and families living with life-threatening or severe advanced illness who are expected to progress toward dying, with the goal of alleviating suffering and promoting QOL. The major components are information sharing, pain and symptom management, advanced care planning, and coordination of care, including psychosocial and spiritual support for patients and their families (American Academy of Hospice and Palliative Medicine, 2003). Palliative care extends the principles of hospice to a broader population that benefits from receiving this care earlier in the illness; therefore, specific therapy is not excluded from palliative care.

This chapter will address palliative care of the older adult with cancer and will discuss many issues facing the older adult and caregivers at the end of life. Issues such as communication, information sharing, advanced care planning, palliative care, and caregiver experiences will be covered. Areas for further research investigating palliative care will be highlighted.

Information Sharing

Information sharing is a reciprocal process and is a critical part of the nursing and advanced practice nurse (APN) role. A patient-centered approach is important when initiating a dialogue and providing education on end-of-life issues. Families of dying patients rated giving timely answers to end-of-life questions and being open in communication as helpful nursing interventions (Steeves & Kahn, 1994). Healthcare professionals should consider the following core principles when having difficult discussions, which are based on the consensus among the specialties of medicine: respect the dignity of the patient and caregiver; be sensitive to and respectful of their wishes; use the most appropriate measures that are consistent with patient choices; and respect their right to refuse treatment care (Cassell & Foley, 1999).

Advanced Care Planning

Advanced care planning helps patients to have control over their health care and makes it easier for healthcare providers and family to follow through with the patients' healthcare wishes. It also provides patients with an opportunity to communicate their philosophy of care with the family and healthcare providers. These serious conversations serve to clarify their understanding of existing conditions, expectations, fears, potential conflicts, and goals of care. Because most patients lose their ability to communicate during the terminal phase, these issues should be discussed early in the disease process and ideally prior to diagnosis. Obtaining information about the patient's wishes through advance directives may prevent future conflict within the family.

Advance directives are legal forms that allow people to state their wishes in the event that they become unable to do so. These documents help to guide medical care choices and are important in giving one control over his or her health care. Two kinds of advance medical directives are available: the durable power of attorney for health care and a living will. The durable power of attorney for health care allows patients to name someone to act on their behalf when they can no longer speak for themselves. This person must be at least 18 years of age and of sound mind. The form documents the decisions patients want the healthcare agent to make for them and allows them to put their desires in their own words. The living will covers only end-of-life decisions when life-support measures such as using a ventilator or artificial nutrition are being considered. The disadvantage of the living will is it does not allow someone else to make healthcare decisions; however, it may be useful when the patient does not have someone to name as a healthcare agent.

Unfortunately, many studies have shown that advance directives often do not influence medical decision making (SUPPORT, 1995). This is usually because one cannot anticipate all possible situations. The medical condition may be complex and uncertain, and some directives lack flexibility. Furthermore, what matters to seriously ill older patients making end-of-life treatment decisions may be different from what was anticipated at the time the advance directive was completed. Most studies on patients' treatment preferences have considered preferences for specific interventions but not the outcomes of the intervention (Emanuel, Barry, Stoeckel, Ettelson, & Emanuel, 1991; Frankl, Oye, & Bellamy, 1989; O'Brien et al., 1995). Few studies have explored end-of-life treatment preferences of those living with a limited life expectancy. Fried and Bradley's (2003) qualitative work with terminally ill older adults found the three major influences on treatment preferences were treatment burden, treatment outcome, and the likelihood of the outcome. The patients' understanding of these outcomes changed over time. Based on these studies, the practice of advanced care planning should include information on treatment burdens, outcomes, and likelihood of these outcomes. Each conversation should be documented. Advanced care planning conversations should be an ongoing dialogue among patients, family members, and healthcare providers. Providing the opportunity to continue talking about decisions after they have been made may reassure patients and families in believing they have made the right choice or clarify if a change in their goals and preferences has occurred. Future research needs to explore the process and outcomes of presenting advance directive information to patients and families.

End-of-Life Treatment Decisions

For the older adult with advanced cancer, multiple options of care may lead to improvement in QOL. Many treatments described in previous chapters, such as chemotherapy, radiation, and surgery, are recognized as an important part of the comprehensive palliation of incurable cancer. Medical treatment decisions often are difficult for the older adult because information about options is complex, and conflicting opinions may exist regarding specific recommendations. The effects of comorbid conditions on prognosis and treatment response and options may be unknown. The uncertainty and unpredictability of the disease course are additional realities that make decision making difficult. The relative value of palliative chemotherapy or supportive care is not well documented. Assessing the patient's understanding of the prognosis, goals, and preferences is the first step. Clarification of the patient's goals should be obtained before information on palliative treatment is provided. Because the ultimate goal of palliative treatment is to maintain or improve QOL, the benefits and risks of treatments need to be considered within this context. Palliative care treatment decisions are based on the ability to relieve or prevent suffering. Numerous decisions exist regarding treatment associated with advanced cancer, including surgery, radiation, chemotherapy, antibiotics, diagnostic testing, code status, nutrition and hydration, and place for end-of-life care.

Palliative Surgery

Palliative surgery has become more common as newer techniques such as laparoscopic procedures, ablation techniques, surgical resections, and new drainage devices have been discovered. Twenty-one percent of all surgical procedures for cancer are performed for palliation (McCahill et al., 2002). The most common cancers that need palliative surgery are lung, colorectal, breast, and prostate, which are also the leading causes of cancer-related deaths (Jemal et al., 2005). The traditional outcome measures of surgery tend to be focused on physiologic response, survival, morbidity, and mortality. Measures of palliative surgical success are undefined and have not been documented in the literature. Functional status, QOL, and symptom relief would be the appropriate outcomes; however, very little has been studied. In the surgical literature from 1990–1996, QOL was examined in only 17% of reports, and pain was measured in only 12% (Miner, Jaques, Tavaf-Motamen, & Shriver, 1999). The difficulty in measuring outcomes of palliative surgery is that the goal often is broad and multifactorial. A better way to document outcomes is to measure the individual patient goal, such as pain relief, symptom avoidance, preservation of or increase in functional status, or improved nutritional status. Currently, the lack of outcome data makes surgical recommendations and decision making difficult for patients with advanced cancer. In addition, healthcare providers should measure the possible effects of invasive techniques that may be advantageous for patients with advanced cancer. The nurse's role in the surgical decision-making process is to educate and share information (see Figure 21-1).

- Enhance the communication between surgeon and patient.
- Help patients to identify their expectations and communicate these to the medical/surgical staff.
- Reinforce and clarify the risk-to-benefit ratio of surgery, and evaluate the patient/family understanding of the issues presented.
- Provide information on nonsurgical symptom management options.
- Provide emotional support for those coping with high-risk outcomes.
- Recognize the difficulty associated with decision making in the setting of advanced disease.

Figure 21-1. Nurses' Role in the Surgical Decision-Making Process

---

Palliative Radiation

Palliative radiation is noncurative and is aimed at relieving or alleviating symptoms such as pain, dyspnea, bleeding, skin/deep tissue metastasis, and impending or actual obstruction. Radiation may be offered to reduce tumor mass or to treat emergencies such as spinal cord compression or superior vena cava obstruction. The primary tumor of non-small cell lung cancer and metastasis to bone and brain are the most commonly treated problems in this setting (Kirkbride & Bezjak, 2002). Isotopes such as strontium-89 may be recommended in the treatment of bone metastases from prostate cancer to treat pain and prevent further lesions. Radical radiation (high intensity and dose) that is traditionally given with curative intent may be used to provide local control of tumor(s) when cure is not possible. Radiation is offered to treat the primary tumor or metastasis if the lesion is causing moderate or severe symptoms and the medical alternatives are not effective, have a high side-effect profile, or are not possible because of coexisting conditions. Patients who are at high risk for developing symptoms and have a good performance status may be offered radiation, although results of one randomized study do not support this approach in patients with lung cancer (Falk et al., 2002). In the palliative setting, often a lower total dose, larger daily fraction sizes, and shorter total treatment times are prescribed to prevent acute side effects such as mucositis, skin reaction, nausea, vomiting, and diarrhea. The expectation is that the patient will tolerate the treatment well, with mild and transient side effects. The decision to offer radiation is based upon objective information about the disease, estimated time of survival, risk-benefit analysis, including all aspects of the patient's well-being, and available radiotherapy resources. The healthcare provider should assist the patient in decision making by offering information on the purpose of treatment, when to expect relief of symptoms, side effects, and time commitment. The nurse can help to guide patients undergoing treatment by providing anticipatory guidance and treatment for acute side effects such as skin erythema or breakdown, nausea and vomiting, diarrhea, dysuria, mucositis, dysphagia, and alopecia.

Research addressing the best dose and course of palliative radiation is in its early stage, resulting in a wide range of possible recommendations. Data are lacking on the specific benefits of radiation on symptom management and QOL because most studies have looked at cure as an end point. Clinical trials aimed at examining dose, fractionation, side effects, symptom relief, and QOL are needed so that healthcare providers can offer the most effective treatment.

Palliative Chemotherapy

Palliative chemotherapy refers to the use of chemotherapy in the treatment of an incurable cancer. The goal is to decrease malignancy-induced symptoms and prolong life through a partial or complete tumor response from either locally advanced or metastatic disease. Although chemotherapy in advanced cancer is given with non-curative intent, the patient still may hope for cure or extension of life. Traditionally, chemotherapy had been prescribed as adjuvant or curative; therefore, most of the research studies only describe tumor reduction (response rate) and length of survival as end points. In the past several years, researchers have designed more studies to describe the impact that chemotherapy has on symptom reduction and QOL. Some clinical trial data are available in selected cancers that chemotherapy may improve QOL and symptom control without impacting survival. Several studies have reported a decrease in pain or other symptoms without objective tumor response in pancreas, breast, and prostate cancers (Ellison & Chevlen, 2002). However, documentation shows that tumor reduction correlates with improvement of symptoms such as pain, mood, and shortness of breath in those with metastatic breast cancer (Geels, Eisenhauer, Bezjak, Zee, & Day, 2000).

Fortunately, the development of new and safer agents and a better understanding of the pharmacologic actions of older agents have allowed safer use in older patients (Balducci & Stanta, 2000). Many studies suggest that older adult patients tolerate some treatments as well as younger patients (Popescu, Norman, Ross, Parikh, & Cunningham, 1999), cope better with chemotherapy, and report less discomfort and anxiety (Ganz, Schag, & Heinrich, 1985). In decision making regarding chemotherapy in the older adult, healthcare providers should consider the tumor type, benefit-to-toxicity ratio, and performance status. A person with a poor performance status of Eastern Cooperative Oncology Group 3 or 4 or a Karnofsky score less than

50% is likely to experience more toxicity than a beneficial response (Buccheri, Ferrigno, & Tamburini, 1996). Healthcare providers should consider the individual patient's needs and related disease factors. It is important to provide the patient and family with accurate and realistic information regarding the probable outcome of chemotherapy, including the expected desired outcomes, risks, and side effects. The safety and effectiveness of the specific chemotherapy also should be outlined. The statistical information regarding efficacy and survival needs to be presented in terms of how it may translate to the individual.

It may be difficult to sort out the patient's goals of chemotherapy; therefore, asking patients what they expect or hope for is important. Younger patients are more likely to undergo chemotherapy for little predicted chance of symptom improvement and life extension (Bremnes, Andersen, & Wist, 1995). Only a few studies on decision making in the older adult with advanced cancer were found. Adults who believed that they were likely to die within six months were less likely to choose life-extending treatment over comfort care (Weeks et al., 1998). Older patients tend to agree to undergo aggressive chemotherapy for palliative purposes but are less willing to trade significant toxicity for increased survival time (Yellen, Cella, & Leslie, 1994). Many patients have difficulty in therapeutic decision making. In one study, 25% of older and sicker men wanted the physician to make all of the treatment decisions (Blanchard, Labrecque, Ruckdeschel, & Blanchard, 1988). When nurses assist patients in decision making on the value of chemotherapy in advanced cancer, the following questions should be directed to the oncologist: What is the response rate of the proposed chemotherapy? What is the median duration of response of the proposed chemotherapy regimen? What is the potential treatment burden? How long must treatment be continued to determine effect? (Weissman, 2000). Practical concerns include length of treatment, impact on family/caregiver schedules and normal routines, travel distance to hospital, and financial reimbursement.

Palliative and supportive care should be ongoing throughout the illness continuum. When chemotherapy is not offered or the patient declines this option, palliative care should continue as a positive active approach to care. Providers should continue to use follow-up care to assess and treat symptoms and reassure patients that the healthcare team will continue to care for them.

Healthcare professionals should continue to use clinical studies to evaluate the clinical benefit response of palliative chemotherapy in order to offer patients more complete information on the benefits of treatment. Because QOL is a very individual and complex issue, further work is required in instrument design to measure the relevant QOL outcomes in the older adult seeking palliative chemotherapy.

Antibiotics

Antibiotics often are used in patients with cancer for treatment of a variety of infections. If the intention of treatment is to increase survival, then the use of antibiotics for the infection is appropriate. Individual factors need to be considered, such as prognosis and treatment goals. If the intention of treatment is palliation, then the decision of starting antibiotics needs to be made on the basis of whether antibiotics will provide comfort or prolong the dying process. Examples of indications for antibiotics for comfort are high fever causing convulsions or mental status changes, reduced cardiac or pulmonary function, history of adverse reaction to fever, or a prolonged fever causing a hypercatabolic state. Providers should consider the side effects of the drug when prescribing these agents.

Pneumonia may occur as a complication of the debilitated state in the older adult with advanced cancer, underlying pulmonary or cardiac disease, or aspiration. When patients with pneumonia are nearing the end of life, nurses should address the issues of starting, continuing, or stopping antibiotics. Nurses should employ extreme sensitivity when explaining the reason for discontinuing or not providing antibiotics to treat infection. When possible, the nurse can address this conversation before the patient enters the terminal phase. Antibiotics should be discontinued in the terminally ill unless they are essential to patient comfort (Working Party on Clinical Guidelines in Palliative Care, 1997). In end-stage disease, antibiotics may be indicated in patients with pneumonia who are experiencing dyspnea, elevated temperature, cough, or congestion, with the goal of improving dyspnea if other measures such as antipyretics, cooling measures, decongestions, and humidifiers are unsuccessful. A workup for infection is not appropriate in end-stage disease.

Diagnostic Testing

Diagnostic testing in the cancer trajectory frequently is done during active treatment and less so during the post-treatment phase. Patients undergoing "watchful waiting" may continue to undergo laboratory tests or scans. When the disease progresses, diagnostic testing may not be appropriate. A specific time is not defined when testing should be stopped, but in extensive disease, healthcare providers should carefully consider performing diagnostic testing. Testing is appropriate if identifying the underlying cause of symptoms is required to direct the course of treatment to alleviate symptoms. If the patient is close to death, treating the symptom based on the likely cause without testing is reasonable. Interventions to provide comfort can be initiated without confirmation of the etiology of the symptom. In general, performing tests in the palliative care setting should be minimal and noninvasive and only be done if the results will provide information to direct interventions to improve comfort. Patient and family education on the issue of discontinuing or not ordering tests is important because their perceptions of the testing process may be one of hope for good news or for the provision of important information needed to keep the patient comfortable or extend survival. The APN can explain the rationale for foregoing tests by reinforcing the concept that tests are not helpful in managing symptoms and may cause discomfort. It is important to reassure the patient and family that daily assessments of the symptom with aggressive symptom management will continue.

Do Not Resuscitate Order

The discussion regarding do not resuscitate (DNR) status is a sensitive issue, and the decision should be medical. Unfortunately, in palliative care practice, patients and families may request cardiopulmonary resuscitation (CPR). They may be expecting more than is possible from medicine or misunderstand the value of CPR (Tadaaki, 1999). Historically, CPR was developed for victims of sudden cardiac or respiratory arrest to be used in drowning, electrical shock, untoward effects of drugs, anesthetic accident, heat block, acute myocardial infarction, or surgery (Talbot, Jude, & Elam, 1965). Between 1960, when closed chest cardiac massage was initiated, until now, it has become standard practice to attempt CPR on patients in the hospital who have a cardiac arrest regardless of the underlying illness, except for those who request not to receive it. Currently, CPR is performed routinely in the absence of a DNR order. The DNR order written by the physician signifies that the patient has refused the procedure. The American Heart Association and American Academy of Sciences at the National Conference on Cardiopulmonary Resuscitation and Emergency Cardiac Care stated the purpose of CPR is the prevention of sudden unexpected death. CPR is not indicated in terminal irreversible illness where death is expected (American Heart Association, 1992). In the patient with advanced metastatic cancer with a limited life expectancy, CPR would offer only a remote chance of survival (Farber-Langendorf, 1991). Survival after CPR to hospital discharge is less than 5% for the older adult and those with serious illnesses (Council Report, 1999).

Typically, the conversation regarding DNR is discussed when a patient is hospitalized, but in the palliative care setting, one should consider having this conversation in the community setting. The need to have the DNR conversation was highlighted in the SUPPORT (1995) study, which showed that although 31% of hospitalized patients asked not to be resuscitated, fewer than half of their physicians had written DNR orders on their charts. Seventy-nine percent of those who died while hospitalized had DNR orders; however, 46% were written two days or less before death. The conversation of the patient's understanding and wishes regarding DNR status should be documented. Patients and families need to be properly informed about the issues that are most important to the decision-making process related to their goal. Hence, the discussion should be focused in the context of their goals of care. Buckman (1992) described six steps in discussing the DNR status (see Figure 21-2).

- Establish the setting. Ensure comfort and privacy, and ask whom the patient would like present.
- Ask the patient and family what they understand about their current health situation and what they have been told.
- Find out what the patient expects will happen in the future.
- Discuss the do not resuscitate order using language that the patient will understand, and provide a clear recommendation against cardiopulmonary resuscitation (CPR) when appropriate. Describe the purpose, risks, and benefits of CPR in detail.
- Respond to emotions.
- Establish and implement a plan.

Figure 21-2. Discussing Do Not Resuscitate Status

Note. Based on information from Buckman, 1992.

By the nature of the specialty, oncology nurses and APNs frequently address the psychological and educational needs of patients and families regarding DNR issues. They are able to reinforce the medical opinion about the efficacy of CPR in their medical situation and clarify that CPR is a treatment that attempts to reverse death and is unlikely to work in their situation. The nurse should explain that in advanced cancer, circulation and breathing stop because of progression of the cancer or its complications and not because of a reversible cardiac or pulmonary condition. The patient and family should be reassured that along with (or in spite of) a DNR order, everything of benefit would be done. Patients should be encouraged to describe what their goals are for the future and what is important; the nurse listens to their thoughts about dying then summarizes and validates the main points. Clarification should be made between what the healthcare providers and the patient expect, and healthcare providers should document the conversation in the medical record and summarize it to the rest of the palliative care team.

Artificial Nutrition and Hydration

When the person with progressive cancer is no longer able to take oral nourishment or fluids, the patient or family may bring up the decision about artificial nutrition and hydration (ANH). Artificial nutrition is any non-oral administration of nutrition, including enteral and IV feedings. Artificial hydration is the administration of fluids by IV, subcutaneous (hypodermoclysis), rectal (proctoclysis), or enteral methods through tube feeding equipment. The decision to initiate, withhold, or withdraw nutrition/hydration may be a difficult choice because of individual beliefs and misconceptions. The current body of clinical research provides some guidance on the use of ANH, but areas of uncertainty and debate remain. The author could not find prospective, randomized, controlled trials on the subpopulation of the older adult with advanced cancer. Methodologic problems with research in this area include a lack of controlled or comparison groups, small sample sizes, and failure to control for confounding variables.

The rationale for providing ANH is to prevent complications, increase survival and comfort, and decrease unpleasant symptoms of malnutrition and dehydration. Healthcare providers should consider if ANH would contribute to these goals. If the decision is to start ANH, providers should identify the specific goal and periodically reevaluate the effectiveness to determine whether to continue or stop ANH.

A common misconception of healthcare providers and patients is that tube feedings will help to prevent aspiration pneumonia. An extensive literature review of the research concluded that tube feedings do not protect against aspiration pneumonia and, in some cases, increase the incidence of aspiration pneumonia in several patient populations, including some older adults with cancer (Finucane & Bynum, 1996).

Patients and surrogate decision makers have cited prolonging life as the reason for choosing tube feeding in terminal situations (Ouslander, Tymchuk, & Krynski, 1993). The evidence regarding the benefits of ANH in survival time in advanced cancer is lacking. Two randomized studies of nutritional support found patients with advanced cancer did not show benefit in survival or QOL (American College of Physicians 1989; Barber, Fearon, & Delmore, 1998). In a prospective study of 150 patients 60 years and older on percutaneous endoscopic gastrostomy tube feedings, patients had a 30-day mortality of 22% and a one-year mortality of 50% (Callahan et al., 2000). Patients with cancer on total parenteral nutrition only demonstrated improvement in survival in 1 of 14 randomized clinical trials (Koretz, 1984).

The effects of malnutrition and dehydration in the patient with terminal cancer are not well documented. Many of the physical symptoms of dehydration seen in healthy subjects also are seen in those with advanced cancer regardless of their hydration and nutritional status (Billings, 1998). Research literature has documented the relationship between thirst and dehydration in the terminally ill. Symptoms of dehydration were uncommon in those at the end of life (McCann, Hall, & Groth-Juncker, 1994). Through an extensive review of textbooks and journal articles, the author has found statements on the frequent hypothetical benefits of terminal dehydration, such as analgesia, decreased respiratory congestion, and less incontinence. The potential risks and complications of tube feedings cited in the literature include the possible need for restraints, infection, pain, aspiration pneumonia, and cost.

Oncology nurses and APNs providing education and counseling on these issues must know and understand the clinical, ethical, and legal implications in foregoing ANH. The challenge for nurses is to be aware of how their own personal biases and beliefs can influence their ability to provide objective information to patients and families. Healthcare providers should clearly communicate and consider the expected outcomes, potential burdens, and appropriate use of ANH relative to the patient's goals. Evaluating the patient's and family's understanding frequently during the conversation helps to clarify misconceptions early. As a patient and family advocate, the APN takes action to ensure that the patient and family understand their legal rights. Once a decision has been made, the next step is to provide reassurance that their values and preferences will be respected. Alternatives to ANH such as aggressive mouth care and the intake of small amounts of food and fluids, as tolerated, may offer comfort to family members. Caregivers should be informed that dehydration and malnutrition are a natural part of the dying process, and they can provide comfort and care with other physical comfort care measures.

Place of End-of-Life Care

Planning and deciding where to spend one's remaining time is dependent upon patient and family preference and available resources. Studies of older adults demonstrate that most patients want to die at home, but only 25% of all deaths take place at home, with 50% in hospitals and 25% in nursing homes (National Hospice and Palliative Care Organization, n.d.). The population surveyed included healthy older adults. Being home allows the patient to be in a familiar environment surrounded by family. The nurse should assess the home situation by considering the physical space and access. The family resources and availability need to be clarified, while assisting members to recognize their limitations if the patients' needs become complicated. For home care to be successful, families need people available to meet the patients' needs. Resources such as professional caregivers available 24 hours a day and a comprehensive homecare service that offers equipment and guidance on patient care are the basic key elements for comprehensive home care for the dying. Providing information on homecare services and coordinating meetings between the family and homecare staff before discharge from the hospital are likely to reduce anxiety and provide continuity of care. When referring or providing information on home hospice care, explaining the philosophy of family-oriented care can reinforce the concept that using this service does not mean giving up on the patient (Schaeffer & Goldstein, 1996). If the family's cultural background reinforces self-sufficiency, this may cause resistance to accepting help from a professional agency or others.

The wishes of those who prefer not to die at home should be respected. Although hospitalized patients frequently experience depersonalization and isolation (Meyer, 1993), a qualitative study of nine patients receiving palliative end-of-life care found that the majority wanted to be cared for in the hospital because they felt safe and trusted staff members (Harstade & Andershed, 2004). In some situations, the illness becomes acute at the time near death, with complex symptoms that may require acute medical care. The older adult may have limited home resources, limited or no family, or the significant other/caregiver may have physical limitations. For some patients, when death is imminent, they may prefer to remain in the hospital because of their familiarity with staff and the security of knowing that they have continuous professional staff caring for them. With the development of palliative care units within some hospitals, the option of receiving end-of-life care in specialized units has become a reality for some.

Assisted living facilities (ALFs) are an alternative to nursing home placement for elders. ALFs provide a range of services, including 24-hour staffing. The advantage of ALFs is provision of a social environment that maximizes residents' autonomy, privacy, and dignity and living accommodations that minimize the need to move (National Center for Assisted Living, 2005). The option of hospice care for terminally ill residents would appear logical. Very little research has focused on the quality of end-of-life care in ALFs. The challenges of providing end-of-life care in ALFs include limited staffing patterns not designed to accommodate the intense, direct care requirements of a dying person; lack of knowledge of the medications used at the end of life; little coordination of services by the hospice and facility and little communication between facility and hospice staff members regarding the resident's changing condition and care needs; and differing views by facility and hospice nurses regarding roles and responsibilities for delegating skilled nursing tasks (Cartwright & Kayser-Jones, 2003). These findings support the need to assess the available resources in the patient's current ALFs early in the illness and to plan accordingly. Further studies on end-of-life care in ALFs are needed so healthcare professionals can determine the magnitude of the issues and consider solutions to the problem.

Nursing homes are a common place of care and site of death. In the United States, one in four people die in a nursing home (Brock & Foley, 1998). Those who chose a nursing home for their place of death felt they did not want to burden their relatives with their care (Harstade & Andershed, 2004). Admission to a nursing home may be indicated if the caregiver is unable to manage the patient at home or if the goal is to obtain rehabilitation prior to going home. For those who decide to remain in the nursing home, the option of receiving hospice care through a contract between the hospice organization and nursing home should be provided.

Hospice care refers to a program, philosophy, and system of reimbursement for terminally ill people. The majority of patients under hospice care live in their own home or in a nursing home, but hospital palliative care units or hospice facilities are available in many cities. To receive Medicare hospice benefits, beneficiaries must be certified by their doctor and the hospice medical director as terminally ill (defined as a life expectancy of six months or less based on disease progression), elect to receive noncurative treatment (may continue to access Medicare benefits for treatment of conditions unrelated to the terminal illness), and sign a statement choosing hospice (Centers for Medicare and Medicaid Services, 2004). The hospice care plan focuses on symptom control, medical and support services, physician and nursing visits, counseling, homemaker services, medical equipment, and medication. Identifying the appropriateness of hospice care for older adult patients can be challenging because prognosticating is not an exact science. The palliative care case manager or APN is in the position to help families to understand more about hospice care, eligibility requirements, and services covered under the Medicare Hospice Benefit. The National Hospice and Palliative Care Organization has a hospice locator program of its members available through a helpline (800-658-8898) or Web site (www.nhpco.org). State hospice associations and state health departments are other ways to find information on Medicare-certified hospice programs.

The Nurse's Role in Decision Making

Investing in conversations with families to help with decision making is a primary (major) function of the palliative care APN. Understanding how patients view the options of treatment, end-of-life care, and place of care is necessary so that any misconceptions or lack of information can be clarified and provided. Listening to their expectations is critical so that the appropriate options can be presented as choices. Assisting with the decision-making process is an ongoing complex nursing process consisting of assessment, planning, intervention, and evaluation. Basic nursing interventions that nurses can provide to help patients and families to make informed decisions already have been described. Research studies should continue to test methods of providing palliative care information and services to the older adult with cancer so that nurses can use evidence-based interventions that provide the best supportive oncology care.

Caregiver Experiences

Family caregiving for the older adult with cancer is common as a result of changes in the healthcare delivery system and the patients'/families' preference to remain at home. In the SUPPORT (1995) study, 55% of patients had family caregiver needs during the course of their terminal illness (Covinsky et al., 1996). The number of terminally ill older adults requiring assistance from family, friends, and paid personnel was a substantial 35%, with 80%–85% of patients receiving the majority of care from unpaid family members (Emanuel et al., 1999). According to the 2000 National Hospice Care Survey, 79.6% of patients in hospice programs were 65 or older, the most common diagnosis was neoplasm, and the mean length of service was 48 days (National Center for Health Statistics, 2002). The hospice survey documented that 84.6% of patients (all age groups) lived with family members, with the primary caregiver being either the spouse (41.8%) or child/child-in-law (32.3%).

The comprehensive care of the older adult includes assistance with personal care, administration of medications, monitoring of condition, skin/wound care, meal preparation, transportation, financial coordination, coordination of healthcare services, management of symptoms, decision making, and providing emotional support to the patient. The dying process in the older adult often consists of long periods of functional dependency, with the need for extensive caregiving from family. Elderly caregivers may have limited physical ability because of their own personal health problems. The younger caregiver may have additional responsibilities such as family/child care or domestic and employment demands. The role of caregiving may be a rewarding and positive experience that many family members choose to assume. However, the toll of the physical, emotional, and psychological demands of this role documented in the research literature should not be ignored. Identifying the positive and negative effects of caregiving will guide the design and testing of interventions aimed at preventing and minimizing the burdens of caregiving.

The major benefit of caregiving is that it allows the patient to remain at home in a familiar environment. The value to the caregiver may vary depending on the individual's goals and situation. Studies have shown that caregiving can provide a feeling of satisfaction, a greater sense of self-worth, personal growth, meaning and purpose in one's life, and gratitude for being able to provide care (Haley, LaMonde, Han, Burton, & Schonwetter, 2003). Caregivers reported feeling closer to their relative, grateful to repay earlier care that they received, increased intimacy, and a positive sense of purpose in this role (Kramer, 1997). Female spouses in the role of caregiver found the experience strengthened the marital relationship, with improved intimacy, communication, and sensitivity to each others' feelings (Gritz, Wellisch, Siau, & Wang, 1990). Numerous other benefits likely exist for patients and caregivers that choose this plan of care, but few studies have qualified or quantified the practical, financial, and personal (individual) advantages.

The numerous detrimental effects of caregiving on QOL are well documented in research spanning over the past several decades. The challenge of caregiving may have a negative impact on physical and mental health, finances, socialization, communication, and employment. Most of the research conducted on caregivers of the older adult has focused on Alzheimer disease and other chronic illnesses, with less attention to the oncology population. The stress associated with caring for someone with cancer may have different effects than caring for those with a nonmalignant disease.

The specific stage and treatment phase of cancer may invoke a variety of challenges. The spouses of newly diagnosed older adult patients with cancer felt prepared for the caregiver role at the initial time of diagnosis (Rusinak & Murphy, 1995). As the disease progresses, caregiver burden tends to increase. Family caregivers of patients receiving palliative care had a lower QOL score and worse physical health than family caregivers of patients receiving curative care (Weitzner, McMillan, & Jacobson, 1999). The psychological strain worsened when cancer metastasized (Sales, Schulz, & Biegal, 1992). Family caregivers of patients receiving home hospice for cancer identified that the need for social, volunteer, and professional support increased as their physical and emotional health suffered (Steele & Fitch, 1996). During the terminal phase, the impact of caregiving in all domains was at its worst (Haley, Ehrbar, & Schonwetter, 1998). These studies indicate that caregiving for a loved one with advanced cancer is often a tremendous psychological and physical strain, worsening over time as the disease progresses.

A major role of the caregiver is to monitor and manage symptoms. The main symptom patients with cancer experience at the end of life is pain. The prevalence of pain is 64%–80% among patients with advanced cancer (Caraceni & Portenoy, 1999). Caregivers are expected to assess, treat, and evaluate the effectiveness and side effects of pain medication. Unfortunately, many caregivers are not given adequate information and training on pain management or may hold erroneous beliefs resulting in needless suffering. The patient's/caregiver's barriers to effective pain management include misconceptions and fears related to pain medication (Ward, Berry, & Misiewicz, 1996). Numerous studies document the negative effects of pain on the patient and family caregiver that cause physical and emotional distress. Caregivers of patients with cancer-related pain had more tension and depressive symptoms than those of pain-free patients (Miaskowski, Kragness, Dibble, & Wallhagen, 1997). However, the healthcare system continues to expect that the caregivers will monitor and manage pain at home. Healthcare providers need to educate caregivers about managing cancer pain and other symptoms in the home.

Comprehensive palliative care programs need to provide support systems to caregivers to help them to cope with the physical and psychological stress associated with the demands of this role. Many programs have been developed to assist the caregiver, including educational classes, support groups, grief therapy, and homecare support programs. Unfortunately, most of these types of programs are not reimbursable and, even if no cost is incurred, the family caregiver may not have the time or energy to attend. Research and program evaluations that document the effectiveness of these programs are more likely to obtain organizational and insurance support than programs that do not demonstrate positive measurable outcomes. For example, the implementation of a cancer pain education program with family caregivers of older adult patients demonstrated improved outcomes for both the patient and caregiver (Ferrell, Grant, Chan, Ahn, & Ferrell, 1995). Caregivers who attended a six-hour caregiver cancer education program felt less overwhelmed, more knowledgeable, and better able to cope with the caregiving role (Robinson et al., 1998). Grief therapy programs for families during the terminal phase of illness improved the psychosocial QOL of caregivers (Kissane, Block, McKenzie, McDowell, & Nitzan, 1998). Although controlled research studies on interventions for cancer caregivers, especially for older adults, have not been widely published, the programs mentioned previously have demonstrated positive outcomes for patients and caregivers.

Practical interventions that the clinician can integrate into clinical practice should be based on nurses' knowledge of caregiver issues and must be applicable within the constraint of the palliative care service delivery system. Establishing rapport and trust with caregivers is the initial step. Recognizing the value and difficulty of their role, as well as including them as part of the healthcare team in decision making, shows respect. A simple example is to ask the caregiver what he or she perceives to be priority problems. Identifying those who are at risk for caregiver burden with specific and sensitive assessment tools can provide vital information to consider when developing a plan of care. Although several family assessment tools are available, the busy clinician needs a brief method to identify those who have limited coping abilities, mental or physical problems, or inadequate resources. Routinely investigating the impact that caregiving has on the individual is important to determine the magnitude of the stress and resultant problems, because issues may change over time. Healthcare providers should explore what has been helpful in mitigating stress and ways to strengthen coping skills. Oncology nurses and palliative care nurse practitioners are in an ideal position to assess the family situation, provide emotional support, teach families about caregiving, provide specific information and advice for caregiving plans, and provide referrals for appropriate resources.

Models of care based on the needs of caregivers are being developed and studied. A pragmatic model discussed by Barrett, Haley, and Sisler (2003) outlined a cost-effective, four-step strategy—CARE: conceptualize the caregiving situation, assess the caregiving situation, respond to assessed needs, and evaluate response and situation. This model of approaching the caregiver can be integrated into every contact with the patient and family so that continuous attention is given to caregiver issues.

Healthcare professionals have the ability to help caregivers to cope with caring for older patients with cancer through direct individual interventions, coordination of care and services, program development, and research. The APN role encompasses helping family caregivers in all of these dimensions. Caregivers depend on nurses for direction and assistance with the management of the older patient with cancer (Hileman, Lackey, & Hassanein, 1992; Reuben, 1997) and can benefit from the nurses' expertise. Caregivers of dying loved ones consistently report that they need more support and information from healthcare professionals (Hudson, Aranda, & Kristjanson, 2004). Research identifying caregiver risk and protective factors will help to improve the conceptual and empirical basis for interventions for family caregivers.

Physical Symptoms

The control of physical symptoms is paramount in palliative nursing care. The common symptoms associated with advanced cancer include pain, dyspnea, bowel obstruction, nausea, anorexia/cachexia, dry mouth/thirst, depression, delirium, skin/wound care, pruritus, and fatigue. The APN needs to have an in-depth knowledge of physical assessment and pharmacology to appropriately address the physical needs of the older adult patient with cancer. Determining the etiology of the symptom helps to direct therapy based on individual circumstances. The APN should have a detailed understanding of the patient's condition before determining a well-thought-out treatment plan. A cookbook approach to symptom management is unacceptable. Practice guidelines on symptom management, which can be helpful as a tool guide, are covered in several nursing and medical textbooks and are beyond the scope of this chapter. Literature searches to determine evidence-based treatment recommendations should be used in palliative care practice, but at this time, the type of data available is limited. Unfortunately, limited evidence-based practice information is available for symptom management in older adults with advanced cancer. Performing research studies on this population is difficult for several reasons. Clinical trials are extremely difficult to perform on people who have a limited life expectancy. The number of subjects in these studies is low. Historically, a bias has existed against administering drugs to older people in general, which makes applying the findings to older adults difficult because drug metabolism and excretion may be altered in older adults and those with comorbid conditions. Most studies examining symptom management in advanced cancer have focused on younger people.

Barriers to Palliative Care in the Older Adult

Barriers to providing palliative care to older adults can be categorized into three main areas: patient/family, professional, and system issues. Patient and family barriers tend to evolve around misconceptions and lack of information. For example, many beliefs held by patients and families contribute to the hesitance to report and use analgesics (Ward & Gatwood, 1994). Lack of compliance, for whatever reason, is detrimental to good symptom management. Elderly caregivers may have difficulty remembering and following through on specific tasks related to their own health issues. Lack of advanced care planning makes it difficult to determine what patients' preferences are toward palliative issues.

Professional impediments to symptom management include educational deficits, misconceptions, and concerns about the use and side effects of medications. Fear and misunderstanding of the regulation of controlled substances also contribute to inadequate symptom management (Murphy-Ende, 2001). Other professional barriers include inappropriate attitudes toward death, ineffective communication about prognosis, unrealistic expectations from treatment, and the failure to recognize the importance of symptom management and psychosocial support (American Society of Clinical Oncology, 1998). Providing optimal palliative care requires healthcare professionals who are dedicated, committed, and educated in this specialty.

System issues include resources and reimbursement. Nursing homes, as noted earlier, are a common place for older adults who are dying of chronic progressive illness to receive end-of-life care. Barriers to end-of-life care in nursing homes include a failure to recognize the futility of curative treatment, difficulties in communication among those making decisions about care, a lack of agreement on the course of care and delayed palliative care measures, rapid staff turnover, nursing shortage, and reimbursement issues (Travis et al., 2002). The Omnibus Budget Reconciliation Act of 1987 developed the primary goal of nursing homes "to attain or maintain the highest practicable physical, mental and psychosocial well-being of each resident" (p. 7). Quality indicators and outcomes based around this goal are incongruent with end-of-life care. The regulatory scrutiny that nursing homes face may influence how they care for residents, especially when a negative outcome such as weight loss or decline in functional status occurs. When a nursing home refers a patient to hospice, it loses reimbursed, skilled nursing home days because Medicare reimbursement is based on residents being categorized into a resource utilization group. For example, the use of tube feeding provides more reimbursement. Access or available palliative services may be limited in certain areas. Palliative care services in hospitals also may be limited because of restrictions in Medicare and insurance reimbursement. For further discussion regarding system barriers and the provision of quality palliative care to older adults, refer to Reb (2003).

Role of the Advanced Practice Nurse in Palliative Care

Patients and families with advanced cancer have complex physical, psychosocial, and spiritual needs. The provision of comprehensive and compassionate palliative care requires expert assessment and critical thinking skills and detailed knowledge about symptom management, physiology, pharmacology, psychology, and communication. Interdisciplinary teams of professionals that provide palliative care include physicians, nurses, social workers, pharmacists, psychologists, chaplains, and other healthcare disciplines. Professional nurses have been the team members who coordinate, direct, and evaluate patients' and families' needs.

The APN is an RN who has completed a master's or doctoral program in a clinical nurse specialist (CNS) or nurse practitioner (NP) program. The CNS or NP may be certified by the American Nurses Credentialing Center (ANCC) in a specialty; may be certified as an Advanced Practice Registered Nurse, Board Certified-Palliative Care Management, through a partnership of the ANCC and the Hospice and Palliative Nurses Association; or may be credentialed as an Advanced Oncology Certified Nurse Practitioner or Advanced Oncology Certified Clinical Nurse Specialist by the Oncology Nursing Certification Corporation (ONCC). With the creation of advanced practice credentialing examinations and graduate palliative care nursing educational programs, the specialty of palliative care APNs is being recognized.

Direct reimbursement for APN services can be obtained from Medicare and insurance companies, and institutions may finance the APN salary based on cost avoidance of unnecessary hospitalizations or intensive care unit days or through efficient use of system resources. The palliative care APN serves as an expert practitioner, consultant, educator, leader, and researcher (Murphy-Ende, 2002). Nurses' involvement in legislative initiatives may contribute to better access, lower cost, and improved QOL. The profession is responsible for establishing and supporting evidence-based care to ensure that the best QOL outcomes are achieved.

Areas for Future Research

The National Cancer Institute and the National Institute on Aging have joined forces to study aging and cancer with research in the following areas: effect of co-morbidity as it relates to treatment and care decisions; the absorption, distribution, metabolism, and excretion of drugs, including radiation; tools to assess the QOL of patients and their caregivers; and pain relief and palliative care that reflect patient and family preferences (Eastman, 2003). The National Institutes of Health and National Institute of Nursing Research have taken the lead in palliative care research in the areas of caregiver issues, symptom management, and methodology issues (National Institute of Nursing Research, 2005). APNs need to document and disseminate the outcomes of their clinical practice, describe the positive effects of their role, and participate in the conduction and dissemination of interdisciplinary research. Research is needed in supporting the role of the nurse in providing cost-effective care, improving access, and promoting clinical excellence in palliative care.

Conclusion

The goal of palliative care for the older adult with cancer is to alleviate suffering and promote QOL. Oncology nurses can play a key role in facilitating and coordinating end-of-life care. Specific areas include education, information sharing, pain and symptom management, and psychosocial and spiritual support for patients and their families/caregivers. With the projected increase in the size of the aging population and cancer incidence in the older adult, further nursing research investigating palliative care issues is critical to develop evidence-based nursing practice.

References

American Academy of Hospice and Palliative Medicine. (2003). *Position statement: Definitions of palliative care and palliative medicine*. Retrieved March 30, 2005, from http://www.aahpm.org/positions/definition.html

American College of Physicians. (1989). Position paper on parenteral nutrition in patients receiving cancer chemotherapy. *Annals of Internal Medicine, 110*, 734–736.

American Heart Association. (1992). Guidelines for cardiopulmonary resuscitation and emergency cardiac care VIII: Ethical considerations in resuscitation. *JAMA, 68*, 2282–2288.

American Society of Clinical Oncology. (1998). Cancer care during the last phase of life. *Journal of Clinical Oncology, 15*, 1986–1996.

Balducci, L., & Stanta, G. (2000). Cancer in the frail patient: A coming epidemic. *Hematology/Oncology Clinics of North America, 14*, 235–250.

Barber, M.D., Fearon, K.C., & Delmore, G. (1998). Should cancer patients with incurable disease receive parenteral or enteral nutritional support? *European Journal of Cancer, 34*, 279–285.

Barrett, J.J., Haley, W.E., & Sisler, L. (2003). Helping family caregivers of elderly cancer patients: The CARE model. In J. Overcash & L. Balducci (Eds.), *The older cancer patient: A guide for nurses and related professionals* (pp. 242–256). New York: Springer.

Billings, J.A. (1998). Dehydration. In A. Berger, R. Portenoy, & D. Weissman (Eds.), *Principles and practice of supportive oncology* (pp. 589–601). Philadelphia: Lippincott-Raven.

Blanchard, C.G., Labrecque, M.S., Ruckdeschel, J.C., & Blanchard, E.B. (1988). Information and decision-making preferences of hospitalized adult cancer patients. *Social Science and Medicine, 27,* 1139–1145.

Bremnes, R., Andersen, K., & Wist, E. (1995). Cancer patients, doctors and nurses vary in their willingness to undertake cancer chemotherapy. *European Journal of Cancer, 31A,* 1955–1959.

Brock, D.B., & Foley, D.J. (1998). Demography and epidemiology of dying in the U.S. with emphasis on death of older persons. *Hospice Journal, 13,* 49–60.

Buccheri, G., Ferrigno, D., & Tamburini, M. (1996). Karnofsky and ECOG performance status scoring in lung cancer: A prospective, longitudinal study of 536 patients from a single institution. *European Journal of Cancer, 32A,* 1135–1141.

Buckman, R. (1992). *How to break bad news: A guide for health care professionals.* Baltimore: Johns Hopkins University.

Callahan, C.M., Haag, K.M., Weinberger, M., Tierney, W.M., Buchanan, N.N., Stump, T.E., et al. (2000). Outcomes of percutaneous endoscopic gastrostomy among older adults in a community setting. *Journal of the American Geriatrics Society, 48,* 1048–1054.

Caraceni, A., & Portenoy, R.K. (1999). An international survey of cancer pain characteristics and syndromes: IASP Task Force on Cancer Pain. *Pain, 82,* 263–274.

Cartwright, J., & Kayser-Jones, J. (2003). End-of-life care in assisted living facilities: Perceptions of residents, families, and staffs. *Journal of Hospice and Palliative Nursing, 5,* 143–151.

Cassell, C.K., & Foley, K.M. (1999). *Principles for care of patients at the end-of-life: An emerging consensus among the specialties of medicine.* New York: Milbank Memorial Fund.

Centers for Medicare and Medicaid Services. (2004). *Hospice manual chapter 2—Coverage of services.* Retrieved March 2004, from http://www.cms.hhs.gov/manuals/21_hospice/hs200.asp

Committee on Care at the End of Life. (1997). Introduction. In M.J. Field & C.K. Cassell (Eds.), *Approaching death. Improving care at the end of life* (pp. 30–31). Washington, DC: National Academies Press.

Council Report. (1999). Council report: Medical futility in end-of-life care. *JAMA, 281,* 937–941.

Covinsky, K.E., Landefeld, C.S., Teno, J., Connors, A.F., Dawson, N., Youngner, S., et al. (1996). Is economic hardship on the families for the seriously ill associated with patient and surrogate care preferences? SUPPORT Investigators. *Archives of Internal Medicine, 156,* 1737–1741.

Eastman, P. (2003, November 10). Renewed warning to cancer care professionals: Don't under treat the elderly. *Oncology Times,* p. 29.

Egan, K.A., & Labyak, M.J. (2001). Hospice care: A model for quality end-of-life care. In B.R. Ferrell & N. Coyle (Eds.), *Textbook of palliative nursing* (pp. 7–26). New York: Oxford University Press.

Ellison, N., & Chevlen, E. (2002). Palliative chemotherapy. In A. Berger, R. Portenoy, & D.E. Weissman (Eds.), *Principles and practice of supportive oncology* (pp. 698–709). Philadelphia: Lippincott-Raven.

Emanuel, E., Fairclough, D., Slutsman, J., Alper, H., Baldwin, D., & Emanuel, L.L. (1999). Assistance from family members, friends, paid caregivers and volunteers in the care of terminally ill patients. *New England Journal of Medicine, 341,* 956–963.

Emanuel, L., Barry, J.J., Stoeckel, J.D., Ettelson, L.M., & Emanuel E.J. (1991). Advanced directives for medical care: A case for greater use. *New England Journal of Medicine, 324,* 889–895.

Falk, S.J., Girling, D.J., White, R.J., Hopwood, P., Harvey, A., Qian, W., et al. (2002). Immediate versus delayed thoracic radiotherapy in patients' with unresectable locally advanced non-small cell lung cancer and minimal symptoms: Randomized controlled trial. *BMJ, 325,* 465.

Farber-Langendorf, K. (1991). Resuscitation of patients with metastatic cancer: Is transient benefit still futile? *Archives of Internal Medicine, 151,* 235–239.

Ferrell, B.R., Grant, M., Chan, J., Ahn, C., & Ferrell, B.A. (1995). The impact of cancer pain education on family caregivers of elderly patients. *Oncology Nursing Forum, 22,* 1211–1218.

Finucane, T.E., & Bynum, J.P. (1996). Use of tube feeding to prevent aspiration pneumonia. *Lancet, 348,* 1421–1424.

Frankl, D., Oye, R.K., & Bellamy, P.E. (1989). Attitudes of hospitalized patients toward life support: A survey of 200 medical inpatients. *American Journal of Medicine, 86,* 645–648.

Fried, R.R., & Bradley, E.H. (2003). What matters to seriously ill older persons making end-of-life treatment decisions: A qualitative study. *Journal of Palliative Medicine, 6,* 237–249.

Ganz, P., Schag, C., & Heinrich, R. (1985). The psychosocial impact of cancer on the elderly: A comparison with younger patients. *Journal of the American Geriatrics Society, 33,* 429–435.

Geels, P., Eisenhauer, E., Bezjak, A., Zee, B., & Day, A. (2000). Palliative effects of chemotherapy: Objective tumor response is associated with symptom improvement in patients with metastatic breast cancer. *Journal of Clinical Oncology, 18,* 2395–2405.

Gritz, E.R., Wellisch, D.K., Siau, J., & Wang, H.J. (1990). Long-term effects of testicular cancer on marital relationships. *Psychosomatics, 31,* 301–312.

Haley, W.E., Ehrbar, L.A., & Schonwetter, R.S. (1998). Family caregiving issues. In L. Balducci, G.H. Lyman, & W.B. Ershler (Eds.), *Comprehensive geriatric oncology* (pp. 805–812). London: Harwood Academic.

Haley, W.E., LaMonde, L.A., Han, B., Burton, A.M., & Schonwetter, R. (2003). Predictors of depression and life satisfaction among spousal caregivers in hospice: Application of a stress process model. *Journal of Palliative Medicine, 6,* 215–224.

Harstade, C.W., & Andershed, B. (2004). Good palliative care: How and where? *Journal of Hospice and Palliative Nursing, 6,* 27–35.

Hileman, J.W., Lackey, N.R., & Hassanein, R.S. (1992). Identifying the needs of home caregivers of patients with cancer. *Oncology Nursing Forum, 19,* 771–777.

Hudson, P.L., Aranda, S., & Kristjanson, L. (2004). Meeting the supportive needs of family caregivers in palliative care: Challenges for health professionals. *Journal of Palliative Medicine, 7,* 19–25.

Jemal, A., Murray, T., Ward, E., Samuels, A., Tiwari, R.C., Ghafoor, A., et al. (2005). Cancer statistics, 2005. *CA: A Cancer Journal for Clinicians, 55,* 10–30.

Kirkbride, P., & Bezjak, A. (2002). Palliative radiation therapy. In A. Berger, R. Portenoy, & D. Weissman (Eds.), *Principles and practice of palliative care and supportive oncology* (2nd ed., pp. 685–697). Philadelphia: Lippincott Williams & Wilkins.

Kissane, D.W., Block, S., McKenzie, M., McDowell, A.C., & Nitzan, R. (1998). Family grief therapy: A preliminary account of a new model to promote healthy family functioning during palliative care and bereavement. *Psycho-Oncology, 7,* 14–25.

Koretz, R.L. (1984). Parenteral nutrition: Is it oncologically logical? *Journal of Clinical Oncology, 2,* 534–538.

Kramer, B.J. (1997). Gain in the caregiving experience: Where are we? What next? *Gerontologist, 37,* 218–232.

McCahill, L.E., Krouse, R., Chu, D., Juarez, G., Uman, G.C., Ferrell, B., et al. (2002). Indications and use of palliative surgery: Results of a Society of Surgical Oncology survey. *Annals of Surgical Oncology, 9,* 104–112.

McCann, R.M., Hall, W.J., & Groth-Juncker, A. (1994). Comfort care for terminally ill patients. The appropriate use of nutrition and hydration. *JAMA, 272,* 1263–1266.

Meyer, C. (1993). End-of-life care: Patients' choices, nurse's challenges. *American Journal of Nursing, 93,* 40–47.

Miaskowski, C., Kragness, L., Dibble, S., & Wallhagen, M. (1997). Differences in mood states, health status, and caregiver strain between family caregivers of oncology outpatients with and without cancer-related pain. *Journal of Pain and Symptom Management, 13,* 138–147.

Miner, T.J., Jaques, D.T., Tavaf-Motamen, H., & Shriver, C.D. (1999). Decision making on surgical palliation based on patient outcome data. *American Journal of Surgery, 177,* 150–154.

Murphy-Ende, K. (2001). Barriers to palliative and supportive care. *Nursing Clinics of North America, 36,* 843–853.

Murphy-Ende, K. (2002). Advanced practice nursing: Reflections of the past, issues for the future. *Oncology Nursing Forum, 29,* 106–112.

National Center for Assisted Living. (2005). *Guiding principles for assisted living.* Retrieved June 19, 2005, from http://www.ncal.org/about/concepts.htm

National Center for Health Statistics. (2002). *National home and hospice care data.* Retrieved June 19, 2005, from http://www.cdc.gov/nchs/about/major/nhhcsd/nhhcsd.htm

National Hospice and Palliative Care Organization. (n.d.). *Means to a better end: A report on dying in America today.* Alexandria, VA: Author. Retrieved June 9, 2005, from http://www.nhpco.org/files/public/MessagesandQAfinal.pdf

National Hospice and Palliative Care Organization. (2004). *An explanation of palliative care.* Retrieved June 9, 2005, from http://www.nhpco.org/i4a/pages/index.cfm?pageid=3657

National Institute of Nursing Research. (2005). *National Institute of Nursing Research.* Retrieved June 19, 2005, from http://ninr.nih.gov/ninr/research/themes.doc

O'Brien, L.A., Grisso, J.A., Maislin, G., La Pann, K., Krotiki, K.P., Greco, P.J., et al. (1995). Nursing home residents' preferences for life-sustaining treatments. *JAMA, 274,* 1775–1779.

Omnibus Budget Reconciliation Act of 1987. (1987). OBRA-87. *Federal Register, 56*(187), 48865–49921.

Ouslander, J.G., Tymchuk, A.J., & Krynski, M.D. (1993). Decisions about enteral tube feeding among the elderly. *Journal of the American Geriatrics Society, 41,* 70–77.

Popescu, R., Norman, A., Ross, P., Parikh, B., & Cunningham, D. (1999). Adjuvant or palliative chemotherapy for colorectal cancer in patients 70 years or older. *Journal of Clinical Oncology, 17,* 2412–2418.

Reb, A.M. (2003). Palliative and end-of-life care: Policy analysis. *Oncology Nursing Forum, 30,* 35–50.

Reuben, D.B. (1997). Geriatric assessment in oncology. *Cancer, 80,* 1311–1316.

Robinson, K.D., Angeletti, K.A., Barg, F.K., Pasacreta, J.V., McCorkle, R., & Yasko, J.M. (1998). The development of a family caregiver cancer education program. *Journal of Cancer Education, 13,* 116–121.

Rusinak, R.L., & Murphy, J.F. (1995). Elderly spousal caregivers: Knowledge of cancer care, perceptions of preparedness, and coping strategies. *Journal of Gerontological Nursing, 21*(3), 33–41.

Sales, E., Schulz, R., & Biegal, D. (1992). Predictors of strain in families of cancer patients: A review of the literature. *Journal of Psychosocial Oncology, 10*(2), 1–26.

Schaeffer, C., & Goldstein, P. (1996). Palliative care. *Continuing Care, 6,* 22–24.

Steele, R.G., & Fitch, M.I. (1996). Needs of family caregivers of patients receiving home hospice care for cancer. *Oncology Nursing Forum, 23,* 823–828.

Steeves, R.H., & Kahn, D. (1994). Family perspectives: Tasks of bereavement. *Quality of Life: A Nursing Challenge, 3*(3), 48–53.

SUPPORT (Study to Understand Prognosis and Preferences for Outcomes and Risks of Treatment). (1995). A controlled trial to improve care for seriously ill hospitalized patients. *JAMA, 274,* 1591–1598.

Tadaaki, S. (1999). Ethical issues. In S.K. Joishy (Ed.), *Palliative medicine secrets* (pp. 208–209). Philadelphia: Hanley & Belfus.

Talbot, J.H., Jude, J.R., & Elam, J.O. (1965). *Fundamentals of cardiopulmonary resuscitation.* Philadelphia: F.A. Davis.

Travis, S.S., Bernard, M., Dixon, S., McAuley, W.J., Loving, G., & McClanahan, L. (2002). Obstacles to palliation and end-of-life care in a long-term care facility. *Gerontologist, 42,* 342–349.

Ward, S., & Gatwood, J. (1994). Concerns about reporting pain and using analgesics: A comparison of persons with and without cancer. *Cancer Nursing, 17,* 200–206.

Ward, S.E., Berry, P.E., & Misiewicz, H. (1996). Concerns about analgesics among patient and family caregivers in a hospice setting. *Research in Nursing and Health, 19,* 205–211.

Weeks, J.C., Cook, E.F., O'Day, S.J., Peterson, L.M., Wenger, N., Reding, D., et al. (1998). Relationship between cancer patients' predictions of prognosis and their treatment preferences. *JAMA, 279,* 1709–1714.

Weissman, D. (2000). *Fast facts and concepts # 014: Palliative chemotherapy.* End of Life/Palliative Education Resource Center. Retrieved May 1, 2005, from http://www.eperc.mcw.edu/fastFact/ff_014.htm

Weitzner, M.A., McMillan, S., & Jacobson, P. (1999). Family caregiver quality of life: Differences between curative and palliative cancer treatment settings. *Journal of Pain and Symptom Management, 17,* 418–428.

Working Party on Clinical Guidelines in Palliative Care. (1997). *Changing gear: Guidelines for managing the last days of life.* London: National Council for Hospice and Specialist Palliative Care Services.

Yellen, S., Cella, D., & Leslie, W. (1994). Age and clinical decision making in oncology patients. *Journal of the National Cancer Institute, 86,* 1766–1779.

CHAPTER 22

Complementary and Alternative Therapies

Georgia M. Decker, RN, MS, CS-ANP, AOCN®

Introduction

National surveys confirm a sustained interest in and use of complementary and alternative medicine (CAM) therapies in the United States and Europe (Eisenberg et al., 1993, 1998). The first of these surveys were not disease or population specific. Although people are learning more about CAM therapies, much remains to be determined about the safety, efficacy, potential benefits, and adverse effects with specific diseases and treatments. A CAM therapy survey reported that patients with cancer who participated in clinical trials used spirituality (94%), imagery (86%), massage (80%), lifestyle, diet, and nutrition (60%), herbal/botanical (20%), and high-dose vitamins (14%) (Sparber et al., 2000). Other surveys reported use of CAM therapies at 50%–83% (Basch & Ulbricht, 2004; Ernst & Cassileth, 1998). At the end of the 1990s, more information was available about the use of CAMs by specific populations with cancer, including cancer site and ethnicity (Ashikaga, Bosompra, O'Brien, & Nelson, 2002; Lengacher et al., 2002; Maskarinec, Shumay, Kakai, & Gotay, 2000; Swisher et al., 2002). Additional data reported CAM use specific to those in urban, suburban, and rural areas and the older adult population (Bennett & Lengacher, 1999; Bernstein & Grasso, 2001; Ernst & Cassileth; Herron & Glasser, 2003; Najm, Reinsch, Hoehler, & Tobis, 2003; Vallerand, Fouladbakhsh, & Templin, 2003).

When compared with non-CAM users, individuals who use CAM are more likely to be female, be better educated, and have higher incomes (Eisenberg et al., 1998). Using a cross-sectional design in females with gynecologic cancer, a recent study reported that characteristics associated with CAM use include annual incomes greater than $30,000, cancer site of origin other than the cervix, and use of CAM prior to cancer diagnosis. Respondents reported their reasons for using CAM as a hope of improved well-being and possible anticancer effects of the particular CAM modalities used (Swisher et al., 2002). Some of the reported reasons for seeking CAM therapies have remained consistent: philosophical similarity (active patient role; natural, less toxic treatments; spiritual elements); personal control over treatment; positive relationship with therapist (time for discussion, including emotional aspects); and increased well-being (Bernstein & Grasso, 2001; Furnham, 1996; Stevinson, 2001). Factors reported as contributing to the decreased use of conventional biomedical medicine in favor of CAM are dissatisfaction with contemporary healthcare systems (ineffective therapies, adverse effects, poor communication), insufficient time with and insufficient access to healthcare professionals, rejection (when antiscience viewpoint is expressed), desperation, and cost of care (Furnham; Stevinson). Authors suggested that the persuasive appeal of CAM is related to a perceived association of CAM with nature, focus on energy forces promoting vitalism, intellectual traditions and sophisticated philosophies, extensive training involving complex systems and concepts, and the likely union of the physical (medical) and spiritual (truth, values, morals) realms (Kaptchuk & Eisenberg, 1998; Stevinson). Patients consistently have expressed a desire to take control of their own health, actively participate in decisions related to health and wellness, and choose treatment plans involving solely conventional biomedical, solely CAM, or a combination of both therapies (Stevinson). With increasing cancer incidence and comorbidities in the older adult, CAM use also may increase in this population. This chapter will provide an overview of CAM therapies and discuss specifically issues related to the use of CAM therapies in the older adult. Recommendations for future research and clinical practice will be presented.

Background

The Office of Alternative Medicine was established in 1992 in response to the continued use of and issues surrounding CAM therapies. It became the National Center for Complementary and Alternative Medicine (NCCAM) in 1998. NCCAM is one of the 27 institutes and centers that make up the National Institutes of Health. NCCAM has four primary focus areas: research (clinical and basic science research), training and career development (predoctoral, postdoctoral, and career researchers), outreach (conferences, educational programs, and exhibits [information clearinghouse]), and integration (scientifically proven CAM practices into conventional medicine) (NCCAM, 2004).

In an effort to increase quality cancer research and information about CAM use, the National Cancer Institute (NCI) established the Office of Cancer Complementary and Alternative Medicine (OCCAM) within the Office of the Director in 1998. OCCAM promotes and supports research within CAM disciplines and therapies as they relate to the prevention, diagnosis, and treatment of cancer, cancer-related symptoms, and side effects of conventional treatment. OCCAM coordinates NCI's CAM research and informational activities, collaboration with other governmental and nongovernmental organizations on cancer CAM issues, and liaisons with health practitioners and researchers regarding cancer CAM issues (OCCAM, 2004; White, 2002a, 2002b).

The White House Commission on Complementary and Alternative Medicine Policy was established in March 2000 to address issues related to access and delivery of CAM, priorities for research, and to identify the need for consumer and health-care professional education. The 10 principles endorsed by this commission are summarized in Figure 22-1. In 2003–2004, the Institute of Medicine (IOM) of the National Academies sponsored seven committee meetings to investigate scientific policy and practice questions that occur from the increasing use of CAM (Jacobson, Workman, & Kronenberg, 2000). The IOM is a nongovernment agency established in 1970 that guarantees unbiased, evidence-based information and advice concerning health and science policy to policy makers, healthcare professionals, and the public (IOM, 2004). The final report of the IOM committees is available and can be found on its Web site (http://www.iom.edu).

- A wholeness orientation in healthcare delivery: Deliver high-quality health care that supports care of the whole person.
- Evidence of safety and efficacy: Use science to generate evidence that protects and promotes public health.
- Healing capacity of a person: Support capacity for recovery and self-healing.
- Respect for individuality: Each person has the right to health care that is responsive, respects preferences, and preserves dignity.
- Right to choose treatment: Each person has the right to choose freely among safe and effective approaches and among qualified practitioners.
- Emphasis on health promotion and self-care: Good health care emphasizes self-care and early interventions for maintaining and promoting health.
- Partnerships in integrated health care: Good health care requires teamwork among patients, healthcare professionals (HCPs), and researchers committed to creating healing environments and respecting diversity of healthcare traditions.
- Education as a fundamental healthcare service: Education about prevention, healthy lifestyles, and self-healing should be part of the curricula of all HCPs and made available to the public.
- Dissemination of comprehensive, timely information: Healthcare quality is enhanced by examination of the evidence on which complementary and alternative medicine systems, practices, and products are based. This information should be widely, rapidly, and easily available.
- Integral public involvement: Input from informed consumers must be incorporated in proposing priorities for healthcare, research, and policy decisions.

Figure 22-1. The White House Commission on Complementary and Alternative Medicine Policy-Guiding Principles

---

Note. From "White House Commission on Complementary and Alternative Medicine Policy," by the White House Commission, 2000. Retrieved February 11, 2005, from http://www.whccamp.hhs.gov/es.html

Defining Complementary and Alternative Medicine

Numerous definitions of CAM describe a broad range of philosophies, approaches, and applications for clinical oncology practice. Table 22-1 provides examples of these definitions. Historically, *alternative* has been used as an umbrella term to describe therapies not taught in U.S. medical schools or provided in U.S. hospitals. This term is no longer accurate because many medical schools include these therapies in their curricula, and some are provided to interested patients in hospitals and cancer centers (Eisenberg et al., 1993). The interchangeable use of the terms *complementary* and *alternative* has led to miscommunications and misunderstandings among healthcare

Table 22-1. Examples of Definitions of Complementary and Alternative Medicine

Source	Definition
Eisenberg et al., 1993	Alternative therapies are those not taught in U.S. medical schools or provided in U.S. hospitals.
Ernst, 2003	Complementary and alternative medicine (CAM) is any approach to improve a health problem that is not used or taught routinely to conventional Western practitioners. Alternative cancer treatments are CAM therapies that reduce tumor burden or replace mainstream medicine.
National Center for Complementary and Alternative Medicine, 2004	CAM is a group of diverse medical and healthcare systems, practices, and products that currently are not considered to be a part of conventional medicine. Complementary medicine is used with conventional medicine. Alternative medicine is used in place of conventional medicine. Integrative medicine combines mainstream and CAM therapies for which scientific evidence of safety and efficacy exists.
Oncology Nursing Society, 2002	CAM involves the interchangeable use of the terms *complementary, alternative,* and *integrative* therapies reflecting what may describe a therapy rather than how it is used. *Complementary* describes a therapy that is used with a conventional therapy, whereas *alternative* describes a therapy that is used "instead of" conventional therapy. *Integrative care* is defined as a combination of complementary and conventional approaches to care.

providers, the public, and patients. *Complementary* and *alternative* are not the same. A therapy is defined by the *intent* with which it is used. A therapy is *alternative* when it is used *instead of* conventional therapy. *Complementary* therapies are those used *in addition to*, or *to complement*, conventional therapy. The more current terms, *integrative* or *integrated*, are preferred because they reflect the use of CAM therapies in combination with conventional treatments (Oncology Nursing Society [ONS], 2004). Using this framework, CAM therapies may be used to reduce the side effects associated with or to improve the patient's tolerance of conventional cancer treatments and improve quality of life.

Early literature refers to seven categories of CAM therapies (see Table 22-2). NCCAM classifies CAM therapies into five domains: (a) alternative medical systems, (b) mind-body interventions, (c) biologically based therapies, (d) manipulative and body-based methods, and (e) energy therapies (NCCAM, 2004). Table 22-2 describes these categories. NCI's OCCAM extended the NCCAM domains with three additional categories: movement therapy, pharmacologic and biologic treatments with a subcategory of complex natural products, and a miscellaneous domain (Lee, 2004b; White, 2002a).

Alternative medical systems are complete systems of theory and practice. *Mind-body medicine* uses a variety of techniques designed to enhance the mind's capacity to affect bodily function and symptoms. *Biologically based therapies* use substances found in nature, including food, herbs, and vitamins. *Manipulative and body-based methods* involve touching the person and are based on manipulation and/or movement of one or more parts of the body. *Energy therapies* involve the use of energy fields and are of two types: biofield therapies that may or may not involve touch and bioelectromagnetic-based therapies.

Table 22-2. Complementary and Alternative Therapy Categories and Major Controversies

Category	Description	Examples	Controversies/Comments
Alternative system of medical care	Stresses prevention of disease and promotion of health, including emphasis on personal responsibility and self-healing	Traditional Chinese medicine Naturopathy Ayurvedic medicine	These systems are a way of being and a way of living. They are not meant to be parceled into individual or separate modalities. Western medicine has begun to incorporate various aspects of these modalities.
Mind-body medicine	Known as behavioral medicine; unites biomedical, behavioral, and psychological strategies for promotion of health	Meditation Guided imagery Visualization Relaxation Spirituality Art therapies Music therapy Biofeedback Yoga	Controversies exist over whether mind-body interventions prolong survival or merely enhance quality of life and a sense of being healed. Imagery and visualization have been used in patients with cancer for relief of treatment- and disease-related symptoms, including pain control. Concerns have been raised about the use of guided imagery in patients with a psychiatric history. The idea that mental efforts can alter the course of cancer has not been proven by research and may induce feelings of guilt and inadequacy in patients whose disease progresses despite best efforts.
Bioelectromagnetic therapies	Based on the use of energy as healing modality	Acupuncture Magnet therapy Cymatics	The contemporary use of magnets has stimulated discussion and research regarding claims that magnets reduce pain and may have health-promoting benefits. Acupuncture (taken from traditional Oriental medicine) has proved to be helpful for various symptoms and now is accepted for pain relief.
Herbal medicine	Based on Doctrine of Signatures, which states that a plant's appearance or characteristics provides a clue to medicinal implications	Herbs may be used as single agents or in combination. Herbs used to treat cancer include Essiac and pau d'arco tea.	Patients believe that "natural means safe" and that "if a little is good, a lot is better." The concern for all patients is possible herb-drug interactions. More information about this issue will become available. To report an adverse event, call 888-SAFE-FOOD or visit the U.S. Food and Drug Administrations's Web site at http://www.fda.gov/medwatch/partner.htm. Because herbs are not regulated or standardized, safety issues must be scrutinized.
Pharmacologic and biologic therapies	Most often used as alternatives and have been described as having the "lure of cure"	Laetrile Shark cartilage Oxidative therapies Antineoplastons PC-SPES (combination of 14 herbs for prostate cancer)	The concern always has been that patients will use these therapies instead of conventional therapies. Because many of the components of these therapies are not known, any risk associated with use as a single agent or in combination has yet to be identified.

(Continued on next page)

Table 22-2. Complementary and Alternative Therapy Categories and Major Controversies *(Continued)*

Category	Description	Examples	Controversies/Comments
Manual healing methods	Usually involve touch and often are viewed as complementary therapies	Reiki Chiropractic Reflexology Massage Therapeutic touch (misnomer because actual touch is not involved)	Although touch usually is desirable, especially in the American culture, the kind of touch has important implications. Controversies related to effect of therapeutic touch have arisen, but it remains a popular complementary therapy.
Diet, nutrition, and lifestyle changes	Use of food or other supplements to prevent and treat illness Appeal to patients because therapies can be initiated immediately and patients have control over them	Macrobiotics Kelley-Gonzales High-dose vitamin therapies Antioxidants	Some controversies are related to risk of malnutrition with restrictive dietary programs, effects of antioxidants and/or vitamins during certain therapies, and effects of soy in certain cancers.

Note. From *Oncology Nursing Secrets* (2nd ed., pp. 144–145), by G.M. Decker and M.J. Cleveland, 2001, Philadelphia: Hanley & Belfus. Copyright 2001 by Elsevier. Reprinted with permission.

Movement therapies are modalities used to improve patterns of bodily movement. *Pharmacologic and biologic therapies* are drugs, vaccines, off-label use of prescription drugs, and other biologic interventions not yet accepted in mainstream medicine. *Complex natural products*, a subcategory of pharmacologic and biologic therapies, consist of crude natural substances and unfractionated extracts from marine organisms used for healing and treatment of disease. The miscellaneous domain includes interventions that have conventional therapeutic applications that generally are not used for cancer treatment but are promoted by cancer CAM practitioners (OCCAM, 2004). Table 22-3 further describes the domains, as defined by OCCAM, and provides examples of those therapies currently in clinical trials (Decker & Lee, 2005).

Complementary and Alternative Medicine and Evidence-Based Practice

NCI's PDQ® Adult Treatment Editorial Board ranks human cancer treatment studies based on the strength of the study's design and statistics and the specific strength of the treatment outcomes. Because randomized controlled clinical trials (double-blinded or non-blinded) are considered the gold standard for study design, this classification has been adapted for CAM clinical trials. Nonrandomized control clinical trials include treatments assigned by an information point, such as date of birth, or any method that would identify the patient to the researcher. Table 22-4 provides examples of CAM clinical trials (NCI, 2004). Case series, population based or nonpopulation based, are

Table 22-3. National Cancer Institute's Office of Cancer Complementary and Alternative Medicine Domains of Complementary and Alternative Medicine: Modalities in Clinical Trials

Domain	Definition	Example(s)	Modality in Clinical Trials (Lee, 2004a, 2004b, 2004c; National Cancer Institute, 2004)
Alternative medical systems	Systems built upon completed systems of theory and practice	Traditional Chinese medicine (acupuncture), Ayurveda, homeopathy, naturopathy, Tibetan medicine	Acupuncture Acupressure Electroacupuncture Traumeel® S
Mind-body interventions	Techniques designed to enhance the mind's capacity to affect bodily function and symptoms	Medication, hypnosis, art therapy, biofeedback, mental healing, imagery, relaxation therapy, support groups, music therapy, cognitive-behavioral therapy, prayer, dance therapy, psychoneuroimmunology, aromatherapy, animal-assisted therapy	Distance healing Exercise-based counseling Group therapy Healing touch Music therapy Spirituality, religiosity Standard counseling Stress management training
Nutritional therapeutics	Assortment of nutrients and nonnutrients and bioactive food components that are used as chemopreventive agents and the use of specific foods or diets as cancer prevention or treatment strategies	Dietary regimens such as macrobiotics, vegetarian, Gerson therapy, Kelley/Gonzalez regimen, vitamins, dietary macronutrients, supplements, antioxidants, melatonin, selenium, coenzyme Q10, ephedrine, orthomolecular medicine	Black cohosh Creatine Curcumin Flax seed Folic acid Fruit and vegetable extracts Garlic Ginger Herbal therapy *Hypericum perforatum* Juven L-carnitine Low-fat diet Lycopene Macrobiotic diet Noni fruit extract Nutritional supplements Pomegranate juice Selenium Soy protein isolate Valerian officinalis Vitamins C and E Zinc sulfate
Manipulative and body-based methods	Methods based on manipulation and/or movement of one or more parts of the body	Chiropractic, therapeutic massage, osteopathy, reflexology	Massage therapy
Energy therapies	Therapies involving the use of energy fields	Qigong, Reiki, therapeutic touch, pulsed fields, magnet therapy	Energy healing Energy therapy Reiki Touch

(Continued on next page)

Table 22-3. National Cancer Institute's Office of Cancer Complementary and Alternative Medicine Domains of Complementary and Alternative Medicine: Modalities in Clinical Trials *(Continued)*

Domain	Definition	Example(s)	Modality in Clinical Trials (Lee, 2004a, 2004b, 2004c; National Cancer Institute, 2004)
Movement therapy	Modalities used to improve patterns of bodily movement	Tai Chi, Feldenkrais, Hatha yoga, Alexander Technique, dance therapy, Qigong, Rolfing, Trager Method, applied kinesiology	–
Pharmacologic and biologic treatments	Drugs, complex natural products, vaccines, and other biologic interventions not yet accepted in mainstream medicine, off-label use of prescription drugs	Antineoplastons, products from honey bees, mistletoe, 714-X, low-dose naltrexone, met-enkephalin, immunoaugmentative therapy, laetrile, hydrazine sulfate, New Castle Virus, melatonin, ozone therapy, thymus therapy, enzyme therapy, high-dose vitamin C	Antineoplastons Mistletoe Pancreatic proteolytic enzymes
Complex natural products	Subcategory of pharmacologic and biologic treatments consisting of an assortment of plant samples (botanicals), extracts of crude natural substances, and unfractionated extracts from marine organisms used for healing and treatment of disease	Herbs and herbal extracts, mixtures of tea polyphenols, shark cartilage, Essiac tea, Cordyceps, Sun Soup, MGN-3	Chinese herbal extract Green tea extract (Polyphenon E) Kanglaite injection Milk thistle Pycnogenol® Shark cartilage Virulizin®
Miscellaneous	Interventions that have conventional therapeutic applications are not generally used for cancer treatment but are promoted by cancer complementary and alternative medicine practitioners	Hyperbaric oxygen	Hyperbaric oxygen

Note. From "Complementary and Alternative Medicine (CAM) Therapies" (6th ed., pp. 593–594), by G. Decker and C. Lee in C.H. Yarbro, M.H. Frogge, and M. Goodman (Eds.), *Cancer Nursing: Principles and Practice,* 2005, Sudbury, MA: Jones and Bartlett. Copyright 2005 by Jones and Bartlett. Adapted with permission.

Table 22-4. Types of Clinical Trials With Complementary and Alternative Medicine (CAM) Examples

Type	Description	Example of Cancer CAM Trial
Prevention trials	Study ways to reduce the risk of developing cancer.	Phase III randomized study of selenium and vitamin E for the prevention of prostate cancer (SELECT trial)
Screening trials	Study ways to detect cancer in people who do not have any symptoms of cancer.	None at this time
Diagnostic	Study tests or procedures that identify cancer earlier.	None at this time
Treatment	Study new therapies or new indications of drugs, vaccines, and approaches to treatment.	Phase II study of supplemental treatment with mistletoe in patients with stage IV non-small cell lung cancer receiving palliative chemotherapy
Supportive care (includes quality of life)	Study ways to improve cancer-related symptoms and quality of life.	Phase II/III randomized study of ginger for chemotherapy-related nausea in patients with cancer
Genetic studies	Study ways in which genetic makeup can affect detection, diagnosis, or treatment response.	None at this time

Note. Based on information from the National Cancer Institute, 2004.

the weakest form of study design. For some CAM modalities, however, case series may be the only means for study. Evidence-based practice is the care of patients using the best available evidence from research to guide clinical decision making.

Levels of evidence in CAM are created in the same manner as in conventional medicine. This process begins with clinical trials involving CAM modalities for the treatment of cancer and cancer-related side effects. Identifying and defining evidence-based practice for certain CAM therapies is a result of the integration of clinical expertise, epidemiologic studies, and anecdotal evidence, a process similar to conventional medicine. Angell and Kassirer (1998) maintained that there cannot be two kinds of medicine—conventional and alternative. Only one type of medicine exists: one that is adequately and rigorously tested and found to be reasonable, safe, and effective. The notion of an evidence-based approach to CAM is still in its genesis. Limited data are available on safety, efficacy, and mechanism of action for many CAM modalities, even as research confirms increasing use in the United States. Recommending CAM remains a challenge for many healthcare professionals. This challenge may increase when conventional therapies are not providing the preferred result and patients request information and/or advice from their healthcare professionals about CAM therapies. The search for CAM therapies is complicated by the amount of information, a significant amount of it inaccurate, that is available from a variety of sources, including well-meaning friends, family, the clerk at the health food store, the neighborhood herbalist, and the Internet. Opinions vary and methods of evaluating therapies differ even among experts. For example, Ernst (2001b) used the "direction of evidence" (clearly positive, tentatively positive, uncertain, tentatively negative, clearly negative) and "weight of evidence" (low, moderate, high) methods, whereas Eisenberg (2001) used "recommend," "tolerate," and "avoid" modalities. Eisenberg (1997) offered an algorithm for physicians advising patients about CAM, and Decker (2005) suggested an algorithm for healthcare professionals advising patients regarding CAM therapies (see Figure 22-2).

Decision Making in the Older Adult With Cancer

Many patients want to participate in medical decision making. A partnering, collaborative relationship is replacing the dated, paternalistic one between physicians and their patients (Pinquart & Duberstein, 2004). Participation in treatment decisions allows patients to reclaim autonomy and a sense of control (Llewelyn-Thomas, McGreal, & Theil, 1995; Truant & Bottorff, 1999). Acquiring and evaluating accurate and sufficient information about a diagnosis and existing treatments is necessary for this process. A variety of other factors will affect this collaborative approach, including the patient's age, educational level, the social structure of the family and the influences of relatives and friends, financial concerns, and insurance coverage. A patient's initial priority needs to focus on a chance of cure and possible spread of disease (Davison, Degner, & Morgan, 1995; Degner et al., 1997). A difference in older patients exists in terms of how much information they seek, the content of information, and the sources of information. Age differences in social network also exist. Older adults may have more friends and family of the same age who have had an experience with cancer (Gattellari, Voigt, Butow, & Tattersall, 2002) and are more likely to have a fatalistic attitude (Powe, 2001).

A demonstrated age difference in locus of control exists, and older adults with cancer are more likely to believe that they lack the ability to influence their illness (Mastaglia & Kristjanson, 2001). Baltes and Staudinger (1996) described age-related differences in coping/control strategies. The older adult is more likely to behave in a passive manner, perhaps believing that helplessness will bring about support from healthcare professionals, family, and friends. Motivational changes are seen in the shift from surviving a set of circumstances to adapting to their situation (Schulz & Heckhausen, 1996). Age-related cognitive weakening limits processing and memorizing information, and therefore the older patient may not seek additional information (Polsky, Keating, Weeks, & Schulman, 2002). Making treatment decisions often is difficult and fraught with anxiety. Feeling forced to make these decisions within a short time interval may diminish a patient's ability to participate in the decision (Elit et al., 2003). Making the decision to integrate a CAM modality can make the entire process more complex.

Brett (2002) described the variability in an individual's response to the subject of CAM modalities. Culture and religion, as well as age, influence a person's perception. These perceptions can change the view of therapy from essential to moderately interested to cynical. For example, older adults with cancer may have concerns about the therapies that involve touch. This can be age-related as well as involving cultural and religious beliefs because aging is intricate and complex and is surrounded by myths and speculation. Holistic nursing acknowledges that patients have personal beliefs about health care and opinions about appropriate processes and outcomes (Goodman, 1995). A patient discussed in the following anecdote exemplified this.

> At the time of our meeting, Edith was 80 years old. She had chronic myalgias and arthralgias related to her diagnoses of osteoporosis and fibromyalgia. Edith is a long-time breast cancer (more than 20 years)

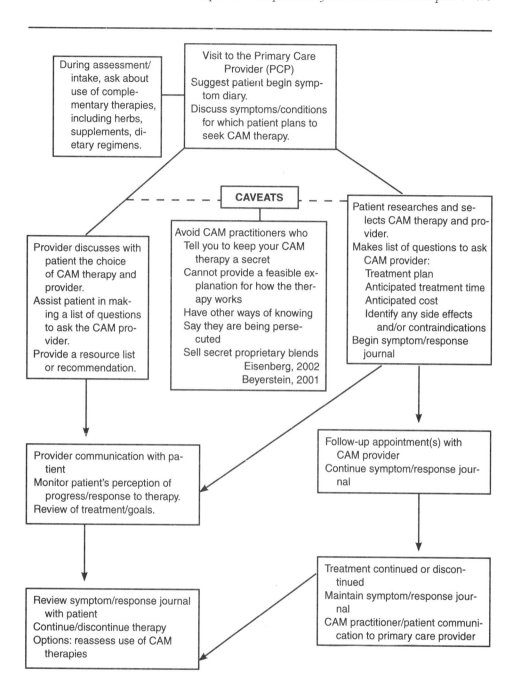

Figure 22-2. Discussing Complementary and Alternative Medicine With Patients

Note. From "Strategies for CAM Program Development" (2nd ed., p. 365), by G. Decker in P. Buchsel and C. Yarbro (Eds.), *Oncology Nursing in the Ambulatory Setting: Issues and Models of Care*, 2005, Sudbury, MA: Jones and Bartlett. Copyright 2005 by Jones and Bartlett. Reprinted with permission.

and colon cancer (15 years) survivor, and her youngest daughter had persuaded her to try Reiki therapy. Edith thought of massage when she heard the word Reiki. At the time of her appointment, Edith was very surprised and relieved to learn that she would be keeping her clothing on during the session. As the Reiki Master positioned herself, it became apparent to Edith that there had been some sort of misunderstanding, and she was fairly certain that this misunderstanding was not hers. The Reiki Master explained the session a second time, and Edith was stunned. She had envisioned a massage session, and she had not heard the differences when they were explained. She politely said that she would "pass" on her gift certificate. She was invited to observe a Reiki session, and she reluctantly agreed. She appeared to be awed when watching the Reiki Master and repeatedly would put her hands between the 'patient' and the hands of the practitioner. She said she was trying to feel the universal energy (see Table 22-5). She ultimately decided to experience Reiki and became increasing enamored with it. Edith is now 84 years young and is a Reiki practitioner working toward becoming a Reiki Master.

Edith exemplifies issues related to CAM use by the older adult with cancer. Cancer incidence typically increases with age. The older adult may have comorbidities as well. A common misconception among CAM users of all ages is that a CAM therapy used for heart conditions or depression cannot/will not have any impact on cancer or cancer therapy. Edith's cancers remained in remission; however, she searched for symptomatic relief from the effects of her comorbidities. Given and Given (1989) reported that despite the fact that most new cancers are diagnosed in those older than 60 years of age, little is known about the biophysical responses of older people to cancer and the effects of cancer therapy. The *graying* of America and the nursing shortage further complicate the issue. Oncology nurses are experts at managing symptoms related to cancer and cancer therapies. ONS (2002) described quality cancer care as including appropriate symptom management as a component of supportive care. ONS developed the Priority Symptom Management project to focus on six symptoms: anorexia, cognitive dysfunction, depression, fatigue, neutropenia, and pain. The therapies most commonly used by nurses who care for patients with cancer include massage, aromatherapy, reflexology, acupuncture, and acupressure. Safe and appropriate use of CAM therapies can enhance conventional approaches to symptom management.

In an early study, Downer et al. (1994) reported that these therapies are used as *complementary*, primarily for musculoskeletal symptoms and stress management. These same authors discovered that even when a chosen complementary therapy had little influence on a patient's illness, he or she still reported satisfaction with that particular therapy. The toxic effects of conventional therapy and a lack of hope caused dissatisfaction with patients. Kassab and Stevensen (1996) reported that misinformation about CAM therapies may arise from word of mouth and speculation (e.g., massage spreads cancer). Opinions vary, even among experts in the field. Recommendations include avoiding deep tissue massage over tumor sites and contiguous lymph glands and over irradiated fields where the skin is fragile (Decker & Cleveland, 2001; Tisserand & Balacs, 1995). Therefore, a decision to use a particular CAM therapy might not be an unequivocal yes or no. The answer might be "not during therapy but okay afterward," "only on the weeks I am NOT receiving chemotherapy," or "you must take a multiple vitamin supplement with this particular therapy."

Table 22-5. Commonly Used Complementary and Alternative Medicine (CAM) Modalities

Domain	Therapy	Description	Strength of Evidence	Contraindications	Opportunities	Practitioners
Alternative medical systems	Acupuncture	Numerous Americans use acupuncture and, in the United States, physicians, dentists, and acupuncturists perform the procedure for a number of health conditions. The foundation of this therapy is that qi (pronounced "chee" and meaning energy) is present at birth and is maintained throughout one's life. Qi flows throughout the body via 12 major pathways known as meridians. Approximately 350 acupoints exist along 12 meridians with additional acupoints that occur outside the meridian pathways. Typically, acupuncture involves insertion of a needle into the skin in a number of specific sites (acupoints) along a meridian. Acupoint stimulation also may be accomplished through the use of electrical current, laser, moxibustion, pressure, ultrasound, and	The diagnostic value of acupuncture has not been established (Ernst, 2001a, 2001b). Although there is no evidence of the physical existence of qi or meridians, evidence exists that the effects of acupuncture are more than placebo (Ernst, 2001a). Opioid peptides, serotonin, and other neurotransmitters are released by acupuncture (Andersson & Lundeberg, 1995; Ernst, 2003; Ernst et al., 1998; Han & Terenius, 1982; Melchart et al., 1999). Acupuncture has been used for pain and other disorders of the musculoskeletal system; headaches; stress; ear, nose, and throat conditions, including sinusitis, tinnitus, and vertigo; allergies; dental pain; addictions; and immune system support. It is commonly used for chronic	"Needling" technique is contraindicated in those patients with severe bleeding disorders or who are at increased risk for infection, as in neutropenia. Treatment for nausea may be an exception (Aikins Murphy, 1998). Some authors suggest that patients with cardiac pacemakers should not be treated with electrical stimulation (Ernst & White, 1997). Caution is advised, and some authors recommend that the first treatment be administered with the patient in a supine position (Ernst, 2001a). Some patients become drowsy, and therefore they should be cautioned to take care when operating	Evidence shows that with accurate diagnosis, acupuncture is safe, and for certain conditions, it may be more effective than placebo when administered by an appropriately trained practitioner (Ernst, 2001a).	In the United States, acupuncturists can be certified in two ways. They can complete a formal, full-time educational program that includes both classroom and clinical hours, or they can participate in an apprenticeship program. Acupuncturists also must complete a "Clean Needle Technique" approved course. Medical doctors with training in acupuncture also can obtain board certification. The National Certification Commission of Acupuncture and Oriental Medicine (NCCAOM) established standards for certification that are accepted by some states for licensure. Some states require medical referral, whereas others allow nonmedical

(Continued on next page)

Table 22-5. Commonly Used Complementary and Alternative Medicine (CAM) Modalities *(Continued)*

Domain	Therapy	Description	Strength of Evidence	Contraindications	Opportunities	Practitioners
Alternative medical systems *(cont.)*	Acupuncture *(cont.)*	vibration. Japanese, Korean, or Chinese variations exist. Health is believed to be a balance of Yin and Yang (opposite forces present in everyone), and disease is a result of imbalance, caused by a blockage or deficiency of energy. Acupuncture theory is based on the belief that stimulating the appropriate acupoints aids the body in the ability to correct any imbalance in the flow of energy. Therefore, balance is restored. Changes in the balance of energy and flow of qi may be identified before disease has developed, and therefore acupuncture has a role in the prevention of illness and maintenance of health. Eastern countries routinely use this treatment, which also has been integrated with allopathic and osteopathic medicine in the United States (Ernst, 2001a; Ernst & Cassileth, 1998).	pain. Conclusive evidence exists that acupuncture is effective in the treatment of dental pain and postoperative nausea (Ernst & Pittler, 1998). Evidence for the use of acupuncture in the treatment of asthma, neck pain, drug dependency, fibromyalgia, migraine and tension headaches, osteoarthritis, and stroke is considered inconclusive by some authors (Ernst, 2001a). Some authors suggest that the evidence is equivocal and/or promising for some indications, including addiction, stroke rehabilitation, postoperative- and chemotherapy-related nausea and vomiting, tennis elbow, carpal tunnel syndrome, and asthma (Mayer, 2000).	machinery. Needles should not be reused, and strict asepsis must be maintained. Side effects may include bleeding, bruising, pain with needling, and worsening of symptoms. Reported adverse events are rare but include pneumothorax and death (Ernst & White).		practitioners to see patients without a referral (www.nccaom. org). A comparison of licensed versus certified acupuncturists is available at www.asny. org. Medical doctors must possess a valid medical license and be certified through the American Academy of Medical Acupuncture (www.medicalacupuncture.org).

(Continued on next page)

Table 22-5. Commonly Used Complementary and Alternative Medicine (CAM) Modalities *(Continued)*

Domain	Therapy	Description	Strength of Evidence	Contraindications	Opportunities	Practitioners
Energy therapies	Qigong	Qigong (pronounced "Chi Kung") means "energy cultivation" and refers to movements that are believed to improve health, longevity, and harmony within oneself and the world (Eichelberger, 2004). Thousands of such movements exist, and Qigong may include any one with the intention of enhancing energy. It is based on four common principles, sometimes referred to as the "secrets" of Qigong: mind (the presence of intention), eyes (the focus of intention), movement (the action of intention), and breath (the flow of intention). Numerous styles exist and may include meditation, exercise, and self-massage (Ernst, 2001a). Mastery in Qigong is the achievement of the ultimate goal—harmonious existence and action in all situations. Mastery does not	There are approximately 100 randomized clinical trials (RCTs) reported in MEDLINE from 1997 to 2004 using Qigong for various conditions. Two trials involved patients with cancer (inspiratory muscle training and relief of breathlessness). Four meta-analyses examined the use of Qigong from 1997 to 2004 for respiratory-related conditions (Corner et al., 1996; Weiner et al., 1997).	Some reported psychosis. It is not known if there was a latent condition (Ernst, 2001a; Wu, 1990).	Yang (2004) has predicted the use of Qigong in the treatment of arthritis. Ernst et al. (1998) suggested the use of Qigong for health promotion, functional disorders, and symptom control.	Because it is considered a form of Chinese medicine, those credentialed in acupuncture and/or Oriental medicine are appropriate practitioners. The National Library of Medicine compiled the Directory of Information Resources Online (DIRLINE) (http://dirline.nlm.nih.gov). It contains information about a variety of health organizations, including CAM associations and organizations.

(Continued on next page)

Table 22-5. Commonly Used Complementary and Alternative Medicine (CAM) Modalities (*Continued*)

Domain	Therapy	Description	Strength of Evidence	Contraindications	Opportunities	Practitioners
Energy therapies (*cont.*)	Qigong (*cont.*)	exhibit as someone knowing everything but rather, regardless of a level of achievement, a willingness to continue learning. Elements that define this level of expertise include curiosity, ease in action, clarity of focus and intention, perseverance, nonattachment, resilience, openness, creativity, responsiveness, and fluid balance. Numerous books and teachers profess to teach the secrets of Qigong and the power of the possibility of its applications. Authors agree that it actually is defined by a person's willingness to practice and experience, that is, the availability to learn (Eichelberger; Ernst, 2001a). There are 24 rules for Qigong practice (Yang, 2004).				

(Continued on next page)

Table 22-5. Commonly Used Complementary and Alternative Medicine (CAM) Modalities (Continued)

Domain	Therapy	Description	Strength of Evidence	Contraindications	Opportunities	Practitioners
Energy therapies *(cont.)*	Reiki	*Reiki* means universal life energy. It is an ancient form of healing. The practitioner is the conduit for the movement of energy. It is the energy, not the healer, that influences healing. In this respect, Reiki differs from other healing systems. That is, energy travels through the healing, not from the healer. Reiki is said to alleviate physical, emotional, and spiritual blockages (Finley, 1992). The five premises of Reiki include an energy of unique properties applicable to physical and psychological conditions; the energy has a source; this source can be tapped; a person can be taught to use this energy; and the effects of this energy are palpable and subjective. The energy is considered pure because the practitioner's faith or religion does not influence it (Finley). The practitioner gently	Reiki is believed to be helpful in the treatment of chronic pain and emotional problems (Ernst, 2001b), decreasing stress and increasing vitality (Finley, 1992). Reiki can be used when massage is not possible or contraindicated (Finley). A significant body of anecdotal literature and two RCTs trials suggest that Reiki may be an effective treatment for fibromyalgia by relieving pain and improving psychological well-being (Finley).	None known (Ernst, 2001a) Use caution in choosing a practitioner.	Reiki appears to have no adverse effects and can eventually be self-administered, making it a low-risk, low-cost, potentially patient-empowering intervention (National Center for Complementary and Alternative Medicine [NCCAM], 2004). NCCAM sponsors clinical trials.	Typically, Reiki is taught in three parts. Reiki I may be the most intense because of the volume of content: history of Reiki; the Reiki hand positions; Reiki symbols, including their names and how to draw and use them for specific conditions; and meditation manifestation. Reiki II is intense in training, using advanced techniques, and includes a review of Reiki I. Reiki III (master) includes a review of previous training and practice and brings to the student knowledge for long-distance healing, scanning techniques, more meditation techniques, and an additional Reiki symbol. Typically, there is a

(Continued on next page)

Table 22-5. Commonly Used Complementary and Alternative Medicine (CAM) Modalities *(Continued)*

Domain	Therapy	Description	Strength of Evidence	Contraindications	Opportunities	Practitioners
Energy therapies *(cont.)*	Reiki *(cont.)*	places his or her hands on the client in a particular series of positions. Typically, five minutes are spent on each of the 12 positions, although this may vary based on the needs of the client. The client remains fully clothed at all times, and no pressure, massage, or manipulation is applied to the client. The environment is kept quiet and soothing, and the client should emerge feeling relaxed. Reiki is considered to be capable of healing anything because it works at very fundamental levels of reality. Even though the capability is there, this is not what always happens. The limits to Reiki seem to be in the recipient's willingness to cast off old habits and patterns, to accept change and healing (Petter, 1997). Ernst (2001a) considered Reiki to be a form of spiritual healing.				Reiki attunement at the end of the course in addition to others during the course. Information regarding Reiki and Reiki practitioners can be found at www.awarinst.com.

(Continued on next page)

Table 22-5. Commonly Used Complementary and Alternative Medicine (CAM) Modalities *(Continued)*

Domain	Therapy	Description	Strength of Evidence	Contraindications	Opportunities	Practitioners
Energy therapies *(cont.)*	Magnetic field therapy	Defined as magnetic fields that are applied to parts of the body that may be permanent or pulsed. Sometimes used in conjunction with acupuncture (Ernst, 2001a). Permanent magnetic fields are sometimes referred to as electromagnets (Whitaker & Adderly, 1999). Some who are enthusiastic about this therapy feel that there is enormous therapeutic potential (Rosenfeld, 1996).	Animal studies have suggested possible application in the treatment of stroke (Grant et al., 1994). Most controlled studies used this for diagnosis, not treatment (Spencer & Jacobs, 1999). Currently, magnets are accepted and incorporated into medical practice in Germany, Japan, Israel, Russia, and approximately 45 other countries for the treatment of arthritis, back pain, bursitis, carpal tunnel syndrome, headaches, and other inflammatory conditions (Whitaker & Adderly, 1999). Growing evidence shows that magnet therapy is an effective approach in the treatment of pain (Rosenfeld, 1996).	Contraindicated during pregnancy and in those with pacemakers, myasthenia gravis, and bleeding disorders (Ernst, 2001a)	Approved by the U.S. Food and Drug Administration for use with nonunion of fractures (Ernst, 2001a; Rosenfeld, 1996)	Used primarily in conjunction with acupuncture or by licensed acupuncturists

(Continued on next page)

Table 22-5. Commonly Used Complementary and Alternative Medicine (CAM) Modalities *(Continued)*

Domain	Therapy	Description	Strength of Evidence	Contraindications	Opportunities	Practitioners
Manipulative body-based method	Reflexology	Reflexology is a therapeutic method that uses a specific type of manual pressure applied to certain areas, or zones, of the feet (and sometimes to the hands or ears) that are believed to correspond to other areas of the body in order to relieve stress and prevent and/or treat physical disorders (Ernst, 2001a). The organs, glands, and other components of the body are believed to be represented on the foot on that side. The feet are examined to assess health and/or detect imbalances that are expressed as tenderness or crepitus. By stimulating these areas with pressure or massage, it is believed that body function can be altered. Reflexology is purported to promote homeostasis, reduce stress, and eliminate toxins. Some believe that because	There is no known neurophysiologic basis for connections between organs or glands and specific areas of the feet. Approximately 20 RCTs were conducted using reflexology for relief from symptoms associated with cancer from 1990–2004. In these studies, reflexology may have included massage and therapeutic touch. Findings included the positive impact reflexology may have on quality of life during a palliative stage of cancer (Hodgson, 2000). Three investigations into the claimed correspondences are known: Reflexologists' diagnoses were no better than chance in identifying medical conditions in one blinded study, whereas in another study, their diagnostic success was better than chance but not clinically significant	Of concern would be conditions of the feet that might worsen or cause pain with applied pressure (e.g., gout, peripheral vascular disease). Ernst (2001a) suggested that reflexology may interfere with some drugs, including insulin. The greatest risk would be if/when a patient used reflexology as an alternative therapy. Reflexology should not be used alone for diagnostic purposes (Ernst, 2001a).	Reflexology probably would cause no harm when provided by an appropriately trained practitioner in an appropriate situation and possibly may help (Ernst, 2001a; Rosenfeld, 1996).	No regulatory system, licensure, or minimum training mandates are needed. Healthcare professionals who may have licensure in areas such as nursing sometimes may use it. Practitioners' background can vary from self-taught to those who attended training courses (Decker, 1999; Ernst, 2001a; Rosenfeld, 1996).

(Continued on next page)

Table 22-5. Commonly Used Complementary and Alternative Medicine (CAM) Modalities *(Continued)*

Domain	Therapy	Description	Strength of Evidence	Contraindications	Opportunities	Practitioners
Manipulative body-based method *(cont.)*	Reflexology *(cont.)*	reflexology involves carring touch, it has impact (Rosenfeld, 1996).	(White, 2002b). Reflexology foot massage may have general health benefits independent of correspondence of the reflex with specific organs. One RCT found reflexology to be superior to placebo reflexology for the treatment of premenstrual symptoms (Oleson & Flocco, 1993). Another RCT showed beneficial effects on blood glucose in diabetics (Wang, 1993). An RCT in patients with multiple sclerosis showed symptomatic improvements; however, the dropout rate was high (Siev-Ner et al., 2003). In a large observational study, 81% of patients with headaches reported themselves helped or cured at three months follow-up (Launso et al., 1999). RCTs have shown no effect on asthma (Petersen et al., 1992).			

(Continued on next page)

Table 22-5. Commonly Used Complementary and Alternative Medicine (CAM) Modalities *(Continued)*

Domain	Therapy	Description	Strength of Evidence	Contraindications	Opportunities	Practitioners
Mind-body interventions	Aromatherapy	Aromatherapy is the controlled use of plant essences for therapeutic purposes (Ernst, 2003). Essential oil is the aromatic essence of a plant in the form of an oil or resin derived from plant leaf, stalk, bark, root, flower, fruit, or seed. The carrier is the diluent used to dilute a concentrated essential oil for application. The neat is the direct application of the essential oil compound (essential oil plus carrier) to the skin. The note is the unique aromatic variable of an essential oil used when blending combinations of essential oil compounds: The top note is bright, the middle note is lingering, and the base note is grounding (Perez, 2003). Essential oils can be applied directly to the skin through a compress or massage, inhaled via a diffuser or steaming water, or added directly to	Published data on dosing, comparative methods of administration, and therapeutic outcomes in the use of essential oils in aromatherapy are limited. In a systematic review of 12 clinical trials, 6 suggested that aromatherapy massage has a relaxing effect (Cooke & Ernst, 2000). Lou s and Kowalski (2002) measured the responses of 17 patients with cancer to humidified essential lavender oil with a positive change noted in blood pressure, pulse, pain, anxiety, depression, and sense of well-being after both the humidified water treatment and lavender treatment. Oliveant et al. (1999) compared drop size between six different essential oils and reported that the bottles differed in their method of delivery and recommended a universal standardization of measure to	Contraindications to the use of essential oils are pregnancy, contagious disease, epilepsy, venous thrombosis, varicose veins, allergies, open wounds or skin sites, and recent surgeries of any type. Essential oils should not be administered orally or applied undiluted on the skin. Possible adverse events associated with the use of essential oils are photosensitivity, allergic reactions, nausea, and headache. Many essential oils have the potential to either enhance or reduce the effects of prescribed medications, including antibiotics, tranquilizers, antihistamines, anticonvulsants, barbiturates, morphine, and	Campbell et al. (2001) offered guidelines for safe integration of aromatherapy in clinical practice: identify certified staff to serve as resources and educators; conduct patient assessment; select essential oils with low known risk potential; choose one supplier with stringent product testing; develop a range of oils and methods of application that can be used consistently; when blending	The practice of aromatherapy can be used in combination with massage therapy and holistic nursing care programs. Certification is available through the National Association for Holistic Aromatherapy (NAHA) Standards of Aromatherapy Training (www.naha.org). Schools must provide 200 hours of training in aromatherapy, essential oil studies, anatomy, and physiology. In addition, students must submit a research paper, 10 case histories, and pass a written examination. Holistic nursing certification is available through the American Holistic Nurses' Certification Corporation (AHNCC) (http://ahna.org/edu/certification.html).

(Continued on next page)

Table 22-5. Commonly Used Complementary and Alternative Medicine (CAM) Modalities (Continued)

Domain	Therapy	Description	Strength of Evidence	Contraindications	Opportunities	Practitioners
Mind-body interven- tions *(cont.)*	Aromatherapy *(cont.)*	bath water. At the present time, there are approximately 150 essential oils (Thomas, 2002). The mechanism of action in the use of essential oils begins with the olfactory sense. After sensing the smell, the limbic system is activated in retrieving learned memories. Essential oils also are absorbed via the dermal route and subcutaneous 'at into the bloodstream. Entry into the body via the oral route into the digestive system is not recommended. Often, aromatherapy is practiced with massage. Aromatherapy massage is used in palliative care settings to improve quality of life for patients with cancer (Ernst, 2001a).	ensure equity and safety in administration. Massage and aromatherapy massage offer short-term benefits for psychological well-being, with the effect on anxiety supported by limited evidence (Fellowes et al., 2004). Evidence is varied as to whether aromatherapy enhances the effects of massage (Fellowes et al.). In 2003, a Cochrane Database was performed involving aromatherapy for dementia (Fellowes et al.).	quinidine (Ernst, 2001a). Cases of potentially serious reactions involving the use of essential oils— were reported in two individuals without known allergies or sensitivities prior to exposure (Maddocks-Jennings, 2004).	oils, consider symptoms, patient allergies, and preference of aroma; obtain a verbal consent; place oil on tissue for patients in semi-private rooms; document outcome of intervention; and avoid vaporizers in clinical settings (Avis, 1999; Campbell et al.; Maddocks-Jennings, 2004).	Requirements include a BSN, continuing education, one year of practice, and passing a written exam. Certification in aromatherapy or holistic nursing does not qualify a nurse to work independently, nor does it necessarily meet institutional requirements for practice (Lee, 2003).
	Meditation	Meditation is a systematic mental focus on particular aspects of an inner or outer experience originally developed within a spiritual context aiming for spiritual	At the time of this publication, no published meta-analysis was available on mindfulness meditation. Between 1973 and 2004, there were 11 RCTs. In	For patients with cancer, mindfulness (and other types of meditation) may offer an opportunity to reduce mood disturbance	Meditation and guided imagery are contraindicated in those people with a history	Trained practitioners may administer this modality in groups or individually.

(Continued on next page)

Table 22-5. Commonly Used Complementary and Alternative Medicine (CAM) Modalities (Continued)

Domain	Therapy	Description	Strength of Evidence	Contraindications	Opportunities	Practitioners
Mind-body interventions *(cont.)*	Meditation *(cont.)*	growth, personal transformation, or a transcendental experience. Transcendental meditation (repeating a mantra with the goal of quieting) and mindfulness meditation (giving spontaneous rise to thoughts, emotions, sensations, and perceptions) are the most extensively researched forms (Astin et al., 2003). Mindfulness meditation is a self-regulatory approach to stress and emotion management (Astin et al.; Ernst, 2001a).	two RCTs using mindfulness meditation involving patients with cancer, it was found to be effective in reducing mood disturbance and stress symptoms in male and female patients (Ernst, 2001a).	and symptoms of stress (Astin et al., 2003; Ernst, 2001a).	of depression, bipolar disorder, and/or schizophrenia.	
Movement therapy	Alexander Technique	Alexander Technique is a psychophysical reeducation process meant to improve postural balance and coordination. The goal is to decrease strain and improve ease of movement. It is based upon three principles: function is affected by use, the organism functions as a whole, and the	Controlled clinical trials demonstrated improved respiratory function in healthy individuals (Astin & Ausubel. 1992). Similar studies have reported improved function in elderly women (Brett, 2002). Patients with Parkinson disease reported improvement in depression and activities of daily living after Alexander	No known contraindications exist, but it does not replace treatment for any medical condition (Ernst, 2001a).	Learning this technique requires time and effort. It may be used as an adjunctive therapy and palliative care (Ernst, 2001a).	Practitioners may be from the arts (e.g., dance, music, movement, theatre) or health care (e.g., nurses, physiatrists, physical therapists).

(Continued on next page)

Table 22-5. Commonly Used Complementary and Alternative Medicine (CAM) Modalities *(Continued)*

Domain	Therapy	Description	Strength of Evidence	Contraindications	Opportunities	Practitioners
Movement therapy *(cont.)*	Alexander Technique *(cont.)*	relationship of the head, neck, and spine are vital to function (Ernst, 2001a). It is believed to improve movement from sitting to standing. It has been used for pain, asthma, osteoarthritis, stress, and headaches (Ernst, 2001a). A series of 30 sessions are recommended to learn basic concepts.	Technique instruction (Stallibrass, 1997). Those with craniomandibular disorders also reported improvement with instruction in the Alexander Technique (Knebelman, 1982).			
Nutritional therapies	Antioxidants	Commonly used antioxidant vitamins (e.g., E, C, beta-carotene) are believed to have health-promoting properties. CoQ10 (Coenzyme Q10, ubiquinone) is an antioxidant found in all living cells and is believed to have potent effects. Patients with cancer typically take antioxidants at doses higher than recommended daily allowances (RDAs) (Ingram, 1994; Van de Creek et al., 1999). Antioxidants act by scavenging free radicals. The most	The antioxidants and cancer therapy debate is not new. The association between beta-carotene and increased risk of lung cancer in smokers is well known (Albanes et al., 1995; Omenn et al., 1996). Some researchers believe that selective inhibition of tumor cell growth is an action of antioxidants and that antioxidants also may promote cellular differentiation with enhanced cytotoxic effects (Conklin, 2000). Ray	Conclusive recommendations as well as contraindications for the patient with cancer have not been established for the category of antioxidants. Contraindications for specific antioxidants are related to those that are known (e.g., beta-carotene, lung cancer risk among smokers). Vitamin C and potential interactions: aluminum antacids,	—	Registered dietitians have a minimum of a bachelor's degree in dietetics. A certified nutrition consultant has education and training in clinical nutrition, and the practitioner may be a nurse or other health-care professional. Caution should be taken when choosing nutrition practitioners to be certain that they have expertise in cancer care as well as knowledge about supplements and nutrition.

(Continued on next page)

Table 22-5. Commonly Used Complementary and Alternative Medicine (CAM) Modalities (Continued)

Domain	Therapy	Description	Strength of Evidence	Contraindications	Opportunities	Practitioners
Nutritional therapies (cont.)	Antioxidants (cont.)	commonly used antioxidant is vitamin C. The debate that surrounds antioxidants and chemotherapy has focused on cancer therapy purposefully creating free radicals through their cytotoxic mechanism, such as alkylating agents, antimetabolites, and radiation therapy. Limited research supports the belief that chemotherapy diminishes total antioxidant status (Durken et al., 2000), but inconsistencies based on cancer site, cancer therapy, research methodologies, patient populations, variability in doses, duration of supplementation, and timing of interventions prevent formulation of conclusions (Ladas et al., 2004).	et al. (2000) suggested that typically recommended doses may be insufficient to cover the higher production of reactive oxygen metabolites. It also has been maintained that inadequate coverage may contribute to malignant cell proliferation (Conklin). Researchers have been concerned that although antioxidants may decrease some kinds of toxicity associated with cancer chemotherapy, the therapeutic benefit of the cancer therapy may be compromised. Ladas et al. (2004) reviewed more than 100 citations on antioxidant status, cancer outcomes, and antioxidant use among patients receiving chemotherapy with or without radiation therapy. Of the 52 that met their research criteria, 31 were observational studies, and 21 were	cyclosporine, statins, calcium channel blockers, protease inhibitors, iron, and vitamin E (Hendler, 2001) Vitamin E and potential interactions: cholestyramine, colestipol, mineral oil, anticonvulsants, anticoagulants, and verapamil (Hendler) Beta-carotene and potential interactions: cholestyramine, colestipol, mineral oil, and orlistat (Hendler)		

(Continued on next page)

Table 22-5. Commonly Used Complementary and Alternative Medicine (CAM) Modalities *(Continued)*

Domain	Therapy	Description	Strength of Evidence	Contraindications	Opportunities	Practitioners
Nutritional therapies *(cont.)*	Antioxidants *(cont.)*		intervention trials. Their findings showed a decline in the total antioxidant status of patients receiving cancer therapy but conflicting and inconsistent results regarding the effect of chemotherapy on antioxidant status in patients receiving cancer therapy (Ladas et al.). Lenzhofer et al. (1983) reported supplementation with vitamin E altered the metabolism of doxorubicin. Some researchers questioned whether this meant decreased treatment efficacy, arguing that adjunctive agents such as mesna and amifostine are used to reduce free radicals and do not appear to interfere with therapeutic benefit (Ladas et al.). Among patients receiving chemotherapy for bone marrow transplant and total-body irradiation, serum vitamin E levels		

(Continued on next page)

Table 22-5. Commonly Used Complementary and Alternative Medicine (CAM) Modalities (*Continued*)

Domain	Therapy	Description	Strength of Evidence	Contraindications	Opportunities	Practitioners
Nutritional therapies (*cont.*)	Antioxidants (*cont.*)		decreased even among those receiving total parenteral nutrition (Jonas et al., 2000). Two randomized studies treating patients with gynecologic cancers with doxorubicin, cyclophosphamide, cisplatin with ftorafur or melphalan and selenium, vitamin E, selenium and vitamin E, or placebo demonstrated increased serum selenium levels but not vitamin E levels after supplementation (Sundstrom et al., 1989). Studies among patients with breast cancer revealed a possible direct effect of selenium supplementation on serum and whole blood selenium (Ladas et al.). RDAs appear to be inadequate for maintaining plasma antioxidant levels in patients receiving high-dose chemotherapy before stem cell transplant (Food and Nutrition Board, 2002).			

(Continued on next page)

Table 22-5. Commonly Used Complementary and Alternative Medicine (CAM) Modalities (Continued)

Domain	Therapy	Description	Strength of Evidence	Contraindications	Opportunities	Practitioners
Nutritional therapies *(cont.)*	Antioxidants *(cont.)*		Antioxidants may have a role in cancer prevention. Holm et al. (1993) and Ingram (1994) suggested that high vitamin C intake prior to diagnosis of breast cancer has a positive effect on mortality. Brawley and Parnes (2000) reported that selenium and vitamin E supplementation may reduce the risk of prostate cancer. Formal conclusions and recommendations could not be reached because of the variability in doses, duration of supplementation, and timing of doses (Ladas et al.).			
	Shark cartilage	Shark cartilage, Carticin, is a derivative of the fin of the hammerhead or spiny dogfish sharks. It has been used because it appeared that sharks did not develop cancers (Lane & Comac, 1992). Using bovine and shark cartilage	Three angiogenic inhibitors have been identified to date. From 1995–2004, seven RCTs used shark cartilage for a variety of conditions. Human studies are limited, and results are reported as inconclusive	There is lack of standardization of available products, including a concern for purity. Shark cartilage is believed to have caused cases of hepatitis (Gotay & Dumitriu, 2000).	Clinical trials are being conducted at this time for those patients who wish to include this in their treatment regimen.	Recommendations for using shark or bovine cartilage should not be made until more conclusive evidence has been established.

(Continued on next page)

Table 22-5. Commonly Used Complementary and Alternative Medicine (CAM) Modalities *(Continued)*

Domain	Therapy	Description	Strength of Evidence	Contraindications	Opportunities	Practitioners
Nutritional therapies *(cont.)*	Shark cartilage *(cont.)*	for the treatment of cancer has been studied for more than 30 years. As a result, numerous commercial products are available.	(National Cancer Institute, 2004). In animal studies, shark cartilage has been administered orally, by injection, through surgically implanted devices, and topically. Miller et al. (1998) reported that a challenge in research is the method of oral administration because the molecules of shark cartilage do not allow for absorption from the intestines. Additional studies are being conducted at this time (National Cancer Institute).			

Conclusion

CAM therapies are widely available, and therefore integration of these therapies into cancer care may be inevitable. Older patients with cancer, similar to their younger counterparts, already are using some of these therapies. The fascination with CAM therapies is that of seeking a therapy that is *natural,* because many equate natural with safe. More information is known about CAM therapies than in the past, but much information is yet to be determined. The use of CAM therapies is on the rise. Decker and Lee (2005) offered suggestions for the scientific and clinical practice communities to safely approach this anticipated trend: (a) collaborate with CAM practitioners to establish a theoretical basis and individualized regimens; (b) assist in the design of methodologically sound trials; (c) perform periodic reviews and meta-analysis; and (d) implement integrated curricula for students and continuing education for established practitioners.

An inclusive, official definition for CAM is not yet available. Liability is a concern if referring to an unlicensed practitioner or recommending a therapy that generally is not accepted by the medical community as a whole. To complicate this matter, some therapists (e.g., massage therapists) are licensed in some states but not in others. Scopes of practice will emerge as an issue as this process advances. Insurers, providers, and consumers also are considering issues related to reimbursement. Consideration of the issue of informed consent is vital. CAM has survived rivalry, conjecture, superstition, and competition, but the shared views of those who are invested and interested will unlock the door to future possibilities. Decker and Lee (2005) suggested that "regulatory arenas that will need to be addressed include informed consent, licensure vs. certification or registration, scopes of practice, malpractice, and professional discipline" (p. 613). In the near future, failure to offer CAM therapies as a component of treatment may be construed as withholding treatment. Considering the established, researched decision-making practices and behaviors of the older adult with cancer, practitioners must become knowledgeable about these therapies. Table 22-6 lists some reliable resources for symptom management information on CAM therapies.

Table 22-6. Common Symptom Management Considerations in Cancer Complementary and Alternative Medicine

Symptom	Traditional Approach(es) and Outcome(s)	Complementary and Alternative Medicine Approach(es) and Outcome(s)
Anorexia	**Hypercaloric feeding via total parenteral nutrition** Ability to increase lean mass, improve quality of life, improve survival benefits, or decrease toxicity of chemotherapy has not been shown. Increase in infections and mechanical complications is reported (Body, 1999).	**Hydrazine sulfate** Inhibition of phosphoenolpyruvate carboxykinase. No normalization of carbohydrate metabolism was reported in cachectic patients with cancer (Kosty et al., 1994; Loprinzi, Goldberg, et al., 1994; Loprinzi, Kuross, et al., 1994).

(Continued on next page)

Table 22-6. Common Symptom Management Considerations in Cancer Complementary and Alternative Medicine *(Continued)*

Symptom	Traditional Approach(es) and Outcome(s)	Complementary and Alternative Medicine Approach(es) and Outcome(s)
Anorexia *(cont.)*	**Glucocorticoids** Limited effect of up to four weeks on appetite, food intake, sensation of well-being, and performance status (Bruera et al., 1985)	**Eicosapentenoic acid (EPA)** Preclinical data show inhibition of lipolysis and muscle protein degradation (Tanaka et al., 1990). Inclusion of EPA increased weight gain, lean body mass, and performance status (Wigmore et al., 1996).
	Progesterones Improvement of appetite, calorie intake, and nutritional status was seen (Mantovani et al., 2001).	**Melatonin** Loss of more than 10% body weight was less common among those treated with melatonin compared to placebo (Lissoni, Paolorossi, Tancini, Ardizzoia, et al., 1996; Lissoni, Paolorossi, Tancini, Barni, et al., 1996)
	Antiserotonergic agents (cyproheptadine) Possess appetite-stimulant effect, decrease diarrhea but do not prevent progressive weight loss (Kardinal et al., 1990)	**Soy** Dietary sources of protein (Grade A: strong scientific evidence) (Natural Medicines, 2004)
	5HT$_3$ receptor antagonists Improve the ability to enjoy food but do not prevent weight loss (Tayek et al., 1986)	**Bromelian** Nutritional supplementation (Grade C: unclear of conflicting scientific evidence) (Natural Medicines)
	Prokinetic agents (metoclopramidc) Relief of anorexia and early satiety with minimal side effects is reported (Davis & Dickerson, 2000).	**Omega-3 fatty acids, fish oil, alpha-linolenic acid** Appetite/weight loss in patients with cancer (Grade D: fair negative scientific evidence) (Natural Medicines)
	Cannabinoids (synthetic tetrahydrocannabinol) Improvement in mood and appetite with either no or some improvement in body weight reported (Nelson et al., 1994)	**Spirulina** Malnutrition (Grade D: fair negative scientific evidence) (Natural Medicines)
	Thalidomide Improvement in well-being, weight gain, insomnia, restlessness, and appetite is reported (Klausner et al., 1996).	**Alfalfa, astragalus, betel nut, black cohosh, blessed thistle, camomile, cranberry, dandelion, devil's claw, essiac, eyebright, fenugreek, ginseng, hawthorn, hops, kava, lavender, oleander, peppermint, sorrel, thyme, turmeric, valerian, white horehound** Appetite stimulant or anorexia (lack sufficient evidence) (Natural Medicines)

(Continued on next page)

Table 22-6. Common Symptom Management Considerations in Cancer Complementary and Alternative Medicine *(Continued)*

Symptom	Traditional Approach(es) and Outcome(s)	Complementary and Alternative Medicine Approach(es) and Outcome(s)
Anorexia *(cont.)*	**Branch-chain amino acids (BCCA)** Improvement in protein accretion and albumin synthesis is reported. Decrease in the severity of cancer-induced anorexia by oral BCCA is reported (Argiles & Lopez-Soriano, 2001; Argiles et al., 2001; Cangiano et al., 1996).	–
Depression	**Antidepressants** Tricyclic antidepressants and selective serotonin reuptake inhibitors demonstrate efficacy in the treatment of depression.	**Acupuncture seems to decrease symptoms of depression.** Randomized controlled trials (RCTs) demonstrated efficacy of electroacupuncture as similar to tricyclic antidepressants (Luo et al., 1985; Lynch et al., 1998). RCTs using nonspecific (sham) acupuncture show conflicting results (Ernst, 2001a). Acupuncture improved the course of depression more than pharmacologic treatment with mianserin alone in an RCT of 70 inpatients with a major depressive episode in three different treatment groups: verum acupuncture, placebo acupuncture, and a control group. All three groups were pharmacologically treated with the antidepressant mianserin (Roschke et al., 2000).
	Counseling/psychotherapy Counseling and psychotherapy are common effective interventions for depression.	Surveys have identified depression as one of the most common reasons for using complementary and alternative medicine. The most popular therapies are exercise, herbal medicine, relaxation, and spiritual healing (Sparber et al., 2000).
		Herbal therapies St. John's Wort (SJW) is effective in the treatment of mild to moderate depression (Ernst, 2001a; Kasper & Dienel, 2002; Stevinson, 2001; Whiskey et al., 2001). The value of SJW in severe depression is questionable (Whiskey et al.).
		Autogenic training When utilized as a single therapy (2x/week x 10 weeks), it resulted in reduction in symptoms similar to psychotherapy alone but not significantly more than with no intervention. Authors warned that autogenic training alone is not recommended as treatment for depression (Krampen et al., 1991).

(Continued on next page)

Table 22-6. Common Symptom Management Considerations in Cancer Complementary and Alternative Medicine *(Continued)*

Symptom	Traditional Approach(es) and Outcome(s)	Complementary and Alternative Medicine Approach(es) and Outcome(s)
Depression *(cont.)*		**Music therapy** Patients with cancer are among those who can benefit from music as a therapy. Music provides unique opportunities and properties that promote well-being. Music has been effective in the treatment of the anxiety and fear associated with a cancer diagnosis and cancer therapy (Burns, 2001; Cassileth et al., 2003; Kwekkeboom, 2003). Music-driven psychoneuroimmunology identifies potential implications for cancer care (Hilliard, 2003; Yamashita & Kato, 2003; Zappa & Cassileth, 2003). **Massage** Massage (daily x five days) was more effective than viewing videos in children and adolescents. Improvements were measured in symptoms of depression, anxiety, sleep, and cortisol levels (Platania-Solazzo et al., 1992). Massage should be used with caution when a patient has a history of abuse, post-traumatic stress disorder, and other psychiatric disorders (Jorm et al., 2002; Moyer et al., 2004; Rexilius et al., 2002). **Exercise** A large body of research considered to be of questionable quality supports the antidepressant effects of exercise. RCTs provide verification of the efficacy of exercise in the treatment of depression. Aerobic and nonaerobic forms of exercise have proved to be effective. Data from three RCTs suggest that aerobic exercise may be as effective as psychological or drug treatment. The exact mechanisms are not known (Crevenna et al., 2003). **Aromatherapy** In a small nonrandomized study (N = 20), the dose of antidepressants was reduced with the use of adjunctive aromatherapy (Komori et al., 1995). Aromatherapy is combined with massage for increased effectiveness in symptom relief for patients with cancer who are experiencing depression (Fellowes et al., 2004; Hadfield, 2001; Jones & Field, 1999).

(Continued on next page)

Table 22-6. Common Symptom Management Considerations in Cancer Complementary and Alternative Medicine *(Continued)*

Symptom	Traditional Approach(es) and Outcome(s)	Complementary and Alternative Medicine Approach(es) and Outcome(s)
Depression *(cont.)*		**Dance and movement therapy** Dance and movement therapy are effective therapeutic interventions in reducing symptoms of depression and improving psychological well-being (Ernst & Cassileth, 1998; Estivill, 1995; Gurley et al., 1984; Ostwald et al., 1994; Pappas et al., 1990). **Relaxation** Three small RCTs have suggested that relaxation training is superior to no treatment and potentially similar to cognitive-behavioral therapy. Although nonspecific effects are difficult to control with relaxation therapy, the evidence is promising (Ernst, 2001a).
Pain	**Surgery** Curative excision or palliative debulking can relieve symptoms of obstruction or compression, improve prognosis, and may increase survival (National Cancer Institute [NCI], 2004). **Antineoplastic therapy** Antineoplastic therapy (chemotherapy, biologic, or hormonal therapy) may provide palliation by reducing tumor burden (Paice, 2004). Chemotherapy is effective in prolonging time to disease progression and survival in patients with advanced colorectal cancer (Simmonds, 2000). **Radiation therapy** Local or whole-body radiation enhances the effectiveness of analgesics and noninvasive therapies to relieve cancer pain. Single injections of beta particle-emitting agents can relieve pain secondary to bony metastases (NCI, 2004). **Nonsteroidal anti-inflammatory drugs (NSAIDs)** NSAIDs appear to be more effective than placebo for cancer pain. Combinations of an NSAID with an opioid have shown either no or slight significant difference compared with either single intervention (McNicol et al., 2004).	**Acupuncture** The National Institutes of Health Acupuncture Consensus Development Panel concluded that acupuncture may be useful for headache and low back pain (Mayer, 2000). **Cognitive-behavioral treatment (CBT)** Standard CBT (five 50-minute sessions) and profile-tailored CBT (based on results from Biobehavioral Pain Profile [measures factors related to pain experience]) showed greater improvement in pain relief than usual care (Dalton et al., 2004). **Chiropractic** Systematic reviews of chiropractic manipulation for back, neck, headache disorders, and nonspinal pain syndromes (excluding headache) failed to demonstrate efficacy (Ernst, 2004). **Massage** RCTs using Swedish massage suggest efficacy for relieving back pain; however, the results were not uniform (Ernst, 2004).

(Continued on next page)

Table 22-6. Common Symptom Management Considerations in Cancer Complementary and Alternative Medicine *(Continued)*

Symptom	Traditional Approach(es) and Outcome(s)	Complementary and Alternative Medicine Approach(es) and Outcome(s)
Pain *(cont.)*	**Opioids** Uncontrolled case series show that chronic pain (not associated with terminal disease) is relieved by a stable nonescalating dose of opioids with minimal risk of addiction. Opioids can induce abnormal pain sensitivity. Prolonged high-dose opioid therapy may have serious adverse sequelae (tolerance, sensitivity, hormonal effects, immunosuppression). Remaining questions include are opioids beneficial over years (versus months), and does the dose of the opioid have an effect on the efficacy and safety of long-term therapy? (Ballantyne & Mao, 2003).	**Relaxation with guided imagery** Relaxation with guided imagery can improve oral mucositis (Pan et al., 2000). Relaxation exercises (e.g., slow rhythmic breathing, touch and massage, reflecting on peaceful past experiences, listening to music) are effective (NCI, 2004).
	Transcutaneous electrical nerve stimulation (TENS) TENS may be effective for the treatment of neuropathic pain (Martin & Hagen, 1997).	**Topical capsaicin** Moderate to poor efficacy in the treatment of chronic musculoskeletal or neuropathic pain. May be useful as an adjunct or sole therapy for pain that is unresponsive to other treatments (Mason, Moore, Derry, et al., 2004).
	Antidepressants Sustained release (SR) of antidepressants suggests efficacy in the treatment of neuropathic pain over placebo. First choice of drug class of antidepressants is uncertain (McQuay et al., 1996).	**Physical modalities** Musculoskeletal pain may be treated with heat, cold, massage, and exercise therapy (NCI, 2004).
	Neurolytic blocks Effective in controlling cancer pain in select patients in addition to pharmacologic therapy. Quality improves when placement is image-guided in collaboration with an interventional radiologist (Kongsgaard et al., 2004).	**Music versus distraction** Lack of definitive findings in RCT using music or distraction for controlling procedural pain versus standard approach (neither music nor distraction) (Kwekkeboom, 2003)
	Topical rubefacients containing salicylates Moderate to poor efficacy in the treatment of musculoskeletal and arthritic pain (Mason, Moore, Edwards, et al., 2004)	**Percutaneous electrical nerve stimulation (PENS)** PENS (acupuncture-like needle probes plus nerve stimulation) is a useful supplement to opioids for the management of bony metastases and pain (Ahmed et al., 1998).

(Continued on next page)

Table 22-6. Common Symptom Management Considerations in Cancer Complementary and Alternative Medicine *(Continued)*

Symptom	Traditional Approach(es) and Outcome(s)	Complementary and Alternative Medicine Approach(es) and Outcome(s)
Pain *(cont.)*	**Bisphosphonates** Bisphosphonates have a role in managing refractory pain from metastases where oncologic or orthopedic intervention is delayed or inappropriate (Mannix et al., 2000).	**Distraction** Distraction via paced auditory serial addition task (mental math) was shown to inhibit pain perception (Terkelsen et al., 2004).

Note. Based on information from Decker & Lee, 2005.

References

Ahmed, H.E., Craig, W.F., White, P.F., & Huber, P. (1998). Percutaneous electrical nerve stimulation (PENS): A complementary therapy for the management of pain secondary to bony metastasis. *Clinical Journal of Pain, 14,* 320–323.

Aikins Murphy, P. (1998). Alternative therapies for nausea and vomiting of pregnancy. *Obstetrics and Gynecology, 91*(1), 149–155.

Albanes, D., Heinonen, O.P., Huttunen, J.K., Taylor, P.R., Virtamo, J., Edwards, B.K., et al. (1995). Effects of alpha-tocopherol and beta-carotene supplements on cancer incidence in the Alpha-Tocopherol Beta-Carotene Cancer Prevention Study. *American Journal of Clinical Nutrition, 62*(Suppl. 6), 1427S–1430S.

Andersson, S., & Lundeberg, T. (1995). Acupuncture—From empiricism to science: Functional background to acupuncture effects in pain and disease. *Medical Hypotheses, 45,* 271–281.

Angell, M., & Kassirer, J.P. (1998). Alternative medicine—The risks of untested and unregulated remedies. *New England Journal of Medicine, 339,* 839–841.

Argiles, J.M., & Lopez-Soriano, F.J. (2001). Insulin and cancer (Review). *International Journal of Oncology, 18,* 683–687.

Argiles, J.M., Meijsing, S.H., Pallares-Trujillo, J., Guirao, X., & Lopez-Soriano, F.J. (2001). Cancer cachexia: A therapeutic approach. *Medical Research Reviews, 21*(1), 83–101.

Ashikaga, T., Bosompra, K., O'Brien, P., & Nelson, L. (2002). Use of complimentary and alternative medicine by breast cancer patients: Prevalence, patterns and communication with physicians. *Supportive Care in Cancer, 10,* 542–548.

Astin, J.A., Shapiro, S.L., Eisenberg, D.M., & Forys, K.L. (2003). Mind-body medicine: State of the science, implications for practice. *Journal of the American Board of Family Practice, 16*(2), 131–147.

Astin, J.H.M., & Ausubel, P. (1992). Enhanced respiratory muscular function in normal adults after lessons in proprioceptive musculoskeletal education without exercise. *Chest, 102,* 486–490.

Avis, A. (1999). Aromatherapy in practice. *Nursing Standards, 13,* 14–15.

Ballantyne, J.C., & Mao, J. (2003). Opioid therapy for chronic pain. *New England Journal of Medicine, 349,* 1943–1953.

Baltes, P.B., & Staudinger, U.M. (1996). *Interactive minds: Life-span perspectives on the social foundation of cognition.* New York: Cambridge University Press.

Basch, E., & Ulbricht, C. (2004). Prevalence of CAM use among U.S. cancer patients: An update. *Journal of Cancer Integrative Medicine, 2*(1), 13–14.

Bennett, M., & Lengacher, C. (1999). Use of complementary therapies in a rural cancer population. *Oncology Nursing Forum, 26,* 1287–1294.

Bernstein, B.J., & Grasso, T. (2001). Prevalence of complementary and alternative medicine use in cancer patients. *Oncology (Huntington), 15,* 1267–1272.

Beyerstein, B.L. (2001). Alternative medicine and common errors of reasoning. *Academic Medicine, 76,* 230–237.

Body, J.J. (1999). The syndrome of anorexia-cachexia. *Current Opinions in Oncology, 11,* 255–260.

Brawley, O.W., & Parnes, H. (2000). Prostate cancer prevention trials in the USA. *European Journal of Cancer, 36*, 1312–1315.

Brett, H. (2002). *Complementary therapies in the care of older people.* Philadelphia: Whurr.

Bruera, E., Roca, E., Cedaro, L., Carraro, S., & Chacon, R. (1985). Action of oral methylprednisolone in terminal cancer patients: A prospective randomized double-blind study. *Cancer Treatment Reports, 69*, 751–754.

Burns, D.S. (2001). The effect of the bonny method of guided imagery and music on the mood and life quality of cancer patients. *Journal of Music Therapy, 38*(1), 51–65.

Campbell, L., Pollard, A., & Roeton, C. (2001). The development of clinical practice guidelines for the use of aromatherapy in a cancer setting. *Australian Journal of Holistic Nursing, 8*(1), 14–22.

Cangiano, C., Laviano, A., Meguid, M.M., Mulieri, M., Conversano, L., Preziosa, I., et al. (1996). Effects of administration of oral branched-chain amino acids on anorexia and caloric intake in cancer patients. *Journal of the National Cancer Institute, 88*, 550–552.

Cassileth, B.R., Vickers, A.J., & Magill, L.A. (2003). Music therapy for mood disturbance during hospitalization for autologous stem cell transplantation: A randomized controlled trial. *Cancer, 98*, 2723–2729.

Conklin, K.A. (2000). Dietary antioxidants during cancer chemotherapy: Impact on chemotherapeutic effectiveness and development of side effects. *Nutrition and Cancer, 37*(1), 1–18.

Cooke, B., & Ernst, E. (2000). Aromatherapy: A systematic review. *British Journal of General Practice, 50*, 493–496.

Corner, J., Plant, H., A'Hern, R., & Bailey, C. (1996). Non-pharmacological intervention for breathlessness in lung cancer. *Palliative Medicine, 10*, 299–305.

Crevenna, R., Zielinski, C., Keilani, M.Y., Schmidinger, M., Bittner, C., Nuhr, M., et al. (2003). Aerobic endurance training for cancer patients. *Wiener Medizinische Wochenschrift, 153*(9–10), 212–216.

Dalton, J.A., Keefe, F.J., Carlson, J., & Youngblood, R. (2004). Tailoring cognitive-behavioral treatment for cancer pain. *Pain Management Nursing, 5*(1), 3–18.

Davis, M.P., & Dickerson, D. (2000). Cachexia and anorexia: Cancer's covert killer. *Supportive Care in Cancer, 8*(3), 180–187.

Davison, B.J., Degner, L.F., & Morgan, T.R. (1995). Information and decision making preferences of men with prostate cancer. *Oncology Nursing Forum, 22*, 1402–1408.

Decker, G. (Ed.). (1999). *An introduction to complementary and alternative therapies.* Pittsburgh, PA: Oncology Nursing Society.

Decker, G. (2005). Strategies for CAM program development. In P. Buchsel & C. Yarbro (Eds.), *Oncology nursing in the ambulatory setting: Issues and models of care* (2nd ed., pp. 355–375). Sudbury, MA: Jones and Bartlett.

Decker, G., & Cleveland, M.J. (2001). Complementary and alternative therapies. In R.A. Gates & R.M. Fink (Eds.), *Oncology nursing secrets* (2nd ed., pp. 144–152) Philadelphia: Hanley & Belfus.

Decker, G., & Lee, C. (2005). Complementary therapies. In M.H. Frogge, C.H. Yarbro, & M. Goodman (Eds.), *Cancer nursing: Principles and practice* (6th ed., pp. 590–620). Sudbury, MA: Jones and Bartlett.

Degner, L.F., Kristjanson, L.J., Bowman, D., Sloan, J.A., Carrier, K.C., ONeil, J., et al. (1997). Information needs and decision making preferences in women with breast cancer. *JAMA, 277*, 1485–1492.

Downer, S.M., Cody, M.M., McCluskey, P., Wilson, P.D., Arnott, S.J., Lister, T.A., et al. (1994). Pursuit and practice of complementary therapies by cancer patients receiving complementary therapies alongside conventional therapies. *BMJ, 309*, 86–89.

Durken, M., Herrnring, C., Finckh, B., Nagel, S., Nielsen, P., Fischer, R., et al. (2000). Impaired plasma antioxidative defense and increased nontransferrin-bound iron during high-dose chemotherapy and radiochemotherapy preceding bone marrow transplantation. *Free Radical Biology and Medicine, 28*, 887–894.

Eichelberger, B. (2004). *A Qigong primer.* Retrieved May 19, 2004, from http://www.acupuncture.com/qigong_tuina/qipri.htm

Eisenberg, D.M. (1997). Advising patients who seek alternative medical therapies. *Annals of Internal Medicine, 127*, 61–69.

Eisenberg, D.M. (2001, February). *Advising patients who seek complementary and alternative medical therapy.* Paper presented by the Complementary and Integrative Medicine: Clinical Update and Implications for Practice conference. Harvard Medical School, Department of Continuing Education, Boston, MA.

Eisenberg, D.M. (2002, March). *Complementary and integrative medicine state of the science and clinical applications.* Syllabus presented at the Complementary and Integrative Medicine: Clinical Update and Implications for Practice conference. Harvard Medical School, Department of Continuing Education, Boston, MA.

Eisenberg, D.M., Davis, R.B., Ettner, S.L., Appel, S., Wilkey, S., Van Rompay, M., et al. (1998). Trends in alternative medicine use in the United States, 1990–1997: Results of a follow-up national survey. *JAMA, 280,* 1569–1575.

Eisenberg, D.M., Kessler, R.C., Foster, C., Norlock, F.E., Calkins, D.R., & Delbanco, T.L. (1993). Unconventional medicine in the United States. Prevalence, costs, and patterns of use. *New England Journal of Medicine, 328,* 246–252.

Elit, L., Charles, C., Gold, I., Gafni, A., Farrell, S., Tedford, S., et al. (2003). Women's perceptions about treatment decision making for ovarian cancer. *Gynecologic Oncology, 88,* 89–95.

Ernst, E. (Ed.). (2001a). *The desktop guide to complementary and alternative medicine: An evidence-based approach.* London: Mosby.

Ernst, E. (2001b). Research into complementary/alternative medicine: An attempt to dispel the myths. *International Journal of Clinical Practice, 55,* 376–379.

Ernst, E. (2003). The current position of complementary/alternative medicine in cancer. *European Journal of Cancer, 39,* 2273–2277.

Ernst, E. (2004). Manual therapies for pain control: Chiropractic and massage. *Clinical Journal of Pain, 20*(1), 8–12.

Ernst, E., & Cassileth, B.R. (1998). The prevalence of complementary/alternative medicine in cancer: A systematic review. *Cancer, 83,* 777–782.

Ernst, E., & Pittler, M.H. (1998). The effectiveness of acupuncture in treating acute dental pain: A systematic review. *British Dental Journal, 184,* 443–447.

Ernst, E., Rand, J.I., & Stevinson, C. (1998). Complementary therapies for depression: An overview. *Archives of General Psychiatry, 55,* 1026–1032.

Ernst, E., & White, A. (1997). Life-threatening adverse reactions after acupuncture? A systematic review. *Pain, 71*(2), 123–126.

Estivill, M. (1995). Therapeutic aspects of aerobic dance participation. *Health Care for Women International, 16,* 341–350.

Fellowes, D., Barnes, K., & Wilkinson, S. (2004). Aromatherapy and massage for symptom relief in patients with cancer. *Cochrane Database of Systematic Reviews, 2,* CD002287.

Finley, S. (1992). Secrets of Reiki: Healing with energy in an ancient tradition. *Body Mind Spirit Magazine, 11*(2), 41–43.

Food and Nutrition Board. (2002). *Dietary reference intakes.* Institute of Medicine of the National Academies. Retrieved August 10, 2005, from http://www.iom.edu/project.asp?id=4574

Furnham, A. (1996). Why do people choose and use complementary therapies? In E. Ernst (Ed.), *Complementary medicine: An objective appraisal* (pp. 71–88). Oxford: Butterworth Heinemann.

Gattellari, M., Voigt, K.L., Butow, P.N., & Tattersall, M.H. (2002). When the treatment goal is not cure: Are patients equipped to make informed decisions? *Journal of Clinical Oncology, 20,* 503–513.

Given, B., & Given, W. (1989). Cancer nursing for the elderly: A target for research. *Cancer Nursing, 12,* 71–77.

Goodman, M. (1995). Patient's views count as well. *Nursing Standard, 9,* 40–55.

Gotay, C.C., & Dumitriu, D. (2000). Health food store recommendations for breast cancer patients. *Archives of Family Medicine, 9,* 613–622.

Grant, G., Cadossi, R., & Steinberg, G. (1994). Protection against focal cerebral ischemia following exposure to a pulsed electromagnetic field. *Bioelectromagnetics, 15,* 205–216.

Gurley, V., Neuringer, A., & Massee, J. (1984). Dance and sports compared: Effects on psychological well-being. *Journal of Sports Medicine and Physical Fitness, 24*(1), 58–68.

Hadfield, N. (2001). The role of aromatherapy massage in reducing anxiety in patients with malignant brain tumours. *International Journal of Palliative Nursing, 7,* 279–285.

Han, J.S., & Terenius, L. (1982). Neurochemical basis of acupuncture analgesia. *Annual Review of Pharmacology and Toxicology, 22,* 193–220.

Hendler, S.S. (2001). *PDR for nutritional supplements.* Montvale, NJ: Thomson Healthcare.

Herron, M., & Glasser, M. (2003). Use of and attitudes toward complementary and alternative medicine among family practice patients in small rural Illinois communities. *Journal of Rural Health, 19,* 279–284.

Hilliard, R.E. (2003). The effects of music therapy on the quality and length of life of people diagnosed with terminal cancer. *Journal of Music Therapy, 40*(2), 113–137.

Hodgson, H. (2000). Does reflexology impact on cancer patients' quality of life? *Nursing Standard, 14*(31), 33–38.

Holm, L.E., Nordevang, E., Hjalmar, M.L., Lidbrink, E., Callmer, E., & Nilsson, B. (1993). Treatment failure and dietary habits in women with breast cancer. *Journal of the National Cancer Institute, 85,* 32–36.

Ingram, D. (1994). Diet and subsequent survival in women with breast cancer. *British Journal of Cancer, 69,* 592–595.

Institute of Medicine. (2004). *Use of complementary and alternative medicine (CAM) by the American public.* Retrieved May 16, 2004, from http://www.iom.edu/project.asp?id=4829

Jacobson, J.S., Workman, S.B., & Kronenberg, F. (2000). Research on complementary/alternative medicine for patients with breast cancer: A review of the biomedical literature. *Journal of Clinical Oncology, 18,* 668–683.

Jonas, C.R., Puckett, A.B., Jones, D.P., Griffith, D.P., Szeszycki, E.E., Bergman, G.F., et al. (2000). Plasma antioxidant status after high-dose chemotherapy: A randomized trial of parenteral nutrition in bone marrow transplantation patients. *American Journal of Clinical Nutrition, 72*(1), 181–189.

Jones, N.A., & Field, T. (1999). Massage and music therapies attenuate frontal EEG asymmetry in depressed adolescents. *Adolescence, 34,* 529–534.

Jorm, A.F., Christensen, H., Griffiths, K.M., & Rodgers, B. (2002). Effectiveness of complementary and self-help treatments for depression. *Medical Journal of Australia, 176*(Suppl.), S84–S96.

Kaptchuk, T.J., & Eisenberg, D.M. (1998). The persuasive appeal of alternative medicine. *Annals of Internal Medicine, 129,* 1061–1065.

Kardinal, C.G., Loprinzi, C.L., Schaid, D.J., Hass, A.C., Dose, A.M., Athmann, L.M., et al. (1990). A controlled trial of cyproheptadine in cancer patients with anorexia and/or cachexia. *Cancer, 65,* 2657–2662.

Kasper, S., & Dienel, A. (2002). Cluster analysis of symptoms during antidepressant treatment with Hypericum extract in mildly to moderately depressed outpatients. A meta-analysis of data from three randomized, placebo-controlled trials. *Psychopharmacology, 164,* 301–308.

Kassab, S., & Stevensen, C. (1996). Common misunderstandings about complementary therapies for patients with cancer. *Complementary Therapies in Nursing and Midwifery, 2,* 62–65.

Klausner, J.D., Freedman, V.H., & Kaplan, G. (1996). Thalidomide as an anti-TNF-alpha inhibitor: Implications for clinical use. *Clinical Immunology and Immunopathology, 81,* 219–223.

Knebelman, S. (1982). The Alexander technique in diagnosis and treatment of craniomandibular disorders. *Basal Facts, 5,* 19–22.

Komori, T., Fujiwara, R., Tanida, M., Nomura, J., & Yokoyama, M. (1995). Effects of aromatherapy with antidepressants. *International Journal of Aromatherapy, 13*(1), 1–2.

Kongsgaard, U.E., Bjorgo, S., & Hauser, M. (2004). Neurolytic blocks for cancer pain—Still a useful therapeutic strategy. *Tidsskrift for den Norske Laegeforening, 124,* 481–483.

Kosty, M.P., Fleishman, S.B., Herndon, J.E., Coughlin, K., Kornblith, A.B., Scalzo, A., et al. (1994). Cisplatin, vinblastine, and hydrazine sulfate in advanced, non-small cell lung cancer: A randomized placebo-controlled, double-blind phase III study of the Cancer and Leukemia Group B. *Journal of Clinical Oncology, 12,* 1113–1120.

Krampen, G., Main, C., & Waelbroeck, O. (1991). Optimizing the learning process in short-term autogenic training by practice protocols. *Zeitschrift fur Klinische Psychologie, 39*(1), 33–45.

Kwekkeboom, K.L. (2003). Music versus distraction for procedural pain and anxiety in patients with cancer. *Oncology Nursing Forum, 30,* 433–440.

Ladas, E.J., Jacobson, J.S., Kennedy, D.D., Teel, K., Fleischauer, A., & Kelly, K.M. (2004). Antioxidants and cancer therapy: A systematic review. *Journal of Clinical Oncology, 22,* 517–528.

Lane, I.W., & Comac, L. (1992). *Sharks don't get cancer.* Garden City Park, NY: Avery Publishing.

Launso, L., Brendstrup, E., & Arnberg, S. (1999). An exploratory study of reflexological treatment for headache. *Alternative Therapies in Health and Medicine, 5*(3), 57–65.

Lee, C.O. (2003). Clinical aromatherapy. Part II: Safe guidelines for integration into clinical practice. *Clinical Journal of Oncology Nursing, 7,* 597–598.

Lee, C.O. (2004a). Clinical trials in cancer part 2. Biomedical, complementary, and alternative medicine: Significant issues. *Clinical Journal of Oncology Nursing, 8,* 670–674.

Lee, C.O. (2004b). *Conventional biomedical and cancer complementary and alternative medicine clinical trials.* Paper presented at the Oncology Nursing Society's Annual Congress, Anaheim, CA.

Lee, C.O. (2004c). Conventional biomedical and cancer complementary and alternative medicine clinical trials part 1: Finding active trials and results of closed trials. *Clinical Journal of Oncology Nursing, 8,* 531–535.

Lengacher, C.A., Bennett, M.P., Kip, K.E., Keller, R., LaVance, M.S., Smith, L.S., et al. (2002). Frequency of use of complementary and alternative medicine in women with breast cancer. *Oncology Nursing Forum, 29,* 1445–1452.

Lenzhofer, R., Ganzinger, U., Rameis, H., & Moser, K. (1983). Acute cardiac toxicity in patients after doxorubicin treatment and the effect of combined tocopherol and nifedipine pretreatment. *Journal of Cancer Research in Clinical Oncology, 106,* 143–147.

Lissoni, P., Paolorossi, F., Tancini, G., Ardizzoia, A., Barni, S., Brivio, F., et al. (1996). A phase II study of tamoxifen plus melatonin in metastatic solid tumour patients. *British Journal of Cancer, 74*, 1466–1468.

Lissoni, P., Paolorossi, F., Tancini, G., Barni, S., Ardizzoia, A., Brivio, F., et al. (1996). Is there a role for melatonin in the treatment of neoplastic cachexia? *European Journal of Cancer, 32A*, 1340–1343.

Llewelyn-Thomas, H.A., McGreal, M.J., & Theil, E.C. (1995) Cancer patients' decision making and trial entry preferences: The effects of framing information about short-term toxicity and long-term survival. *Medical Decision Making, 15*, 4–12.

Loprinzi, C.L., Goldberg, R.M., Su, J.Q., Mailliard, J.A., Kuross, S.A., Maksymiuk, A.W., et al. (1994). Placebo-controlled trial of hydrazine sulfate in patients with newly diagnosed non-small cell lung cancer. *Journal of Clinical Oncology, 12*, 1126–1129.

Loprinzi, C.L., Kuross, S.A., O'Fallon, J.R., Gesme, D.H., Jr., Gerstner, J.B., Rospond, R.M., et al. (1994). Randomized placebo-controlled evaluation of hydrazine sulfate in patients with advanced colorectal cancer. *Journal of Clinical Oncology, 12*, 1121–1125.

Louis, M., & Kowalski, S.D. (2002). Use of aromatherapy with hospice patients to decrease pain, anxiety, and depression and to promote an increased sense of well-being. *American Journal of Hospice and Palliative Care, 19*, 381–386.

Luo, H.C., Jia, Y.K., & Li, Z. (1985). Electro-acupuncture vs. amitriptyline in the treatment of depressive states. *Journal of Traditional Chinese Medicine, 5*(1), 3–8.

Lynch, E.P., Lazor, M.A., Gellis, J.E., Orav, J., Goldman, L., & Marcantonio, E.R. (1998). The impact of postoperative pain on the development of postoperative delirium. *Anesthesia and Analgesia, 86*, 781–785.

Maddocks-Jennings, W. (2004). Critical incident: Idiosyncratic allergic reactions to essential oils. *Complementary Therapies in Nursing and Midwifery, 10*(1), 58–60.

Mannix, K., Ahmedzai, S.H., Anderson, H., Bennett, M., Lloyd-Williams, M., & Wilcock, A. (2000). Using bisphosphonates to control the pain of bone metastases: Evidence-based guidelines for palliative care. *Palliative Medicine, 14*, 455–461.

Mantovani, G., Maccio, A., Massa, E., & Madeddu, C. (2001). Managing cancer-related anorexia/cachexia. *Drugs, 61*, 499–514.

Martin, L.A., & Hagen, N.A. (1997). Neuropathic pain in cancer patients: Mechanisms, syndromes, and clinical controversies. *Journal of Pain and Symptom Management, 14*, 99–117.

Maskarinec, G., Shumay, D.M., Kakai, H., & Gotay, C.C. (2000). Ethnic differences in complementary and alternative medicine use among cancer patients. *Journal of Alternative and Complementary Medicine, 6*, 531–538.

Mason, L., Moore, R.A., Derry, S., Edwards, J.E., & McQuay, H.J. (2004). Systematic review of topical capsaicin for the treatment of chronic pain. *BMJ, 328*, 991.

Mason, L., Moore, R.A., Edwards, J.E., McQuay, H.J., Derry, S., & Wiffen, P.J. (2004). Systematic review of efficacy of topical rubefacients containing salicylates for the treatment of acute and chronic pain. *BMJ, 328*, 995.

Mastaglia, B., & Kristjanson, L.J. (2001). Factors influencing women's decisions for choice of surgery for stage I and stage II breast cancer in western Australia. *Journal of Advanced Nursing, 35*, 836–847.

Mayer, D.J. (2000). Acupuncture: An evidence-based review of the clinical literature. *Annual Review of Medicine, 51*, 49–63.

McNicol, E., Strassels, S., Goudas, L., Lau, J., & Carr, D. (2004). Nonsteroidal anti-inflammatory drugs, alone or combined with opioids, for cancer pain: A systematic review. *Journal of Clinical Oncology, 22*, 1975–1992.

McQuay, H.J., Tramer, M., Nye, B.A., Carroll, D., Wiffen, P.J., & Moore, R.A. (1996). A systematic review of antidepressants in neuropathic pain. *Pain, 68*(2–3), 217–227.

Melchart, D., Linde, K., Fischer, P., White, A., Allias, G., Vickers, A., et al. (1999). Acupunctures for recurrent headaches: A systematic review of randomized controlled trials. *Cephalalgia, 19*, 779–786.

Miller, D.R., Anderson, G.T., Stark, J.J., Granick, J.L., & Richardson, D. (1998). Phase I/II trial of the safety and efficacy of shark cartilage in the treatment of advanced cancer. *Journal of Clinical Oncology, 16*, 3649–3655.

Moyer, C.A., Rounds, J., & Hannum, J.W. (2004). A meta-analysis of massage therapy research. *Psychology Bulletin, 130*(1), 3–18.

Najm, W., Reinsch, S., Hoehler, F., & Tobis, J. (2003). Use of complementary and alternative medicine among the ethnic elderly. *Alternative Therapies in Health and Medicine, 9*(3), 50–57.

National Cancer Institute. (2004). *PDQ® cancer information and summaries: Complementary and alternative medicine.* Retrieved April 13, 2004, from http://www.cancer.gov/cancertopics/pdq/cam

National Center for Complementary and Alternative Medicine. (2004). *Understanding complementary and alternative medicine (CAM).* Retrieved May 8, 2004, from http://nccam.nih.gov/

Natural Medicines. (2004). *Natural Medicines comprehensive database.* Retrieved May 19, 2004, from http://www.naturaldatabase.com/

Nelson, K., Walsh, D., Deeter, P., & Sheehan, F. (1994). A phase II study of delta-9-tetrahydrocannabinol for appetite stimulation in cancer-associated anorexia. *Journal of Palliative Care, 10*(1), 14–18.

Office of Cancer Complementary and Alternative Medicine. (2004). *NCI CAM history and the role of OCCAM.* Retrieved May 8, 2004, from http://www.cancer.gov/cam/cam/_at_nci.html

Oleson, T., & Flocco, W. (1993). Randomized controlled study of premenstrual symptoms treated with ear, hand, and foot reflexology. *Obstetrics and Gynecology, 82,* 906–911.

Olleveant, N.A., Humphris, G., & Roe, B. (1999). How big is a drop? A volumetric assay of essential oils. *Journal of Clinical Nursing, 8,* 299–304.

Omenn, G.S., Goodman, G.E., Thornquist, M.D., Balmes, J., Cullen, M.R., Glass, A., et al. (1996). Effects of a combination of beta carotene and vitamin A on lung cancer and cardiovascular disease. *New England Journal of Medicine, 334,* 1150–1155.

Oncology Nursing Society. (2002). *Quality cancer care.* Retrieved June 14, 2005, from http://www.ons.org/publications/positions/QualityCancerCare.shtml

Oncology Nursing Society. (2004). *The use of complementary and alternative therapies in cancer care.* Retrieved June 14, 2005, from http://www.ons.org/publications/positions/Complementary Therapies.shtml

Ostwald, P.F., Baron, B.C., Byl, N.M., & Wilson, F.R. (1994). Performing arts medicine. *Western Journal of Medicine, 160*(1), 48–52.

Paice, J.A. (2004). Pain. In C.H. Yarbro, M.H. Frogge, & M. Goodman (Eds.), *Cancer symptom management* (3rd ed., pp. 77–96). Sudbury, MA: Jones and Bartlett.

Pan, C.X., Morrison, R.S., Ness, J., Fugh-Berman, A., & Leipzig, R.M. (2000). Complementary and alternative medicine in the management of pain, dyspnea, and nausea and vomiting near the end of life. A systematic review. *Journal of Pain and Symptom Management, 20,* 374–387.

Pappas, G.P., Golin, S., & Meyer, D.L. (1990). Reducing symptoms of depression with exercise. *Psychosomatics, 31*(1), 112–113.

Perez, C. (2003). Clinical aromatherapy. Part I: An introduction into nursing practice. *Clinical Journal of Oncology Nursing, 7,* 595–596.

Petersen, L.N., Faurschou, P., Olsen, O.T., & Svendsen, U.G. (1992). Foot zone therapy and bronchial asthma—A controlled clinical trial. *Ugeskrift for Laeger, 154,* 2065–2068.

Petter, F.A. (1997). *Reiki fire.* Twin Lakes, WI: Lotus Light Publications.

Pinquart, M., & Duberstein, P.R. (2004). Information needs and decision-making processes in older cancer patients. *Critical Reviews in Oncology/Hematology, 51,* 69–80.

Platania-Solazzo, A., Field, T.M., Blank, J., Seligman, F., Kuhn, C., Schanberg, S., et al. (1992). Relaxation therapy reduces anxiety in child and adolescent psychiatric patients. *Acta Paedopsychiatrica, 55*(2), 115–120.

Polsky, D., Keating, N.L., Weeks, J.C., & Schulman, K.A. (2002). Patient choice of breast cancer treatment: Impact on health state preferences. *Modern Care, 40,* 1068–1079.

Powe, B.D. (2001). Cancer fatalism among elderly African-American women: Predictors of the intensity of the perceptions. *Journal of Psychosocial Oncology, 19*(3/4), 85–95.

Ray, S.D., Patel, D., Wong, V., & Bagchi, D. (2000). In vivo protection of DNA damage associated apoptotic and necrotic cell deaths during acetaminophen-induced nephrotoxicity, amiodarone-induced lung toxicity, and doxorubicin-induced cardiotoxicity by a novel IH636 grape seed proanthocyanidin extract. *Research Communications in Molecular Pathology and Pharmacology, 107*(1–2), 137–166.

Rexilius, S.J., Mundt, C., Erickson, J., Megel, M., & Agrawal, S. (2002). Therapeutic effects of massage therapy and handling touch on caregivers of patients undergoing autologous hematopoietic stem cell transplant [Online exclusive]. *Oncology Nursing Forum, 29,* E35–E44.

Roschke, J., Wolf, C., Muller, M.J., Wagner, P., Mann, K., Grozinger, M., et al. (2000). The benefit from whole body acupuncture in major depression. *Journal of Affective Disorders, 57*(1–3), 73–81.

Rosenfeld, I. (1996). *Dr. Rosenfeld's guide to alternative medicine.* New York: Knopf.

Schulz, R., & Heckhausen, J. (1996). A lifespan model of successful aging. *American Journal of Psychology, 51,* 702–714.

Siev-Ner, I., Gamus, D., Lerner-Geva, L., & Achiron, A. (2003). Reflexology treatment relieves symptoms of multiple sclerosis: A randomized controlled study. *Multiple Sclerosis, 9*, 356–361.

Simmonds, P.C. (2000). Palliative chemotherapy for advanced colorectal cancer: Systematic review and meta-analysis. Colorectal Cancer Collaborative Group. *BMJ, 321*, 531–535.

Sparber, A., Bauer, L., Curt, G., Eisenberg, D., Levin, T., Parks, S., et al. (2000). Use of complementary medicine by adult patients participating in cancer clinical trials. *Oncology Nursing Forum, 27*, 623–630.

Spencer, J., & Jacobs, J. (Eds.). (1999). *Complementary and alternative medicine. An evidence-based approach.* St. Louis, MO: Mosby.

Stallibrass, C. (1997). An evaluation of the Alexander technique for the management of disability in Parkinson's disease—A preliminary study. *Clinical Rehabilitation, 11*, 8–11.

Stevinson, C. (2001). Why patients use complementary and alternative medicine. In E. Ernst (Ed.), *The desktop guide to complementary and alternative medicine: An evidence-based approach* (pp. 395–403). Chicago: Harcourt.

Sundstrom, H., Korpela, H., Sajanti, E., & Kauppila, A. (1989). Supplementation with selenium, vitamin E and their combination in gynaecological cancer during cytotoxic chemotherapy. *Carcinogenesis, 10*, 273–278.

Swisher, E.M., Cohn, D.E., Goff, B.A., Parham, J., Herzog, T.J., Rader, J.S., et al. (2002). Use of complementary and alternative medicine among women with gynecologic cancers. *Gynecologic Oncology, 84*, 363–367.

Tanaka, Y., Eda, H., Fujimoto, K., Tanaka, T., Ishikawa, T., & Ishitsuka, H. (1990). Anticachectic activity of 5'-deoxy-5-fluorouridine in a murine tumor cachexia model, colon 26 adenocarcinoma. *Cancer Research, 50*, 4528–4532.

Tayek, J.A., Bistrian, B.R., Hehir, D.J., Martin, R., Moldawer, L.L., & Blackburn, G.L. (1986). Improved protein kinetics and albumin synthesis by branched chain amino acid-enriched total parenteral nutrition in cancer cachexia. A prospective randomized crossover trial. *Cancer, 58*, 147–157.

Terkelsen, A.J., Andersen, O.K., Molgaard, H., Hansen, J., & Jensen, T.S. (2004). Mental stress inhibits pain perception and heart rate variability but not a nociceptive withdrawal reflex. *Acta Physiologica Scandinavica, 180*, 405–414.

Thomas, D.V. (2002). Aromatherapy: Mythical, magical, or medicinal? *Holistic Nursing Practice, 16*(5), 8–16.

Tisserand, R., & Balacs, T. (1995). *Essential oil safety: A guide for healthcare professionals.* New York: Churchill Livingstone.

Truant, T., & Bottorff, J.L. (1999). Decision making related to complementary therapies: A process of regaining control. *Patient Education and Counseling, 38*, 131–142.

Vallerand, A.H., Fouladbakhsh, J.M., & Templin, T. (2003). The use of complementary/alternative medicine therapies for the self-treatment of pain among residents of urban, suburban, and rural communities. *American Journal of Public Health, 93*, 923–925.

Van de Creek, L., Rogers, E., & Lester, J. (1999). Use of alternative therapies among breast cancer outpatients compared with the general population. *Alternative Therapies in Health and Medicine, 5*(1), 71–76.

Wang, X.M. (1993). Treating type II diabetes mellitus with foot reflexology. *Zhongguo Zhong Xi Yi Jie He Za Zhi, 13*, 536–588.

Weiner, P., Man, A., Weiner, M., Rabner, M., Waizman, J., Magadle, R., et al. (1997). The effect of incentive spirometry and inspiratory muscle training on pulmonary function after lung resection. *Journal of Thoracic and Cardiovascular Surgery, 113*, 552–557.

Whiskey, E., Werneke, U., & Taylor, D. (2001). A systematic review and meta-analysis of Hypericum perforatum in depression: A comprehensive clinical review. *International Clinical Psychopharmacology, 16*, 239–252.

Whitaker, J., & Adderly, B. (1999). *The pain relief breakthrough.* Boston: Little, Brown and Company.

White, J.D. (2002a). Complementary and alternative medicine research: A National Cancer Institute perspective. *Seminars in Oncology, 29*, 546–551.

White, J.D. (2002b). The National Cancer Institute's perspective and agenda for promoting awareness and research on alternative therapies for cancer. *Journal of Alternative and Complementary Medicine, 8*, 545–550.

Wigmore, S.J., Ross, J.A., Falconer, J.S., Plester, C.E., Tisdale, M.J., Carter, D.C., et al. (1996). The effect of polyunsaturated fatty acids on the progress of cachexia in patients with pancreatic cancer. *Nutrition, 12*(Suppl. 1), S27–S30.

Wu, C.Y. (1990). Spontaneous dynamic qigong and mental disorders. *Chinese Journal of Modern Developments in Traditional Medicine, 10,* 497–498.

Yamashita, A., & Kato, S. (2003). Music therapy used on a patient in the terminal stage of cancer who narrated a tale based on her fantasy. *Psychiatria et Neurologia Japonica, 105,* 787–794.

Yang, J.M. (2004). *A brief history of QiGong.* Retrieved May 10, 2004, from http://www.acupuncture.com/qigong_tuina/qigonghistory.htm

Zappa, S.B., & Cassileth, B.R. (2003). Complementary approaches to palliative oncological care. *Journal of Nursing Care Quality, 18*(1), 22–26.

CHAPTER 23

Spiritual Care of the Older Adult With Cancer

Marilyn Tuls Halstead, RN, PhD, and
Holly C. Nilsson, BA, RN

Introduction

Although many older adults are enjoying healthy, active lifestyles for a longer period of time, maintaining this lifestyle is a common concern. Older adults face a myriad of emotions and questions related to the aging process, chronic illness, and existential concerns. Decisions involving loss of independence and changes of lifestyle, including giving up one's home, weigh heavily on their minds. Familiar sources of support may live far away, be ill, or be facing death themselves. On the other hand, older adults may accept the idea that illness is part of the aging experience. Throughout their lives, they discovered and practiced familiar coping strategies that enable them to effectively deal with problems.

In either case, living well for a longer time or facing the problems of illness and death, spirituality is a source of comfort and strength for many older adults (Idler et al., 2003; Weaver, Flannelly, & Flannelly, 2001). For example, in most cultural frameworks, prayer is a widely utilized practice that occurs more frequently as individuals age (Levin & Taylor, 1997).

Older adults define health as multidimensional and holistic: Health is composed of mind, body, and spirit (Armer & Conn, 2001). Thus, spiritual health is a significant factor in providing holistic care (see Table 23-1). Spiritual and religious practices engender healing emotions such as hope, forgiveness, love, and peace and decrease other more negative emotions such as depression, despair, and hostility (Larson, Larson, Puchalski, & Koenig, 2000a, 2000b; Mueller, Plevak, & Rummans, 2001). In fact, some caregivers and care receivers describe spirituality as the most important aspect of their lives (Theis, Biordi, Coeling, Nalepka, & Miller, 2003). Because of this phenomenon, nurses should examine the literature about spirituality and

Table 23-1. Spiritual Care Rationales

Rationale for Inclusion of Spirituality in a Care Plan	Examples
Spirituality may be an important factor in the patient's understanding of disease.	Illness as punishment for real or imagined failures; excessive guilt
Religious beliefs may influence decision making.	End-of-life care; treatment cessation decisions; use of blood products
Spirituality may be a preferred coping style for the individual.	Prayer or meditation promotes relaxation.
Spirituality is an important aspect of holistic care.	Quality-of-life models

Note. Based on information from Puchalski, 2001.

older adults so that they may better understand healthy spirituality and the role it plays in their patients' lives.

Meisenhelder and Chandler (2002) examined three measures of spirituality: frequency of prayer, importance of faith, and religious coping for correlation with attributes of mental and physical health. The three measures correlated with positive mental health in a community-based population of older adults. The researchers discovered that only importance of faith had independent relevance; thus, the study indicated that the *attitude* of the individual toward faith had a greater impact on health than the *frequency* of behaviors, such as prayer.

Because spirituality often is important to older adults, nurses have a responsibility to provide spiritual care. Furthermore, nurses ascribe to the concept of wholeness, meaning that the individual patients' needs are recognized to be an interdependent relationship of physical, emotional, and spiritual aspects. Spiritual care of older adults with cancer remains an accepted part of holistic nursing care. Nonetheless, basic assumptions and implications may impact spiritual caregiving (see Table 23-2).

This chapter will examine the relationship of spirituality and ill older adults, define spirituality, identify indicators of spiritual well-being as well as indicators of spiritual need, explain the relationship of spirituality and religious expression, look at spiritual development, and discuss ways to enhance spiritual caregiving through improved communication, assessment, and spiritual care interventions. In addition, spiritual self-care for the nurse will be addressed.

Review of Literature

Spirituality and Ill Older Adults

Several researchers developed programs to investigate the role of spirituality, religion, and coping with illness. Research studies of spirituality include qualitative and quantitative methodologies, surveys, and descriptive, correlational, and interventional designs. It is generally agreed that more interventional research is needed.

Table 23-2. Selected Assumptions of Spirituality

Assumptions	Implications
A spiritual nature is part of being human.	Ethical holistic care requires care of the human spirit.
Spirituality is personal and is expressed in a variety of culturally appropriate ways, including, but not limited to, religious expression.	Assessment of spirituality incorporates more than religious affiliation. Cultural values influence spiritual expression.
Acknowledgment of spiritual need may arise at any time.	Nurses must be familiar with assessment, diagnosis, intervention, and evaluation of spirituality.
Joy is a spiritual emotion.	Humor can be a spiritual intervention.
Sharing spiritual concerns is a personal decision.	Sensitivity and gentleness are important aspects of quality nursing care.
Not all individuals are aware of or able to articulate spiritual concerns.	Resources should be available to enable exploration of spirituality (if so desired by the patient).
Healing and spiritual growth are possible in difficult circumstances without intervention.	Acknowledgment and support of spirituality should be offered with the recognition that listening may be all that patients desire or need.

Note. Based on information from the Spiritual Care Workgroup, 1990.

Although it is not within the scope of this chapter to rigorously review each of the studies, in general, researchers agree that older adult patients are likely to use spiritual coping strategies when facing illness (Koenig, 1999; Pargament, 1997). Koenig's and Pargament's research programs are basically descriptive and interventional in design. However, criticisms of their programs include the fact that some studies have mostly religious people in the sample. Nonetheless, religious and spiritual coping strategies are rated as highly effective, especially for individuals who are more religiously committed and involved in religious practices (Pargament).

Similarly, Meisenhelder and Chandler (2002) used a mailed survey (N = 271; 56% response rate) to examine the relationship of attitudinal and behavioral measures of spirituality with physical and mental health outcomes. The researchers found that all three outcome measures (prayer, faith, and religious coping) correlated strongly with positive mental health. Additionally, older adults with poor physical functioning tended to pray more often than those who had higher physical functioning scores. Similarly, Rajagopal, MacKenzie, Bailey, and Lavizzo-Mourey (2002) tested the effectiveness of prayer in relieving anxiety and minor depression in older adult residents (N = 22) of a continuing care facility. Anxiety scores decreased significantly, and a trend was noted toward decreased depression. If residents continued the prayer intervention, depression scores decreased further. Depression scores increased if the intervention was discontinued.

A frequent criticism of the research about spirituality and health is that the participants are primarily middle class Caucasian women. Dingley and Roux (2003) sought to address this gap in a qualitative study of inner strength in older Hispanic women with chronic illness. Researchers recruited Hispanic women who were 60 years of age or older and living with chronic illness. The data revealed that inner strength included several interrelated dimensions. The women drew strength from the past, focused on possibilities, were supported by others, knew their purpose in life, and nurtured their spirit. Although the population in this study was not specifically patients with cancer, knowledge of this study can help oncology nurses to practice spiritual care in the Hispanic population with greater sensitivity. Studies that deal more specifically with older adults with cancer will be discussed in the next section.

Spirituality and Older Adults With Cancer

Few research studies focus on spirituality and older adults with cancer. One study examined the correlation between spiritual well-being and demands of illness in people with colorectal cancer (Fernsler, Klemm, & Miller, 1999). Demands of illness are defined as events that individuals experience in response to health problems, including dealing with physical symptoms; finding personal meaning of the illness; coping with family functioning, social relationships, and self-image; monitoring symptoms, self, and others; and handling treatment issues. This study population consisted of 21 people older than age 66 (17% of the total sample), and the demands of illness scores were lower in the older age group than in younger age groups. No significant differences were found in spiritual well-being scores among the older age group than in other age groups.

Review of Literature—Summary

Obviously, a need exists for further research in the area of spiritual health and older adults with cancer. At the present time, nurses can conclude that spirituality and religious coping strategies are important for many older adults. Furthermore, although the empirical data support a relationship among spirituality, religious coping, and health, more theoretical and empirical verification would explicate the nurse's role in supporting spiritual health. Intervention studies, although difficult to conduct, would further the state of the science and facilitate evidence-based practice. Currently, several research studies, including intervention trials, are in place that will aid in the goal of evidence-based practice. Interventions include meaning-focused psychotherapy with the goal of enhancing psychospiritual well-being and quality of life, relaxation using healing touch, yoga and meditation, mindfulness-based art therapy, spirituality counseling for weight management in African American women, prayer, and distant healing (defined as mental intention, including prayer, energy healing, and spiritual healing, on behalf of one person to benefit another at a distance) (Clinical Trials, n.d.; National Center for Complementary and Alternative Medicine, 2005). Spiritual transformation is another area of interest for researchers (Metanexus Institute, n.d.). Notably, an obvious problem for researchers interested in the overarching concept of spirituality is that of a clear definition of terms.

Spirituality Defined

As noted, the concept of spirituality is addressed in the nursing literature. Yet a common, unifying definition of spirituality currently is not available. In fact, Draper and McSherry (2002) argued that because of the inability of nurses to universally agree on a definition of spirituality, the concept of spirituality should not be considered as part of the nursing realm of care. Supportive listening and communication through touch and presence would be provided not as spiritual care but as an integration throughout holistic care. Other nurse authors disagree with this position, stating that to ignore the concept of spirituality in nursing practice is to ignore an expanding body of research literature (in nursing as well as in other disciplines) that describes the relationship of spiritual well-being and health (Swinton & Narayanasamy, 2002). Acknowledging that diversity exists within the realm of spirituality enables nurses to explore this rich arena of nursing practice, thereby strengthening practice (Swinton & Narayanasamy).

"Spirituality is similar to the clouds we see in the sky. They seem so clear and distinct to us as we gaze at them from the ground, but if we could reach out and touch a cloud, we could not grab hold of one at all. Our hands would be filled with the essence of a cloud, with all the elements that make up a cloud, but it would no longer be visible" (Meraviglia, 1999, p. 18). Exactly how, then, can spirituality be defined? Nurses have grappled with this issue for many years (see Table 23-3).

Table 23-3. Definitions of Spirituality

Author	Definition
Colliton, 1981	"... the life principle that pervades a person's entire being, including volitional, emotional, moral-ethical, intellectual, and physical dimensions, and generates a capacity for transcendent values" (p. 492).
Dossey & Guzzetta, 2000	"A unifying force of a person; the essence of being that permeates all of life and is manifested in one's being, knowing, and doing; the interconnectedness with self, others, nature, and God/Life Force/Absolute/Transcendent" (p. 7).
Hungelmann et al., 1985	Harmonious interconnectedness among self, others, nature, and the Ultimate Other that transcends time. It is a dynamic and integrative growth process that leads to ultimate meaning and purpose in life.
Meraviglia, 1999	"The experiences and expressions of one's spirit in a unique and dynamic process reflecting faith in God or a supreme being; a connectedness with oneself, others, nature or God; and an integration of all human dimensions" (p. 18).
Narayanasamy, 1999	"... is rooted in an awareness which is part of the biological makeup of the human species. Spirituality is therefore present in all individuals and it may manifest as inner peace and strength derived from perceived relationship with a Transcendent God/an Ultimate Reality, or whatever an individual values as supreme. The spiritual dimension evokes feelings which demonstrate the existence of love, faith, hope, trust, awe, and inspirations; therein providing meaning and a reason for existence" (pp. 274–275).
Reed, 1992	"Spirituality refers to the propensity to make meaning through a sense of relatedness to dimensions that transcend the self in such a way that empowers and does not devalue the individual. This relatedness may be experienced intrapersonally (as a connectedness within oneself), interpersonally (in the context of others and the natural environment), and transpersonally (referring to a sense of relatedness to the unseen, God, or power greater than the self and ordinary resources)" (p. 350).

(Continued on next page)

Table 23-3. Definitions of Spirituality *(Continued)*

Author	Definition
Shelly & Miller, 1999	Christian spirituality is "the whole person in dynamic relationship with God through Jesus" that impels one to "nurture that relationship in contemplation, community and compassion for others. Rather than seeking a vague inwardness or manipulating to the spirit world, spirituality leads us to a mature faith and a life of service" (p. 96).
Stoll, 1989	"Spirituality involves a vertical dimension (i.e., a person's relationship with God, the transcendent, supreme values) and a horizontal dimension (i.e., which 'reflects' and 'fleshes out' the supreme experiences of one's relationship with 'God through one's beliefs, values, life-style, quality of life, and interactions with self, others, and nature')" (p. 7).

Because of the fact that spirituality is an intensely personal phenomenon, the underlying world view must be explicated. Simplistically, Eastern and Western world views are the underpinnings of spiritual preferences. Energy-based theories and definitions often are reflective of the Eastern world view, whereas relationship-based theories reflect Western philosophical viewpoints (Halstead & Mickley, 1997). For example, blocking the life-giving energy or flow of chi may cause distress or illness in Eastern philosophical traditions. Restoration of chi or balance, therefore, is a useful treatment for many who adhere to this philosophy. In a Western world view, a relationship with a higher power or deity, relationships with others and self, and harmony with nature promote or restore health of body, mind, and spirit. These philosophical views are the basis of values and ethical behaviors. Thus, holistic, sensitive, and ethical nursing care requires the nurse to be aware of individual preferences.

In many ways, defining spirituality is similar to defining pain: It is what the patient says it is. If spirituality is as individualized as pain, a universally accepted definition would be difficult to obtain. Thus, the importance of careful assessment of patients and self to ascertain spiritual definitions is emphasized. Additionally, this approach facilitates the ethical practice of spiritual care: respect for the patient's belief system, autonomy of the individual to choose a belief system, and refusing to impose one's own belief system on another (proselytizing). Careful assessment will provide information necessary to determine the individual's spiritual need. To achieve this, the nurse must be knowledgeable of the characteristics of spiritual health.

Indicators of Spiritual Well-Being

In spite of the difficulty with defining spirituality, generally accepted characteristics of spiritual well-being exist. The National Interfaith Coalition on Aging (1975) made one of the first attempts to elucidate these characteristics. This group suggested that spiritual well-being is the "affirmation of life in a relationship with God, self, community and environment that nurtures and celebrates wholeness" (p. 1). Ellison (1983) built upon this definition by postulating that spiritual well-being is a nonphysical dimension of awareness that does not exist in isolation. Furthermore, transcendence is an important aspect of human life (Ellison). Transcendence is built upon the need for commitment to a purpose that brings forth meaning in life.

If spiritual well-being consists of wholeness, interdependence, transcendence, commitment to a purpose, and finding meaning in life's experiences, what are some of the characteristics one might look for in a spiritually healthy person? Spiritual health is dynamic and, as such, exists on a continuum of health and illness. Therefore, individuals are not consistently spiritually well or spiritually unwell. Rather, spiritual health is a flow between healthy and less healthy.

Hood-Morris (1996) conceptualized a spiritual well-being model as a dynamic, integrated, unfolding growth process. Key attributes of the concept include harmonious interconnectedness, creative energy, and faith in a power greater than self. Enablers of attributes such as love, trust, contemplation, meditation, prayer, and pivotal events result in actualization of spiritual well-being, producing specific outcomes such as hope, fulfillment, and meaning (see Figure 23-1). As spiritual well-being becomes actualized, the individual's ultimate purpose is understood, spiritual virtues are acquired, and humankind benefits. Yet, many individuals do not consistently possess these characteristics, perhaps more often during periods of stressful illness. Therefore, nurses must identify and document spiritual needs.

• Development of guiding values	• Self-transcendence	• Gentleness
• Surpassing problems	• Peace	• Kindness
• Inner healing	• Hope	• Appreciation
• Finding meaning	• Joy	• Forgiveness
• Nurturing wholeness	• Warmth	• Empathy
	• Fulfillment	

Figure 23-1. Outcomes of Spiritual Well-Being

Note. Based on information from Hood-Morris, 1996.

Indicators of Spiritual Need

If spiritual well-being is a dynamic concept, then each person experiences varying levels of spiritual need. For the older adult, retirement, loss of friends and loved ones, health issues, fixed incomes, loss of independence, and confronting death are challenges that may bring on a period of increased spiritual need (Berggren-Thomas & Griggs, 1995). Although these challenges also may result in spiritual growth, spiritual needs should be recognized so that nurses can assist with meeting these needs, thereby facilitating spiritual growth.

Highfield and Cason (1983) were among the first nurse researchers to investigate nurses' recognition of spiritual needs in patients with cancer. They based their exploratory study on Clinebell's (1966) theoretical framework of religious-existential need. In this framework, spiritual needs consist of the following: to find meaning and purpose in life, to receive love, to give love, and to have a sense of hope and creativity. Respondents (N = 35) indicated that nurses recognize relatively few spiritual needs. The nurse only consistently identified the need to receive love as a spiritual need.

Ross (1997) examined hospitalized British older adults' perception of spiritual needs in a pilot study. Although the small sample precludes generalization, the older adults identified categories of spiritual needs, including religious need, making sense of life, love and belonging needs, needs related to death and the dying experience, and the need for integrity or moral standing. A few of the patients identified the need for forgiveness. Two felt that they had never experienced any spiritual needs. Interestingly, none of the four patients who identified the need for meaning in life had ever talked to anyone about this need.

If nurses and patients have difficulty recognizing spiritual need, is it possible to assist the patient in meeting these needs? Is this problem related to the definition of terms? If spirituality and religion are not the same or are related in some way, does a developmental process occur as one ages? How does spirituality develop across the life span? How is it best to communicate about the highly personal area of spirituality?

The Relationship Between Spirituality and Religion

Spirituality is part of the holistic person. If one agrees with that statement, all human beings have a spiritual nature. Indeed, Florence Nightingale assumed that spiritual care was part of nursing's domain (Burkhardt & Nagai-Jacobson, 2002; O'Brien, 1999). Yet many nurses, when assessing the spiritual domain, ask only about religious practices. Are the two concepts related? All people are not religious; therefore, how can spirituality be part of the holistic human being?

Discussion on this topic could go on forever. Is knowledge of religion necessary for nurses to carry out their sensitive spiritual care of older adults with cancer (see Lewis, 2001, for additional discussion)? Maybe not in the clinical arena. While assuming that not all people are religious yet all people have a spiritual nature, perhaps the most acceptable conceptualization is to think of spirituality as a broad, overarching framework. Religion could be conceptualized as a way that many individuals express their spirituality. Religious expression can be either healthy (i.e., contributes to an overall sense of well-being) or not healthy (i.e., detracts from a sense of well-being, such as an overwhelming feeling of guilt). Certainly, if spirituality is a highly personal aspect of human life, nurses should allow individuals to tell them their conceptualization of spirituality. If they define their spirituality as having a strongly religious connotation, nurses should accept that as their personal definition. Berggren-Thomas and Griggs (1995) said, "An approach to spiritual care that sees each individual as being on a unique spiritual journey and views nurses as persons who can enhance that journey is more realistic and holistic and less arrogant" (p. 9). Accepting an individual's unique, personal definition of terms will enable healthcare providers to become fellow travelers in the patients' journey as it develops over the life span.

Spiritual Development

Human development takes place in the context of society and human relationships. Viewed as a connecting essence of being, spirituality flows and develops throughout the life span. Although various theorists examine spirituality over the life span, they generally agree that spiritual development usually does not reach the highest level. For example, if adverse life situations such as sexual abuse occurred over time in an individual's life, spiritual development may not progress beyond the level expected of a much younger person. Older adults with dementia may regress to previous levels of spiritual development. Therefore, all levels of spiritual development should be presented in a text about older adults. The literature presents various descriptions of the developmental nature of spirituality.

Fowler (1981), a Christian theologian, described spiritual development as a theory of growth in faith. Fowler's stages of faith development begin in infancy and progress through predictable stages (see Figure 23-2). Life's experiences influence transition to higher levels of development. Therefore, earlier stages of spiritual development may become apparent in the older adult (see examples in preceding paragraph).

- Stage 0—Undifferentiated faith
- Stage 1—Intuitive-projective faith
- Stage 2—Mythical-literal faith
- Stage 3—Synthetic-conventional faith
- Stage 4—Individuating-reflective faith
- Stage 5—Conjunctive faith
- Stage 6—Universalizing faith

Figure 23-2. Stages of Faith

Note. Based on information from Fowler, 1981.

Faith is a dynamic existential stance or a way of finding or giving meaning to the conditions of people's lives. Dynamics of faith underlie four constructs: self, others, world, and ultimate environment. Therefore, faith is intimately connected with personhood (Fowler, 1981). For Fowler, faith is related to the person throughout the life span. In undifferentiated faith (stage 0), the individual has no concept of right or wrong or convictions to guide behavior. Foundations for faith development are laid through trust and a relationship with the primary caregiver. If the ratio of trust to mistrust is favorable, hope emerges.

Stage 1 is labeled intuitive-projective faith. Although this level of faith development usually is associated with early childhood, dependent, powerless adults may revert to this level of development. For example, the adult with dementia may enjoy singing hymns learned in childhood without being able to understand the meaning of the words. At this stage, the individual imitates the behaviors or gestures of others without any understanding of basic, underlying concepts. Physical size and visible symbols of authority determine who should be obeyed. The virtue of will becomes apparent. Moral judgment is in the beginning stages. The individual hears a judging voice, an internalized caretaker and/or parental injunctions (Fowler, 1981).

In stage 2, or mythical-literal faith, people have a strong interest in religion and are able to articulate a basic level of understanding about faith. Moral judgment is dependent on a set of rules or guidelines (Fowler, 1981). Some adults may not progress beyond this level of development.

Stage 3 (synthetic-conventional faith) results in further moral development. The individual identifies third person perspectives that define justice in a given situation. Actions are considered right if they conform to the expectations of significant others (Fowler, 1981). Often people do not advance to higher levels of spiritual development as defined by Fowler. If one matures further in faith, social systems and conscience relate to stage 4 or individuative-reflective faith. Duty is related to the legal requirements. This stage results in individual contemplation and evaluation of the values important in previous levels of faith.

In stage 5 (conjunctive faith), the individual recognizes the relativity of most social rules and laws. Commitment to the greatest good for the greatest number of people becomes the standard. One is able to look beyond self-satisfaction and prioritization of the self (Fowler, 1981).

Although only a few people attain stage 6 (universalizing faith) according to Fowler (1981), the individual in this stage is committed to principles of justice that are universally valued, such as the golden rule. Billy Graham, Mother Teresa, and Gandhi are examples of those attaining this level of faith (Fowler).

Nurses should aim to tailor their spiritual care interventions according to the assessed level of spiritual development (Hart & Schneider, 1997). Although Hart and Schneider's work refers to children, information about interventions for adults who may be at a lower stage of spiritual development because of life circumstances is presented. Interventions may be presented if they are provided in a respectful way that does not demean the older adult. For example, spiritual care for the individual at stage 0 centers on attending to needs in a timely manner. Concerns require active listening, reassurance of adequacy of caretaking skills, and use of a religious support system. Individuals at stage 1 might need reassurance that God is not punishing them, limit setting, and behavioral examples of love, acceptance, and caring from caretakers in their environment. For stage 2, caregivers should assess for thoughts that cause anxiety, such as punishment by a deity. Appropriate, concrete explanations for religious rituals and behaviors are necessary. Promoting the use of prayer is appropriate. Care of those at stage 3 requires openness and acceptance. Unbiased answers to questions encourage participation in religious rituals and stimulate personal thinking. Continuation or development of honest, trusting relationships is the key in this stage (Hart & Schneider). The outcome is that by relating to the person's stage of faith development, nurses are enabled to communicate more efficiently about spiritual concerns.

Communicating About Spirituality

As previously stated, spirituality is an intensely personal phenomenon. As such, spiritual care requires great sensitivity on the part of the nurse. Communication about spiritual concerns must convey acceptance and respect for the individual's belief system. Constant vigilance on the part of the nurse as communication occurs identifies the nurse's feelings and responses to the patient's revelations. If acceptance and respect are conveyed, the patient will feel free and empowered to continue the discussion. Conversely, if the nurse's attitude and nonverbal communication exhibit a sense of disrespect or lack of understanding, the patient may cut off the communication.

One easy way to begin communication is by observing cues in the patient's environment. Cards, books, religious jewelry or medals, photos, or pictures on the wall often denote something that has great meaning for the patient. These types of objects lend themselves to opening a discussion of spiritual concerns. Patients appreciate the fact that the nurse notices such objects and understands that they are given permission to speak of meaningful parts of their lives. This "giving permission" may open the floodgates, as patients begin to talk about meaningful aspects of their lives.

As the conversation progresses, the nurse must pay special attention to the nuances of the communication. Observance of body language, words that indicate reluctance to continue the conversation, or difficulty expressing needs or feelings must be handled with gentle probing, redirecting, or even discontinuing the specific area of conversation. Communicating in such a way will enable the nurse to connect with the older adult in a healthy, spiritual relationship.

Connecting

The concept of connecting is vital to spiritual caregiving. By its very nature, Western conceptualization of spirituality involves relationship. Walton (1996) stated that all human relationships may develop into spiritual relationships. Furthering this idea, Goldberg (1998) described spirituality as connection. Goldberg looked at themes that were identified as part of the concept of spirituality, including meaning, presencing, empathy, hope, love, touch, and healing—terms related to either physical or emotional/spiritual relationships. However, separating the persona into two distinct components is not applicable to human beings. Thus, the term *connection* was chosen to describe the concept of spirituality.

Similarly, in a grounded theory study of spiritual well-being in healthy older adults, harmonious interconnectedness was the basic social process (Hungelmann, Kenkel-Rossi, Klassen, & Stollenwerk, 1985). How do nurses establish a spiritual relationship or connection with older adults and then foster this sense of connectedness within older adults?

First, nurses must be in touch with their own spiritual nature (intrapersonal relationship). The nature of spiritual relationships is recognition of one's own spirit that acknowledges and reaches out to another. By recognizing one's own spirituality, one can begin to acknowledge another's spiritual nature. Nurses must be cognizant of any dehumanizing attitudes and behaviors that impede spiritual relationships (Walton, 1996). Approaching patients nonjudgmentally and honestly begins the spiritual relationship.

As the relationship develops and trust is established, patients are encouraged to share more personal information (interpersonal relationship). The nurse then can gather more information about the patients' relationship with God, a higher power, or nature (transpersonal). If issues are blocking these relationships, they can be brought to light and examined (Reed, 1992). Referral to a professional pastoral care chaplain or counselor may be necessary in some cases.

Nurses should not expect intense spiritual relationships to occur with every encounter or with all patients. Personality conflicts will impede spiritual relationships, and often certain patients are easier to get along with or develop a more intimate relationship. Sometimes, nurses or patients simply cannot put forth the emotional energy that is required for this type of relationship. Nonetheless, spiritual relationships often become landmark "cases" for the nurse, providing a sense of accomplishment, wonder, and even awe for those involved. O'Brien (1999) called this experience "standing on holy ground." Spiritual relationships are enhanced as nurses examine their own values and personal experiences with spirituality.

Values Clarification

Discomfort or difficulty expressing spiritual concerns may indicate a need to explore or clarify one's values. Taylor, Highfield, and Amenta (1999) found in a sample of oncology and hospice nurses (N = 819) that personal spirituality predicted nurses' ability and comfort level in providing spiritual care. Thus, the process of examining one's own feelings about spiritual care is important. For further discussion, please see the section on the nurse's spiritual self-care that appears later in this chapter.

For a variety of reasons, older adults also may have difficulty discussing spirituality. Thinking about spiritual concerns when life is progressing without major problems can be difficult. However, when illness strikes, many people begin to think about what is important in their lives and death or the dying process (Lewis, 2001). Hence, it is a good time to bring up the topic of spirituality. As patients are given permission to talk about the meaningful aspects of their lives, spiritual concerns (or satisfactions) may be discovered. This can be a therapeutic process.

For those individuals who may need or desire to think more deeply about their lives, the process of a spiritual life review is an excellent beginning. Spiritual life review allows individuals to discover that their life has depth and meaning and that they are leaving a legacy to younger generations. Other factors that are important to them, but perhaps go unrecognized, include unresolved conflicts, unfinished business, and excessive guilt that may emerge in the process of life review (Eliopoulos, 2001). For older adults who are not spiritually minded, those who recently have become aware of their spirituality, or those who are struggling with difficult issues of guilt, forgiveness, abandonment, or previous sexual abuse, spiritual life review may elicit the need for in-depth, professional psychological or spiritual counseling. If this is the case, the nurse must be prepared to refer the patient to appropriate professionals.

How, then, do nurses go about the process of life review for the purpose of values clarification? One way to begin is by asking about music, photographs, or scrapbooks that are part of the individual's environment. Significant historical events (e.g., Depression, World War II) that took place during the individual's lifetime are another way to begin discussion. Questions about coping skills that helped in a difficult time also elicit helpful responses.

Once the individual identifies areas that give life meaning, the nurse should further explore these areas. Assessment may reveal that the patient is experiencing difficulties in one or more aspects of psychospiritual health, such as anger, the need to forgive or be forgiven, or fear. How does the nurse approach a patient with these difficulties?

The Angry Patient

One of the major psychosocial tasks for older adults is finding integrity in their lives. To live with integrity means living according to cherished values. Spiritual values such as love, peace, connectedness, and joy are impossible to achieve in an atmosphere of anger and hostility. Perhaps some of these values become more important as one ages. How often do hospice nurses hear the complaint, "I wish I had spent more time with my family instead of working overtime"? Thus, for some individuals, unfinished business remains at the end of life. Unfinished business can take the form of anger or depression (anger turned inward).

Furthermore, the diagnosis of cancer brings out anger in some patients. The anger may be focused on the healthcare system or individuals providing care. Others exemplify their worst behavior toward the spouse or other loved ones. Some patients become angry with God. Pargament (1997) found that individuals who reported dissatisfaction with God, religious professionals, and/or congregations also reported lower levels of mental health, negative mood, and less positive resolution to problems. Pargament pointed out that anger at God may be the initial coping strategy. Careful assessment, active listening, and acceptance encourage the patient to work through this anger in a positive way. Cathartic change becomes the goal.

Facilitating Forgiveness

Examination of personal values, particularly religious values, may identify areas that require reconciliation before integrity can be achieved. Reconciliation cannot occur without seeking and accepting forgiveness. Hebl and Enright (1993) proposed a series of conditions that the offended party must work through before forgiveness can be claimed (see Figure 23-3). Reconciliation is a distinct concept and does not always accompany forgiveness. However, forgiveness is a necessary precedent for reconciliation (Festa & Tuck, 2000).

- A deep hurt elicits resentment.
- A moral right for resentment—offended party overcomes resentment.
- Development of a new response, such as compassion, empathy, or love
- New response occurs without obligation for positive emotions.

Figure 23-3. Forgiveness

Note. Based on information from Hebl & Enright, 1993.

Research in the discipline of psychology pinpoints the importance of forgiveness for mental health. Mauger et al. (1992) conducted a study about forgiveness in a group (N = 237) of outpatient counseling patients. The researchers found that deficits in forgiveness of self and of others correlated significantly with increased rates of depression, anxiety, and other psychopathologies. Other psychologists looked for a link between the conditions of resentment and forgiveness. They discovered that development of empathy for the one who committed the offense is a necessary link (McCullough, Worthington, & Rachal, 1997).

A grounded theory study described the process of forgiveness in a group of hospice patients with cancer (Mickley & Cowles, 2001). Although not all participants were older adults, the mean age was 62.5. For many of the respondents in this study, cancer was the impetus to identifying priority values and change behaviors. The basic social psychological problem identified was tension brought about by an offense that created conflict between the individual's value system and anger or bitterness. The process of relieving the tension incorporated a series of four phases. The first phase was enduring the incident. In this phase, the offended party finds it difficult to forgive or may refuse to forgive. Following this phase, the individual begins to experience escalating tension between refusing to forgive and personal values. For example, it may not seem possible to forgive the offense, but the individual's values mandate forgiveness. Over time, the individual begins to gain perspective on the situation and asks the question, "How would the situation change if I forgave the offense?" The fourth phase, achieving resolution, occurs as forgiveness is enabled (Mickley & Cowles). Forgiveness is a process that occurs over time.

The nurse facilitates the forgiveness process through active listening and maintaining a nonjudgmental attitude. The nurse assists the patient in identifying priority values, exploring alternative behaviors, and carefully considering the potential benefits and losses associated with offering forgiveness (Festa & Tuck, 2000; Mickley & Cowles, 2001).

The Fearful Patient

All nurses come into contact with some patients who require sensitive attending skills because of fear. Some older adults are paralyzed by what some healthcare providers may consider to be an excessive level of fear. Fear can come from feelings of alienation or result in separation from God, others, the self, or even nature (Burkhardt & Nagai-Jacobson, 2002). Perhaps fear is caused by previous life experiences with cancer. In the not-too-distant past, cancer implied a certainty of painful, disfiguring treatment, extensive suffering, and death. Chemotherapy meant enduring extended bouts of vomiting. Radiation meant severely burned skin. Other patients become consumed with fear of death. For some, God is a vengeful being imposing severe punishment on those who committed certain acts, held "bad" thoughts, or omitted certain behaviors.

Assessment of the patient's belief system helps to pinpoint the cause of the fear. Although active listening helps the patient to work through these fears, referral to a professional pastoral counselor may be required.

Summary

Specific situations provide unique challenges for the nurse in spiritual caregiving. Although in many settings nurses attend to patients' needs around the clock and therefore are often primary spiritual caregivers, they may feel unequipped to handle long-standing, deep theologic struggles. Similarly, caring for patients with differing religious backgrounds may seem challenging. Yet nurses have skills that can be developed and honed to meet these needs. The rewards that accompany spiritual caregiving reinforce the nurses' desire to provide spiritual care and give satisfaction in their work experience.

Other situations may require the assistance of a pastoral care or other mental health professional. Examples of deep spiritual conflicts include excessive guilt or fear, feeling that cancer is a punishment for real or imagined sin, an inability to give or receive forgiveness, and suicidal ideation. Most healthcare organizations have board certified pastoral care professionals and other mental healthcare professionals on staff who are willing to receive referrals or are aware of professionals from specific religious groups that can meet a patient's needs. Conducting a thorough assessment will identify individual patients in need of these services.

Spiritual Assessment

Having established a relationship that encourages open communication, the caregiver is able to thoroughly assess the patient's spiritual resources or needs. Many assessment tools or questions are found in the literature of various healthcare disciplines (Anandarajah & Hight, 2001; Dossey, Keegan, Guzzetta, & Kolkmeier, 1995; Dudley, Smith, & Millison, 1995; Farran, Fitchett, Quiring-Emblen, & Burck, 1989; Hicks, 1999; Maugans, 1996; Puchalski & Romer, 2000; Stoll, 1979; Taylor, 2002).

The majority of assessment tools are not specific for older adults or for patients with cancer. However, one nurse author wrote about spiritual assessment for older adult nursing home residents (Hicks). Taylor (2002), an oncology clinical nurse specialist, designed a spiritual assessment tool for use with any population. In the next section, common themes among the tools will be examined, and a tool designed for self-administration by older adult patients with cancer will be presented.

Common Themes

Although some authors were conscious of the variations in defining spirituality, all of them attempted to differentiate, at least to some degree, spiritual and religious themes. All of the tools asked questions about the individual's interpretation of God/higher power, faith/ritual practices, or community of faith. Several authors examined the importance of the individual's belief system. Another recurring theme was the relationship of the individual's beliefs and illness. Only three asked about terminal events planning or death. Other themes that occurred less frequently were meaning and purpose, love, sources of strength, hope, spiritual needs, and need to give or receive forgiveness.

Considering the number of older Americans who profess a belief in a Supreme Being and associate with a community of believers, nurses should assess the individual's religious preferences, if any. It is necessary to ask individuals to rate the importance of these resources in their lives. Understanding older adults' thoughts about the relationship of their beliefs to the cancer diagnosis is equally valuable information. Is the diagnosis a punishment? Does the illness cause isolation? Are they unable to practice cherished religious rituals or remain a part of their religious community?

Other areas of assessment that are particularly important for older adults include thoughts about death and terminal illness planning. Do their religious views impact their expectations for care? Do they want a religious professional to be notified of impending death? Do they have a sense of "unfinished business"? The need to give and receive love, sources of strength and hope, and forgiveness issues are other areas of consideration.

Self-Administered Tool

If assessment of spiritual health is an important part of care for the older adult with cancer, the tool should be easily understood and provide valuable information for the time-stressed nurse. The nurse needs a tool that could be self-administered or administered verbally. Figure 23-4 presents a tool the first author recently developed for clinical use based on a review of the spirituality literature. Currently, no reliability or validity testing results are available for the tool.

Promoting Spiritual Health Throughout the Cancer Trajectory: A Case Study Approach

Spiritual needs likely will vary as the older adult with cancer progresses through the cancer trajectory, even if cure is a distinct possibility. Yet spiritual care may not be provided or even offered by professional spiritual caregivers (Halstead & Hull, 2001).

1. Do you consider yourself spiritual or religious?
   a. Spiritual
   b. Religious
   c. Neither
   d. Both

2. If you are spiritual, how important is your spirituality to you? Put a mark on the line between VERY IMPORTANT and NOT IMPORTANT AT ALL.

   _____

   NOT IMPORTANT AT ALL   VERY IMPORTANT

3. If you are religious, how important is your religion to you? Put a mark on the line between VERY IMPORTANT and NOT IMPORTANT AT ALL.

   _____

   NOT IMPORTANT AT ALL   VERY IMPORTANT

4. If you believe in God, what is God like? Please circle all that apply.

   a. Loving   i. Far away   p. Punishing
   b. Protector   j. Accepting   q. Unforgiving
   c. Just   k. Judgmental   r. Forgiving
   d. Angry   l. One   s. Other_____
   e. Shepherd   m. Many   _____
   f. Holy   n. Caring
   g. Answers prayer   o. Humiliating
   h. Guide

5. Do you belong to a community of faith? If so, please list the community. _____
   _____

6. How important is your community of faith to you? Put a mark on the line between VERY IMPORTANT and NOT IMPORTANT AT ALL.

   _____

   NOT IMPORTANT AT ALL   VERY IMPORTANT

7. Would you like us to notify someone in your faith community if you become seriously ill? If so, who? _____
   _____

8. Has your faith helped you face your illness? Yes_____No_____
   Please explain. _____
   _____

9. What gives your life meaning and/or purpose? Please circle all that apply.

   a. Family   j. Writing in my journal   s. Yoga
   b. Friends   k. Gardening   t. Meditating
   c. Home   l. Exercising   u. Being alone
   d. Possessions   m. Sports   v. Helping others
   e. Movies   n. Eating   w. Pet
   f. Nature   o. My car   x. Nothing
   g. God   p. Photography   y. Other_____
   h. Books   q. Church
   i. Music   r. Prayer

Figure 23-4. Self-Administered Spiritual Assessment Tool for Older Adults With Cancer
(Continued on next page)

10. What are your sources of strength and comfort?

    _____

    _____

11. What helps you cope with life's difficulties? _____

    _____

    _____

12. Does your illness interfere with the practice of religious rituals? Yes_____No_____

    If yes, what rituals? _____

    _____

13. Do you feel loved? Yes_____No_____

    If yes, by whom? _____

    _____

    _____

14. Are you able to give love? Yes_____No_____

    If yes, whom do you love? _____

    _____

    _____

15. Do you think you should forgive someone for something? Yes_____No_____

    Please explain. _____

    _____

    _____

16. Do you feel that you need forgiveness for something? Yes_____No_____

    Please explain. _____

    _____

    _____

17. Do you have spiritual needs? Yes_____No_____

    Would you like to talk to someone about your needs? Yes_____No_____

    If so, what are your needs? _____

    _____

    _____

18. Do you have any religious or spiritual concerns, rituals, desires, or needs related to care at the
    end of life? Yes_____No_____

    Please explain. _____

    _____

    _____

    _____

Figure 23-4. Self-Administered Spiritual Assessment Tool for Older Adults With Cancer *(Continued)*

Figure 23-5 contains a list of spiritual care interventions that may assist the nurse or other healthcare professional in facilitating spiritual care interventions.

To help nurses to assess and plan spiritual care, researchers attempted to describe the process of spiritual development in individuals with cancer (Halstead & Hull, 2001; Taylor, 2000). Although results in these grounded theory studies may not be generalizable, several interesting factors emerged. For women with cancer, most of whom were expected to survive their illness, a period of greater spiritual need was

• Presence	• Touch	• Imagery
• Prayer	• Humor	• Dream work
• Music	• Reminiscence	• Relaxation
• Art	• Values clarification	• Ritual
• Journaling	• Anticipatory guidance	• Intentional listening
• Bibliotherapy (sacred readings)	• Meditation	• Stories
	• Nature	

Figure 23-5. Spiritual Care Interventions

experienced during the treatment phase of their illness. Gradually, as their needs were met and treatment issues resolved, these women noticed that they had changed. Spiritual growth occurred. Women who were older at the time of their diagnosis described less spiritual distress at diagnosis and throughout treatment. These women indicated that health problems were more likely at their age; therefore, the illness did not seem out of the realm of the expected (Halstead & Hull). In the following section, two very different case studies will be presented. Spiritual care assessment, diagnoses, and interventions will be presented as they relate to the specific cases.

Case Study A: Mrs. M

Mrs. M, a 67-year-old Japanese American female, is diagnosed with ovarian carcinoma. Her family emigrated from Japan in 1948, settling in the San Francisco area. Her parents rapidly adjusted to life in the United States and worked hard to educate their children. Mrs. M married another Japanese American, creating enduring social ties to other Japanese Americans. Although the M's desired to have a family, Mrs. M was not able to conceive in spite of seeking medical assistance through a fertility clinic in the area. Mrs. M is highly educated and works as an engineer. She does not belong to any religious group and does not consider spirituality to be an important part of her life, much to the dismay of her mother, a devout Buddhist.

Diagnosis

Mrs. M noticed that she was having continual bouts of indigestion, a decreased appetite, and gradual change in her bowel habits over the past several months. She was somewhat worried about these symptoms but told no one and did not see a doctor because of her demanding schedule at work and several big projects that were coming due. She did not make an appointment until her symptoms progressed to severe abdominal pain. Her healthcare provider evaluates her and recommends further testing to rule out cancer. When she tells her husband and mother that they are testing her for cancer, they are shocked and immediately concerned. Mrs. M brushes this off and does not let herself become too concerned because of all of her other responsibilities. She is completely shocked when she receives the diagnosis of ovarian cancer. All she can think of is the work she has to do and how she cannot afford to take a break. She worries that her mother and husband will be angry that she did not seek medical treatment sooner. She will not let herself think about death and the possible ramifications of her disease. She decides she must be strong and stoic for her family's sake and to get through this with dignity.

Spiritual assessment in this phase is difficult because of the brief interactions with the nurse in the outpatient setting, the new relationship with the patient, and the patient's initial acceptance of the diagnosis. Mrs. M seems to be a very private person who does not display emotion easily. She is polite and matter-of-factly answers initial questions. After asking "What helped you to cope in the past?" Mrs. M responds, "I can deal with anything. My family immigrated to San Francisco at the end of WWII, and I endured a lot of prejudice and hate. You learn to be strong and hold your head high, trusting your family and friends for support. I am also a minority female in a male-dominated profession, and I know how to work hard and endure opposition to succeed. My husband and I were not able to have children. We have experienced heartache before and are stronger because of it." Mrs. M also states that she has no religious affiliation. She comments that her mother is a devout Buddhist, and she respects her mother's faith because it helps her but that she personally does not need such a crutch.

Mrs. M seems to cope by taking all responsibility herself. She is interested in learning about her disease and getting treated quickly. Interventions that are appropriate at this time include providing information, answering questions, conveying unconditional positive regard, building rapport and connecting with the patient, encouraging participation of family during visits, applying cultural sensitivity, and not delving too deeply or too fast.

Treatment

Mrs. M's surgery included hysterectomy, bilateral salpingo-oophorectomy, omenectomy, selective biopsies, lymphadenectomy, and tumor debulking. Results revealed macroscopic peritoneal metastases beyond the pelvis measuring less than 2 cm (stage IIIB). Mrs. M chooses aggressive chemotherapy to treat her remaining disease.

Following surgical recovery, Mrs. M is placed on a chemotherapeutic regimen of paclitaxel 135 mg/m^2 over 24 hours and cisplatin 75 mg/m^2 every 21 days. The primary toxicity that Mrs. M developed was neutropenia. Despite aggressive treatment with antiemetics, Mrs. M endures mild nausea and vomiting. Additional side effects include alopecia, stomatitis, and mild paresthesia in a glove and stocking distribution.

In the hospital environment, the staff does not assess spirituality except to ask religious preference. Mrs. M's mother is continually present and does not speak much English. The staff comment about Mrs. M's stoicism and assume she is just "weird." Her husband is not around very often, and Mrs. M seems to miss him. One night, a nurse cares for her frequently and connects with Mrs. M while everyone else is sleeping. Mrs. M begins to ask the nurse questions about her disease, her prognosis, the pain, and how to make out a will. She expresses anger over never being able to have children and her sense of loss because of her hysterectomy. She tells the nurse that this is the first time in her life she has had time to sit and think. She expresses her desire to focus her energy on things that are meaningful. Her mother thinks Buddhism is meaningful, but Mrs. M does not think that is for her. The nurse asks what is meaningful for Mrs. M. She responds by saying, "I don't know anymore." She used to think her work was, but now she realizes there must be something more. She wants her family to know she cares for them. She also expresses her fear of dying. Many spiritual needs manifest themselves in these exchanges (the need to find meaning and purpose in life, to have a sense of hope, and to give and receive love).

The nurse uses presence and advanced awareness (listening with full attention, intuition, and something greater than self to make insightful responses) to allow exploration of thoughts and fears (Taylor, 2002). She asks questions to encourage reminiscence and uses touch to let her know she is loved. The nurse brings Mrs. M a journal one night and says she can use it to write her thoughts, reflections, frustrations, and fears. Journaling is a safe way to express concerns and anger that one may be unwilling to express to others. It also can help to clarify feelings and serves as a form of therapeutic release. Mrs. M uses the journal and begins to find that her writings are an exploration of what she really believes and what is most important to her. She finds she is able to have more open discussions with her husband and mother about these things as a result.

Mrs. M also begins to explore different forms of meditation to help her to relax and rid herself of her worries when they arise. The focus on breathing is important to many types of meditation. Inspiration and expiration are the essence of life and influence one's overall spirit (Taylor, 2002). She allows her mother to teach her some of her own rituals and seems comforted by them and enjoys sharing this bond.

As she goes through outpatient chemotherapy, Mrs. M begins to read books about different religions to find out what she believes. Her husband reads these with her, and they like to discuss them together. The night nurse visits her in the clinic occasionally, and Mrs. M really appreciates this. At this time, she is beginning to move along the continuum toward spiritual wellness, as she is open to receive love and care from those around her and explore her meaning and purpose in life. She even asks her nurse to pray for her as she searches and copes with treatments and plans for the future.

Recurrence

During six cycles of chemotherapy, Mrs. M develops a belief and trust in God as a Supreme Being. Although the specifics of this still are being worked out, she has a newfound peace about her that grants the ability to express her worries and fears, to live life at a less hurried pace, and to pray to a higher power for comfort. Although her belief in one higher power is in conflict with her mother's belief system, they reach an understanding and mutually respect one another's beliefs and are not filled with tension. Mrs. M does not fear death as she did before and has strengthened and deepened her relationships with those she cares for most.

Unfortunately, after six cycles of chemotherapy, Mrs. M suffers a recurrence. When she receives the news of her recurrence, she is understandably upset. However, she openly discusses her grief with her loved ones, prays and meditates for guidance, and decides to discontinue treatments.

Upon follow-up in the clinic, Mrs. M appears as a woman with much more spiritual wholeness than when initially diagnosed. When asked how news of her recurrence changed her life plans and goals, she smiles and says, "Sometimes life doesn't go according to plan." She continues to work part time from home but is no longer consumed with her work. She enjoys gardening, reading, and continues to write in her journal. Her husband also cut back his hours at work but still travels extensively. Mrs. M meditates with her mother and tries to find meaning in each day.

Interventions appropriate during these visits include providing information and resources for end-of-life care, advanced awareness, and encouraging participation in activities meaningful to the patient.

During one clinic visit, Mrs. M completes the Self-Administered Spiritual Assessment Tool (see Figure 23-4). The results indicate that Mrs. M is at a moderate level of spiritual well-being and progressing toward spiritual wellness.

End of Life

A year later, Mrs. M decides to enter hospice care. Her primary caretaker was her mother, as her husband's job required extensive travel. The family believes that hospice care will relieve some of the burden on her mother and prepare the family for the death event at home. She relishes the moments of prayer she has with the hospice nurse and asks the nurse to write down some thoughts for her in her journal. She is still somewhat unsure of what will happen after she dies, but accepts the comfort of others. Her mother meditates with her and is thankful for the help and care of the nurses. Interventions appropriate at this time include presence, intentional listening of family members, incorporating patient and family wishes for death, communication with patient and family religious leaders, and prayer.

Case Study B: Mr. B

Following a routine physical exam, Mr. B, a 72-year-old male, is notified that his prostate-specific antigen (PSA) level is elevated and that his prostate gland is enlarged. He is scheduled for a biopsy, and the results indicate a prostate malignancy. He is married to his lifelong sweetheart. As lifelong members of a Christian denomination, spirituality is very important to them.

Diagnosis

In the diagnostic phase, assessing spiritual needs is difficult because of the brief interactions that take place in outpatient settings. However, a brief assessment, including questions such as, "What helped you to cope with difficult situations in the past?" or "What support systems exist for you and your family at this time?" will give patients permission to discuss spiritual concerns if they desire. Brief assessments such as these may be therapeutic in themselves. Interventions such as presence, active listening, touch, and identifying areas of strength and support often are helpful.

Treatment

Mr. B chooses to have a radical prostatectomy because he wants the "cancer out." The surgeon reassuringly states that the cancer was found in the early stage. Mr. B's daughter, an oncology nurse, is willing to come from out of state to be with her parents at the time of the surgery.

Mr. B's surgery is scheduled for June 9. The surgery seems to take longer than expected. Finally, Mr. B's wife and daughter are notified that he is in his room. During the first post-op night, Mr. B's blood pressure is low, and he requires several units of packed red blood cells. The surgeon informs the family that Mr. B had "some bleeding in the OR." His daughter is upset by the lack of communication with the medical and nursing team.

After four days of recovery complicated by inadequate pain management and hypokalemia, the surgeon tells Mr. B and his family that "a few cancer cells were found in one peritoneal lymph node." He feels that it will be less than two years before the cancer will return. He recommends immediate treatment with hormonal therapy. The family struggles with the pathology findings and the treatment options. The Bs, their extended family, and friends pray for guidance from God as they make treatment choices. He is placed on the prayer list at his church. The pastor provides spiritual care interventions such as presence, reading the Bible, and prayer. Mrs. B is included in the interventions.

Mr. B goes through staging tests and waits for the results. As the staging is completed, Mr. and Mrs. B find solace in their religious faith. Favorite scripture passages, prayer, and the fact that others in their religious community are praying for them help them to face the future.

They decide to seek additional opinions from a medical oncologist and their internist. Both of these physicians identify watchful waiting as a treatment alternative to immediate hormonal therapy. The Bs opt for this treatment approach.

In the hospital environment, no one assesses Mr. B's spirituality except to ask his religious preference. The family has individual and family times of prayer and scripture readings. The pastor of the Bs' church keeps in close contact. The religious community keeps in touch through the telephone, cards, and brief visits. Spiritual needs are much different and more intense at this time. Mr. B is understandably worried, but worry is a conflicting emotion for him. To him, worry carries connotations of a lack of faith and trust in God's care. His spiritual/emotional conflict becomes a vicious cycle of worry, depression, and guilt.

Mr. B's homecare nurse creates a "God's Worry Box" for him. She covers a shoebox with wrapping paper, cuts a hole in the cover, and supplies Mr. B with a pad of paper and pencil. His instructions are to write out his worry whenever a disturbing thought occupies his mind. Then he is to drop the worry into "God's Worry Box." Of course, the worry box may contain the same worries multiple times, but this in itself helps the individual to identify patterns of concerns and enables the individual to express concerns confidentially. The identified patterns can be addressed more systematically when a plan of spiritual care is in place. The worry box becomes a form of prayer. Eventually, after a period of time, Mr. B may decide to open the box and reread the worries, thereby seeing that God answered his prayers and provided for his needs throughout his illness experience.

Suggested Interventions

If patients are angry or disillusioned, journaling is another way to express anger without fears of judgment or retaliation. Writing a letter to God is another form of prayer. Pastoral counselors often remind their clients that it is important to let God know inner feelings and conflicts, even those that are perceived as negative, because "God can take it." Older adults may be reluctant to do so, but writing their thoughts out becomes a safe alternative.

Music may be profoundly helpful for those who cannot express emotions. Music interventions must be tailored to individual preferences (Halstead & Roscoe, 2002). Anger can be released through "drumming" with the tempo. Making up lyrics to songs such as "Down by the Riverside" and other simple methods become a safe (and sometimes even fun) way to express emotions. Anxieties can be controlled through focused breathing exercises as one listens to calm, steady rhythms. Lyrics of religious songs often are a reminder of God's presence and caring in difficult times (Halstead

& Roscoe). The Bs found solace in reading the Psalms. The Psalms are full of emotion and easily can be matched to the individual's needs.

Watchful Waiting

As time moves forward and Mr. B's PSA levels remain low, his spiritual/emotional conflicts decrease. Their legal papers are updated on a regular basis, and they enjoy an active lifestyle, including travel. Mr. B faces heightened anxiety as he periodically awaits PSA results, but overall, his worries are less oppressive.

After 10 years, their home is sold, and they make plans to move closer to their daughter. However, shortly after the sale of their home, the daughter is diagnosed with breast cancer. This new crisis interjects another spiritual dilemma. Mr. B feels that "I did OK, but my mother and sister died of breast cancer." He reminds himself that cancer does not always result in death. Some of the feelings surrounding his own experience with cancer return. Although he has to work through these feelings, he is able to cope because "I know that God will be with us. Even in the deaths of other family members, God was with us." He realizes that over time, events in the past prepared him to face whatever was ahead. Mr. B states, "The older I get, the more I realize God has been with me throughout my life."

Spiritual interventions such as talking with his wife, family members, and friends help him to face his daughter's illness as well as the uncertainties of moving to a new community. Prayers, scripture readings, and reflecting on the past are helpful as well.

After a year, Mr. B's nurse asks him to complete the Self-Administered Spiritual Assessment Tool (see Figure 23-4). The results indicate that Mr. B is at a high level of spiritual well-being. The Bs are grateful that their nurse demonstrated knowledge of spiritual care. They wondered how oncology nurses could be in such an "emotionally difficult" profession. They concluded that their nurse seemed to know how to care spiritually for herself as well as her patients. In the next section, the oncology nurse's need for spiritual self-care will be discussed. The concept of compassion fatigue will be examined, followed by a look at interventions for spiritual self-care.

Spiritual Self-Care for the Nurse

Oncology Nurses and Compassion Fatigue

Nurses, in general, and oncology nurses, in particular, choose their career paths because of the opportunity for personal fulfillment, intellectual stimulation, and/or an innate capacity to care for others (Henry & Henry, 2004; Medland, Howard-Ruben, & Whitaker, 2004). However, these qualities become an occupational hazard in the form of compassion fatigue. Those who experience compassion fatigue often are the brightest and best nurses or those with extra sensitivity (Menninger, 1996).

What exactly do we mean by compassion fatigue? Compassion is thought of as the capacity to care or the capacity to be filled with loving kindness, patience, humility, and altruism. Compassion fatigue, therefore, results in a stunting or loss of these qualities in an individual who normally exhibits them. It is a malaise of spirit that occurs when the human spirit is faced with the reality that individuals are powerless to change (Vander Zyl, 2002). Compassion fatigue consists of physical, emotional, and spiritual parameters. Symptoms of compassion fatigue are listed in Figure 23-6. Researchers across disciplinary lines agree that spiritual and religious activities are important for prevention and treatment of compassion fatigue (Henry & Henry, 2004; Koenig, 1999; Medland et al., 2004; Pendleton & Poloma, 1991).

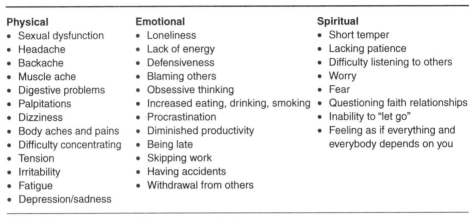

Physical
- Sexual dysfunction
- Headache
- Backache
- Muscle ache
- Digestive problems
- Palpitations
- Dizziness
- Body aches and pains
- Difficulty concentrating
- Tension
- Irritability
- Fatigue
- Depression/sadness

Emotional
- Loneliness
- Lack of energy
- Defensiveness
- Blaming others
- Obsessive thinking
- Increased eating, drinking, smoking
- Procrastination
- Diminished productivity
- Being late
- Skipping work
- Having accidents
- Withdrawal from others

Spiritual
- Short temper
- Lacking patience
- Difficulty listening to others
- Worry
- Fear
- Questioning faith relationships
- Inability to "let go"
- Feeling as if everything and everybody depends on you

Figure 23-6. Symptoms of Compassion Fatigue

Selected Interventions for Spiritual Self-Care

Work Environment

Beyond the time pressures and dealing with multiple losses, it is said, "Nurses eat their young." In other words, nurses do not provide a supportive environment that nurtures and allows individual team members to develop. How do nurses move away from this negativity to become healers for others and themselves? The first strategy is awareness of the problem. But far too often, nurses accept the status quo as an unchangeable reality. Awareness must include a good hard look at internal resources as well as the resources available within the institution. What are the values of the institution? What is the mission statement? How does this problem detract from the mission of the institution? Am I contributing to the problem? Who seems to be aware/unaware of this problem? Who is in denial that a problem exists? If my energies were used for change rather than complaining about the problem, would it make a difference? Although advocating for the team and self is difficult for those who are struggling with compassion fatigue, it often is the best way to raise consciousness about the problem.

Community building is a valuable protective mechanism against compassion fatigue. Strategies to increase sense of community include interdisciplinary gatherings, granting permission to "have fun" at work, providing spiritual care for staff members, allowing time to grieve after a difficult death, creating staff awareness of positive coping strategies, emphasizing the "gifts" that each individual brings to the work situation, and creating opportunities for increased social support (Henry & Henry, 2004; Medland et al., 2004). Promotion of self-care strategies is the beginning of an effective change in the workplace environment.

Individual Self-Care

One of the first steps in self-care is identifying the reasons that one became a nurse (Henry & Henry, 2004). Do you have special talents or gifts that enable you (or enabled you at one time) to be an effective caregiver? Do you view your profession as a calling or vocation? Is your work a way for you to find meaning or purpose in life? Do you have realistic expectations of yourself? What do you enjoy the most (and the least) about your work? Is your work a way to make money, or is it more than that? What is your philosophy of nursing? How does your philosophy of nursing match your personal philosophy of life? What are the values that are most important for you?

Journaling is one way to uncover truths about inner thoughts and emotions. For some, it becomes a form of therapeutic prayer. Try answering the questions in the preceding paragraph in a journal. Make a list, stretch your memory, and force yourself to identify strengths and/or noble desires. Review the cases or patients that provided satisfaction throughout your career. Try to remember that NO ONE relates to every patient in a special way, but all nurses can find one or more special patients who make them glad to be a nurse.

Meditation and prayer are two strategies that are mentioned frequently in the nursing literature. Both are purported to have health benefits; both are practiced in many cultures and/or religious frameworks (Dossey, 1996; Koenig, 1999; Levin, 1996; Pendleton & Poloma, 1991). The literature lacks an explicit description of the types of prayer and meditation. In spite of this obvious gap, evidence is strong enough to conclude that prayer and meditation effectively decrease stress in the general population (see Figure 23-7). However, intervention studies that examine the effectiveness of these strategies in nurses are scarce.

- Koenig (1999): Multiple, randomized studies in a variety of populations
- Matthews (1998): Multiple, randomized studies in a variety of populations
- Dossey (1996): Multiple studies in a variety of populations
- Pargament (1997): Multiple studies of religious coping in a variety of populations
- King et al. (2000): Two studies of use and effectiveness of prayer and meditation by RNs
- Schoenberger et al. (2002): Population included physicians, nurses, and occupational and physical therapists

Figure 23-7. Research Programs Supporting Health Benefits of Prayer and Meditation

---

Part of the problem is that prayer and meditation are strategies that take time—a commodity that is scarce for most nurses. Are there forms of prayer and meditation that are effective, beginning strategies? In this section, several forms of prayer and meditation will be presented.

Meditation

Several types of meditative practices involve time frames that may be acceptable for nurses on the go (see Figure 23-8). The goals are to interrupt the stress, reframe the problem, and find a brief period of relaxation and stillness.

- Relaxation/guided imagery
- Mindfulness meditation
- Dzogchen meditation
- Meditative arts

Figure 23-8. Meditative Practices

Nurses are familiar with the strategies of relaxation and guided imagery and teach them to their patients. Unfortunately, teaching them is easier than practicing them. Nurses should try to take a moment or two for deep-breathing exercises when tasks seem overwhelming.

In mindfulness meditation, methods such as yoga, Zen meditation, and others may require a class or instructive video. Simpkins and Simpkins (1997) described a simple exercise: Think about a situation you are trying to master, possibly related to your job or home life. Carefully review what you need to do. Visualize it as clearly as possible. Keep your mind on the situation itself as you address it moment by moment. Pressures from time, other people, and goals are secondary, outside of the circle of your focus. When you remain fully present in the situation that you are finding stressful, you may discover that your worries take on less importance and even become background materials.

Dzogchen meditation is a meditative strategy that does not necessarily require a large block of time (Das, 2000). Das emphasized the importance of having fun while meditating. It is practiced with the eyes and ears open. Four types of meditation exist: breathing exercises, the Ah chant, skygazing, and chanting sacred words, such as the "Om Mani Padme Hung." Ideally, the meditator practices outdoors in a comfortable, yoga position.

Meditative arts include methods such as journaling, sound meditation using chanting, Tibetan singing bowls, or singing (Taize chants, favorite hymns, and other music that relaxes).

Prayer

Prayer is defined individually. Although all religious groups have some type of prayer practice, it is not always connected to a specific religious practice. Dossey (1996) defined prayer as "intention plus love." For Billy Graham (cited in Galli & Bell, 1999), prayer is "the rope that pulls God and man together, but it doesn't pull God down to us; it pulls us up to him." There are many forms of prayer (see Figure 23-9).

- Colloquial or conversational prayers
- Petitioning prayer
- Meditative prayer
- Ritual prayer

Figure 23-9. Prayer Typology

Note. Based on information from Poloma & Gallup, 1991.

Colloquial or conversational prayer (Poloma & Gallup, 1991) is more an attitude of prayer or sensing God's presence throughout the day. It involves finding God in the ordinary moments of life (Brother Lawrence, 1982). Prayer can be an angry outpouring of emotion, either verbal or on paper (O'Brien, 2003). The prayer of helplessness admits that one cannot do it all alone (Marshall, 1975). As this fact is admitted to God, people allow God's resources to become active in their lives. The prayer of relinquishment occurs when answers are not apparent. This prayer is the giving up of self-will. It is a powerful prayer that opens the spirit to more than one can see in the situation. It is not resignation. Resignation steels itself for the worst. Relinquishment is opening oneself to accept willingly whatever a loving God sends. It is full of hope (Marshall).

Petitioning Prayer

Petitioning prayer (Poloma & Gallup, 1991) is a form of prayer that many people frequently use. While practicing it, people ask God for a special type of help or response. Sometimes it takes the form of "emergency prayer." This prayer often is practiced when one gets into a situation and needs help quickly (I face a "difficult stick"; I can't seem to find the right words to communicate effectively). Sometimes when people are emotionally exhausted, the Jesus prayer ("Lord Jesus Christ, you are merciful to me"), repeated over and over again, allows them to regroup. O'Brien (2003) presented a prayer for compassionate caregiving. Through this prayer, God enables people to go the extra mile so that they can demonstrate His care for the ill. At the end of the day, prayer may enable people to leave their thoughts of work and other obligations. One method is to listen to music, including lullabies, classical, Native American flute, or favorite religious songs.

Meditative Prayer

Obviously, meditative prayer (Poloma & Gallup, 1991) closely resembles meditative strategies described earlier. For the purposes of this chapter, meditative prayer will be differentiated according to Keating's (1992) description. Keating stated that meditative prayer is different from meditation as practiced by proponents of Eastern philosophies in that the intention is different. In Eastern philosophies, the intent is to empty oneself of all reality. In meditative prayer, the intent is to fill the self with God. The transformation involves being more like Christ rather than more like our true selves. In meditative prayer, the Holy Spirit heals the roots of self-centeredness.

Centering prayer is a specific method of preparing for the gift of contemplation. In centering prayer, the individual assumes a comfortable position, chooses a sacred word of one or two syllables, and gently introduces the word into the imagination, as if laying a feather on a piece of cotton. When other thoughts intrude, individuals should return to their sacred word, accept the stillness and silence, and listen for God's voice.

In contemplative prayer, the practitioner uses centering prayer. Following a period of centering, God initiates conversation (if the person consents) that results in a divine union with God. Practitioners should use contemplative prayer twice daily for a minimum of 20 minutes (Galli & Bell, 1999; Keating, 1992).

Lectio Divina is an ancient method of listening for God (Galli & Bell, 1999). The prayer begins with the step of Lectio: A passage from a spiritual book is read aloud until a particular word or phrase is noticed in a new way. The practitioner then stops reading. In Meditatio, the phrase is read over and over, emphasizing a different word each time. The goal is to let the words sink into the practitioner's mind and heart. In Oratio, the word or phrase is repeated until the person is ready to stop and listen in silent prayer. The person should listen for the special meaning at this time. He or she can ask God a question, such as, "Lord, what burden am I carrying that I could let go of?" The practitioner can end the time by simply enjoying God's presence.

Ritual Prayer

Ritual prayers usually are prayers of a specific religious group, although individuals also can compose a special prayer for themselves and use it as a ritual practice (Poloma & Gallup, 1991).

In Jewish traditions, prayer is both communal and individual, although communal prayer is considered the essence of Jewish prayer life (Olitzky & Judson, 2002; Steinsaltz, 2000). Gathering together as a community in prayer can extend oneself beyond individual suffering. The idea of Sabbath and participation in Holy Days is psychologically healthy.

It is caring for the soul. In individual prayer, the Hebrew term *tefillah* is understood as an activity done to the self. As one reflects on the personal spiritual journey, one is reaching out to God for guidance through prayer. *Kavanah*, or intention, is the spontaneous form of prayer. Kavanah is what the individual brings to the prayer experience—emotions, state of mind, individual life journey. Similarly, blessings throughout the day stimulate awe and awareness of God's presence. "Praised are You . . . who made me free; who opens the eyes of the blind; who clothes the naked; who causes those who stoop to stand straight; who releases the bonds of those who are constrained," or "Praised are you, Adonai, Our God, Sovereign of the universe, who has placed such beauty in the world," or the *Amidah:* "Heal us God, and we will be healed; save us, and we will be saved."

Catholic traditions pray the Rosary. Each step of the Rosary is a meditative prayer ("A Detailed Guide to Praying the Rosary," n.d.). The prayer is incorporated of eight steps with specific prayers at each step. For example, step III involves praying the "Hail Mary" ("Hail Mary, full of grace, the Lord is with thee, blessed art thou amongst women and blessed is the fruit of thy womb, Jesus. Holy Mary Mother of God, pray for us sinners now and at the hour of our death"). While praying, people meditate on the three virtues of faith, hope, and love. The Rosary concludes with another prayer, the Salve Regina.

Other religious traditions also have ritual prayers. Praying the Psalms is a favorite suggested by Galli and Bell (1999). Simply reading a Psalm and reflecting on its meaning is one method. Adopting a Psalm as a personal prayer is another way. Practitioners can read the Psalm as if they are thanking God, petitioning God, or even arguing with God.

Prayer and meditation are time-tested strategies that are healing, protective, and stress reducing. Practicing these types of strategies may take a period of trial and error, but the benefits are known. People should try different methods until they find the right strategy.

Conclusion

As individuals age, spirituality often becomes more important than at earlier stages in life. Spirituality is a dynamic concept, and spiritual health may fluctuate from day to day. Indicators of spiritual health and spiritual need are presented in the chapter. Although spiritual development occurs throughout the life span, older adults with cognitive deficits may revert to earlier stages of development. More research is needed in this area.

Spiritual assessment is the basis for spiritual care. Spiritual interventions in older adults who are angry, fearful, or depressed are discussed. Spiritual interventions must be tailored to overall physical, emotional, and spiritual health.

Before nurses can address spiritual needs in their patients, they must be aware of their own spiritual health. Interventions for nurses' spiritual development and spiritual health maintenance are important for prevention of compassion fatigue in the nurse.

References

Anandarajah, G., & Hight, E. (2001). Spirituality and medical practice: Using the HOPE questions as a practical tool for spiritual assessment. *American Family Physician, 63,* 81–88.

Armer, J., & Conn, V. (2001). Exploration of spirituality and health among diverse rural elderly individuals. *Journal of Gerontological Nursing, 27,* 28–37.

Berggren-Thomas, P., & Griggs, M.J. (1995). Spirituality in aging: Spiritual need or spiritual journey. *Journal of Gerontological Nursing, 21,* 5–10.

Brother Lawrence. (1982). *The practice of the presence of God.* Springdale, PA: Whitaker House.

Burkhardt, M.A., & Nagai-Jacobson, M.G. (2002). *Spirituality: Living our connectedness.* Albany, NY: Delmar.

Clinebell, H. (1966). *Basic types of pastoral counseling: New resources for ministering to the troubled.* Nashville, TN: Abingdon Press.

Clinical Trials. (n.d.). *Linking patients to medical research.* Retrieved October 23, 2004, from http://www.clinicaltrials.gov/ct/action/getstudy

Colliton, M. (1981). The spiritual dimension of nursing. In I. Beland & J. Passos (Eds.), *Clinical nursing* (4th ed., pp. 492–501). New York: Macmillan.

Das, L.S. (2000). *Natural meditation: A Tibetan Buddhist practice for clearing the mind and opening to effortless awareness* [Video]. Louisville, CO: Sounds True.

A detailed guide to praying the Rosary. (n.d.). Retrieved June 30, 2005, from http://www.catholic.net/

Dingley, C., & Roux, G. (2003). Inner strength in older Hispanic women with chronic illness. *Journal of Cultural Diversity, 10,* 11–22.

Dossey, B., & Guzzetta, C. (2000). Holistic nursing practice. In B. Dossey, L. Keegan, & C. Guzzetta (Eds.), *Holistic nursing: A handbook for practice* (3rd ed., pp. 5–26). New York: Aspen.

Dossey, B., Keegan, L., Guzzetta, C., & Kolkmeier, L. (1995). *Holistic nursing: A handbook for practice* (2nd ed.). New York: Aspen.

Dossey, L. (1996). *Prayer is good medicine: How to reap the healing benefits of prayer.* New York: HarperCollins.

Draper, P., & McSherry, W. (2002). A critical view of spirituality and spiritual assessment. *Journal of Advanced Nursing, 39,* 1–2.

Dudley, J., Smith, C., & Millison, M. (1995). Unfinished business: Assessing the spiritual needs of hospice clients. *American Journal of Hospice and Palliative Care, 12,* 30–37.

Eliopoulos, C. (Ed.). (2001). *Gerontological nursing* (5th ed.). Philadelphia: Lippincott.

Ellison, C. (1983). Spiritual well-being: Conceptualization and measurement. *Journal of Psychology and Theology, 11,* 330–340.

Farran, C., Fitchett, G., Quiring-Emblen, J., & Burck, J. (1989). Development of a model for spiritual assessment and intervention. *Journal of Religion and Health, 28,* 185–193.

Fernsler, J., Klemm, P., & Miller, M. (1999). Spiritual well-being and demands of illness in people with colorectal cancer. *Cancer Nursing, 22,* 134–140.

Festa, L.M., & Tuck, I. (2000). A review of forgiveness literature with implications for nursing practice. *Holistic Nursing Practice, 14,* 77–86.

Fowler, J. (1981). *Stages of faith: The psychology of human development and the quest for meaning.* San Francisco: Harper & Row.

Galli, M., & Bell, J. (1999). *The complete idiot's guide to prayer.* Indianapolis, IN: Alpha Books.

Goldberg, B. (1998). Connection: An exploration of spirituality in nursing care. *Journal of Advanced Nursing, 27,* 836–842.

Halstead, M., & Hull, M. (2001). Struggling with paradoxes: The process of spiritual development in women with cancer. *Oncology Nursing Forum, 28,* 1534–1545.

Halstead, M., & Mickley, J. (1997). Attempting to fathom the unfathomable: Descriptive views of spirituality. *Seminars in Oncology Nursing, 13,* 225–230.

Halstead, M.T., & Roscoe, S.T. (2002). Restoring the spirit: Music as an intervention for oncology nurses. *Clinical Journal of Oncology Nursing, 6,* 332–336.

Hart, D., & Schneider, D. (1997). Spiritual care for children with cancer. *Seminars in Oncology Nursing, 13,* 263–270.

Hebl, J., & Enright, R. (1993). Forgiveness as a psychotherapeutic goal with elderly females. *Psychotherapy, 30,* 658–667.

Henry, J., & Henry, L. (2004). Self-care begets holistic care. *Reflections on Nursing Leadership, 30,* 26–27.

Hicks, T. (1999). Spirituality and the elderly: Nursing implications with nursing home residents. *Geriatric Nursing, 20,* 144–146.

Highfield, M., & Cason, C. (1983). Spiritual needs of patients: Are they recognized? *Cancer Nursing, 6,* 187–192.

Hood-Morris, L. (1996). A spiritual well-being model: Use with older women who experience depression. *Issues in Mental Health Nursing, 17,* 439–455.

Hungelmann, J., Kenkel-Rossi, E., Klassen, L., & Stollenwerk, R. (1985). Spiritual well-being in older adults: Harmonious interconnectedness. *Journal of Religion and Health, 24,* 147–153.

Idler, E., Musick, M., Ellison, C., George, L., Krause, N., Ory, M., et al. (2003). Measuring multiple dimensions of religion and spirituality for health research. *Research on Aging, 25,* 327–365.

Keating, T. (1992). *Open heart, open mind: The contemplative dimension of the gospel.* New York: Continuum International.

King, M., Pettigrew, A., & Reed, C. (2000). Complementary, alternative, integrative: Have nurses kept pace with their clients? *Dermatology Nursing, 12,* 41–48.

Koenig, H. (1999). *The healing power of faith: Science explores medicine's last great frontier.* New York: Simon and Schuster.

Larson, D., Larson, S., Puchalski, C., & Koenig, H. (2000a). Patient spirituality in clinical care: Clinical assessment and research findings—Part I. *Primary Care Reports, 6,* 165–172.

Larson, D., Larson, S., Puchalski, C., & Koenig, H. (2000b). Patient spirituality in clinical care: Clinical assessment and research findings—Part II. *Primary Care Reports, 6,* 173–180.

Levin, J. (1996). How prayer heals: A theoretical model. *Alternative Therapies in Health and Medicine, 2,* 66–73.

Levin, J.S., & Taylor, R.J. (1997). Age differences in patterns and correlates of the frequency of prayer. *Gerontologist, 37,* 75–88.

Lewis, M. (2001). Spirituality, counseling, and elderly: An introduction to the spiritual life review. *Journal of Adult Development, 8,* 231–240.

Marshall, C. (1975). *Adventures in prayer.* Old Tappan, NJ: Chosen Books.

Matthews, D. (1998). *The faith factor: Proof of the healing power of prayer.* New York: Viking.

Maugans, T. (1996). The SPIRITual history. *Archives of Family Medicine, 5*(1), 11–16.

Mauger, P., Perry, J., Freeman, T., Grove, D., McBride, A., & McKinney, K. (1992). The measurement of forgiveness: Preliminary research. *Journal of Psychology and Christianity, 11,* 170–180.

McCullough, M.E., Worthington, E.L., & Rachal, K.C. (1997). Interpersonal forgiving in close relationships. *Journal of Personality and Social Psychology, 73,* 321–336.

Medland, J., Howard-Ruben, J., & Whitaker, E. (2004). Fostering psychosocial wellness in oncology nurses: Addressing burnout and social support in the workplace. *Oncology Nursing Forum, 31,* 47–56.

Meisenhelder, J.B., & Chandler, E.N. (2002). Spirituality and health outcomes in the elderly. *Journal of Religion and Health, 41,* 243–252.

Menninger, W.W. (1996). Practitioner, heal thyself: Coping with stress in clinical practice. *Bulletin of the Menninger Clinic, 60,* 197.

Meraviglia, M.G. (1999). Critical analysis of spirituality and its empirical indicators: Prayer and meaning in life. *Journal of Holistic Nursing, 17,* 18–33.

Metanexus Institute. (n.d.). *Spiritual transformation. Scientific research program.* Retrieved June 30, 2005, from http://www.metanexus.net/spiritual_transformation/index.html

Mickley, J., & Cowles, K. (2001). Ameliorating the tension: Use of forgiveness for healing. *Oncology Nursing Forum, 28,* 31–37.

Mueller, P., Plevak, D., & Rummans, T. (2001). Religious involvement, spirituality, and medicine: Implications for clinical practice. *Mayo Clinical Proceedings, 76,* 1225–1235.

Narayanasamy, A. (1999). ASSET: A model for actioning spirituality and spiritual care education and training in nursing. *Nurse Education Today, 19,* 274–285.

National Center for Complementary and Alternative Medicine. (2005). *NCCAM-funded research for fiscal year 2004.* Retrieved October 24, 2004, from http://nccam.nih.gov/research/extramural/awards/2004/index.htm

National Interfaith Coalition on Aging. (1975). *Spiritual well-being: A definition.* Bethesda, MD: U.S. Department of Health and Human Services.

O'Brien, M.E. (1999). *Spirituality in nursing: Standing on holy ground.* Sudbury, MA: Jones and Bartlett.

O'Brien, M.E. (2003). *Prayer in nursing.* Sudbury, MA: Jones and Bartlett.

Olitzky, K., & Judson, D. (Eds.). (2002). *The rituals and practices of a Jewish life: A handbook for personal spiritual renewal.* Woodstock, VT: Jewish Lights Publishing.

Pargament, K. (1997). *The psychology of religion and coping: Theory, research, and practice.* New York: Guilford Press.

Pendleton, B.F., & Poloma, M.M. (1991). The effects of prayer and prayer experiences on measures of general well-being. *Journal of Psychology and Theology, 19,* 71–83.

Poloma, M., & Gallup, G. (1991). *Varieties of prayer: A survey report.* Philadelphia: Trinity Press.

Puchalski, C. (2001). Spirituality and health: The art of compassionate medicine. *Hospital Physician, 37,* 30–36.

Puchalski, C., & Romer, A. (2000). Taking a spiritual history allows clinicians to understand patients more fully. *Journal of Palliative Medicine, 3,* 129–137.

Rajagopal, D., MacKenzie, E., Bailey, C., & Lavizzo-Mourey, R. (2002). The effectiveness of a spiritually-based intervention to alleviate subsyndromal anxiety and minor depression among older adults. *Journal of Religion and Health, 41,* 153–166.

Reed, P. (1992). An emerging paradigm for the investigation of spirituality in nursing. *Research in Nursing and Health, 15,* 349–357.

Ross, L. (1997). Elderly patients' perceptions of their spiritual needs and care: A pilot study. *Journal of Advanced Nursing, 26,* 710–715.

Schoenberger, N.E., Matheis, R.J., Shiflett, S.C., & Cotter, A.C. (2002). Opinions and practices of medical rehabilitation professionals regarding prayer and meditation. *Journal of Alternative and Complementary Medicine, 8,* 59–69.

Shelly, J., & Miller, A. (1999). *Called to care: A Christian theology of nursing.* Downer's Grove, IL: InterVarsity Press.

Simpkins, C.A., & Simpkins, A.M. (1997). *Living meditation: From principle to practice.* Boston: Charles E. Tuttle.

Spiritual Care Workgroup. (1990). Assumptions and principles of spiritual care. *Death Studies, 14,* 75–81.

Steinsaltz, A. (2000). *A guide to Jewish prayer.* New York: Schocken Books.

Stoll, R. (1979). Guidelines for spiritual assessment. *American Journal of Nursing, 79,* 1574–1577.

Stoll, R. (1989). Spirituality and chronic illness. In V. Carson (Ed.), *Spiritual dimensions of nursing practice* (pp. 180–216). Philadelphia: Saunders.

Swinton, J., & Narayanasamy, A. (2002). Response to: 'A critical view of spirituality and spiritual assessment' by P. Draper and W. McSherry (2002) *Journal of Advanced Nursing, 39,* 1–2. *Journal of Advanced Nursing, 40,* 158–162.

Taylor, E.J. (2000). Transformation of tragedy among women surviving breast cancer. *Oncology Nursing Forum, 27,* 781–788.

Taylor, E.J. (2002). *Spiritual care: Nursing theory, research and practice.* Upper Saddle River, NJ: Prentice Hall.

Taylor, E.J., Highfield, M.F., & Amenta, M. (1999). Predictors of oncology and hospice nurses' spiritual care perspectives and practices. *Applied Nursing Research, 12,* 30–37.

Theis, S., Biordi, D., Coeling, H., Nalepka, C., & Miller, B. (2003). Spirituality in caregiving and care receiving. *Holistic Nursing Practice, 17,* 48–55.

Vander Zyl, S. (2002). Compassion fatigue and spirituality. *Nursing Matters, 13,* 4, 14.

Walton, J. (1996). Spiritual relationships. *Journal of Holistic Nursing, 14,* 3.

Weaver, A., Flannelly, L., & Flannelly, K. (2001). A review of research on religious and spiritual variables in two primary gerontological nursing journals: 1991–1997. *Journal of Gerontological Nursing, 27,* 47–54.

CHAPTER 24

Legal and Ethical Issues

Alice S. Kerber, MN, RN, AOCN®

Introduction

How many times have you, as a medical professional or adult child of an older parent, found yourself questioning treatment decisions that seem wrong or caring for family members who struggle with ethical dilemmas associated with advancing illness and care decisions? Every day, healthcare providers (HCPs) face ethical issues that conflict with personal and professional values and obligations. Most HCPs entered the profession to provide comfort and care to individuals while valuing patient participation in decision making and respecting patients' privacy, wishes, and quality of life. In caring for patients, especially the older adult with a lifetime of experiences to share and appreciate, connections develop. Situations leading to the potential for moral distress and legal and ethical issues arise. The purpose of this chapter is to provide an approach to managing some ethical and legal issues that commonly occur when caring for older adults. The chapter will present the scope of the problem with the projected increases in the older adult population and in the cancer incidence in this age group as well as associated values and conflicts that exist in caring for the older adult. A case study scenario and decision-making model will illustrate and enhance the definition, application, and discussion of some legal and ethical principles in the care of the older adult with cancer. Implications for nursing and research also will be discussed.

Cancer and the Older Adult

By the year 2030, 20% of the population in the United States will be 65 or older. The median age at the time of cancer diagnosis is 68 years. Because of population growth and aging, the absolute number of patients with cancer is expected to double from 1.3 million to 2.6 million between 2000 and 2050 (Boyle, 2003). Consequently, an increasing number of HCPs will be caring for older adults with cancer. Advances in technology have expanded available options for cancer diagnosis, treatment, and symptom management. HCPs face critically ill patients, limited resources that necessitate balancing and prioritizing care, distant or absent family members, and decreased length of hospitalization. The efficient use of resources in the hospital, community, and among HCPs is essential to meet the needs of older adults with cancer (O'Donnell, 2004).

Regardless of age, race, gender, creed, or financial situation, individuals are entitled to appropriate medical care. The older adult often encounters covert discrimination in the healthcare system, which can be seen as denial or limitation of services. For example, there is limited availability of geriatric training for medical students, even though older adults comprise a significant proportion of their patients (Balducci & Yates, 2000; Robinson, 1994). Barriers to care can include paternal (physician or other HCP), familial (family), and institutional (facility) systems. As an individual ages and physical limitations escalate, the duty to do good (beneficence) often competes with the preservation of self-determination (autonomy) (Haley, 2003; Monagle, 1998; Pence, 2004). Historically, a paternalistic model has been the norm with the physician or HCP at the center of the decision-making process. This model was particularly evident in oncology and remains the case to some extent today (Beauchamp & Childress, 2001; Graber, 1998; Monagle; Pence). However, the emergence of patient autonomy over traditional paternalism and the involvement of several outsiders in previously private decisions between the patient and HCP reflect some of the factors leading to the rise in ethical issues in advancing illness (American Cancer Society, 2004; Ersek, Scanlon, Glass, Ferrell, & Steeves, 1995; Ferrell & Rivera, 1995; Gruber, 1998; O'Donnell, 2004).

Ageism in the healthcare management of the older adult with cancer is substantiated in several ways, including limited representation of older adults in clinical trials, provider attitudes about the intensity of care, and symptom and disease management. Hutchins, Unger, Crowley, Coltman, and Albain (1999) compared 16,396 patients with breast cancer with the general population in a Southwest Oncology Group clinical trial. Findings suggested that incidence data for clinical trial participation were the same for those younger than age 65, but researchers identified significant underrepresentation in those older than age 65. In another study of the effect of less than definitive care on breast cancer outcomes, Lash, Silliman, Guadagnoli, and Mor (2000) found that older women consistently received less than definitive care and were more likely to have disease recurrence identified at death. In a review of published reports of investigations and treatment of cancer in older adults, Turner, Haward, Mulley, and Selby (1999) noted discrepancies between cancer incidence in the older adult and the amount of investigational opportunities and treatment. The study also noted that some older adult patients could tolerate cancer treatment as well as younger patients, reinforcing the need for a consistent method of minimizing generalizations within this population. As a result of these and other study findings, future clinical trial recommendations include increased representation of this high-risk population (Hutchins et al.; Jaklitsch et al., 1999; Lash et al.) and more age-based studies in order to explain responses to cancer treatment and determine more individualized management strategies (Ault, 2003; Balducci & Yates, 2000; Dale, 2003; Ershler, 2003). Careful assessment and consideration of the unique physical, emotional, and spiritual needs and values of older adults would facilitate informed decision making by all parties.

Current recommendations by the National Comprehensive Cancer Network (NCCN, 2005) include the use of a comprehensive geriatric assessment (CGA) tool for older adults with cancer (Balducci & Yates, 2000; NCCN). Functional status, comorbid conditions, and personal and social resources must be considered in order to provide appropriate, individualized care. Many older adults have physical, social, cultural, or financial limitations or restrictions that affect their ability to fully understand, seek out, and receive comprehensive health care. Certain reversible conditions such as depression may be discovered during a CGA. Addressing and treating such conditions can facilitate cancer treatment and improve quality of life.

By 2030, an estimated 80% of long-term care will be provided in the home (Binstock, 1998; Ershler, 2003; Given & Given, 1996; Glajchen, 2004; Graber, 1998; Stone & Kemper, 1989). Technologic advances have provided opportunities for prolongation of life and transition of cancer to a chronic disease; however, receiving high-tech care at home increases stressors not only for the care recipient but also for all members of the household (Nevidjon, 2004; Pence, 2004). More than 13 million adults in the United States who have older adult parents are potentially providers of long-term care, financial assistance, and emotional support. As the children become the caregivers and the parents become the care recipients, the potential for conflict increases. Adult children who have relied on their parents for personal support find themselves supporting their parents. The role reversal can be painful and may involve conflicting values and obligations among patients, families, and HCPs.

Cancer has become a chronic illness often associated with conflicts concerning quality of life, family dynamics, communication patterns, life-sustaining treatment, and palliative care. The goal of nursing is to provide care in a compassionate and individualized manner. Patients, family members, and caregivers often experience distress related to ethical issues and decision making during the cancer trajectory (Erlen, 2001; Jameton, 1993). As a result, sensitivity to value conflicts in decision making in advanced illness is important, especially in the areas of communication and disclosure (Elger & Harding, 2002; O'Donnell, 2004). Advances in technology and information gathering and limitations on inpatient care have increased family and other informal caregivers' participation in seeking out HCPs who encourage shared decision making. However, lack of time and attitudes still undermine shared decision making (White, Keller, & Horrigan, 2003). As a result, difficult decisions will continue to increase, and HCPs must be prepared to take a more assertive role in guiding and supporting patients, families, and colleagues.

Ethical and Legal Principles

Ethics is a study of patterns of values and norms based on personal history, morals, and beliefs. It is a branch of philosophy also called moral philosophy. Ethics offers a critical, rational, defensible, systematic, and intellectual approach to determining what is best or "right" in a difficult situation. Many laws are based on four ethical principles that include beneficence, autonomy, nonmaleficence, and justice (see Table 24-1). The law reflects societal views and essentially attempts to legislate morality. Both ethics and the law offer guidance in deciding the "right" thing to do. Ethical principles are universal and seem very general, but, when understood in the light of a particular person's situation and existing legal statutes, can guide the moral decision-making process (Beauchamp & Childress, 2001; Flynn, 1997; Monagle, 1998; Pence, 2004).

Table 24-1. Definitions of Ethical Principles

Principle	Definition	Application
Autonomy	Independent deci-sion making	Advocate for expressed desires and preferences; initiate early intervention with use of resources and progressive care; support sense of identity and independence; educate about treatment and care options.
Beneficence	Duty to act in the best interest of the patient	Promote good outcomes; consider options and expecta-tions. Advocate for disease and treatment information; support decision making; and include the patient and family in the process.
Nonmaleficence	Duty to do no harm	Follow standards and guidelines to avoid excessive or unnec-essary care. Support patient decisions about treatment alter-natives; provide palliative care and symptom management.
Justice	Distributing ben-efits, risks, and costs fairly	Promote equality in individual welfare; support fair alloca-tion of resources and access to care based on medical criteria.

Note. Based on information from Beauchamp & Childress, 2001.

Addressing Ethical and Legal Dilemmas in the Older Adult

Ethics are based on value systems, which are specific to the individual. A consistent method for developing and selecting options can be helpful in minimizing distress arising from moral dilemma or conflict (Duhamel & Dupuis, 2004; Monagle, 1998; Rowe, 2004). Strategies to address these problems include appreciating the holistic needs of the older person with cancer and focusing on goals of care and shared decision making. Principles of bioethics and various legal concepts can guide in this endeavor. Charon (2004) stated that ethics include the possession of the "set of skills required to recognize, absorb, interpret and be moved by the stories one reads or hears" (p. 862). Relating to the patient on a personal level and truly hearing his or her story is the best approach to understanding the unique needs of that individual. Engaging significant others in the conversation also can help to promote understand-ing and participation (Becchetti, 2003).

A number of models are available to guide ethical decision making (see Table 24-2). Indications for choosing a model include user-friendliness, time constraints, and personal preference. For example, the Quadrant Model (Jonsen, Siegler, & Winslade, 2002) addresses four basic areas to review when confronted with an ethi-cal situation, including medical indications, patient preferences, quality of life, and contextual features. Regardless of the model selected, it is vital to consider the best interest of the individual, caregiver issues, the obligations of the HCPs, contributing factors, and the environment.

Case Study and Discussion

The case study describes an older adult male as he finds his life changing from one of independent living among his circle of friends, family, and community to his

Table 24-2. Examples of Models for Ethical Decision Making

Model	Description
Quadrant Model (Jonsen et al., 2002)	Information is compiled in four basic areas: medical indications, patient preferences, quality of life, and contextual features.
Bioethical decision model (Thompson & Thompson, 1992)	Information is compiled using a 10-step formula (similar to the nursing process) in which the user is asked to review the situation, gather additional information, identify ethical issues, identify personal and professional values, identify the values of key individuals, identify any value conflicts, determine who should make decisions, identify the range of actions and anticipated outcomes, decide and implement a course of action, and evaluate the results.
Ethics case analysis (Bioethics Consultation Group, 1992)	Burdens and benefits of the decision are viewed from the perspective of each interested party and then ranked by relevance to the patient. All principal players are considered.

reluctant acceptance of lifestyle changes resulting from a steady deterioration of health and functional status. The depicted ethical dilemma of conflicting values is common in this population as he, his family, and HCPs attempt to balance his desire for independence while complying with personal and professional obligations to support his safety and best interests. The ethical principles of autonomy and beneficence will be discussed as they apply to the case study, highlighting issues of communication and decision making in advanced illness.

Case Study

Mr. K is an 82-year-old man who lives alone in his home since his wife of 53 years died five years ago. He is independent in activities of daily living and active in his church and with friends. In recent months, macular degeneration has made it increasingly difficult to drive after dark. He has five adult children, one of whom lives in a neighboring town with her husband and two children. The others live in cities on the same coast and visit throughout the year.

Mr. K has a history of prostate cancer, which was treated with radiation therapy 10 years ago. He also has a history of hypertension, chronic obstructive pulmonary disease, and peripheral vascular disease. He recently has developed renal insufficiency, which his primary care physician attributes to probable prostate cancer progression. No specific treatment of the possible metastases has been recommended, as he has no physical complaints at this time.

On his way home from church one evening, Mr. K runs off the road and totals his car, but survives with only a broken wrist (dominant hand) and a bruised body and ego. A friend meets him at the emergency room and then takes him home. Mr. K calls his daughter in the morning and asks that she come help him to get things organized. They set up a plan for her to come over on a daily basis to assist him. He agrees to allow his nearby daughter durable power of attorney for financial matters only. Thus begins a change in both of their lifestyles, as Mr. K can no longer drive, write his name, or perform routine hygiene.

Mr. K is concerned about his physical limitations and is distressed at this new level of dependence he is experiencing. His arm heals, but his automobile insurance company refuses to insure him, so he no longer has his accustomed mobility. His neighbors (also in their 80s) help him with his daily activities and drive him to the doctor and grocery store. In his mind, life has settled into relative normalcy. Issues for his family are the desire to comply with his wishes and promote his independence while ensuring his safety.

Mr. K's daughter calls her sister, an oncology nurse, and tells her that their father "isn't acting right" and is sometimes confused. The neighbor mentions that during a recent office visit, the doctor told him that Mr. K's lab results were a little "out of kilter" and that adjustments had been made in his medications. The oncology nurse/daughter comes to town, speaks with the physician, and finds out her father's sodium is low and calcium is high (both of which can contribute to changes in behavior and mentation). She stays until Mr. K and his repeat tests show improvement. The daughters have a sense of impending doom but are hesitant to suggest any change to their father. They discuss the situation with their siblings, who agree to visit soon, not thinking anything dramatic is happening as their father has recovered from similar problems in the past.

The oncology nurse/daughter gets home on Friday evening and her sister calls Sunday morning. Mr. K is in the hospital, having fallen in the kitchen the night before. This is a pivotal event for the family because tests now confirm bone metastases and further deterioration of his kidney function. Mr. K receives medication for acute pain related to the fall, but the medical team does not initiate discussion about the advancing illness and potential treatment and supportive care options.

The entire family now recognizes that Mr. K cannot go back home to live alone and begins to discuss options among themselves. Attempts to include Mr. K in the discussion are unsuccessful, as he does not want to consider any options but returning to his home and declines attending a planned conference with the family and hospital case manager. At the daughters' request, the primary care physician mentions to Mr. K that he may need to think of other options after this hospitalization, but Mr. K does not respond positively to his suggestion.

During the care conference, the hospital case manager suggests that the family visit assisted living facilities with progressive care options in the area. When the oncology nurse/daughter reviews the conference suggestions with Mr. K, he becomes angry, insisting they had not mentioned this conference to him and declares they are planning his life without his input. After a cool down period, Mr. K acknowledges that he might have forgotten, as he did not want to attend anyway. Mr. K, a former chemical engineer, "list maker," and independent individual, sits with his oncology nurse/daughter and makes a list of desirable qualities to look for in the potential living facilities.

Eventually, Mr. K chooses to move to a small assisted living facility located within a mile of his home and church. His children had investigated several locations, one of which was closer to the nearby daughter, but opted for this one because of its size, location, services, his preferences, and "gut feeling." At his request, the house is kept as he left it. He has planned for retirement, does not want to live with his children, and calculates that he has enough money to manage both the house and assisted living quarters for the next five years. The family moves his favorite chair and some personal items to his new room.

Mr. K keeps up with his friends, who continue to drive him to appointments and church services, and slowly becomes acclimated to his new living arrangements. He grows to enjoy sharing stories with one of the staff members but gradually seems to lose interest in going too far from his bed. All five children visit during the late summer. One evening they go out to dinner and he later mentions that it "didn't seem to sit well." He goes to bed feeling sick and, in the middle of the night, he wakes up with chest pains and shortness of breath and is taken back to the hospital.

Mr. K had a myocardial infarction. He is in congestive heart failure, but is stabilized within 24 hours. His children talk with the physician and case manager about what they believe are their father's preferences concerning resuscitation and end-of-life care. Mr. K is discouraged about needing continuous oxygen and the pain in his back is getting worse. He does not want to take too much pain medicine, but he cannot find a comfortable position, and it is getting harder to breathe. He still has not signed the papers about the living will, but he states he is getting very weary of all these problems and maybe it is time to get some rest. Any exertion, mental or physical, is just too much. After discussion with Mr. K and his daughter, the primary care physician writes the do not resuscitate (DNR) order in the chart.

All five children call that week, and Mr. K has his weekly visit with his priest. Mr. K is feeling better and plans to go back to the assisted living facility in the morning. As he is talking to his younger son on Wednesday, Mr. K mentions seeing his wife and mother (both dead years ago) that evening. His son is surprised by this and questions Mr. K, who says he must have been dreaming or just thinking about them.

The chest pain comes back during the night, and Mr. K calls for some pain medication. The nurse tells him she will be there soon but will be delayed with an emergency. She can send someone else. He says he can wait. When she goes to the room, he is dead.

Discussion

Ethical dilemmas stem from a conflict between values and obligations. In an effort to adhere to what is believed to be in the best interest of the patient, professional and societal obligations and expectations may be encountered, which may lead to moral distress or immobilization. The Quadrant Model (Jonsen et al., 2002) was selected as an example of how a model can guide ethical decision making about the living arrangements described in the case study (see Figure 24-1). These and other decisions are guided by general ethical principles, such as autonomy and beneficence, and can be applied to the case study. As in real life, ethical principles are not absolute, often overlap, and assume different priorities. The following discussion will further expand on the ethical principles of autonomy and beneficence and incorporate relevant legal issues with some applications from the case study.

Autonomy

Autonomy: auto = self; nomos = law, governance

Autonomy is defined as self-rule, self-determination, free choice, and independent decision making. Autonomy is a sense of control of life and self and supports

Medical indications

Based on current and past medical history, how can the patient benefit from medical and nursing care while avoiding harm?

Active treatment for Mr. K's bony metastases has not been discussed. Comorbidities include hypertension, chronic obstructive pulmonary disease, renal insufficiency, congestive heart failure, and peripheral vascular disease. He has a recent history of a fractured wrist as a result of a motor vehicle accident and has been hospitalized since a fall at his home. He takes multiple medications and requires continuous oxygen. He would benefit from being in assisted living where his medications, pain management, oxygen, nutrition, and physical care would be monitored. The potential for injury from another fall would be minimized.

Patient preferences

Is the right to choose being respected?

Mr. K would rather be home, but does not want live-in assistance or to live with his children. Although initially reluctant to consider other options, he finally agrees to participate in the decision process concerning the choice of an assisted-living facility based on his list of preferences.

Considering that Mr. K is experiencing intermittent cognitive impairment, which impacts his decision-making capacity, a surrogate decision maker should be identified and included in the discussion.

Quality of life

What is the patient's assessment of his quality of life? Can the patient be expected to return to a desirable style of life based on his values? Is palliative care being incorporated into the care plan?

Based on Mr. K's values and preferences, assisted living is the more desirable situation, as he is now unable to drive and is dependent on others. He will still see friends and family, but his meals will be prepared; he will have company and physical assistance. Palliative care, including symptom management, is the goal throughout the illness trajectory, but this has not been discussed with all principal parties (Mr. K, family, and healthcare provider). Pain management is limited to as-needed meds. Palliative chemotherapy, bisphosphonates, or radiation options have not been discussed with the patient or family. Deteriorating renal function may be a contributing factor for decisions about foregoing certain treatments.

Contextual features

What environmental issues (family, facility, financial, cultural, access) impact the situation?

Paternalism, support of family, friends, staff, spirituality, stoicism, and independence of patient are all factors to consider. The most important issue for Mr. K and his family is the proximity of home, church, friends, doctor, and family to the assisted living facility, which allows him to maintain his connections with life and some sense of control. Mr. K has sufficient financial resources to manage his living arrangements.

Figure 24-1. Application of the Quadrant Model of Ethical Decision Making

principles of confidentiality, informed consent, and advance directives (Beauchamp & Childress, 2001; Graber, 1998; Monagle, 1998; Pence, 2004). Autonomy involves two conditions: (a) freedom from controlling influences and (b) capacity for independent action. The obligations of the HCP related to autonomy are to be truthful, provide respect and confidentiality, obtain consent, and assist with decision making (O'Donnell, 2004). Human beings strive for control of self and, although illness and age can cause this ability to be diminished, the desire for independence may remain. Erikson (1964) described the stage of development for the older adult as that of ego integrity versus despair. According to Erikson, achievement of this stage requires reflection upon and acceptance of one's life accomplishments in order to attain a sense of fulfillment. As the individual ages, he has the right to expect to be treated with dignity and allowed some control of his life (American Cancer Society, 2004; Sheridan, 2000).

As illustrated in the case study, the HCP and family are concerned for Mr. K's safety because of his history of a recent fall and intermittent periods of confusion. They feel he is not able to live alone. Mr. K wants to remain independent and continue to live alone. He refuses to participate in a family conference and rejects initial suggestions from his physician to consider alternative living arrangements. Additional involvement and communication from the HCP would help to better prepare Mr. K during this transition. Discussing the patient's values and wishes and frank discussions of Mr. K's advancing illness and likely complications would improve communication and assist in the decision-making process.

Several legal constructs also affect care and decision making for the older adult and are supported by the ethical principle of autonomy. These include informed consent, competency, and advance directives.

Informed Consent

Autonomy establishes the right of the patient to determine the nature of his or her medical care. Respect for autonomy is the moral basis for the legal notion of informed consent. A corollary to informed consent is the right of a competent adult to refuse or receive treatment (Birke, 2004; Hetzler, Marting, Powell, & Scott, 2004).

By definition, consent is a legal process used to promote patient autonomy. Informed consent includes a discussion about the specific nature, purpose, risks, and benefits of intervention, alternatives, and an option of no treatment prior to implementing a proposed treatment. Informed consent is required when some degree of risk exists and is followed by explicit agreement or refusal. Procedurally, informed consent is a formal process that institutions require before permitting procedures and usually requires patient or surrogate written consent. Ethically, informed consent is the autonomous authorization of a medical intervention. Legally, informed consent is a conversation between a patient and HCP about a proposed treatment, nontreatment, alternative treatments, and risks and benefits of each. Simple consent is an explanation of a low-risk intervention, followed by patient agreement or refusal (implied or expressed). Other elements are present when appropriate (risk, benefit, alternatives) (Birke, 2004; Whitney, McGuire, & McCullough, 2003).

In the case study, had treatment and supportive care options and goals of care been discussed, Mr. K and his family would have been better prepared to make informed decisions and to anticipate complications of his advanced illness. For example, Mr. K may have benefited from earlier initiation of supportive and palliative care, such as home health care, visiting nurses, or hospice referral. The physician chose to treat only those symptoms as mentioned by Mr. K. Without a discussion of all the burdens and benefits of care options and understanding on his part, Mr. K did not have the opportunity to make a choice or give informed consent.

Competency and Capacity

Competency and capacity are similar concepts used in determining the ability of an adult to make decisions about and manage personal affairs. Competency is a legal decision based on capability and is determined by the courts. Capacity is the basis for informed consent and is the responsibility of the HCP to determine four factors: understanding of treatment benefits and risks, appreciation of the situation, reasoning, and consistent expression of choice or decision (Beauchamp & Childress, 2001; Birke, 2004; Hetzler et al., 2004). The patient's capacity for decision making is often a key concern in ethical dilemmas arising in the older adult with advanced illness (O'Donnell, 2004). HCPs often assess decision-making capacity to guide medical treatment, choice of living arrangements, or assist in competency determination. However, capacity is a fragile entity in the older person and subject to fluctuations because of a variety of events or situations, such as medications, illness, complications of progressive disease, or time of day. The ability to make independent decisions also may vary depending on the task or situation being discussed (Birke).

As in the case of Mr. K, the capacity of an individual may change during the day, shift, or hour based on emotions, mentation, treatment status, level of understanding, and complexity of decision. When his electrolytes were abnormal, Mr. K became confused. During his hospitalization, he denied knowledge of any request for his participation in decisions and became disproportionately angry. He later admitted delayed recollection exemplifying that a change of environment can lead to disorientation in the older adult. Mr. K had multiple issues—illness, electrolyte imbalance, trauma, change in environment, sensory overload, and probable sleep deprivation—all of which contributed to his questionable and fluctuating decision-making capacity. Despite some intermittent periods of confusion, Mr. K was able to make decisions after receiving guidance from his HCP and daughter.

Advance Directives

The Patient Self-Determination Act (PSDA) of 1991 is the first federal legislation to address the rights of healthcare decision making and the rights of the individuals to refuse or accept treatment and execute advance directives. The PSDA requires many Medicare and Medicaid providers (hospitals, nursing homes, hospice programs, home health agencies, and health maintenance organizations) to give adult individuals, at the time of inpatient admission or enrollment, particular information about their rights under state laws governing advance directives, including (a) the right to participate in and direct their own healthcare decisions, (b) the right to accept or refuse medical or surgical treatment, (c) the right to prepare an advance directive, (d) information on the provider's policies that govern the utilization of these rights. The act also prohibits institutions from discriminating against a patient who does not have an advance directive. The PSDA further requires institutions to document patient information and provide ongoing community education on advance directives.

The moral obligation of supporting patients' rights to self-determination and doing no harm includes recognizing the need to give appropriate care as well as abide by patients' desires. *Advance directives* is the general term for a variety of written documents recognized under state law that allow competent individuals to make healthcare decision-making plans prior to future incapacity, including terminal illness. For example, a *living will* is a written document addressed to the HCP reflecting the expressed desires of the patient concerning life-sustaining treatment.

Ideally, situations involving health care should be driven by shared decision making between the patient and HCP. However, in cases of incapacitation, another person may be designated to make decisions on behalf of the person or act as a surrogate and represent his or her best interests. The surrogate gives or refuses consent to treatment options recommended by the HCP, who has the obligation to provide information and guidance. *Durable power of attorney for health care* is a written document that covers all types of healthcare decisions. A surrogate is identified who will make decisions based on patient (principle) desires, which may be in writing or based on prior knowledge of the patient's values and preferences. *Durable power of attorney for finances* is a written document in which the patient gives authority to an individual to make financial decisions. This document may be general or specific (Birke, 2004; Hetzler et al., 2004).

Most institutions are meticulous in distributing the information, but as reflected in the case study, not as efficient in facilitating their completion. Earlier communications by the physician and other HCP may have facilitated more timely decisions regarding advance directives. Mr. K would have benefited from early intervention and education about advance directives and the goals of care. Frank discussion of his values and preferences prior to a crisis event might have helped the family to better prepare for his declining health (American Bar Association, 2004; Ascension Health, 2004; Birke, 2004; Hetzler et al., 2004). The delay in finalizing Mr. K's wishes seems to imply that Mr. K may not have fully understood the potential complications of his advancing illness. Further, Mr. K also may have been too overwhelmed and in need of additional time to consider this decision. HCP discussions focusing on the goals of care and incorporating Mr. K's priorities would likely facilitate the decision-making process.

Beneficence

Beneficence: bene = well; facere = to do

Beneficence is defined as the duty to "do good" or active kindness. HCPs have the duty or moral obligation to provide compassionate, appropriate, culturally sensitive care in an environment supportive of the patient. Establishing meaningful connections with the patients and family allows them to feel more secure and comfortable in the environment. Beneficence is to act in the best interest of the patient while considering the benefits of treatment against the costs and risks. Because values determine the assessment of costs, benefits, and risks (Beauchamp & Childress, 2001), they need to be considered in decisions about care. Therefore, beneficence may involve spending extra time with the patient and family to provide information and reassurance and to assess the patient's values and preferences. In cases where autonomy is compromised and a surrogate is designated, the surrogate is mandated to act in what is believed to be the patient's best interest considering previously stated values and goals.

Although advance directives are associated with the domain of autonomy or self-determination, early discussion and support by a trusted HCP is a beneficent act. Unfortunately, many HCPs are uncomfortable with such discussions because of emotional response, lack of time, or discomfort with the topic (Bradley et al., 2001; Feldman, Novack, & Gracely, 1998). For example, in a content analysis of documents produced during the SUPPORT (Study to Understand Prognosis and Preferences for Outcomes and Risks of Treatment) study, investigators found that nurses delivering the intervention felt inadequately prepared in grief theory and also perceived that they could not bring the patients and families to a state of readiness (Murphy, Price, Stevens, Lynn, & Kathryn, 2001). Various authors suggested the need for retraining and mentoring to guide HCPs in overcoming these difficulties (Bradley et al.; Reb, 2003; Weiner & Cole, 2004).

The principle of beneficence often competes with the principle of respect for autonomy, particularly in the older adult (e.g., when the patient makes a decision that the HCP believes is not in his or her best interest). Whether autonomy of patients should have priority over beneficence has become a central issue in ethics (see Beauchamp & Childress, 2001, for further discussion). From a legal perspective, the wishes of the competent patient cannot be overridden, even in what others consider his or her best interest (Beauchamp & Childress; Graber, 1998; Hetzler et al., 2004; Monagle & Thomasma, 1998; Pence, 2004). However, discussions focusing on patient values and goals of care may help to resolve these conflicts and guide the patient and family in the decision-making process. The care plan should reflect an understanding of the patient's and family's preferences, goals, needs, and available resources. An ongoing discussion facilitates communication and patient involvement in decision-making because preferences or goals of care may change as the disease progresses (Ingham, 2000).

As portrayed in the case study, Mr. K's functional status deteriorated rapidly after his accident and also was reflective of progression of his prostate cancer. Beneficence was germane as he and his children tried to balance his desire for independence with their concern for his best interests (safety, physical care, quality of life). Mr. K's concept of best interest was to go home and continue to live alone, but the family and HCP had serious doubts about his safety and ability to care for himself in light of his advancing illness. The physician gave little direction or information to the family, perhaps in the interest of patient confidentiality. The hospital case manager involved the family in decision making about options for living arrangements, but, unfortunately, Mr. K refused to participate. As Mr. K's mental status began to fluctuate, the family was left with little direct guidance about his wishes.

In the case of Mr. K, his physician did not pursue further treatment for his metastatic disease but provided some pain management. In view of Mr. K's multiple health problems, this may have been the best course to "do no harm," but this was not clearly communicated to the patient or his family. By not discussing the plan with the family, they were deprived of the opportunity to support each other and their father more effectively. Had the situation been understood before his accident, they may have been able to access homecare assistance and perhaps avoid the subsequent fall and Mr. K's sense of being a burden as they hurriedly relocated him to an assisted living facility. Although Mr. K's fluctuating mental status was an impeding factor, ongoing communications with both patient and family would help to minimize distress, provide an opportunity for explicit understanding of Mr. K's preferences, and perhaps facilitate the family's recognition of the limited time they had to share with him (Brennan, 2004).

Nursing Care Issues

Ethical issues are complex, and the best course of action may not always be clear. Difficulties lie in morally valid but conflicting duties, obligations, and choices. Senge (1994) described a Ladder of Influence, stating that beliefs affect what data are identified as important. Therefore, when considering an ethical dilemma or experiencing distress, nurses should recognize the impact of personal beliefs, values, and biases on the situation and consider other perspectives before making a decision. Input from objective others such as ethics team members, social workers, and other experienced colleagues is essential (Pence, 2004; Thomasma, 2001) and will guide nurses in supporting patients and families in the decision-making process.

The healthcare system provides limited support to caregivers. Medicare reform is needed for case management and supportive care options other than hospice (Bogardus, Geist, & Bradley, 2004; McCabe, 1993; Pence, 2004; Reb, 2003). HCPs play an essential role in assisting this expanding group of informal caregivers. An early trust relationship can be invaluable when the time comes to discuss end-of-life and other difficult issues in advancing illness (Duhamel & Dupuis, 2004; Haley, 2003). No easy recipe exists for the right thing to say at any given time, but the patient and family will recognize and appreciate practical suggestions and the sense of connection, compassion, and respect (Coyle & Sculco, 2004; Duhamel & Dupuis; Rowe, 2004).

Although ethical decision making is integrated into most nursing programs, many nurses believe they are not adequately prepared to guide patients and families (Duhamel & Dupuis, 2004; Scanlon, 1994). An environment in which autonomy, professional practice, and collaboration are valued can minimize moral distress related to seemingly unworkable problems (Erlen, 2001). For that reason, the Joint Commission on Accreditation of Healthcare Organizations (JCAHO) requires that any HCP or family be able to request an ethics consultation within his or her institution for assistance both in evaluating the decision-making and problem-resolving capacity of an individual and to protect the patient's rights (JCAHO, 2002).

When patients, families, surrogates, HCPs, or other involved parties are uncertain or in conflict regarding value-laden issues related to health care, an ethics consult may be helpful. Ethics committees can act as resources in triage, facilitate decision making, and provide guidance as an objective observer (O'Donnell, 2004). Too often, the request for the input from the ethics committee is retrospective. In the current high-tech environment, involved parties may be better served by the early identification of and intervention with high-risk patients or families, rather than waiting until the crisis is imminent or has occurred. Figure 24-2 provides a list of general suggestions for ethical situations that may facilitate initial recognition and decision making.

---

1. Ask yourself the right questions.
    a. Consider the facts. Find relevant research.
    b. Identify what values are at risk. Describe the values of the patient, family, healthcare provider, staff, institution, and society that apply to the presenting dilemma.
    c. Define the principal conflict between the identified values and professional norms and beliefs.
2. List the possible courses of action.
    a. Which values and ethical principles does each course embody or violate?
    b. What is the burden and benefit of each course of action?
3. Make a decision and defend the course of action that the decision implies.
4. Evaluate the outcome for all involved.
5. Share yourself and your feelings with colleagues.
    a. Develop a trusting and supportive work group.
    b. Discuss the issues before they become overwhelming.
    c. Recognize that everyone identifies with some patients more than others, making objectivity more difficult.

Figure 24-2. General Suggestions for Ethical Decision Making

Note. Based on information from Beauchamps & Childress, 2001; Cassells et al., 2003.

Advocacy

HCPs have unique opportunities in patient advocacy as well as the fundamental responsibility to adhere to national, state, and institutional standards of the profession (Oncology Nursing Society [ONS], 2005). The International Council of Nurses (2000) Code of Ethics provides a framework of ethical standards for the professional nurse in relation to people, practice, the profession, and colleagues. Involvement of nurses and other HCPs in multidisciplinary ethics committees, assisting in clarifying issues concerning access to care, communications, quality of life, and support to patient, family, and colleagues can generate personal and professional growth. The caregiver can help to translate the story told by the patient into basic ethical principles before conclusions are made. Maximizing resources such as professional and institutional guidelines, ethics committees, and collegial relationships facilitates the inclusion of all principal players and increases the likelihood of acceptable and appropriate resolution for the patient (Belde, Kinlaw, Kraweicki, & Trotochaud, 2004; Brody, 1997).

Education

The HCP is the primary resource for the patient and family in terms of information gathering and reality-based understanding. Assistance in navigating the healthcare system and locating reliable educational and community resources are ways to guide the patient and family in the decision-making process. The preferred decision is that which is best for the patient with consideration of his or her particular wants and needs but must be put in perspective with the burdens (to a family unit) or risks (physical or emotional harm) involved. Honest discussion of the goals of care and assessment of values and preferences based on understanding and trust will minimize confusion and unrealistic expectations (Cassell, 1982, 1991; Thomasma, 1987, 2001). From a legal perspective, the wishes of the competent patient cannot be overridden even in what others consider his or her best interest; so early and clear communication is critical (Beauchamp & Childress, 2001; Graber, 1998; Hetzler et al., 2004; Monagle & Thomasma, 1998; Pence, 2004).

Research Priorities

Legal and ethical conflicts will continue to exist and present themselves to HCPs on a daily basis. With heightened awareness of the dynamics of aging, better communications, and early recognition of value-laden conflicts, HCPs can be better prepared to participate in the resolution of these issues. Priorities for research include age-based studies to more accurately represent this population and guide cancer care; practical educational offerings for HCPs concerning communication, conflict resolution, and ethical decision making; and directed studies of the impact of early identification and intervention with patients and families at high risk for ethical conflict.

Conclusion

In caring for the older adult with cancer, oncology nurses will face ethical and legal issues on a daily basis because of the projected increase in the aging population with cancer and the complexity in caring for an individual with numerous physical and social issues. As the case study depicted, the older adult may possess comorbidities and functional impairments that can impact oncology treatment decisions. In addition, social factors such as limited resources and family and caregiver support must be incorporated into the plan of care. An awareness of ethical and legal principles and thorough, ongoing discussion regarding the patient's condition, treatment options, and advanced directives will facilitate shared decision making among the HCP, patient, and caregivers. Focusing on the goals of care and sensitivity to the patient's and family's values will enhance quality, evidence-based care for this unique population. With this approach, ethical and legal dilemmas may be minimized.

The author wishes to acknowledge the support, review, and comments of her family, Kathleen Kinlaw, M. Div., Director, Center for Ethics, and Program Director, Health Sciences Ethics at Emory University, Atlanta, GA, and Patricia O'Donnell, DSW, LICSW, Director, Center for Ethics, Inova Health System, Springfield, VA.

References

American Bar Association. (2004). *Law for older Americans. Health care advance directives.* Retrieved November 30, 2004, from http://www.abanet.org/publiced/practical/patient_self_determination_act.html

American Cancer Society. (2004). *Cancer facts and figures, 2004.* Atlanta, GA: Author.

Ascension Health. (2004). *Healthcare ethics. Patient self-determination act.* Retrieved November 30, 2004, from http://www.ascensionhealth.org/ethics/public/issues/patient_self.asp

Ault, A. (2003). Older cancer patients should be offered full treatment range. *Lancet, 362,* 808.

Balducci, L., & Yates, J. (2000). General guidelines for the management of older patients with cancer. *Oncology, 14,* 221–227.

Beauchamp, T.L., & Childress, J.F. (2001). *Principles of biomedical ethics* (5th ed.). New York: Oxford University Press.

Becchetti, R. (2003). Difficult conversations. *Oncology Issues, 18,* 36–39.

Belde, D., Kinlaw, K., Kraweicki, N., & Trotochaud, K. (2004, September). *Advanced workshop in ethics case consultation.* Symposium conducted by Healthcare Ethics Consortium of Georgia, Atlanta.

Binstock, R.H. (1998). Older people and long term care: Issues of access. In J. Monagle & D. Thomasma (Eds.), *Health care ethics: Critical issues for the 21st century* (pp. 177–188). Gaithersburg, MD: Aspen.

Bioethics Consultation Group. (1992). *Forming a moral community: A resource for healthcare ethics committees.* Berkeley, CA: General Printing.

Birke, M. (2004). Elder law, Medicare, and legal issues in older patients. *Seminars in Oncology, 31,* 282–292.

Bogardus, S.T., Geist, D.E., & Bradley, E.H. (2004). Physicians' interactions with third-party payers: Is deception necessary? *Archives of Internal Medicine, 164,* 1841–1844.

Boyle, D.A. (2003). Cancer in the elderly: Key facts. *Oncology Supportive Care Quarterly, 2,* 6–21.

Bradley, E.H., Cherlin, E., McCorkle, R., Fried, T.R., Kasl, S.V., Cicchetti, D.V., et al. (2001). Nurses' use of palliative care practices in the acute setting. *Journal of Professional Nursing, 17,* 14–22.

Brennan, J. (2004). *Cancer in context: A practical guide to supportive care.* New York: Oxford University Press.

Brody, H. (1997). Who gets to tell the story? Narrative in postmodern ethics. In H.L. Nelson (Ed.), *Stories and their limits: Narrative approaches to bioethics* (pp. 18–30). New York: Routledge Press.

Cassell, E.J. (1982). The nature of suffering and the goals of medicine. *New England Journal of Medicine, 306,* 639–645.

Cassell, E.J. (1991). *The nature of suffering and the goals of medicine.* New York: Oxford University Press.

Cassells, J.M., Jenkins, J., Lea, D.H., Calzone, K., & Johnson, E. (2003). An ethical assessment framework for addressing global genetic issues in clinical practice. *Oncology Nursing Forum, 30,* 383–390.

Charon, R. (2004). Narrative and medicine. *New England Journal of Medicine, 350,* 862–864.

Coyle, N., & Sculco, L. (2004). Expressed desire for hastened death in seven patients living with advanced cancer: A phenomenologic inquiry. *Oncology Nursing Forum, 31,* 699–706.

Dale, D.C. (2003). Poor prognosis in elderly patients with cancer: The role of bias and undertreatment. *Journal of Supportive Oncology, 1*(Suppl. 2), 11–17.

Duhamel, F., & Dupuis, F. (2004). Guaranteed returns: Investing in conversations with families of patients with cancer. *Clinical Journal of Oncology Nursing, 8,* 68–70.

Elger, B.S., & Harding, T.W. (2002). Should cancer patients be informed about their diagnosis and prognosis? Future doctors and lawyers differ. *Journal of Medical Ethics, 28,* 258–296.

Erikson, E.H. (1964). *Childhood and society* (2nd ed.). New York: Norton.

Erlen, J.A. (2001). Moral distress: A pervasive problem. *Orthopaedic Nursing, 20,* 76–80.

Ersek, M., Scanlon, C., Glass, E., Ferrell, B.R., & Steeves, R. (1995). Priority ethical issues in oncology nursing: Current approaches and future directions. *Oncology Nursing Forum, 22,* 803–807.

Ershler, W.B. (2003). Cancer: A disease of the elderly. *Journal of Supportive Oncology, 1*(Suppl. 2), 5–10.

Feldman, D.S., Novack, D.H., & Gracely, E. (1998). Effects of managed care on physician-patient relationships, quality of care, and the ethical practice of medicine: A physician survey. *Archives of Internal Medicine, 158,* 1626–1632.

Ferrell, B.R., & Rivera, L.M. (1995). Ethical decision making in oncology: A case study approach. *Cancer Practice, 3,* 94–99.

Flynn, E.P. (1997). *Issues in medical ethics.* Kansas City, MO: Sheed & Ward.

Given, B., & Given, C.W. (1996). Family caregiver burden from cancer care. In R. McCorkle, M. Grant, M. Frank-Stromberg, & S.B. Baird (Eds.), *Cancer nursing: A comprehensive textbook* (2nd ed., pp. 93–109). Philadelphia: Saunders.

Glajchen, M. (2004). The emerging role and needs of family caregivers in cancer care. *Journal of Supportive Oncology, 2,* 145–155.

Graber, G.C. (1998). Basic theories in medical ethics. In J. Monagle & D. Thomasma (Eds.), *Health care ethics: Critical issues for the 21st century* (pp. 515–526). Gaithersburg, MD: Aspen.

Gruber, A. (1998). Social systems and professional responsibility. In J. Monagle & D. Thomasma (Eds.), *Health care ethics: Critical issues for the 21st century* (pp. 392–397). Gaithersburg, MD: Aspen.

Haley, W. (2003). Family caregivers of elderly patients with cancer: Understanding and minimizing the burden of care. *Journal of Supportive Oncology, 1*(Suppl. 2), 25–29.

Hetzler, D., Marting, A., Powell, P., & Scott, C. (2004, November). *Healthcare ethics and the law.* Symposium conducted by Healthcare Ethics Consortium of Georgia, Atlanta.

Hutchins, L.F., Unger, J.M., Crowley, J.J., Coltman, C.A., & Albain, K.S. (1999). Under representation of patients 65 years of age or older in cancer-treatment trials. *New England Journal of Medicine, 341,* 2061–2068.

Ingham, J. (2000). End-of-life considerations in breast cancer patients. In J. Harris, M. Lippman, M. Morrow, & C. Osborne (Eds.), *Diseases of the breast* (2nd ed., pp. 967–983). Philadelphia: Lippincott Williams & Wilkins.

International Council of Nurses. (2000). *The ICN code of ethics for nurses.* Geneva, Switzerland: Author.

Jaklitsch, M.T., Bueno, R., Swanson, S.J., Mentzer, S.J., Lukanich, J.M., & Sugarbaker, D.J. (1999). New surgical options for elderly lung cancer patients. *Chest, 116,* 480–485.

Jameton, A. (1993). Dilemmas of moral distress: Moral responsibility and nursing practice. *Association of Women's Health Obstetric and Neonatal Nurse's Clinical Issues in Perinatal and Women's Health Nursing, 4,* 542–551.

Joint Commission on Accreditation of Healthcare Organizations. (2002). *Comprehensive accreditation manual for hospitals.* Oakbrook Terrace, IL: Author.

Jonsen, A.R., Siegler, M., & Winslade, W.J. (2002). *Clinical ethics: A practical approach to ethical decisions in clinical medicine* (5th ed.). New York: McGraw Hill.

Lash, T.L., Silliman, R.A., Guadagnoli, E., & Mor, V. (2000). The effect of less than definitive care on breast carcinoma recurrence and mortality. *Cancer, 89,* 1739–1747.

McCabe, M.S. (1993). The ethical context of healthcare reform. *Oncology Nursing Forum, 20*(Suppl. 10), 35–43.

Monagle, J. (1998). Ethically responsible creativity—friendship of an understanding heart: A cognitively affective model for bioethical decision making. In J. Monagle & D. Thomasma (Eds.), *Health care ethics: Critical issues for the 21st century* (pp. 566–577). Gaithersburg, MD: Aspen.

Monagle, J., & Thomasma, D. (Eds.). (1998). *Health care ethics: Critical issues for the 21st century.* Gaithersburg, MD: Aspen.

Murphy, P.A., Price, D.M., Stevens, M., Lynn, J., & Kathryn, E. (2001). Under the radar: Contributions of the SUPPORT nurses. *Nursing Outlook, 49,* 238–242.

National Comprehensive Cancer Network. (2005). *Senior adult oncology guidelines.* Retrieved September 26, 2005, from http://www.nccn.org/professionals/physician_gls/PDF/senior.pdf

Nevidjon, B. (2004). Managing from the middle: Integrating midlife challenges of children, elder parents, and career. *Clinical Journal of Oncology Nursing, 8,* 72–75.

O'Donnell, P. (2004). Ethical issues in end-of-life care: Social work facilitation and proactive intervention. In J. Berzoff & P.R. Silverman (Eds.), *Living with dying: A handbook for end-of-life healthcare practitioners* (pp. 171–187). New York: Columbia University Press.

Oncology Nursing Society. (2005). *Statement on the scope and standards of oncology nursing practice.* Pittsburgh, PA: Author.

Pence, G.E. (2004). *Classic cases in medical ethics* (4th ed.). New York: McGraw Hill.

Reb, A.M. (2003). Palliative and end-of-life care: Policy analysis. *Oncology Nursing Forum, 30,* 35–50.

Robinson, B. (1994). *Ageism.* Retrieved September 6, 2004, from http://ist-socrates.berkeley.edu/~aging/ModuleAgeism.html

Rowe, M. (2004). Words and our way with them. *Journal of Supportive Oncology, 2,* 301.

Scanlon, C. (1994). Survey yields significant results. *American Nurses Association Center for Ethics and Human Rights Communiqué, 3,* 1–3.

Senge, P.M. (1994). *The fifth discipline fieldbook.* New York: Doubleday.

Sheridan, C. (2000). Ethical dimensions in cancer care. In B. Nevidjon & K. Sowers (Eds.), *A nurse's guide to cancer care* (pp. 469–478). Philadelphia: Lippincott Williams & Wilkins.

Stone, R., & Kemper, P. (1989). Spouses and children of disabled elders: How large is a constituency for long term care reform? *Milbank Quarterly, 67,* 485–506.

Thomasma, D.C. (1987). Ethical and legal issues in the care of the elderly cancer patient. *Clinics in Geriatric Medicine, 3,* 541–547.

Thomasma, D.C. (2001). Ethical issues in cancer nursing practice. In C.H. Yarbro, M.H. Frogge, M. Goodman, & S.L. Groenwald (Eds.), *Cancer nursing: Principles and practice* (4th ed., pp. 1741–1759). Sudbury, MA: Jones and Bartlett.

Thompson, J.E., & Thompson, H.O. (1992). *Bioethical decision-making for nurses.* Lanham, MD: University Press of America.

Turner, N.J., Haward, R.A., Mulley, G.P., & Selby, P.J. (1999). Cancer in old age: Is it adequately investigated and treated? *BMJ, 319,* 309–313.

Weiner, J.S., & Cole, S.A. (2004). Three principles to improve clinician communication for advance care planning: Overcoming emotional, cognitive, and skill barriers. *Journal of Palliative Care Medicine, 7,* 817–827.

White, M.K., Keller, V., & Horrigan, L.A. (2003). Beyond informed consent: The shared decision making process. *Journal of Clinical Outcomes Management, 10,* 323–328.

Whitney, S.N., McGuire, A.J., & McCullough, L.B. (2003). A typology of shared decision making, informed consent, and simple consent. *Annals of Internal Medicine, 140,* 54–59.

CHAPTER 25

Older Adults and Cancer Survivorship

Kimberly Christopher, PhD, RN, OCN®

Background Information on the Older Adult Population and Cancer Incidence

The U.S. population older than 65 is growing (Cope, 2003). In 2000, the estimate for all adults 65 and older was 35 million, or 13% of the total U.S. population. By 2030, the projected estimate for this group is 70 million, or 20% of the total population (Bottomley & Lewis, 2003; U.S. Census Bureau, 2004; Yancik & Ries, 2000). In 1998, minorities 65 years and older were estimated to compose 16% of the older adult population. By 2030, these minority groups are projected to compose 25% of the total population (Bottomley & Lewis). Consider these demographic changes another way. From 1998–2030, the older adult white population will increase by 78%. However, the older adult minority population will increase by 226% (Bottomley & Lewis).

Cancer Incidence and Survivors

The median age of occurrence of all types and sites of cancer is 68 years. Sixty percent of all cancers occur in adults older than age 65. An individual older than 65 is 11 times more likely to be diagnosed with cancer than one younger than 65. The National Cancer Institute estimated that as of 2001, approximately 9.8 million Americans are living with a history of cancer (Office of Cancer Survivorship, National Cancer Institute, 2004). Of the 9.8 million survivors, an estimated 60% or six million are adults 65 years or older (American Cancer Society, 2005; Rowland, Aziz, Tesauro, & Feuer, 2001).

This chapter will address several areas. Examples of different perspectives on survivors and survivorship are described first. An overview of social theories of human development and the stress process framework then are described within the psychosocial context of the survivorship experience. The current research evidence on older adults and survivorship is reviewed, including psychosocial issues, coping and adaptation, quality of life (QOL), health promotion interventions, and predictors of survivorship outcomes. Finally, future directions in age-focused research are discussed, and areas for potential further work are identified.

What Is Survivorship and Who Are the Survivors?

Perspectives on survivorship vary depending on one's point of view. Points of view include those of the researcher, clinician, personal experience, and family member. Examples of definitions include that of Susan Leigh (1994), founding member of the National Coalition for Cancer Survivorship (NCCS), who stated, "Survivorship is the dynamic and ongoing process of an individual living with, through, and beyond cancer . . ." (p. 784) and nurse researcher Dr. Jody Pelusi (2001), who stated, "Survivorship is the accumulation of physical, psychological, sexual, and spiritual responses to change that evolved from diagnosis and treatment of cancer" (p. 266). One accepted definition of cancer survivor does not exist. The common medical definition of cancer survivor is a person treated for cancer and who is disease-free for a designated number of years, typically five years. NCCS defined a survivor as a person diagnosed with cancer, from the time of diagnosis, and for the remainder of life (Leigh). Survivors also are characterized by length of time from diagnosis. For example, researchers investigate the specific experiences of short, intermediate, and long-term survivors. Short-term survivorship is considered less than two years, intermediate is from two to five years, and long-term survivorship is greater than five years (Schag, Ganz, Wing, Sim, & Lee, 1994). The next section will address the survivorship experience as conceptualized within the frameworks of developmental stages and the stress process framework.

Aging Theories: Overview of Social Theories of Human Development and the Stress Process Framework

Understanding older adults' survivorship experiences is best accomplished within the context of the aging process (O'Connor & Blesch, 1992). Although many theories on aging exist, the social theories of human development and the stress process framework of coping and adaptation provide a holistic context for potentially understanding how older adults live and cope with cancer. Three social theories of development and the stress process framework of coping and adaptation are briefly reviewed (see Table 25-1).

Social Theories of Human Development

Life Stage Theories

According to life stage perspective theories, most individuals will progress through a set of sequential developmental stages (Kart & Kinney, 2001). The three primary characteristics of the life stage perspective are (a) a fixed order in progression exists from one stage to the next; (b) stages are qualitatively different; and (c) success

Table 25-1. Aging Theories: Overview of Social Theories of Human Development

Social Theories	Primary Characteristics of Development	Example of Theorist
Life stage theories	1. Progression through developmental stages occurs in a fixed order. 2. Stages are qualitatively different. 3. Success in each stage impacts transition to the next stage.	Erikson
Life span theories	1. Development is a lifelong process. 2. Development is multidirectional and includes positive and negative changes. 3. Development is characterized by intraindividual variability. 4. Development is embedded within historical context, including social and cultural conditions.	Neugarten
Life course theories	1. Developmental transitions are socially created, recognized, and shared. 2. Social norms and definitions influence transitions. 3. Individuals shape their life course through their choices and behaviors.	Hagestad and Neugarten

in each stage will, in part, impact transition to the next stage (Kastenbaum, 1995). Erik Erikson's Theory of Psychosocial Development is an example of the life stage perspective. The perspective has both strengths and limitations. Its strength is recognizing development as an ongoing process. Its limitations, however, are assuming development proceeds in one direction, not accounting for individual differences in progression, and tying development to chronologic age (Bush & Simmons, 1990).

Life Span Theories

The life span perspective theories were developed in response to life stage theories (Kart & Kinney, 2001). The life span perspective's objective is to describe age-related behavioral changes from birth to death (Baltes & Goulet, 1970). According to these theories, behavior change results from the interaction of the individual and social characteristics (Kart & Kinney). Baltes and Graf (1996) identified the characteristics of the life span perspective theories. Development is (a) a lifelong process, (b) multidirectional, (c) composed of both positive and negative changes, (d) characterized by intraindividual variability in development, (e) embedded within a historical context, and (f) dependent on many contextual factors, including social and cultural conditions. Finally, a multidisciplinary approach is essential to understand the process of development. An example of the life span perspective theory is Neugarten's (1973) work on how both biologic and social events influence life cycle changes.

Life Course Theories

Age-related transitions that are socially created, recognized, and shared are the basis for life course perspective theories (Hagestad & Neugarten, 1985). These theories examine how social norms and definitions influence role changes and transitions in the life course (Kart & Kinney, 2001). Aging is a lifelong process influenced by social processes. The life course perspective "emphasizes the timing by which individuals and families make their transitions into and out of various roles and developmental tasks in relation to social time clocks" (Hareven, 1996, p. 31). Moreover, individuals' life courses are shaped by the choices they make and the behaviors they choose (Elder, 1998).

The three perspectives are not mutually exclusive. However, they differ in terms of amount of change possible, abruptness of the change, direction, universality, and origin of change (Kart & Kinney, 2001). How an individual manages stressors or challenges also may impact progression through the developmental stages. The Stress Process Framework is a model that can be useful in conceptualizing the impact of stressors and life events within the survivorship experience.

The Stress Process Framework, Coping, and Adaptation

The stress process framework hypothesizes that the timing of challenges, the individual's unique biography, and social and historical contexts of that person influence how an individual deals with challenges (stressors) (Pearlin & Skaff, 1995). The framework has three main components: stressors/undesirable life events, moderators, and outcomes (Kart & Kinney, 2001).

Stressors/Undesirable Life Events

Older adults experience life events less frequently than younger adults (Ensel, 1991). Moreover, older adults generally are less stressed by events when they occur (Cox, 2001; Hoyer & Roodin, 2003; Murrell, Norris, & Grote, 1988). Normative life events, those that are anticipated and planned for, often are less stressful even if they occur "off-time" (Murrell et al.). However, a great variability exists in older adults' appraisals of stressful events (Kart & Kinney, 2001). Older adults' life events involve losses in roles and/or status (Pearlin & Skaff, 1995). The most common life events are health-related and loss of a spouse or partner (Ensel).

Moderators

Coping, social support, and a sense of mastery are the internal and external resources that older adults use to deal with stressors (Pearlin & Skaff, 1995). Coping includes both problem-focused coping (behavioral strategies) and emotion-focused coping (cognitive/emotional strategies) (Lazarus & Folkman, 1984). Problem-focused coping is "action-oriented" and uses behavioral strategies to change the stressful situation and solve the problem (Carroll-Johnson, Gorman, & Bush, 1998). For example, an individual may seek information, may change his or her behavior, or change his or her environment. Emotion-focused coping is passive and includes the cognitive processes that influence emotional responses to the stressful situation (Carroll-Johnson et al.). Emotional coping includes ranges of responses such as anger, denial, projection, avoidance, and seeking meaning from the situation. Social support includes the instrumental and/or emotional assistance that family members and friends provide (Pearlin & Skaff). Mastery is the extent to which people can control what happens to them (Pearlin & Skaff). A sense of mastery buffers people from the negative consequences of stressors and also enables people to activate coping efforts and to engage social support (Pearlin & Skaff).

Outcomes

The stress process framework investigates the impact of stressors and moderators on outcomes (Kart & Kinney, 2001). The most frequently examined outcomes include life satisfaction, morale, depression, and functional abilities (Pearlin & Skaff, 1995). Although the majority of older adults maintain positive well-being and functioning, the relationships among stressors, moderators, and outcome variables are complex (Kart & Kinney).

Framing Survivorship in the Context of Aging Theories

Drawing from the previously described aging theories and the stress process framework, older adults potentially face a number of key developmental issues. First, changes occur in interpersonal relationships because of the deaths of a spouse, friends, siblings, and other relatives. Older adults need to find new and meaningful roles after employment status changes. Many older adults will enter full-time retirement. However, an increasing number will work part-time in the same or a new capacity. Older adults also will confront potential health changes. For some, health may decline. For others, this is a time to begin or increase health promotion activities (e.g., walking clubs) or to engage in recreational activities such as golf, tennis, and bicycle riding. In addition, many older adults are in the process of recognizing and accepting that most of their life span has been lived. For example, a diagnosis of cancer may be framed as "cancer in the context of a 'life mostly lived'" (Kagan, 2004).

How older adults have coped with previous stressors and undesirable events will, in part, influence their capacity to cope and adapt after a cancer diagnosis. Their sense of mastery and personal control, along with the availability of social and caregiver support, will influence their ability to cope and adapt as survivors. Additional medical problems and lifestyle choices also will impact survivorship. For example, comorbidities such as arthritis, cardiac disease, diabetes, and vision and hearing deficiencies may have a negative impact on QOL in survivorship. Also, being willing and able to change behaviors and having the resources needed to make changes have the potential to improve survivorship. Activities such as exercise, weight management, adhering to screening measures, and appropriate self-management of chronic conditions will improve survivors' QOL. An overview of research on survivorship in older adults is presented in the next section.

Overview of the Current State of Research on Older Adult Cancer Survivors

To date, a paucity of research exists on older adults with cancer. Even less research is available on older adults and their survivorship experience. Much of the survivorship research to date has focused on White, middle-aged, middle-class adults, particularly breast cancer survivors. As the age of the U.S. population continues to shift, the number of older adults living with cancer will be unprecedented. Empirical evidence that identifies the unique experiences and needs of older adult survivors is essential. Increased funding for basic, clinical, and translational research investigating this population is necessary (Oncology Nursing Society [ONS] & Geriatric Oncology Consortium [GOC], 2004). Several agencies and organizations recognize the need for additional funds and research. For example, the mission of the Office of Cancer

Survivorship is to develop and support a research agenda that explores the short- and long-term physical and psychological effects of cancer and its treatment across all age groups (Office of Cancer Survivorship, National Cancer Institute, 2004). ONS and GOC stressed the need for research with older adults. In a 2004 ONS membership survey, doctorally prepared members ranked research on older adults (#1) and survivorship (#19) in the top 20 priority topics (Berger et al., 2005). In addition, ONS has funded at least six research proposals on survivorship through its small grants program (Ferrell, Verani, Smith, & Juarez, 2003). These proposals, however, have not focused on older adults. Although neither the National Institute on Aging (NIA) nor the National Institute of Nursing Research (NINR) identify "older adult survivorship" as a specific priority research area, each institute has research goals aimed at positively impacting older adults. Specifically, NIA's strategic research goals aim to improve older adults' QOL by focusing on physical and mental health and enhancing social roles (NIA, 2001). NINR's scientific goals include a commitment to promising avenues of research on chronic illness, specifically self-management activities and health promotion activities, and also QOL issues, cultural considerations, and health disparities (NINR, 2005). The hope is that large organizations such as ONS, NIA, and NINR will increasingly focus their research goals and funding priorities on older adults living with cancer.

Review of Research on Older Adult Cancer Survivors

This systematic review was undertaken to describe research that addresses older adult cancer survivors (aged 65 and older). The review included searching Medline (medical) and CINAHL (nursing and allied health) research databases for cancer survivorship research reports of studies published from 1995–2004. Inclusion criteria were studies with men and women 65 years of age and older or studies with a mean age of 65 years or older. Key search terms were survivorship, cancer survivorship, survivors, older adults, and elders. An analysis of references cited in those reports identified further research. In addition, abstracts from the National Cancer Institute and the American Cancer Society's survivorship conference in 2004 were reviewed. Unfortunately, very few studies focused on older adults. Abstracts that identified the study subjects as 60 years of age and older or a sample mean age of 60 years of age or older were included. Because no agreement exists on the age definition of older adulthood, and both 60 and 65 are used as the lower limit, 60 years of age was used in order to include as many of the survivorship conference abstracts as possible.

In general, the research with older adult survivors investigates three broad areas: psychosocial issues, coping and adaptation, and QOL; health promotion activities; and predictors of survivorship outcomes (see Table 25-2). Much of the current research evidence is based on descriptive and correlational study designs. However, interventional studies are increasing. As a result, the number of randomized clinical trials that compare and identify the differences in outcomes between groups also will increase. Having more randomized studies will increase and strengthen the evidence on which the care of older adult survivors is based. In addition, a need exists for further psychometric research (process of developing instruments, scales, or tools used to collect data) to determine whether the measurement instruments developed with middle-aged adults are appropriate for use with older adults.

Table 25-2. Research Studies Focusing on the Older Adult With Cancer

Category	Author/Year	Purpose	Study Design	Sample Characteristics (Size, age range, mean/[SD], disease types, mean years of survivorship/range or years since diagnosis/range or years since active treatment/range)	Outcomes
Psychosocial issues: Coping and adaptation and quality of life (QOL)	Bowman et al., 2003	Explore factors related to appraisal of cancer experience.	Descriptive Correlational Survey interview	321 58–95 72/(7.5) Breast, colorectal, prostate Mean years of survivorship, > 10/ range 3–34	1. Being older and being African American were associated with being less likely to perceive cancer as a stressful life event. 2. Survivors who perceived family members as stressed appraised their cancer experience as more stressful.
	Benyamini et al., 2003	Determine if history of cancer affects perception of current symptoms and disease and reaction to symptoms.	Descriptive Exploratory Compared three group interviews	108 77–78 all groups Not available Melanoma, prostate, breast, colon, uterine/ovarian, other Not available	1. Cancer survivors (CS) felt more vulnerable to cancer. 2. CS were less confident that symptoms from arthritis were because of arthritis and were more likely to call healthcare provider (HCPS). for confirmation and reassurance. 3. CS called HCPS for reassurance when they experienced ambiguous signs and symptoms.
	Deimling, Kahana, et al., 2002	Test conceptual model factors contributing to general psychological distress and symptoms of post-traumatic stress.	Descriptive Hypothesis testing Survey interview	180 Not available 72/(7.7) Breast, colorectal, prostate Time since active treatment, five or more years	1. Findings demonstrated low levels of anxiety and hostility. 2. Approximately 25% of the sample had scores indicating levels of clinical depression. 3. No significant differences were observed in distress outcome by cancer type, race, or gender. 4. Strongest predictor of depression and post-traumatic stress disorder "hyper-arousal" was current cancer-related symptoms.

(Continued on next page)

Table 25-2. Research Studies Focusing on the Older Adult With Cancer *(Continued)*

Category	Author/Year	Purpose	Study Design	Sample Characteristics	Outcomes
	Ramsey et al., 2002	Evaluate general health status and several dimensions of illness.	Descriptive Mailed survey	227 Not available 74/(8.9) Colorectal Time since diagnosis, five or more years	1. Summary measures of health-related QOL rated high. 2. Responses are not associated with stage of disease or time since diagnosis. 3. Decreased QOL was associated with continued symptoms, especially diarrhea. 4. Depression was more prevalent among respondents than the general population.
	Deimling et al., 2004	Describe extent to which cancer and treatment effects combined with comorbidities influence health, physical functioning, and perceptions of disability burden.	Descriptive Correlational	321 Not available Not available 60 years or older Breast, prostate, colorectal Time since diagnosis, five or more years	1. Approximately 40% of sample reported one symptom because of cancer or treatment, and 10% reported three or more symptoms. 2. Pain was the most common symptom, and 21% of those reporting pain attributed it to cancer.
	Haley et al., 2004	Determine if survivorship is associated with decreased well-being among older women with a history of breast cancer compared to women with no history.	Interview	127 Not available Not available 70 years or older Breast Time since diagnosis, one or more years	1. No difference in depressive symptoms between groups 2. Survivors had higher levels of depressed and anxious mood, lower levels of positive psychological states and social support, and more negative social interactions. 3. Survivors reported poorer function on six of eight subscales of the Medical Outcomes Study Health Survey Questionnaire (SF-36).
Health promotion interventions	Demark-Wahnefried et al., 2003	To test an intervention that aimed to improve overall diet and physical activity	Randomized Controlled trial Intervention	158 Not available 72/(4.9) Breast, prostate Time since diagnosis, up to 18 months	1. Background provided on methodology, recruitment process, and data analysis 2. Study is in process; results not available

(Continued on next page)

Table 25-2. Research Studies Focusing on the Older Adult With Cancer (*Continued*)

Category	Author/Year	Purpose	Study Design	Sample Characteristics	Outcomes
	Damush et al., 2004	To test an intervention to increase physical activity and determine the effects on cancer-specific and generic health-related QOL	Intervention pilot one-group Pre-/post-test design	34 50–77 60/Not available Breast Time since diagnosis, up to 24 months	1. Barriers to exercise decreased, frequency of exercise and exercise self-efficacy improved after completion of self-management program 2. Study is in process; results not available
Predictors of survivorship outcomes	Mandelblatt et al., 2003	Test hypotheses 1. Breast conservation treatment resulted in better postsurgical health. 2. Axillary node dissection is a risk for long-term impairment. 3. Satisfaction with breast cancer care is associated with perceptions of process of care.	Descriptive Hypotheses testing	1,812 Not available 73/(5.0) Breast Time since diagnosis, three to five years	1. Axillary dissection was the only surgical treatment that affected outcomes. 2. Having arm problems had a consistent negative effect on all outcomes. 3. Processes of care were most important determinants of long-term QOL. 4. Study participants expressed desire to participate in decision-making process. 5. Participation in decision making may impact long-term QOL.
	Wichmann et al., 2001	Investigated possibility that gender differences existed in the outcomes of curative colorectal cancer resection	Descriptive Hypotheses testing	894 Not available 65/(0.4) Colorectal Time since diagnosis, up to 10 years	1. Disease-free and overall survival were significantly longer in women when compared with men.

(Continued on next page)

Table 25-2. Research Studies Focusing on the Older Adult With Cancer (Continued)

Category	Author/Year	Purpose	Study Design	Sample Characteristics	Outcomes
	Deimling, Schaefer, et al., 2002	1. Describe long-term health challenges in terms of health problems, concerns, and determine any racial differences. 2. Determine if problems are related to gender, treatment factors, or type of cancer. 3. Determine best predictors of current health problems and health perceptions.	Descriptive Correlational	180 Not available 72/Not available Breast, colorectal, prostate Mean years since diagnosis, 10.7/5–34	1. Overall sample reported fairly good health and low levels of symptoms attributable to cancer. 2. Best predictor of health perceptions were functional health problems for both White and African American groups. 3. African Americans reported higher levels of health difficulties with comorbid conditions and functioning than Whites. 4. African Americans rated their overall health lower than Whites. 5. African Americans are less likely to worry about second cancers than Whites.
	Yang et al., 2004	Describe factors associated with long-term survivor's prognosis and QOL.	Descriptive Survey	148 Not available Not available Mean age at diagnosis 65 years, study conducted 5 years post-diagnosis Lung Time since diagnosis, 5 or more years	1. Analysis is ongoing. 2. Preliminary findings indicate that the overall sample had fairly good health despite some physical and psychological problems.

Research on Psychosocial Issues, Coping and Adaptation, and Quality of Life

Appraisal of the Cancer Experience by Older Long-Term Survivors

A descriptive, correlational study explored factors related to the appraisal of the cancer experience in 321 randomly selected older adults who were five or more years post-treatment for breast, colorectal, or prostate cancer (Bowman, Deimling, Smerglia, Sage, & Kahana, 2003). The mean age was 72, and 37% of the sample was African American. Trained interviewers collected structured survey data in a two-hour face-to-face interview. Findings indicated that being older and African American were associated with being less likely to perceive cancer as a stressful life event, and those subjects who perceived their family as stressed appraised their cancer experience as more stressful.

Beliefs about family distress modified survivors' stress appraisal. Clinical interventions are needed to address how survivors feel about illness, how survivors perceive others' feelings about their illness, and survivors' and family members' need to share their thoughts and feelings on how they are affected by cancer.

Living With the Worry of Cancer: Health Perceptions and Behaviors of Older Adults With Self, Vicarious, or No History of Cancer

Another study explored whether a history of cancer affected older people's perception of current symptoms and disease and their reactions to current symptoms (Benyamini, McClain, Leventhal, & Leventhal, 2003). This descriptive, exploratory study was composed of a convenience sample of 108 retirement community residents, all of whom reported having osteoarthritis. Study participants were predominately White, affluent, and educated, with a mean age of 77. The sample included three groups: those with a history of cancer, those who lived with someone with cancer, and those with no cancer experience. Data were collected in face-to-face interviews in participants' homes. Findings indicated that cancer survivors felt more vulnerable to cancer. Other findings included that when cancer survivors experienced an episode of arthritis, they were less confident that the cause was arthritis and more likely to call the healthcare provider (HCP), and when cancer survivors experienced ambiguous signs and symptoms, they called the HCP for reassurance.

Findings suggest that a history of cancer affects not only QOL and fears of recurrence but also daily living with additional chronic illness. Therefore, HCPs need to be aware of cancer survivors' heightened vigilance and need for continuing reassurance about cancer and other diseases. Health counseling should be delivered in a way that is sensitive to survivors' special concerns.

Cancer Survivorship and Psychological Distress in Later Life

The purpose of another study was to test a conceptual model of contributing factors of general psychological distress and symptoms of post-traumatic stress disorder (PTSD) (Deimling, Kahana, Bowman, & Schaefer, 2002). Face-to-face survey interviews were conducted with 180 White and African American survivors who were 60 years of age or older and were five or more years post-treatment. Study findings demonstrated low levels of anxiety and hostility in this sample.

No significant differences were found in distress outcome by cancer type, race, or gender. The strongest predictor of depression and PTSD "hyper-arousal" was current cancer-related illness symptoms.

These data suggest that fears of recurrence do not decrease with time. Therefore, cancer survivors experiencing long-term symptoms also should be monitored for depression and hyper-arousal symptoms, such as impaired concentration and sleep disturbances.

Quality of Life in Long-Term Survivors of Colorectal Cancer

A study's objectives were to evaluate general health status and several cancer-specific dimensions of illness (Ramsey, Berry, Moinpour, Giedzinska, & Andersen, 2002). The sample included 227 men and women, mean age 74, who were at least five years after a colorectal cancer diagnosis. Participants completed a mailed survey that elicited data on general QOL and colon cancer–specific issues. Study findings showed that respondents rated summary measures of health-related QOL as relatively high. Responses were not associated with stage of disease or time since diagnosis. Decreased QOL was associated with continued symptoms, particularly diarrhea. Depression was more prevalent among respondents than the general population. However, diarrhea was not associated with depression scores.

These data demonstrate high health-related QOL in older adults five or more years post-diagnosis. Findings also suggest that long-term problems with symptoms of diarrhea decrease QOL, and depression is a potential mental health problem. Therefore, healthcare professionals should evaluate long-term survivors for persistent symptoms.

Post-Treatment Health and Functioning of Older Adult, Long-Term Cancer Survivors

The purpose of this descriptive correlational study was to describe the extent to which cancer and its treatment effects combined with comorbidities to influence health, physical functioning, and perceptions of disability burden (Deimling, Bowman, Sterns, & Wagner, 2004). Three hundred and twenty-one adults, 60 years of age and older who were long-term survivors of breast, prostate, or colorectal cancer, were randomly selected from a cancer registry. Study results determined that approximately 40% of the sample reported at least one symptom because of cancer or treatment, and 10% reported three or more symptoms. Adults reported pain most commonly, and 21% of those reporting pain attributed it to cancer. More specifically, more than 40% of breast cancer survivors and almost 20% of prostate cancer survivors reported pain. In addition, correlational analyses showed that being African American and/or female was associated with more current symptoms and greater functional difficulty. Regression analysis showed that comorbid health conditions were the single best predictor of functional difficulties and disability burden. These findings suggest that older adults continue to experience cancer-related symptoms, and African Americans and women are at greater risk.

Psychological, Social, and Health Impact of Breast Cancer Survivorship in Older Women

The purpose of this study was to determine if survivorship was associated with decreased well-being among older women with breast cancer (Haley et al., 2004). A total of 127 women, who were 70 years or older and were survivors for at least one year, were identified from a cancer registry. Researchers selected a comparison group of 147 demographically similar women with no history of cancer. Both groups were interviewed and data collected on psychological distress, positive psychological states, social support, and health-related QOL.

T-test statistics comparing the groups determined no difference in depressive symptoms; however, survivors experienced higher levels of depressed and anxious mood. Survivors had lower levels of positive psychological states and social support and more negative social interactions. Survivors also reported poorer function than the comparison group on six of eight subscales on the Medical Outcomes Study Health Survey Questionnaire short form (SF-36). These data suggest that some older female breast cancer survivors experienced sustained subclinical effects in some areas, including mood changes, decreased life satisfaction, physical functioning, vitality, and role-emotional functioning. However, length of time since completion of treatment may influence outcomes. Future studies should carefully consider time since treatment was completed.

Summary of Psychosocial Issues, the Coping and Adjustment Process, and Quality-of-Life Research

Although the current, limited evidence on survivors' psychological issues, coping and adjustment process, and QOL is primarily based on descriptive correlational research, study findings suggest that older adult survivors have a range of experiences and outcomes. Survivors' adjustment may be affected by their family members' experiences of stress as the family adjusts to the survivor living with cancer. Older adult survivors' ability to cope may vary by ethnic group, gender, and age. Some data suggest that ethnic group and gender also may be associated with increased risk of symptoms and functional difficulty and that a history of cancer may impact older adults' ways of coping with other chronic diseases. In current studies, older adults generally reported high QOL. However, persistent cancer-related symptoms had a negative impact on QOL. Survivors may have difficulty with depression, mental concentration, and sleep or be at risk for subclinical problems such as depressed mood. More research is needed with large, random samples and ethnically diverse older adult survivors.

Health Promotion Interventions

The following two studies investigated the extent to which health promotion interventions such as exercise and diet impacted the QOL of older adult survivors. Unfortunately, very little research has focused on health promotion activities and interventions for these survivors. Health promotion research is an important area for future investigation.

Leading the Way in Exercise and Diet: Intervening to Improve Functions Among Older Breast and Prostate Cancer Survivors

The purpose of this study was to test an intervention that aimed to improve overall diet and physical activity (Demark-Wahnefried et al., 2003). The experimental group received tailored educational workbooks and a telephone counseling program based on stage of readiness, whereas the control group received mailed workbooks and telephone counseling in other health-related areas. One hundred and fifty-eight men and women with a mean age of 72 and a mean of 10 months after breast or prostate cancer diagnosis were enrolled in this randomized controlled trial. The article provided background information on the methodology, including study goals, the recruitment process, and the data analysis process. The goal is to improve understanding of how tailored interventions for diet and exercise are or are not effective in a sample of older adult survivors. The authors described this work as translational research between clinically based research and public health. If such tailored interventions are shown to be effective, more large-scale diet and exercise interventions should be planned using these models.

Increasing Exercise and Health-Related Quality of Life Among Older Women Surviving Breast Cancer

The purpose of this pilot intervention study was to increase physical activity and determine the effects on cancer-specific and generic health-related QOL (Damush, Perkins, & Miller, 2004). The study used principles of self-management as guided by the Social Cognitive Theory. The study included 34 women with a mean age of 60 who were treated for breast cancer within the previous two years. Baseline measures of health-related QOL, fatigue, physical activity, sleep deprivation, and physical performance were obtained. The intervention included three group classes on self-management and three follow-up telephone calls. Assessment measures were repeated at six months.

Findings indicated that barriers to exercise decreased and frequency of exercise and exercise self-efficacy improved. In addition, physical and psychosocial functioning, sleep, and fatigue improved. These findings suggest that a self-management program is effective for increasing activity and improving health-related QOL.

Summary of Health Promotion Interventions

Although more research is needed in the area of health promotion interventions, this area offers exciting opportunities to improve older adult survivors' QOL. Determining the extent to which self-management principles and interventions to improve exercise levels and diet are successful will increase the understanding of self-management as a process and identify behavioral interventions that have a positive impact.

Predictors of Survivorship Outcomes

The following section will describe research findings from four studies that investigated predictors of survivorship outcomes.

Predictors of Long-Term Outcomes in Older Breast Cancer Survivors

This hypothesis testing study included a random cross-sectional national sample of women 67 years of age or older diagnosed with stage 1 or 2 breast cancer within the past three to five years (Mandelblatt et al., 2003). The hypotheses tested were

(a) breast conservation treatment results in better post-treatment physical and mental health; (b) axillary node dissection places women at moderate risk for long-term impairment of arm motion and leads to lower physical function; and (c) satisfaction with breast cancer care is associated with perceptions of the process, not actual treatment. Findings demonstrated axillary dissection was the only surgical treatment that affected outcomes, and that having arm problems had consistent, negative independent effect on all outcomes. After axillary dissection, processes of care were the most important determinant of long-term QOL, not actual therapy. Women who perceived high levels of ageism or felt they had no choice with regard to treatment reported more bodily pain, lower mental health, and less general satisfaction. These factors, plus perceived racism, resulted in decreased satisfaction with the medical care system.

Based on these findings, women need education and counseling on treatment choices. Study participants expressed a desire to be involved in the decision-making process, and participation in this process may impact long-term QOL. Clinicians' personal values, beliefs, and/or biases about age and race also potentially impact their patients' outcomes.

Gender Differences in Long-Term Survival of Patients With Colorectal Cancer

Using prospective analysis of a database of patients with colorectal cancer, this study investigated the possibility that gender differences existed in disease-related outcomes of curative colorectal cancer resection (Wichmann et al., 2001). Statistically significant gender differences were observed. Women had disease-free and overall survival rates that were higher than those for men. Further research is needed to determine if differences are related to gender-specific immune function or to other gender-related local or systemic factors. Although these findings have limited clinical application at this time, they may begin to explain why women with colorectal cancer have better outcomes than men.

Racial Differences in the Health of Older Adult Long-Term Cancer Survivors

The purpose of this descriptive correlational study was to describe (a) the long-term survivors' health challenges in terms of health problems, concerns, and perceptions and determine if racial differences were present; (b) determine if problems were related to gender, treatment factors, or type of cancer; and (c) determine best predictors of current health problems and health perceptions (Deimling, Schaefer, Kahana, Bowman, & Reardon, 2002). The study used in-person interviews with 180 survivors 58 years of age or older who were 5–34 years post-treatment. Sixty participants were African American. Findings indicated that generally most survivors reported low levels of symptoms attributable to cancer and most reported fairly good health. Neither group perceived their health as seriously compromised by cancer and its treatment. African Americans reported higher levels of health difficulties with comorbid conditions and functioning and rated their overall health as lower. It was not clear, however, if African Americans' poor health was linked to the cancer experience, continuing sequelae, both, or poorer health in general. African Americans also were less likely to worry about second cancers. For both groups, the best predictors of health perceptions were functional health problems.

Characteristics of Long-Term Lung Cancer Survivors

This descriptive study investigated factors associated with long-term lung cancer survivors' prognosis and QOL (Yang et al., 2004). Of the 347 survivors surveyed, 148 returned the questionnaire that included measures on general health, performance status, symptoms, diet, and spiritual well-being. Results indicated that 97% of these survivors reported fairly good overall health. Sixteen percent reported worsening health compared to one year earlier. Other findings indicated that 90% had an Eastern Cooperative Oncology Group Performance Status (ECOG-PS) score of 0–1, 50% scored highly energetic, 33% reported limited social engagement, 25% reported emotional problems, and 73% reported very good or best spiritual well-being. Although this sample of long-term lung cancer survivors experienced some physical and psychological difficulties, the majority had fairly good overall health.

Summary of Predictors of Survivorship Outcomes

Consistent with previous research evidence, predictors of older adult survivorship outcomes are primarily based on descriptive correlational research. However, these studies identify factors that need further investigation. For example, research findings suggest that survivorship outcomes vary by ethnic group and gender. Further, physical health, mental health, and satisfaction with health care were impacted when older adults perceived ageism among healthcare professionals. Comorbid conditions also had a greater impact on the survivorship experience than the cancer itself. Findings also suggest that functional health status predicted survivors' health perceptions. More well-designed studies are needed to determine the full extent to which these variables and others predict survivorship outcomes.

Future Directions in Age-Focused Research

Theoretical Models of Quality of Life

Although many theoretical models of QOL exist, they all generally conceptualize QOL as a sense of well being in several domains: physical, psychological, social, and spiritual (Cella & Tulsky, 1990; Ferrans, 1996; Taylor, Jones, & Burns, 1995). The conceptual model by Ferrell and Dow (1997) incorporated these four domains and identified important subcategories/concepts within each domain. The model also demonstrated the interrelationship among the four domains. Ferrell and Dow's model was based on extensive work with cancer survivors. However, the survivors were mainly middle-aged adults and survivors of women's cancers. The challenge of healthcare professionals is to determine the extent to which this model or others is appropriate for older and multicultural adults who survive a range of cancers.

Areas for Future Research

Underexplored Cancers

Healthcare professionals should increase their knowledge of survivorship in older adults through the conduct of systematic research. Research is needed on underexplored cancers in older adults, including lung, colorectal, breast, ovarian, prostate, lymphomas, myeloma, and other cancers. Increasingly, researchers are focusing on the long-term impact of surviving cancer. Investigators should focus not only on the problems but also on successful outcomes. For example, what are the positive survivorship outcomes and how are they achieved?

Culture and Survivorship

Much research is needed in the area of culture and survivorship. Studies on middle-aged adults' responses to cancer are not uniform across ethnic groups (Aziz & Rowland, 2002). Prior experiences, mores, and cultural beliefs affect middle-aged adults' survivorship. Therefore, to posit that minority older adults' experiences also will vary is reasonable. Minority/ethnic group experiences need to be described, and the influence of culture on older adults' survivorship also should be explicated and better understood. Specifically, research needs to address how culture influences beliefs about cancer cause and recurrence, surveillance, monitoring, chronic illness, and health promotion. This research is needed before culturally appropriate interventions to improve survivorship can be designed and implemented (Aziz & Rowland).

Health Promotion and Chronic Illness

As cancer increasingly is considered a chronic illness, innovative models of care that include health promotion activities as part of the self-management program are essential. Health promotion activities will facilitate achieving the goal of older adult survivors living long, satisfying lives while managing chronic illness. Further, interdisciplinary collaboration among clinicians, educators, and researchers could facilitate the development and testing of new health promotion models (Chiverton, Votava, & Tortoretti, 2003).

Several examples of current work provide a basis for further investigation in this area. Recommendations for designing health promotion programs and education materials for community dwelling older adults should be evaluated to determine their appropriateness for older adult cancer survivors. One example includes Davidhizar, Eshler, and Moody's (2002) work based on *Healthy People 2010* objectives. Older adults' ability to perform activities of daily living (ADL) and instrumental ADL will impact their QOL. Cognitive function is necessary to perform ADL and instrumental ADL. Therefore, educational interventions designed to improve memory, attention, and concentration, such as McDougall's (2001) pilot study to improve memory efficacy, should be replicated in large samples of cancer survivors. The physical, psychological, and cognitive benefits of regular exercise are well documented (Anderson & Jakicic, 2003; Bartlett, 2003; Courneya et al., 2003; Emery, Hauck, Shermer, Hsiao, & MacIntyre, 2003; Hung et al., 2004; Kennedy, Haykowsky, Daub, Van Lohuizen, & Knapik, 2003; Steffen et al., 2001). Nurse scientists have investigated and identified the benefits of exercise programs for older adults with chronic illness (Banks-Wallace & Conn, 2002; Conn, Valentine, & Cooper, 2002; Resnick, 2004; Rosenberg & Resnick, 2003). Research was conducted with cancer survivors who were primarily middle aged (Blanchard et al., 2003; Courneya & Friedenreich, 1997; Courneya et al., 2003), and research was extended to focus also on older adults (Courneya et al., 2004).

Several oncology nurses also suggested a number of research areas to focus on to ensure that survivors live healthy and complication-free lives (Cope, 2003; Ferrell et al., 2003; Taylor et al., 2001). Although Cope addressed pediatric survivors, it was striking the extent to which her suggestions are applicable to older adult survivors. For example, a 75-year-old woman successfully treated for breast cancer may live for 20 or more years. Therefore, maximizing her QOL, as well as that of other older adult survivors, is important. Cope suggested to continue to identify new and emerging late effects; create high-risk survivor profiles; offer medical and nursing education programs on risks, management, and surveillance; encourage participation in prospective, controlled trials of risk reduction and health promotion; and offer multidisciplinary health promotion and lifestyle approaches to wellness, including nutrition, exercise, and social activities/interaction. Ferrell et al. and Taylor et al. (2001) stressed the need to determine the extent to which advanced practice oncology nurses can meet the complicated health needs of older cancer survivors and impact their health by monitoring health status, continuing surveillance for recurrent or new cancers, addressing rehabilitation issues, and facilitating palliative care. Ferrell et al. also stressed the general need for more funding to support research on older adult survivors. Oncology nurses and healthcare colleagues are challenged to address these areas and determine additional areas for investigation to ensure that older adult cancer survivors live long and meaningful lives.

Conclusion

The projected increase in the aging population will bring special challenges in caring for the growing number of older adult cancer survivors. The survivorship experience can be framed within the context of the aging process considering the unique challenges and transitions experienced across the aging continuum. Social theories of human development and the stress process framework of coping and adaptation may provide a context for how older adults cope with cancer. Only limited research exists on older adults and their survivorship experience. Further research is needed to address common cancers in this population, QOL issues, cultural influences, and health promotion interventions. Oncology nurses have identified various research priorities, including surveillance for late effects and new cancers, healthcare provider education, multidiciplinary health promotion activities, rehabilitation, and palliative care. Ongoing and future collaborative research efforts will contribute to the evidence base to improve healthcare and survivorship outcomes in the older adult population.

References

American Cancer Society. (2005). *Cancer facts and figures, 2005*. Retrieved June 22, 2005, from http://www.cancer.org/docroot/STT/stt_0.asp

Anderson, R., & Jakicic, J. (2003). Physical activity and weight management: Building the case for exercise. *Physician and Sports Medicine, 31*(11), 39–45.

Aziz, N., & Rowland, J. (2002). Cancer survivorship research among ethnic minority and medically under-served groups. *Oncology Nursing Forum, 29,* 789–800.

Baltes, P., & Goulet, L. (1970). Status and issues of a life-span developmental psychology. In L.R. Goulet & P. Baltes (Eds.), *Life-span developmental psychology* (pp. 3–21). New York: Academic.

Baltes, P., & Graf, P. (1996). Psychological aspects of aging: Facts and frontiers. In D. Magnusson (Ed.), *The lifespan development of individuals: Behavioral, neurobiological and psychosocial perspectives* (pp. 427–460). New York: Cambridge University Press.

Banks-Wallace, J., & Conn, V. (2002). Interventions to promote physical activity among African American women. *Public Health Nursing, 19,* 321–335.

Bartlett, S. (2003). Motivating patients toward weight loss: Practical strategies for addressing overweight and obesity. *Physician and Sports Medicine, 31*(11), 29–36.

Benyamini, Y., McClain, C., Leventhal, E., & Leventhal, H. (2003). Living with the worry of cancer: Health perceptions and behaviors of elderly people with self, vicarious, or no history of cancer. *Psycho-Oncology, 12,* 161–172.

Berger, A.M., Berry, D.L., Christopher, K.A., Greene, A.L., Maliski, S., Swenson, K.K., et al. (2005). Oncology Nursing Society year 2004 research priority survey. *Oncology Nursing Forum, 32,* 281–290.

Blanchard, C., Baker, F., Denniston, M., Courneya, K., Hann, D., Gesman, D., et al. (2003). Is absolute amount in exercise or change in exercise more associated with quality of life in adult cancer survivors? *Preventive Medicine, 37,* 389–395.

Bottomley, J., & Lewis, C. (2003). *Geriatric rehabilitation* (2nd ed.). Upper Saddle River, NJ: Prentice Hall.

Bowman, K., Deimling, G., Smerglia, V., Sage, P., & Kahana, B. (2003). Appraisal of the cancer experience by older long-term survivors. *Psycho-Oncology, 12,* 226–238.

Bush, D., & Simmons, R. (1990). Socialization processes over the life course. In M. Rosenberg & R.H. Turner (Eds.), *Social psychology: Sociological perspectives* (pp. 133–164). New Brunswick, NJ: Transaction Publishers.

Carroll-Johnson, R., Gorman, L., & Bush, N. (Eds.). (1998). *Psychosocial nursing care along the cancer continuum.* Pittsburgh, PA: Oncology Nursing Society.

Cella, D., & Tulsky, D. (1990). Measuring quality of life today: Methodological aspects. *Oncology, 4,* 29–38.

Chiverton, P., Votava, K., & Tortoretti, D. (2003). The future role of nursing in health promotion. *American Journal of Health Promotion, 18,* 192–194.

Conn, V., Valentine, J., & Cooper, H. (2002). Interventions to increase physical activity among aging adults: A meta-analysis. *Annals of Behavioral Medicine, 24,* 190–200.

Cope, D. (2003). Length of survival time increases risk for related effects. *Clinical Journal of Oncology Nursing, 7,* 19.

Courneya, K., & Friedenreich, C. (1997). Relationship between exercise pattern across the cancer experience and current quality of life in colorectal cancer survivors. *Journal of Alternative and Complementary Medicine, 3,* 215–226.

Courneya, K., Mackey, J.R., Bell, G.J., Jones, L.W., Field, C.J., & Fairey, A.S. (2003). Randomized controlled trial of exercise training in postmenopausal breast cancer survivors: Cardiopulmonary and quality of life outcomes. *Journal of Clinical Oncology, 21,* 1660–1668.

Courneya, K., Vallance, J., McNeely, M., Karvinen, K., Peddle, C., & Mackey, J. (2004). Exercise issues in older cancer survivors. *Critical Reviews in Oncology/Hematology, 51,* 249–261.

Cox, H. (2001). *Later life. The realities of aging* (5th ed.). Upper Saddle River, NJ: Prentice Hall.

Damush, T., Perkins, A., & Miller, K. (2004, June). *Increasing exercise and HRQOL among older women surviving breast cancer.* Abstract presented at the National Cancer Institute's *Cancer Survivorship. Pathways to Health After Treatment* conference, Washington, DC.

Davidhizar, R., Eshler, J., & Moody, M. (2002). Health promotion for aging adults. *Geriatric Nursing, 23,* 28–34.

Deimling, G., Bowman, K., Sterns, S., & Wagner, L. (2004, June). *The post-treatment health and functioning of older adult, long-term cancer survivors.* Abstract presented at the National Cancer Institute's *Cancer Survivorship. Pathways to Health After Treatment* conference, Washington, DC.

Deimling, G., Kahana, B., Bowman, K., & Schaefer, M. (2002). Cancer survivorship and psychological distress in later life. *Psycho-Oncology, 11,* 479–494.

Deimling, G., Schaefer, M., Kahana, B., Bowman, K., & Reardon, J. (2002). Racial differences in the health of older adult long-term cancer survivors. *Journal of Psychosocial Oncology, 20*(4), 71–94.

Demark-Wahnefried, W., Morey, M., Clipp, E., Pieper, C., Snyder, D., Sloane, R., et al. (2003). Leading the way in exercise and diet (Project LEAD): Intervening to improve function among older breast and prostate cancer survivors. *Controlled Clinical Trials, 24,* 206–223.

Elder, G. (1998). The life course as developmental theory. *Child Development, 69,* 1–12.

Emery, C., Hauck, E., Shermer, R., Hsiao, E., & MacIntyre, N. (2003). Cognitive and psychological outcomes of exercise in a one-year follow-up study of patients with chronic obstructive pulmonary disease. *Health Psychology, 22,* 598–604.

Ensel, W. (1991). "Important" life events and depression among older adults. *Journal of Aging and Health, 3,* 546–566.

Ferrans, C. (1996). Development of a conceptual model of quality of life. *Scholarly Inquiry for Nursing Practice: An International Journal, 10,* 293–304.

Ferrell, B., & Dow, K. (1997). Quality of life among long-term cancer survivors. *Oncology, 11,* 565–571.

Ferrell, B., Virani, R., Smith, S., & Juarez, G. (2003). The role of oncology nursing to ensure quality care for cancer survivors: A report commissioned by the National Cancer Policy Board and Institute of Medicine [Online exclusive]. *Oncology Nursing Forum, 30,* E1–E11.

Hagestad, G., & Neugarten, B. (1985). Age and the life course. In R. Binstock & E. Shanas (Eds.), *Handbook of aging and the social science* (2nd ed., pp. 35–61). New York: Van Nostrand Reinold.

Haley, W., Robb, C., Balducci, L., Extermann, M., Perkins, E., Bergman, E., et al. (2004, June). *Psychological, social, and health impact of breast cancer survivorship in older women.* Abstract presented at the National Cancer Institute's *Cancer Survivorship. Pathways to Health After Treatment* conference, Washington, DC.

Hareven, T. (1996). Life course. In J. Birren (Ed.), *Encyclopedia of gerontology: Age, ageing, and the aged* (Vol. 2, p. 31). San Diego, CA: Academic.

Hoyer, W., & Roodin, P. (2003). *Adult development and aging* (5th ed.). Boston: McGraw Hill.

Hung, C., Daub, B., Black, B., Welsh, R., Quinney, A., & Haykowsky, M. (2004). Exercise training improves overall fitness and quality of life in older women with coronary artery disease. *Chest, 126,* 1026–1031.

Kagan, S. (2004). Gero-oncology nursing research. *Oncology Nursing Forum, 31,* 293–299.

Kart, C., & Kinney, J. (2001). *The realities of aging. An introduction to gerontology* (6th ed.). Boston: Allyn and Bacon.

Kastenbaum, R. (1995). Life course. In G.L. Maddox (Ed.), *The encyclopedia of aging* (2nd ed., pp. 553–556). New York: Springer.

Kennedy, M., Haykowsky, M., Daub, B., Van Lohuizen, K., & Knapik, G. (2003). Effects of a comprehensive cardiac rehabilitation program on quality of life and exercise tolerance in women: A retrospective analysis. *Current Control Trials in Cardiovascular Medicine, 4,* 1.

Lazarus, R., & Folkman, S. (1984). *Stress, appraisal, and coping.* New York: Springer.

Leigh, S. (1994). Cancer survivorship: A consumer movement. *Seminars in Oncology, 21,* 783–786.

Mandelblatt, J., Edge, S., Meropol, N., Senie, R., Tsangaris, T., Grey, L., et al. (2003). Predictors of long-term outcomes in older breast cancer survivors: Perceptions versus patterns of care. *Journal of Clinical Oncology, 21,* 855–863.

McDougall, J. (2001). Memory improvement program for elderly cancer survivors. *Geriatric Nursing, 22,* 185–190.

Murrell, S., Norris, F., & Grote, C. (1988). Life events in older adults. In L. Cohen (Ed.), *Life events and psychological functioning: Theoretical and methodological issues* (pp. 96–122). Newbury Park, CA: Sage.

National Institute of Nursing Research. (2005). *Mission statement.* Retrieved April 13, 2004, from http://ninr.nih.gov/ninr/research/diversity/mission.html

National Institute on Aging. (2001). *Research goal A: Improve health and quality of life of older people.* Retrieved November 9, 2004, from http://www.nia.nih.gov/AboutNIA/StrategicPlan/Research GoalA.htm

Neugarten, B.L. (1973). Personality change in later life: A developmental perspective. In C. Eisdorfer & M. Powell-Lawton (Eds.), *The psychology of adult development and aging* (pp. 311–335). Washington, DC: American Psychological Association.

O'Connor, L., & Blesch, K. (1992). Life cycle issues affecting cancer rehabilitation. *Seminars in Oncology Nursing, 8,* 174–185.

Office of Cancer Survivorship, National Cancer Institute. (2004). *Estimated U.S. cancer prevalence counts.* Retrieved July 20, 2004, from http://dccps.nci.nih.gov/ocs/prevalence/

Oncology Nursing Society & Geriatric Oncology Consortium. (2004). *Oncology Nursing Society and Geriatric Oncology Consortium joint position on cancer care in the older adult.* Retrieved April 10, 2004, from http://www.ons.org/publications/positions/Geriatric.shtml

Pearlin, L., & Skaff, M. (1995). Stress and adaptation in late life. In M. Gatz (Ed.), *Emerging issues in mental health and aging* (pp. 97–123). Washington, DC: American Psychological Association.

Pelusi, J. (2001). The past sets the stage for the future: Follow-up issues facing long-term cancer survivors. *Seminars in Oncology Nursing, 17,* 263–267.

Ramsey, S.D., Berry, K., Moinpour, C., Giedzinska, M., & Andersen, M.R. (2002). Quality of life in long-term survivors of colorectal cancer. *American Journal of Gastroenterology, 97,* 1228–1234.

Resnick, B. (2004). Encouraging exercise in older adults with congestive heart failure. *Geriatric Nursing, 25,* 204–211.

Rosenberg, H., & Resnick, B. (2003). Exercise interventions in patients with chronic obstructive pulmonary disease. *Geriatric Nursing, 24,* 90–95.

Rowland, J.H., Aziz, N., Tesauro, G., & Feuer, E.J. (2001). The changing face of cancer survivorship. *Seminars in Oncology Nursing, 17,* 236–240.

Schag, C., Ganz, P., Wing, S., Sim, M., & Lee, J. (1994). Quality of life in adult survivors of lung, colon, and prostate cancer. *Quality of Life Research, 3,* 127–141.

Steffen, P., Sherwood, A., Gullette, E., Georgiades, A., Hinderliter, A., & Blumenthal, J. (2001). Effects of exercise and weight loss on blood pressure during daily life. *Medicine and Science in Sports and Exercise, 33,* 1635–1640.

Taylor, E., Jones, P., & Burns, M. (1995). Quality of life. In I.M. Lubkin (Ed.), *Chronic illness: Impact and intervention* (3rd ed.). Sudbury, MA: Jones and Bartlett.

Taylor, J., Hobbie, W., Carlino, H., Deatrick, J., Fergusson, J., & Lipman, T. (2001). Describing the value of specialized distance education in pediatric oncology nursing. *Journal of Pediatric Oncology Nursing, 18,* 26–36.

U.S. Census Bureau. (2004). *Population estimates.* Retrieved July 10, 2004, from http://www.census.gov/popest/estimates.php

Wichmann, M., Muller, C., Hornung, M., Lau-Werner, U., Schildberg, F., & the Colorectal Cancer Study Group. (2001). Gender differences in long-term survival of patients with colorectal cancer. *British Journal of Surgery, 88,* 1092–1098.

Yancik, R., & Ries, L. (2000). Aging and cancer in America: Demographic and epidemiologic perspectives. *Hematology/Oncology Clinics of North America, 14,* 17–23.

Yang, P., Sugimura, H., Ebbert, F., Nichols, C., Marks, S., Kelemen, L., et al. (2004, June). *Characteristics of long-term lung cancer survivors.* Abstract presented at the National Cancer Institute's *Cancer Survivorship. Pathways to Health After Treatment* conference, Washington, DC.

Index

The letter f *after a page number indicates that relevant content appears in a figure; the letter* t, *in a table.*

Q